Mosby's

COMPREHENSIVE

PEDIATRIC

Emergency Care

Revised Edition

Barbara Aehlert, RN, BSPA

Southwest EMS Education, Inc.
Phoenix, Arizona/Pursley, Texas

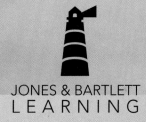

JONES & BARTLETT
LEARNING

World Headquarters
Jones & Bartlett Learning
5 Wall Street
Burlington, MA 01803
978-443-5000
info@jblearning.com
www.jblearning.com

Jones & Bartlett Learning books and products are available through most bookstores and online booksellers. To contact
Jones & Bartlett Learning directly, call 800-832-0034, fax 978-443-8000, or visit our website, www.jblearning.com.

Production Credits
Chief Executive Officer: Ty Field
President: James Homer
SVP, Editor-in-Chief: Michael Johnson
SVP, Chief Marketing Officer: Alison M. Pendergast
Executive Publisher: Kimberly Brophy
Executive Acquisitions Editor—EMS: Christine Emerton
Vice President of Sales, Public Safety Group: Matthew Maniscalco
Director of Sales, Public Safety Group: Patricia Einstein
Production Editor: Tina Chen
Director of Marketing: Alisha Weisman
VP, Manufacturing and Inventory Control: Therese Connell
Director of Photo Research and Permissions: Amy Wrynn
Printing and Binding: Courier Companies
Cover Printing: Courier Companies

ISBN: 978-1-284-03807-1

6048

Printed in the United States of America
16 15 14 13 12   10 9 8 7 6 5 4 3 2 1

To
My daughters, Andrea and Sherri
For the beautiful young women you have become

Preface

This book is designed for use by healthcare professionals including Pediatricians, Family Practice Physicians, Anesthesiologists, Emergency Physicians, Nurses, Paramedics, and Respiratory Therapists.

Each chapter contains instructional objectives followed by a review of the critical elements related to the subject. A sp-question pretest and posttest are provided in addition to short quizzes at the conclusion of each chapter. Answers and rationales are provided for all questions in this text.

With the help of the text reviewers, every effort has been made to provide information that is consistent with current research and resuscitation guidelines. However, the reader is advised to consult expert opinion articles and guidelines for more authoritative advice. In clinical practice, it is essential to confirm all medication doses, indications, and contraindications before use. The author and publisher assume no responsibility or liability for loss or damage resulting from the use of information contained within.

If you have suggestions about how this book could be improved, please contact me through my web site address shown below.

Barbara Aehlert, RN, BSPA
http://www.swemsed.com

Acknowledgments

I would like to thank:

Linda Honeycutt for providing the resources necessary for an undertaking of this magnitude.

Laura Bayless and Katherine Tomber for their kindness and extraordinary talents in taking "plain" pages and making them a user-friendly final product. Jeff Somers for his professionalism, attention to detail, and patience while making final changes to this book.

The text reviewers for their thorough review of the content. Your comments were most helpful in shaping the material covered in this book.

Andrea Legamaro, RN, for her assistance with the instructor test bank that accompanies this text.

Jeanne Shepard, CEP, and Sherri Aehlert for their assistance with the instructor scenarios.

Ed and Pat Tirone for graciously providing photos of their daughters Kimberly and Sarah.

Gregg Rich, Tim Eiman, and Ralph M. Shenefelt of the American Safety & Health Institute. It is a pleasure working with you.

Publisher's Acknowledgments

The editors wish to acknowledge and thank the many reviewers of this book, who devoted countless hours to intensive review. Their comments were invaluable in helping develop and fine-tune the manuscript.

David A. Boer, NREMT-P, MBA
Program Director, Emergency Medical Services for Children
University of South Dakota School of Medicine
Sioux Falls, South Dakota

Joanne McCall, RN, MA, CEN, FNE
Emergency Department Nurse Educator
Providence Hospital & Medical Centers
Novi, Michigan

Michelle M. McLean, BSEE, MD
Synergy Medical Education Alliance
Saginaw, Michigan

Laraine Yakowich Moody, MSN, RN, CPNP
Pediatric Nurse Practitioner
Children's Hospital of Michigan
Detroit, Michigan

Catharine L. Shaner, MD, FAAP
Pediatric Advisor
American Safety & Health Institute
Holiday, Florida

A. Keith Wesley, MD
Emergency Medicine Physician
Chippewa Valley Emergency Care
Eau Claire, Wisconsin

Contents

Contents

Pretest

Questions

1. Which of the following lists conditions that affect the upper airway?
   A) Bacterial tracheitis, epiglottitis, bronchiolitis.
   B) Bronchiolitis, croup, asthma.
   C) Asthma, bronchiolitis, pneumonia.
   D) Croup, epiglottitis, bacterial tracheitis.

2. Systemic complications of vascular access include:
   A) Phlebitis.
   B) Cellulitis.
   C) Hematoma formation.
   D) Catheter-fragment embolism.

3. A child with signs of cyanosis, diminished breath sounds with minimal chest excursion, and an inadequate respiratory rate is exhibiting signs of:
   A) Hyperthermia.
   B) Hypovolemia.
   C) Respiratory failure.
   D) Early respiratory distress.

4. In the pediatric patient, cardiac arrest is most often due to:
   A) Hypothermia.
   B) Acid-base imbalance.
   C) Respiratory failure.
   D) Sepsis.

5. For which of the following conditions is calcium administration appropriate?
   A) Hypoglycemia.
   B) Supraventricular tachycardia.
   C) Hyperkalemia.
   D) Tricyclic antidepressant overdose.

6. The tracheal dose of epinephrine for an infant or child is:
   A) 0.1 mg/kg (0.1 mL/kg) of 1:1000 solution.
   B) 0.01 mg/kg (0.1 mL/kg) of 1:10,000 solution.
   C) 0.02 mg/kg of 1:1000 solution.
   D) 0.04 mg/kg of 1:10,000 solution.

7. Suctioning of the newly born infant should be limited to _____ per attempt.
   A) 3 to 5 seconds.
   B) 5 to 10 seconds.
   C) 10 to 15 seconds.
   D) 15 to 30 seconds.

8. The peak incidence of sudden infant death syndrome occurs at age:
   A) 1 to 2 months.
   B) 2 to 4 months.
   C) 6 to 8 months.
   D) 10 to 12 months.

9. You are a paramedic called to a private residence for a 6-month-old infant with difficulty breathing. Upon arrival, the infant's mother is frantic. Mom states she went to check on the napping infant and found him blue and not breathing. She picked up the infant and ran to the phone to call 9-1-1. The infant began spontaneously breathing while she was on the phone. You find the infant awake and alert with normal color and vital signs for age. Mom is uncertain if her baby requires transport to the hospital. Your best course of action will be to:
   A) Allow the mother to refuse further care. The infant is in no obvious distress at this time.
   B) Contact Child Protective Services.
   C) Explain your concerns regarding the infant's reported color change and apneic episode and encourage the mother to permit transport for physician evaluation.
   D) Remain on the scene until the mother has made a follow-up appointment with the infant's pediatrician.

10. Select the **incorrect** statement regarding human poisoning exposures.
    A) Ingestion is the most common route of entry for toxic exposure.
    B) Most pediatric poisoning exposures involve children < 6 years of age.
    C) Most pediatric toxic exposures involve a single substance.
    D) The majority of pediatric toxic exposures are intentional.

Questions 11 through 18 refer to the following scenario.

An apneic and pulseless 6-year-old boy is brought by ambulance to the Emergency Department. EMT-Basics report the child was the front-seat passenger of a vehicle involved in a rollover crash. The child was not restrained. Examination confirms the child is apneic and pulseless with contusions noted on the anterior chest and open fractures of both femurs. Chest compressions are being performed and the child is being ventilated with 100% with a bag-valve-device.

11. Positive-pressure ventilation should be provided at a rate of:
    A) 8 to 12 breaths/minute.
    B) 10 to 14 breaths/minute.
    C) 14 to 30 breaths/minute.
    D) 12 to 20 breaths/minute.

The cardiac monitor has been applied and reveals the following rhythm:

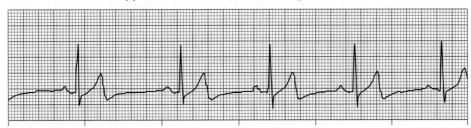

12. The rhythm displayed is:
    A) Sinus bradycardia.
    B) Ventricular fibrillation.
    C) Complete AV block.
    D) Supraventricular tachycardia.

13. Despite the rhythm observed on the cardiac monitor, the child is unresponsive, apneic, and pulseless. This clinical situation is called:
    A) Asystole.
    B) Ventricular fibrillation.
    C) Pulseless electrical activity.
    D) Pulseless ventricular tachycardia.

14. List four possible reversible causes of this clinical situation.

    Hypothermia   Pulmonary Embolus
    Hypoxia   Toxin
    Acidosis
    Tension Pneumo

15. In addition to other injuries, physical examination of this child revealed anterior chest contusions. Select the correct statement regarding thoracic trauma and the pediatric patient.
    A) Children are more likely to sustain rib fractures than adults are.
    B) A pulmonary contusion/laceration is the most common thoracic injury seen in children.
    C) Thoracic trauma in children is associated with a low mortality rate.
    D) A pulmonary contusion is a life-threatening injury that is readily recognized in the pediatric trauma patient.

16. A first-line medication used in the management of this clinical situation is:
    A) Atropine.
    B) Dopamine.
    C) Epinephrine.
    D) Sodium bicarbonate.

17. The first-line medication given in the management of this clinical situation is used to:
    A) Decrease myocardial contractility.
    B) Increase systemic vascular resistance.
    C) Decrease heart rate.
    D) Increase myocardial oxygen consumption.

18. Despite the interventions performed thus far, the child's cardiac rhythm remains unchanged. A pulse is not present. Should defibrillation be performed? *most Definitely! no!* *PEA*

19. Which of the following statements is true regarding the use of the Glasgow Coma Scale (GCS)?
    A) The GCS is used to assess the patient's verbal response, motor response, and pupillary reactivity.
    B) When assigning a score using the GCS, the maximum possible score is 13.
    C) When using the GCS, the minimum possible score is 3.
    D) The GCS is used to assess the patient's verbal response, motor response, and capillary refill.

20. Pediatric rhythm disturbances may be categorized as normal for age, fast, slow, or absent/pulseless. List three examples of rhythm disturbances found in the absent/pulseless rhythm category.
    PEA
    Vfib
    Vtach

21. Which of the following formulas may be used to approximate the correct uncuffed endotracheal tube size in a child 1 to 10 years of age?
    A) Age in years/2 + 12.
    B) 70 + (2 × age in years).
    C) (16 + age in years)/4.
    D) 90 + (2 × age in years).

22. A 5-year-old girl is unresponsive, apneic, and pulseless. The child is being ventilated with a bag-valve-mask and 100% oxygen. Chest compressions are being performed. The cardiac monitor reveals ventricular fibrillation. Which of the following interventions should be performed next?
    A) Establish vascular access and administer epinephrine 0.01 mg/kg.
    B) Defibrillate with 2 J/kg.
    C) Perform synchronized cardioversion with 1 J/kg.
    D) Establish vascular access and administer amiodarone 5 mg/kg.

23. Which of the following statements is **incorrect** regarding pediatric defibrillation?
    A) Damp skin and air pockets beneath hand-held paddles or self-adhesive defibrillation pads increase transthoracic resistance and may cause an uneven delivery of current.
    B) Initial management of pulseless VT or VF includes CPR and defibrillation.
    C) Pediatric paddles or self-adhesive pads should be used when defibrillating patients up to 1 year of age; however, adult paddles should be used when performing synchronized cardioversion.
    D) Alcohol-soaked pads should never be used during defibrillation.

24. Which of the following statements is correct regarding alternatives for failed or difficult pediatric tracheal intubation?
    A) Performing a needle cricothyrotomy is an acceptable alternative.
    B) Performing a surgical cricothyrotomy is generally contraindicated until age 18 years.
    C) Blind nasotracheal intubation is generally contraindicated until age 14 years.
    D) Insertion of an age-appropriate or size-appropriate laryngeal mask airway (LMA) is contraindicated.

25. Management of a tension pneumothorax in the pediatric patient may necessitate needle decompression of the chest. This is accomplished using an over-the-needle catheter inserted:
    A) In the fifth intercostal space in the midaxillary line, just above the sixth rib.
    B) In the fifth intercostal space in the midaxillary line, just below the sixth rib.
    C) In the second intercostal space in the midclavicular line, just above the third rib.
    D) In the second intercostal space in the midclavicular line, just below the third rib.

26. Select the **incorrect** statement regarding sinus tachycardia.
    A) Sinus tachycardia is a normal compensatory response to the need for increased cardiac output or oxygen delivery.
    B) In sinus tachycardia, the heart rate is usually more than 220 beats/minute in infants or 200 beats/minute in children.
    C) The onset of a sinus tachycardia occurs gradually.
    D) Patient management includes treatment of the underlying cause that precipitated the rhythm.

27. A 2-year-old boy appears to be choking. You find the child responsive, but cyanotic. He is unable to cough or speak. Initial interventions in this situation should include:
    A) Performing a blind finger sweep to remove the obstruction.
    B) Alternating 5 back blows with 5 chest thrusts.
    C) Performing direct laryngoscopy to visualize the obstruction.
    D) Informing the child that you are going to help him, and then performing abdominal thrusts.

28. Which of the following is NOT a desirable feature of a bag-valve-mask device?
    A) A clear mask.
    B) A compressible, self-refilling bag.
    C) Availability in adult and pediatric sizes.
    D) Pop-off (pressure release) valve.

29. A 3-year-old child weighing 15 kilograms requires tracheal intubation.
    A) What type of blade should be used? MAC
    B) What size laryngoscope blade should be used? 2
    C) What size tracheal tube should be used? 4
    D) Should you use a cuffed or uncuffed tracheal tube for this child? uncuffed
    E) When the tracheal tube has been inserted to the proper depth, what is the cm marking that should appear at the patient's lips? 12 cm

30. A 44-pound child presents with fever, irritability, mottled color, cool extremities, and a prolonged capillary refill time. The appropriate initial fluid bolus for administration to this child is:
    A) 100 mL of normal saline over 30 to 60 minutes.
    B) 200 mL of 5% dextrose in water in less than 20 minutes.
    C) 400 mL of normal saline or Ringer's lactate in less than 20 minutes.
    D) 800 mL of normal saline or Ringer's lactate infused over 30 to 60 minutes.

31. Select the **incorrect** statement regarding the use of cricoid pressure.
    A) Cricoid pressure is used to minimize the risk of choking in a conscious infant or child.
    B) Cricoid pressure occludes the esophagus by displacing the cricoid cartilage posteriorly.
    C) Cricoid pressure is applied using one fingertip in infants and the thumb and index finger in children.
    D) Cricoid pressure may result in tracheal obstruction in infants if excessive pressure is used.

32. List the four essential questions to ask in the initial emergency management of a pediatric patient with a dysrhythmia.

    _____

    _____

    _____

    _____

Questions 33 through 35 pertain to the following scenario.

You are called to see an 18-month-old child with difficulty breathing. Mom reports the child has had a cough and cold for the past two days and appears worse today. You note the child is cyanotic and appears limp in his mother's arms. His respiratory rate is rapid and shallow. Intercostal retractions are visible and wheezing is audible without a stethoscope.

33. From the information provided, complete the following documentation regarding the Pediatric Assessment Triangle.
    A) Appearance: _Limp w/ retractions_
    B) Breathing: _Shallow rapid_
    C) Circulation: _Cyanotic_

34. Your initial assessment reveals a patent airway. The child's respiratory rate is 60/min. Auscultation of the chest reveals wheezes bilaterally. A weak brachial pulse is present at a rate of 194 beats/min. The skin is cyanotic. Capillary refill is 2 to 3 seconds; temperature is 101.8° F; and the pulse oximeter reveals a SpO_2 of 80%. This child's presentation is most consistent with:
    A) Respiratory distress.
    B) Respiratory failure.
    C) Respiratory arrest.
    D) Cardiopulmonary arrest.

35. Is this child sick or not sick? Describe your approach to the initial management of this patient.
    Sick — Duonebs (?) + O_2 @ 15 Lpm

36. The child's condition worsens. Central cyanosis persists despite assisted ventilation with 100% oxygen. The child's respiratory rate is now 8 to 14/min and shallow. The cardiac monitor reveals narrow QRS complexes at a rate of 32/min. You are unable to palpate a peripheral pulse, but a weak central pulse is present. An IV has been established. You should now:
    A) Begin chest compressions and give epinephrine.
    B) Give atropine.
    C) Continue to monitor the child closely for signs of deterioration.
    D) Give adenosine.

37. Select the **incorrect** statement.
    A) Hypotension is an early sign of shock in a child.
    B) The diastolic blood pressure is usually two-thirds of the systolic pressure.
    C) A child may be in shock despite a normal blood pressure.
    D) Blood pressure is one of the least sensitive indicators of adequate circulation in children.

38. The presence of compensated shock can be identified by:
    A) Assessment of heart rate, ECG rhythm, and skin temperature.
    B) Assessment of the presence and strength of peripheral pulses, mental status, and pupil response to light.
    C) Assessment of heart rate, presence and strength of peripheral pulses, and the adequacy of end-organ perfusion.
    D) Assessment of end-organ perfusion, ECG rhythm, and pupil response to light

Questions 39 through 45 refer to the following scenario.

A 3-year-old is found barely responsive by her babysitter. The babysitter was distracted "for just a minute" by a telephone call and lost track of the child. The child was found on the ground just outside the garage door. The patient's skin looks flushed and she is laboring to breathe. You note secretions are draining from the patient's mouth and she has been incontinent of urine. The child is unaware of your presence.

39. From the information provided, complete the following documentation regarding the Pediatric Assessment Triangle.
    A) Appearance: _Unaware of presence_
    B) Breathing: _Labored + secretions_
    C) Circulation: _Flushed skin_

40. Based on the information provided, your FIRST intervention should be to:
    A) Establish vascular access.
    B) Suction the airway.
    C) Perform a secondary (head-to-toes) survey.
    D) Perform tracheal intubation.

41. For each of the following, record the estimated values for a 3-year-old child.
    A) Weight:
    B) Respiratory rate:
    C) Heart rate:
    D) Blood pressure:

42. Your assessment reveals the child will open her eyes and withdraw in response to a painful stimulus but makes incomprehensible sounds. Her Glasgow Coma Scale score is:
    A) 6.
    B) 8.
    C) 10.
    D) 12.

43. The child's respiratory rate is 44/min, heart rate is 158/min, and blood pressure is 80/60. Her skin is warm and moist. Her pupils are equal and reactive at 2 mm. Auscultation of her lungs reveals bilateral diffuse wheezes. Excessive oral secretions are present. These findings are most consistent with the _Cholinergic_ toxidrome.

44. Further questioning of the babysitter reveals that the child may have been out of sight for 20 to 30 minutes before she was found. The babysitter recalls having seen an open bottle of white liquid on the floor of the garage. As you continue interviewing the babysitter, a coworker tells you that he smells garlic on the child's breath. This child was most likely exposed to:
    A) An organophosphate.
    B) Camphor.
    C) Ethylene glycol.
    D) Gasoline.

45. You are instructed to administer atropine to this patient. Which of the following statements is correct?
    A) Question the order. Atropine is indicated for symptomatic bradycardias. This patient is not bradycardic.
    B) Administer the atropine as instructed. Atropine is being ordered in this situation to increase the patient's blood pressure.
    C) Question the order. Although atropine may be used in situations such as this, the patient is tachycardic. Atropine is contraindicated if a tachycardia is present.
    D) Administer the atropine as instructed. In this situation, atropine is being given to dry the patient's airway of secretions.

46. When administering medications by means of a tracheal tube you should:
    A) Continue chest compressions throughout administration of the medication.
    B) Insert a needle through the wall of the tracheal tube to administer the medication.
    C) Temporarily stop chest compressions, instill the medication down the endotracheal tube, flush the drug with 5 mL of normal saline, ventilate 5 times with a bag-valve-mask, then resume CPR.
    D) Temporarily stop chest compressions, instill the medication down the tracheal tube, ventilate the patient for a minimum of 5 minutes with a bag-valve-mask device to ensure the drug is dispersed through the alveoli, and then resume CPR.

47. Medications used to maintain cardiac output include:
    A) Midazolam, epinephrine, and naloxone.
    B) Lorazepam, midazolam, and naloxone.
    C) Diazepam, dopamine, and dobutamine.
    D) Dopamine, epinephrine, and dobutamine.

48. The term "conscious sedation" is equivalent to:
    A) Minimal sedation/analgesia.
    B) Moderate sedation/analgesia.
    C) Deep sedation/analgesia.
    D) General anesthesia.

49. Indications for the use of amiodarone include:
    A) Asystole.
    B) Severe bradycardia.
    C) Ventricular fibrillation.
    D) Sinus tachycardia.

50. The single most common cause of injury in children is:
    A) Motor vehicle crashes.
    B) Falls.
    C) Pedestrian injuries.
    D) Firearm-related injuries.

Pretest Answers

1. D. Pneumonia, asthma, and bronchiolitis are conditions that affect the lower airway. Croup, epiglottitis, and bacterial tracheitis are conditions that affect the upper airway.

2. D. Systemic complications of vascular access include sepsis, fluid overload/electrolyte imbalance, hypersensitivity reactions, air embolism, catheter-fragment embolism, and pulmonary thromboembolism. Local complications include pain and irritation, cellulitis, phlebitis, thrombosis, bleeding, hematoma formation, inadvertent arterial puncture, infiltration and extravasation, and nerve, tendon, ligament, and/or limb damage.

3. C. A child with signs of cyanosis, diminished breath sounds with minimal chest excursion, and an inadequate respiratory rate is exhibiting signs of respiratory failure. Signs of respiratory failure include the findings of respiratory distress with any of the following additions or modifications: sleepy, intermittently combative, or agitated; increased respiratory effort at sternal notch, absent or significantly decreased breath sounds, marked use of accessory muscles, retractions; head bobbing, grunting, gasping; central cyanosis despite oxygen administration; poor peripheral perfusion; mottling; marked tachycardia (bradycardia is a late sign), decreased muscle tone, decreased level of consciousness or response to pain; inadequate respiratory rate, effort, or chest excursion, or tachypnea with periods of bradypnea; slowing to bradypnea/agonal breathing.

4. C. In children, cardiopulmonary arrest is usually the result of respiratory failure or shock that progresses to cardiopulmonary failure with profound hypoxemia and acidosis, and eventually cardiopulmonary arrest.

5. C. Calcium administration is appropriate for documented or suspected hyperkalemia, ionized hypocalcemia, hypermagnesemia, or calcium channel blocker toxicity. If calcium **chloride** 10% is used, give 20 mg/kg (0.2 mL/kg) slowly IV/IO. If calcium **gluconate** 10% is used, give three times the dose of calcium chloride (i.e., 60 mg/kg [0.6 mL/kg]) slowly IV/IO.

6. A. Because epinephrine is supplied in different dilutions, it is important to ensure selection of the correct concentration before administering this medication. The tracheal dosage of epinephrine for an infant or child is 0.1 mg/kg (0.1 mL/kg) of **1:1000** solution. This dose is 10 times the recommended initial IV/IO dose (0.01 mg/kg [0.1 mL/kg] of **1:10,000** solution).

7. A. Suctioning of the newly born infant should be limited to 3 to 5 seconds per attempt.

8. B. The peak incidence of sudden infant death syndrome is 2 to 4 months.

9. C. The infant has experienced an Apparent Life-Threatening Event (ALTE). These events can involve any of the following: apnea, color change (cyanosis, pallor, or erythema), marked change in muscle tone (limpness), choking, or gagging. The infant should be transported and evaluated by a physician.

10. D. In 2002, more than 50% (51.6%) of human poisoning exposures occurred in children younger than 6 years; more than 30% occurred in children younger than 3 years. The majority of pediatric toxic exposures are unintentional, occur in the home, and involve only a single substance. Cosmetics and personal care products are the substances most frequently involved in pediatric exposures involving children <6 years. Death due to unintentional poisoning in young children is uncommon due to increased product safety measures (e.g., child-resistant packaging), increased poison prevention education, early recognition of exposure, and improvements in medical management.

11. D. Positive-pressure ventilation for infants and children should be provided at a rate of 12 to 20 breaths/minute (1 breath every 3 to 5 seconds). Each breath should be given over 1 second.

12. A. The rhythm shown is a sinus bradycardia.

13. C. Despite the presence of an organized rhythm on the monitor that you would expect to produce a pulse, the child is pulseless. This situation is called pulseless electrical activity (PEA). Many conditions may cause PEA. PEA has a poor prognosis unless the underlying cause can be rapidly identified and appropriately managed.

14. Possible reversible causes of PEA include hypoxemia (give oxygen), hypovolemia (replace volume), hypothermia (use simple warming techniques), hyper-/hypokalemia and metabolic disorders (correct electrolyte and acid-base disturbances), cardiac tamponade (pericardiocentesis), tension pneumothorax (needle decompression), toxins/poisons/drugs (give antidote/specific therapy), and thromboembolism.

15. B. The most common thoracic injuries seen in children are pulmonary contusion/laceration (53%), pneumothorax/hemothorax (38%), rib/sternal fractures (36%), cardiac (5%), diaphragm (2%), major blood vessel (1%). In children, thoracic trauma is associated with a high mortality rate. The greater elasticity and resilience of the chest wall in children makes rib and sternum fractures less common than in adults; however, force is more easily transmitted to the underlying lung tissues, resulting in pulmonary contusion, pneumothorax, or hemothorax. A pulmonary contusion is a potentially life-threatening injury that is frequently missed due to the presence of other associated injuries.

16. C. Epinephrine is a first-line medication used in the management of PEA.

17. B. Epinephrine stimulates alpha, beta-1, and beta-2 receptors. Effects of alpha receptor stimulation result in constriction of the arterioles in the skin, mucosa, kidneys, and viscera → increased systemic vascular resistance. These effects are beneficial in cardiac arrest because blood is shunted to the heart and brain. Effects of beta-1 receptor stimulation include increased force of contraction (+ inotropic effect) and increased heart rate (+ chronotropic effect). These effects result in increased myocardial workload and oxygen requirements. Stimulation of beta-2 receptors results in relaxation of bronchial smooth muscle.

18. No. Although the patient has no pulse, *organized* electrical activity is visible on the cardiac monitor. Defibrillation is used to terminate *disorganized* cardiac rhythms, such as ventricular fibrillation. The shock attempts to deliver a uniform electrical current of sufficient intensity to simultaneously depolarize ventricular cells, including fibrillating cells, causing momentary asystole. This provides an opportunity for the heart's natural pacemakers to resume normal activity.

19. C. The Glasgow Coma Scale is used to assess a patient's level of responsiveness by evaluating best verbal response, best motor response, and eye opening. The minimum possible score is 3, maximum possible score 15. When caring for an infant or child, use the GCS that has been modified for pediatric use.

20. Absent/pulseless rhythms include 1) pulseless ventricular tachycardia, in which the ECG displays a wide QRS complex at a rate faster than 120 beats/min, 2) ventricular fibrillation, in which irregular chaotic deflections that vary in shape and amplitude are observed on the ECG but there is no coordinated ventricular contraction, 3) asystole, in which no cardiac electrical activity is present, and 4) pulseless electrical activity (PEA), in which electrical activity is visible on the ECG but central pulses are absent.

21. C. Uncuffed endotracheal tube size may be estimated using the following formula for children 1 to 10 years of age: (16 + age in years)/4. Some systems use the formula (age in years/4) + 4 = mm ID.

22. B. The definitive treatment for ventricular fibrillation (VF) or pulseless ventricular tachycardia (VT) is defibrillation. When pulseless VT or VF is present, defibrillation takes priority over attempts to establish vascular access or administration of medications. Synchronized cardioversion is not indicated for VF.

23. C. When performing manual defibrillation, the same size paddle or self-adhesive pad should be used for both defibrillation and cardioversion. The largest size paddle that allows good skin contact but maintains separation between the two paddles is preferred. Infant paddles should be used for patients up to 1 year of age or 10 kg. Larger paddles may be used as long as contact between the paddles is avoided. Adult paddles should be used for patients older than 1 year or weighing more than 10 kg. Some pediatric-ready automated external defibrillators (AEDs) require the use of pediatric pads for children less than 8 years of age. Follow the AED manufacturer's instructions. Damp skin and air pockets beneath hand-held paddles or self-adhesive defibrillation pads increase transthoracic resistance and may cause an uneven delivery of current. Initial management of pulseless VT or VF includes CPR and delivery of three serial shocks in rapid succession without pausing to check for the presence of a pulse between each shock (assuming the rhythm is unchanged). Do not use alcohol-soaked pads for defibrillation - they may ignite!

24. A. Alternatives for failed or difficult pediatric tracheal intubation include:
    A) Combitube: only if over 4 feet tall.
    B) Laryngeal mask airway (LMA) for age: acceptable.
    C) Blind nasotracheal intubation: contraindicated until age 10 years.
    D) Needle cricothyrotomy: acceptable.
    E) Surgical cricothyrotomy: contraindicated until age 10 years.

25. C. Management of a tension pneumothorax in the pediatric patient may necessitate needle decompression of the chest. This is accomplished using an over-the-needle catheter inserted in the second intercostal space in the midclavicular line, just above the third rib.

26. B. Sinus tachycardia is a normal compensatory response to the need for increased cardiac output or oxygen delivery. In sinus tachycardia, the heart rate is usually less than 220 beats per minute in infants or 180 beats per minute in children. Onset of the rhythm occurs gradually. The ECG shows a regular, narrow QRS complex rhythm that often varies in response to activity or stimulation. P waves are present before each QRS complex. The history given typically explains the rapid heart rate (i.e., pain, fever, volume loss due to trauma, vomiting, or diarrhea). Patient management includes treatment of the underlying cause that precipitated the rhythm (e.g., administering medications to relieve pain, administration of fluids to correct hypovolemia due to diarrhea).

27. D. Inform the child that you are going to help him, then administer abdominal thrusts until the object is expelled or the child becomes unresponsive. A blind finger sweep should not be performed in an infant or child, and is never appropriate in a responsive choking victim. A blind finger sweep may push the foreign body into the airway, causing further obstruction. Back blows and chest thrusts are appropriate maneuvers to relieve foreign body airway obstruction in infants, not children. Although direct laryngoscopy may ultimately be necessary, it is not performed before attempting less invasive methods of relieving the obstruction.

28. D. The BVM used for resuscitation should have either no pop-off (pressure-release) valve or a pop-off valve that can be disabled during resuscitation. Some resuscitation situations require higher than normal ventilatory pressure, such as near-drowning, CPR, pulmonary edema, asthma, partial upper airway obstruction, or initial resuscitation of the newly born. To effectively ventilate a patient in these situations, the ventilatory pressure needed may exceed the limits of the pop-off valve. Thus, a pop-off valve may prevent generation of sufficient tidal volume to overcome the increase in airway resistance.

29. Tracheal intubation of a 3-year-old, 15 kg child:
   A) A straight or curved blade may be used.
   B) A size 2 laryngoscope blade should be used.
   C) A 5.0 mm tracheal tube should be used. Be sure to have a 4.5 mm and 5.5 mm immediately available.
   D) Use an uncuffed tracheal tube for this child. In the hospital setting, a cuffed or uncuffed tube may be used.
   E) When the tracheal tube has been inserted to the proper depth, the 14 to 15 cm marking should appear at the patient's lips.

30. C. Administer a bolus of 20 mL/kg of isotonic crystalloid solution (NS or LR) over 5 to 20 minutes. 44 pounds = 20 kilograms. For this child, the appropriate initial fluid bolus is 400 mL of normal saline or Ringer's lactate.

31. A. Cricoid pressure (also called the Sellick maneuver) is used only in unresponsive patients and is usually applied by an assistant during positive-pressure ventilation.

32. The initial emergency management of pediatric dysrhythmias requires a response to four important questions:
    A) Is a pulse (and other signs of circulation) present?
    B) Is the rate within normal limits for age, too fast, too slow, or absent?
    C) Is the QRS wide (ventricular in origin) or narrow (supraventricular in origin)?
    D) Is the patient sick (unstable) or not sick (stable)?

33. Pediatric Assessment Triangle (first impression) findings:
    A) Appearance: Awake but appears limp.
    B) Breathing: Respirations are rapid and shallow; audible wheezing is present; increased work of breathing evident.
    C) Circulation: Skin is cyanotic; no evidence of bleeding.

34. B. This child's presentation is most consistent with respiratory failure. The presence of tachypnea and tachycardia reflects compensatory mechanisms that are attempting to increase cardiac output. However, these mechanisms will fail (signifying the onset of cardiopulmonary failure) as oxygen demand increases and the child tires. Aggressive treatment is essential.

35. This child is sick. Move quickly. Open the airway and suction if necessary. Correct hypoxia by giving high-flow oxygen. Begin assisted ventilation if the patient does not improve. Provide further interventions based on assessment findings.

36. A. If there is no improvement after approximately 30 seconds of effective assisted ventilation and the child's heart rate is less than 60 beats/min with signs of poor perfusion, begin chest compressions and give epinephrine. If the bradycardia persists, consider atropine and pacing. Adenosine is contraindicated in this situation because the patient is bradycardic. Adenosine is used to **slow** the heart rate in supraventricular tachycardia (SVT).

37. A. Hypotension is a late sign of shock in a child. Tachycardia and signs of poor perfusion such as pale, cool, mottled skin occur earlier and are more reliable indicators than hypotension.

38. C. The presence of compensated shock can be identified by evaluation of heart rate, the presence and volume (strength) of peripheral pulses, and the adequacy of end-organ perfusion (Brain - assess mental status, skin - assess capillary refill, skin temperature, and kidneys - assess urine output).

39. Pediatric Assessment Triangle (first impression) findings:
    A) Appearance: barely responsive, incontinent of urine, unaware of your presence.
    B) Breathing: increased work of breathing evident.
    C) Circulation: Skin is flushed; no evidence of bleeding.

40. B. The presence of secretions draining from the mouth of a child that is unaware of your presence requires **immediate** intervention. Clear the airway with suctioning.

41. "Normal" values for a 3-year-old child:
    A) Weight: 14 kg (31 lb.).
    B) Respiratory rate: 24 to 40.
    C) Heart rate: 90 to 150.
    D) Blood pressure: BP > 70.

Refer to the tables and formulas in Chapter 3 if you need to review this information.

42. B. The patient's Glasgow Coma Scale score is 8.

Eyes:	To pain	2
Verbal:	Incomprehensible sounds	2
Motor:	Withdraws from pain	4

See page 64 to review the Glasgow Coma Scale.

43. This patient's physical findings are most consistent with the *cholinergic* toxidrome.

44. A. The patient's physical findings and additional information regarding the events surrounding the exposure strongly suggest organophosphate exposure.

45. D. Atropine is the antidote for the muscarinic effects of organophosphate exposure. The goal of atropine administration in this situation is drying of airway secretions to maintain oxygenation and ventilation. Tachycardia is NOT a contraindication to its use.

46. C. When administering medications by means of a tracheal tube, temporarily stop chest compressions, instill the medication down the tube, flush the drug with 5 mL of normal saline, ventilate 5 times with a bag-valve-mask, then resume CPR.

47. D. Dopamine, epinephrine, and dobutamine are medications used to maintain cardiac output. Midazolam (Versed), lorazepam (Ativan), and diazepam (Valium) are benzodiazepines used for sedation. Naloxone (Narcan) is an opioid (narcotic) antagonist.

48. B. Sedation is dose-dependent continuum from minimal sedation to general anesthesia. Individual patient responses to a given dosage of a drug vary. Because of this variation in patient response, the American Society of Anesthesiologists (ASA) prefers the term "sedation-analgesia" and the American College of Emergency Physicians (ACEP) uses the term "procedural sedation" instead of "conscious sedation."

49. C. Amiodarone may be used in the treatment of pulseless VT/VF and perfusing tachycardias - particularly ectopic atrial tachycardia, junctional ectopic tachycardia, and ventricular tachycardia.

50. B. Falls are the single most common cause of injury in children.

1

Chain of Survival and Emergency Medical Services for Children

Case Study

A 3-year-old is found floating face down in the family pool. The child's distraught mother says she last saw the child about 15 minutes ago. Mom removed the child from the pool and then called 9-1-1. She is performing cardiopulmonary resuscitation (CPR) per the emergency medical service (EMS) dispatcher's instructions via the phone. Police officers are the first to arrive on the scene. They begin CPR after confirming that the child is unresponsive, apneic, and pulseless.

With what frequency do pediatric out-of-hospital cardiac arrest victims survive? What prevention measures could have been implemented to prevent this tragic situation?

Objectives

1. Identify the links in the Pediatric Chain of Survival.
2. Explain the purpose of the Emergency Medical Services for Children (EMSC) program.
3. Define the terms *primary prevention*, *secondary prevention*, and *tertiary prevention* as they relate to injury prevention.

Pediatric Chain of Survival

In adults, sudden nontraumatic cardiopulmonary arrests are usually the result of underlying cardiac disease. In children, causes of nontraumatic cardiopulmonary arrest include bronchospasm, congenital cardiac abnormalities, dysrhythmias, foreign body aspiration, gastroenteritis, seizures, sepsis, drowning, sudden infant death syndrome (SIDS), and upper and lower respiratory tract infection, among other causes.

The Pediatric Chain of Survival represents a sequential series of events to assess, support, or restore effective ventilation and circulation to the infant or child experiencing a respiratory or cardiorespiratory arrest. The sequence consists of four important steps (Figure 1-1):

The importance of prevention is reflected in the links of the Pediatric Chain of Survival.

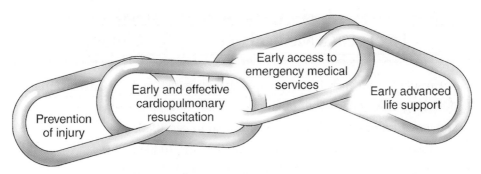

Figure 1-1   The Pediatric Chain of Survival.

- Prevention of illness or injury
- Early CPR
- Early EMS activation
- Early advanced life support (ALS)

Note that activating EMS is delayed until after a trial of early CPR. This is based on the higher likelihood of respiratory conditions and lower likelihood of ventricular fibrillation as the cause of cardiopulmonary arrest in the pediatric patient.

Pediatric out-of-hospital cardiac arrest patients rarely survive. In a study published in 1999,[1] researchers found that there were only five survivors of 300 pediatric out-of-hospital cardiac arrests, a survival rate of 1.7%. The researchers assessed the care given and found that the weak link was the lack of bystander and, especially, parental CPR.

The Role of Emergency Care Professionals in Caring for the Ill or Injured Child

Emergency care of children and families requires specific knowledge, equipment, skills, and resources. A child's physiologic response to a critical illness or injury differs from an adult's for such conditions as shock and prolonged respiratory distress. The causes of catastrophic events, such as cardiopulmonary arrest, are different from those in adults. In children, the signs and symptoms of distress may be subtle.

The impact of an injured or acutely ill child is devastating not only for the child but also for the child's family and the emergency care provider. When treating the child, we must remember to treat the family. Psychological and emotional management of the family is important at this critical time.

Emergency Medical Services for Children

The EMS system resulted from military experiences that demonstrated that survival could be greatly enhanced through appropriate triage, pre-hospital care, and timely transport. Early EMS systems (mid to late 1960s and early 1970s) focused on providing rapid intervention for sudden cardiac arrest in adults and rapid transport for motor vehicle crash victims. Because these systems focused on adult care, outcomes for adults in emergencies improved dramatically, whereas the specialized needs of children experiencing a medical emergency went largely unrecognized. As a result, the equipment, training, experience, and expertise of prehospital personnel were often less developed to meet the needs of children.

In the mid 1970s, this weakness in the EMS system began to be recognized. Healthcare professionals including pediatric surgeons, pediatricians, emergency physicians, and other concerned groups worked to ensure that the special needs of children were integrated into the EMS system. Their efforts remained unfunded until Congress enacted legislation in 1984 (Public Law 98-555) authorizing the use of federal funds for EMSC.

EMSC efforts have improved the availability of child-size equipment in ambulances and emergency department (EDs). EMSC has initiated hundreds of programs to prevent injuries and has provided thousands of hours of training to EMTs, paramedics, and other emergency medical care providers.

The EMSC program is designed to reduce child and youth mortality and morbidity sustained due to severe illness or trauma. It aims to

- Ensure state-of-the-art emergency medical care for the ill or injured child and adolescent
- Ensure that pediatric service is well integrated into an EMS system backed by optimal resources
- Ensure that the entire spectrum of emergency services, including primary prevention of illness and injury, acute care, and rehabilitation, is provided to children and adolescents, as well as adults.

Current goals of the EMSC program include the following:

- Include pediatric issues in all aspects of clinical care
- Improve and expand pediatric emergency care education systems
- Promote and strengthen pediatric EMS research and evaluation
- Enhance EMS human resource development
- Include pediatric components in the development of EMS information systems
- Ensure that integration of health services meets children's needs
- Promote institutionalization of EMSC through legislation and regulation

The federal EMSC program defines the population of children to include those from birth to 21 years of age.

- Include pediatric protocols in medical direction for all EMS agencies
- Develop broad-based support for prevention activities
- Ensure universal public access to the emergency care system for all children and their families
- Improve pediatric EMS through public education

EMSC has funded grants to focus on special pediatric EMS system development issues that are of regional or national concern. These grants have addressed such topics as quality improvement, the development of multimedia EMS training materials, managed care, and children with special healthcare needs.

EMSC grantees have developed many elements of a model EMSC system, including the following:

- Prehospital protocols for triage and treatment of children as distinct from adults
- Curricula for prehospital and ED staff addressing the differences between children and adult patients
- Standards for hospital facilities accepting pediatric patients

Scope

The EMSC program is responsible for a broad spectrum of services including prevention, early recognition of problems, initial stabilization of infants and children, and rehabilitative care.

EMSC encompasses seven phases of child and family services:

1. Prevention
2. System access
3. Field treatment (prehospital response)
4. Transport
5. ED (stabilization) care
6. Inpatient services (definitive care)
7. Rehabilitation (physical therapy, occupational therapy, social services)

Prevention Programs

Epidemiology of Pediatric Illness and Injury

Use of the term *accident*, which implies an unpredictable or unavoidable event, is being replaced with the term *injury* to more accurately reflect the nature of the problem.

Pediatric injuries are a major public health concern. In the United States, more than 20,000 children die each year from injuries. As a cause of death, pediatric injuries outrank all childhood diseases combined.

Children are at higher risk for injury than adults and are more likely to be seriously affected by the injuries they suffer. The American Academy of Pediatrics estimates that for each of these deaths, there are 16 injuries that require hospitalization and 381 injuries that require some form of outpatient treatment. Each year, roughly one in four children will suffer an injury serious enough to require a visit to an ED.

Childhood Injury Facts: How Frequently Are Children Injured?

- Each year in the United States, emergency departments treat more than 200,000 children ages 14 and younger for playground-related injuries.
- Children, especially those under age 6, are more likely to have unintentional poisonings than older children and adults.

- Among children ages 0 to 14 years, traumatic brain injuries (TBI) result in an estimated 400,000 emergency department visits each year.
- Children ages 4 years and younger are among those at highest risk for residential fire deaths and injuries.

From the National Center for Injury Prevention and Control. http://www.cdc.gov/ncipc/factsheets/children.htm Accessed 10/4/04.

Two criteria by which the significance of childhood injuries can be measured are death and **morbidity**. Although death is the worst possible outcome, injuries cause widespread morbidity, which results in the need for medical care and an inability to perform normal daily activities.

The type, number, and severity of pediatric injuries in a given area depend partly on regional characteristics.

- Geography (type of terrain, average response times for emergency care)
- Climate and weather conditions (temperature extremes, violent storms)
- Population density (crime rates, 9-1-1 coverage, availability of medical services)
- Population traits (ethnic backgrounds, education levels)
- Age also influences injury rates and patterns

Unintentional injuries are the leading killer of children aged 14 years and younger.

Primary prevention involves measures that can be applied in advance to reduce the likelihood that an injury will occur, such as installing a pedestrian overpass at a dangerous intersection. *Secondary prevention* includes interventions that will help prevent or minimize an injury while it happens, such as the use of bicycle helmets. Prehospital professionals, nurses, pediatricians, emergency physicians, and pediatric emergency medicine specialists must promote primary and secondary prevention to address the pediatric injury problem effectively. *Tertiary prevention* includes measures to lessen the severity of an injury and improve the patient's outcome *after* the injury has occurred, such as advanced trauma care and rehabilitation. Tertiary prevention cannot change the fact that the victim is injured, and it cannot help those whose injuries are too severe for them to be saved.

Successful injury prevention requires an approach that incorporates the "Four E's": education, enforcement, environmental modification, and engineering.

Understanding Injury Prevention

Healthcare professionals play an important role in injury prevention.

The "Four E's" of injury prevention: education, enforcement, environmental modification, and engineering.

Enforcement is viewed by some as interference with individual rights, which may result in resistance to new legislation.

- Education attempts to bring about positive behavioral changes by informing various groups about the existence of hazards and explaining ways to reduce or prevent the injuries these hazards may cause.
- Enforcement attempts to reduce dangerous behaviors through legislation that requires individuals, manufacturers, and local governments to comply with certain safety practices. Examples include mandatory seat belt and helmet laws, handgun control, zoning codes that require fences around private swimming pools, and safety regulations governing the manufacture of children's toys.
- Environmental modifications target social issues and physical features within a community that contribute to injury patterns. Examples include providing free smoke detectors or bike helmets to low-income families.
- Engineering involves technological changes that make products or the environment safer. Examples include childproof caps for medications and household solvents.

The most effective prevention strategies combine methods from multiple categories from the "Four E's." For example, a legislative change might combine environmental modification, enforcement, and education strategies to increase public acceptance.

Pediatric Equipment

The Injury Prevention Program (TIPP) is an educational program initiated by the American Academy of Pediatrics (AAP) for parents of children newborn through 12 years old to help prevent common injuries from motor vehicles, drowning, firearms, falls, bicycle crashes, pedestrian hazards, burns, poisoning, and choking.

Age-related safety sheets and rotating injury-specific TIPP sheets in conjunction with national safety campaigns are available on the AAP website (http://www.aap.org/family/tippmain.htm).

When caring for the pediatric patient, treatment interventions are usually based on the weight of the child. As a result, a range of age-appropriate and size-appropriate equipment (including bags and masks, tracheal tubes, and intravenous [IV] catheters) must be readily available for use in pediatric emergencies. The equipment and supplies must be logically organized, routinely checked, and readily available.

Studies have documented unreliability at estimating children's weights, a high rate of errors made when performing drug calculations, and a loss of valuable resuscitation time secondary to computing drug dosages and selecting equipment.

Length-based resuscitation tapes (Figure 1-2) are one example of a system that may be used to estimate weight by length and simplify selection of the medications and supplies needed during the emergency care of children. In the example shown, the tape assigns children to a color zone on the basis of their length. Appropriate resuscitation medication doses and equipment sizes are listed on the tape, as well as abnormal vital signs, fluid calculations, and energy levels recommended for defibrillation. If the child is taller than the tape, standard adult equipment and medication dosages are used.

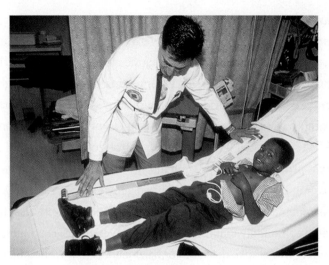

Figure 1-2   A length-based resuscitation tape is used to quickly estimate a child's height and to determine equipment needs and medication doses.

Treatment Protocols and Practice Guidelines

Treatment protocols and procedures specific to the pediatric patient are essential and should be developed to guide and maintain consistency in the delivery of emergency care. As protocols are developed, prevention, access, prehospital care, ED care, inpatient services, and rehabilitation must be considered.

Prehospital

Prehospital management of the pediatric patient necessitates the development and implementation of protocols for pediatric triage, transport, and treatment. Medical direction guidelines for the management of pediatric patients should exist for basic life support (BLS) and ALS prehospital providers. These guidelines may exist in off-line protocols or online medical direction.

Appropriate prehospital triage of the pediatric patient requires knowledge of community levels of pediatric care, available transport methods, and skill in pediatric assessment. Pediatric triage protocols should include hospital bypass criteria. The National Association of EMS Physicians has developed pediatric field treatment protocols for prehospital professionals. They are available online at *www.naemsp.org*.

Emergency Departments

Because caregivers often take an ill or injured child directly to the ED, it is essential that EDs and hospitals provide treatment that conforms to the recognized level of care with appropriate equipment, trained personnel, patient care guidelines, and an organized system of care response.

Minimum voluntary requirements endorsed by the American College of Emergency Physicians (ACEP), American Academy of Pediatrics, and a task force sponsored by the federal EMSC program were published in 2001. These guidelines outline necessary resources for pediatric emergency care in all EDs and address stabilization and transfer of selected patients to specialized pediatric centers (e.g., pediatric trauma centers, pediatric critical care centers).

When a child requires specialized care, agreements should exist between hospitals to facilitate transfer of the child and ensure a smooth and rapid transition. Children who experience a major complication or disability because of their illness or injury should be linked to rehabilitation services as early as possible.

Primary Care Providers

Children should have a designated primary care provider for preventive health services and management of healthcare conditions before they become emergencies. These primary care providers should be prepared to manage potential emergencies in their office setting until prehospital professionals are able to respond.

Identifying the Ill or Injured Child

Public Information and Education

Parents and other guardians, such as childcare providers, day care workers, and baby sitters need to know how to do the following:

- Distinguish emergent and nonemergent events
- Perform emergency first aid procedures
- Contact the child's physician
- Access the emergency care system
- Authorize emergency care and provide essential information to emergency care professionals

Emergency Care Professionals

Emergency care professionals

- Must be trained and competent in the care of pediatric patients. Support personnel from respiratory therapy, radiology, laboratory, and other departments should be oriented to the care of the pediatric patient.
- Must be able to recognize the signs that indicate a child's condition is becoming potentially life threatening. This requires understanding that there are differences in anatomic and physiologic characteristics and in cognitive, emotional, and psychosocial responses in pediatric age groups.

Essential knowledge for emergency care professionals includes growth and development, pediatric triage and acuity level identification, pediatric assessment and intervention techniques, common pediatric disease and injury processes, and prevention strategies as they relate to the infant, child, and adolescent.[2]

Children account for a small number of the total patients treated by emergency care professionals. Therefore there are frequently insufficient opportunities to use pediatric assessment and life-saving skills. Because skill decay is rapid, frequent practice sessions and refresher training are extremely important to maintaining preparedness.

Case Study Resolution

Pediatric out-of-hospital cardiac arrest patients rarely survive. Among children ages 1 to 4 years, most drownings occur in residential swimming pools. Most young children who drown in residential swimming pools were last seen in the home, had been out of sight less than 5 minutes, and were in the care of one or both parents at the time.

Primary prevention measures applicable in this situation include the use of a pool fence and a self-latching and locking gate surrounding the entire pool area and ensuring that the caregivers know how to swim. Parents, other relatives, and neighbors should be taught CPR. These individuals should also be taught that **constant** supervision of children is necessary, particularly around water.

As a healthcare professional, you play a vital role in the Chain of Survival. By working together, we can increase the pediatric patient's chance of survival.

Web Resources

- www.aap.org (American Academy of Pediatrics)
- www.ems-c.org (Emergency Medical Services for Children)
- www.naemsp.org (National Association of EMS Physicians)
- www.ashinstitute.org/public education.asp (American Safety & Health Institute)

References

1. Sirbaugh PE, Pepe PE, Shook JE, et al. A prospective, population-based study of the demographics, epidemiology, management, and outcome of out-of-hospital pediatric cardiopulmonary arrest. *Ann Emerg Med* 1999;33:174–184.
2. Emergency Nurses Association. *ENPC Provider Manual.* Park Ridge, IL: Emergency Nurses Association, 1998.

Chapter Quiz

1. The efforts of the _____ _____ _____ _____
   _____ program have improved the availability of child-size equipment in ambulances and
   emergency departments, initiated hundreds of programs to prevent injuries, and provided thousands of
   hours of training to emergency medical care providers.

2. True or False: The upper age limit of a child, as defined by the federal EMSC program, is 14 years of age.

3. List the seven phases of child and family services encompassed by the EMSC program.
   1. _____
   2. _____
   3. _____
   4. _____
   5. _____
   6. _____
   7. _____

4. Which of the following correctly reflects the sequential steps in the pediatric Chain of Survival?
   A) Early EMS activation, early ALS, prevention of illness or injury, early CPR.
   B) Early CPR, prevention of illness or injury, early ALS, early EMS activation.
   C) Early ALS, early EMS activation, early CPR, prevention of illness or injury.
   D) Prevention of illness or injury, early CPR, early EMS activation, early ALS.

5. _____ prevention involves measures that can be applied in advance to reduce the
   likelihood that an injury will occur. _____ prevention includes interventions that will help
   prevent or minimize an injury while it happens. _____ prevention includes measures to
   lessen the severity of an injury and improve the patient's outcome *after* the injury has occurred.

6. List the "Four E's required for successful injury prevention.
   1. _____
   2. _____
   3. _____
   4. _____

Chapter Quiz Answers

1. The efforts of the <u>Emergency Medical Services for Children</u> (EMSC) program have improved the availability of child-size equipment in ambulances and emergency departments, initiated hundreds of programs to prevent injuries, and provided thousands of hours of training to emergency medical care providers.

2. False. The Federal EMSC program defines the population of children to include those from birth to 21 years of age.

3. The seven phases of child and family services encompassed by the EMSC program are:
   1. Prevention.
   2. System access.
   3. Field treatment (prehospital response).
   4. Transport.
   5. Emergency department (stabilization) care.
   6. Inpatient services (definitive care).
   7. Rehabilitation (physical therapy, occupational therapy, social services).

4. D. The pediatric Chain of Survival represents a sequential series of events to assess, support, or restore effective ventilation and circulation to the child experiencing a respiratory or cardiorespiratory arrest. The sequence consists of four important steps: 1) Prevention of illness or injury, 2) Early CPR, 3) Early EMS activation, and 4) Early ALS.

5. <u>Primary</u> prevention involves measures that can be applied in advance to reduce the likelihood that an injury will occur. <u>Secondary</u> prevention includes interventions that will help prevent or minimize an injury while it happens. <u>Tertiary</u> prevention includes measures to lessen the severity of an injury and improve the patient's outcome *after* the injury has occurred.

6. Successful injury prevention requires an approach that incorporates the "Four E's": *E*ducation, *E*nforcement, *E*nvironmental modification, and *E*ngineering.

Growth and Development

2

Case Study

A 5-year-old boy has been struck by a car. He apparently ran into the street and was struck by a car traveling at 20 to 30 miles per hour. He was thrown about 15 feet, striking his head on the pavement after landing on his left hip and side.

Is the child's reported behavior consistent with his age? What strategies will you use for interacting with this child?

Objectives

1. Identify key growth and developmental characteristics of infants and children and their relevance to emergency care.
2. Identify key anatomic and physiologic characteristics of infants and children and their relevance to emergency care.
3. Describe techniques for successful assessment of infants and children.
4. Recognize the emotional dependence of the infant/child on his/her caregiver.
5. Describe techniques for successful interaction with families of acutely ill or injured infants and children.

Pediatric Age Classifications

- Newly born: neonate in the first minutes to hours following birth
- Neonate: Birth to 1 month
- Infant: 1 to 12 months of age
- Toddler: 1 to 3 years of age
- Preschooler: 4 to 5 years of age
- School age: 6 to 12 years of age
- Adolescent: The period between the end of childhood (beginning of puberty) and adulthood (18 years of age)
  - Highly child-specific (male child 10 to 16 years, average 13 years; female child 7 to 16 years, average 11 years)

- May also be defined as early (puberty), middle (middle school/high school), and late (high school/college age)

Developmental Characteristics, Common Fears, and Emergency Care Implications

- Cognitive milestones: Perceptual information from five sophisticated senses with smell, touch, and taste most adultlike
- Language milestones: Cries for multiple reasons including pain, hunger, too hot/too cold, dirty diaper
- Anatomic and physiologic considerations
  - At birth, the neonate's head accounts for one fourth of the body length and one third of the body weight. Because of the neonate's large occiput, it is very easy to either hyperextend or flex the neck, compromising the airway.
  - At birth, the ribs are mainly composed of cartilage and project at right angles from the vertebral column. As a result, the rib cage is more circular than that in adults.
  - Muscle mass makes up about 25% of birth weight.
  - Cranial bones are soft and separated by sutures. Membranous spaces (fontanelles) between the cranial bones allow expansion of the skull to accommodate brain growth. Vaginal delivery often causes molding of the neonate's skull, during which the cranial bones may shift and overlap. The skull resumes its appropriate size and shape within days.
  - The neonate's body, particularly the shoulders and back, may be covered with lanugo (fine, silky hair). Most of this hair is shed within 10 to 14 days.
  - Neonates are obligatory nose breathers. Complete or partial obstruction often results in respiratory distress.
  - Neonates are predisposed to hypothermia because of their small mass, large ratio of surface area to weight, and poor development of the subcutaneous fat layer of the skin.
  - Limited glycogen stores predispose the neonate to hypoglycemia.
- Physical milestones
  - Birth weight regained by 2 to 3 weeks of age
  - Reflex movements controlled by spinal cord and used for survival (sucking) or protection (eye blink)
  - Cannot roll or sit up (Figure 2-1)
  - Can grasp finger placed in palm but does not reach for objects

Birth to 1 month

The periods presented are averages. Some children may achieve developmental milestones earlier or later than the average but still be within the normal range.

To decrease the likelihood of sudden infant death syndrome (SIDS), instruct caregivers to place the infant on his or her back when sleeping.

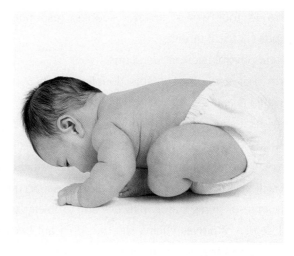

Figure 2-1 At 1 month, an infant is unable to sit upright.

- Demonstrates **Moro reflex** after loud hand clap: straightens elbows and opens arms, then flexes elbows in a hugging motion
- Social and emotional milestones
  - Alert when awake; little facial expression
  - Startles to sound, but does not turn to sound
  - Prefers to look at faces, but cannot follow objects
  - Soothed by calm, continuous speech
- Emergency care implications
  - Observe the baby before making contact
  - Keep in caregiver's arms if possible
  - Handle patient gently, but firmly, supporting head and neck
    - **Do not shake or jiggle the baby**
    - A one-per-second swaying motion is comforting
  - Perform least invasive parts of the examination first
  - Keep baby warm; warm anything that touches baby such as hands, stethoscope, blankets; keep the baby covered when not being examined
  - Speak softly and smile
  - Allow baby to suck on pacifier for comfort
  - Avoid loud noises, bright lights, and abrupt, jerky movements

Infant (1 to 12 months)

- Cognitive milestones: Looks, listens, smells, touches, and tastes to learn about the world
- Language milestones: Prespeech (0 to 10 months)
  - Cooing and babbling (2 to 3 months)
  - Babbling and blows raspberries (4 to 6 months)
  - Begins imitating word sounds ("ma ma" "da da") (6 to 8 months)

- Says two to four words, imitates sounds, responds to simple commands (10 to 12 months)
- Anatomic and physiologic considerations
  - The birth weight of most infants doubles within 5 months and triples within a year.
  - The three fetal shunts (ductus venosus, foramen ovale, and ductus arteriosus) normally close at birth or shortly thereafter.
  - Infants younger than 6 months are obligate nose breathers. Any degree of obstruction (e.g., swelling of the nasal mucosa, accumulation of mucus) can result in respiratory difficulty and problems with feeding.
  - A small degree of airway edema can be significant because of the small diameter of the airway, resulting in disproportionately higher resistance to airflow than in an adult.
  - An infant's vocal cords are more cartilaginous than an adult's and easily damaged.
  - An infant's chest wall is thin and the bony and cartilaginous rib cage is soft and pliant. Breathing is predominantly a result of diaphragmatic movement. Impaired movement of the diaphragm such as that due to gastric distention can significantly affect ventilation. Because of an infant's thin chest wall, transmitted breath sounds make it difficult to localize a problem area.
  - Infants in the first 3 months of life have an immature immunologic system and are more susceptible than an older infant or child to severe infections and to infections by unusual organisms.
  - Salivation starts at about 3 months. Drooling continues until the infant's swallowing reflex is more coordinated.
  - The midpoint in the height of an infant is the umbilicus, whereas the midpoint of an adult occurs at the symphysis pubis.
  - Infants have a higher circulating blood volume (about 75 mL/kg) compared with that of an adult (55 to 75 mL/kg).
  - The anterior and posterior fontanelles are membranous spaces formed where four cranial bones meet and intersect. Pulsations of the fontanelle reflect the heart rate. The posterior fontanelle is triangular and usually closes by 2 months of age. In most infants, the anterior fontanelle closes between 7 and 14 months of age. A bulging anterior fontanelle may be due to crying, coughing, vomiting, or increased intracranial pressure (ICP) due to a head injury, meningitis, or hydrocephalus. A depressed anterior fontanelle is seen in dehydrated or malnourished infants.
  - Subcutaneous fat reaches a maximum thickness in children 9 months of age.[1] This is reflected in the difficulty in placing a peripheral intravenous line at this age.

- An infant's abdomen is protuberant due to poorly developed abdominal muscles. The liver is proportionately larger in the abdominal cavity compared with the liver of an adult.
  - Underdeveloped cervical ligaments, relatively weak neck muscles, and anteriorly wedged cervical vertebrae make an infant susceptible to extreme hyperflexion and hyperextension of the neck and greater head motion when subjected to acceleration–deceleration forces.[2]
- Physical milestones

Gross-motor development begins with holding head up and progresses to rolling, sitting, creeping, crawling, standing, and walking. Fine-motor development starts with reaching and bringing objects to the mouth and then focuses on pincher grasp as manual exploration replaces oral. Red flags for weakness or spasticity include listing to one side after 3 months, frog-leg posturing, scissoring, pulling directly to a stand instead of a sit (at 4 months), bunny hopping, persistent toe-walking, and hand dominance before 18 months.

  - Control of eye muscles, lifts head when on stomach (2 to 3 months)
  - Flexion of extremities and Moro reflex begin to decrease, localizes sounds, control of head and arm movements, purposeful grasping/reaching for objects, rolls over (4 to 6 months)
  - Control of trunk and hands, sits without support, creeps (7 to 9 months)
  - Control of legs and feet, stands, crawls, opposition of thumb and forefinger (10 to 12 months)
- Social and emotional milestones
  - Can fix and follow on moving objects, smiles at a face, may be soothed by rocking (2 to 3 months) (Figure 2-2)
  - Turns to sound, recognizes caregiver, distinguishes between familiar persons and strangers, enjoys being cuddled (4 to 6 months)
  - Emotional attachment to primary caregiver, protests separation from primary caregiver, begins developing fear of strangers (7 to 9 months)
  - Responsive to own name, fear of strangers, curious, waves good-bye, gives and takes objects, understands "no!" (10 to 12 months)
- Common fears
  - Separation from primary caregiver
  - Stranger anxiety (crying or being wary of strangers)
- Emergency care implications
  - Observe the infant before making contact
  - Keep infant on caregiver's lap during physical examination if possible
  - Handle patient gently, but firmly, supporting head and neck
    - **Do not shake or jiggle the infant**

Foreign body airway obstruction risk begins at approximately 6 months.

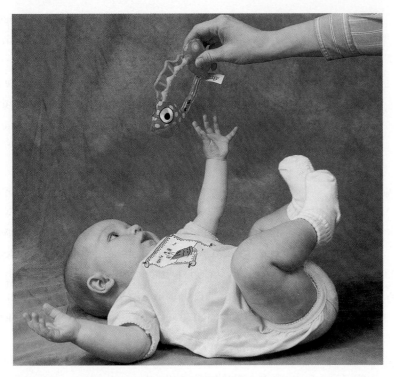

Figure 2-2   A 3-month-old infant focuses on a visual object and reaches toward it.

- Keep caregiver in sight if possible to decrease separation anxiety and involve caregiver in care of infant whenever possible
- Return infant to caregiver as soon as possible after procedures; allow caregiver to comfort
- Perform least invasive parts of the examination first
- Keep infant warm, warm anything that touches the infant (e.g., hands, stethoscope), and keep the environment warm
- Speak softly and smile; touch, rock, hold, cuddle if possible
- Examine from toes to head
- Provide comfort measures (e.g., pacifier)
- Distract with keys, penlight, musical toy in the infant's field of vision
- Persistent crying, irritability, or inability to console or arouse patient may indicate physiologic distress

Toddler (1 to 3 years)

Development of language (verbal intelligence) and problem-solving skills (nonverbal intelligence) are key to this stage. Object permanence (an object still exists when it is not in view) begins. Causality (actions produce a certain effect) is understood and used to produce desired results.

- Cognitive milestones
  - Obeys limited commands, repeats a few words, feeds self (1 to 1½ years).
  - Says words, phrases, and simple sentences, understands simple

directions, identifies simple pictures, likes to look at books, short attention span, avoids simple hazards (2 years).

- ◦ Says short sentences, tells simple stories, uses words as tools of thought, wants to understand environment, answers questions, plays make-believe with dolls, animals, and people; may recite few nursery rhymes, can count to 10 but may get the numbers out of sequence, can recall a two-step instruction ("Go find the ball and bring it to me"), improvement in memory skills (3 years).

- Language milestones
  - ◦ 10 to 18 months
    - ▪ Naming period: people and objects have labels
    - ▪ Follows simple commands with gestures
  - ◦ 18 to 24 months
    - ▪ Word combination period
      - • Two-word to three-word sentences
      - • Uses "I," "me," and "you"
    - ▪ Understands physical relationships ("on," "in," "under")
  - ◦ Strangers can understand child's speech at age 3

- Anatomic and physiologic considerations
  - ◦ Trachea is small and short; may result in intubation of the right mainstem bronchus or inadvertent extubation.
  - ◦ Thin chest wall allows for easily transmitted breath sounds; easy to miss a pneumothorax or misplaced tracheal tube because of transmitted breath sounds.
  - ◦ The chest grows at a faster rate than the cranium; at some time between 6 months and 2 years, both measurements are about the same. After age 2, the chest circumference is greater than the head circumference.[3]
  - ◦ Increased risk of head injuries from falls and motor vehicle crashes because of higher center of gravity.
  - ◦ Children younger than 3 years are much less likely to have serious injuries than older children who fall the same distance. It is thought that younger children may better dissipate the energy transferred by the fall because they have more fat and cartilage and less muscle mass than older children.[4]
  - ◦ Higher incidence of multiple-organ injury from trauma than adults because kinetic injury is dissipated into a smaller mass.
  - ◦ On auscultation, breath sounds are louder and harsher than in an adult because of the child's relative lack of musculature and subcutaneous tissue overlying the thorax.
  - ◦ The young child is particularly prone to temperature extremes because thermoregulatory controls are not completely developed.

- Body surface area is larger than in an adult, predisposing the child to increased heat loss through radiation, convection, and conduction.
- Physical milestones
  - Walks alone, climbs stairs, runs, may learn bowel and bladder control
  - At age 2, a child is 50% of his or her adult height.
  - Toddlers are prone to injury.
- Social and emotional milestones
  - Temper tantrums (1 to 3 years)
  - Upset when separated from primary caregiver, beginning a sense of personal identity and belongings, possessive, enjoys physical affection (1½ to 2 years)
  - Imitates adults and playmates (Figure 2-3), greater sense of personal identity, beginning to be adventuresome, understands concept of "mine" and "his/hers" (2 to 3 years)
  - Separates easily from primary caregiver by age 3
- Common fears
  - Being left alone
  - Interacting with strangers
  - Interruptions in usual routine
  - Losing control
  - Getting hurt (e.g., falls, cuts, abrasions)

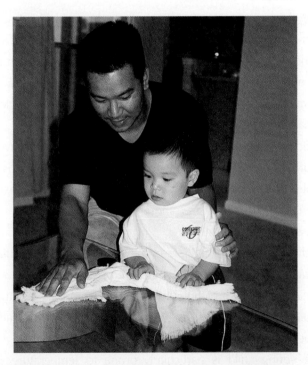

Figure 2-3 Mimicking adults and playmates is common during toddlerhood.

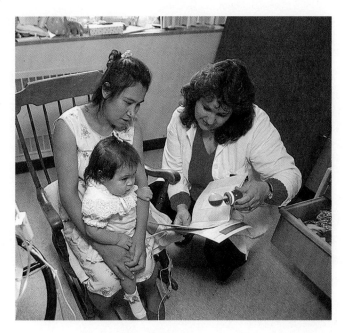

Figure 2-4   When possible, examine the child in an upright position and assume a position at his or her level.

Toddlers will often use a transitional object such as a blanket, doll, stuffed animal, or toy to help them feel secure.

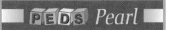

Because a child expects his or her caregiver to protect them, do not ask a caregiver to restrain a child or participate in any way other than to comfort the child.

- Emergency care implications: examine as for infant plus
  - Encourage child's trust by gaining cooperation of caregiver
  - Try not to separate child from the caregiver (Figure 2-4)
  - Address the child by name
  - Smile and speak in calm, quiet tone
  - Allow child to participate in care when possible
  - Respect modesty; keep child covered if possible and replace clothing promptly after examining each body area
  - Allow the child to hold transitional objects (Figure 2-5)
  - Explain that illness or injury is not the child's fault
  - Reassure child if a procedure will not hurt
  - Do not show needles, scissors unless necessary
  - Avoid procedures on the dominant hand/arm
  - Avoid covering the child's face
  - Involve caregiver in treatment whenever possible
  - Persistent irritability and inability to console or arouse patient may indicate physiologic distress
  - Foreign body airway obstruction continues to be a risk

Preschooler (3 to 5 years)

- Cognitive milestones
  - Highly imaginative
  - Fears pain and disfigurement

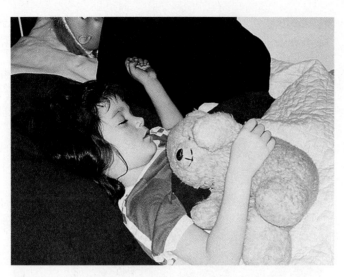

Figure 2-5   A toddler will often use a transitional object such as a blanket, doll, stuffed animal, or toy to help them feel secure.

- ◦ Beginning to know difference between fact and fiction (lying), interested in environment; can reliably explain where pain is located (5 years)
- ◦ Thinks in absolutes (things are "good" or "bad"; a cut either hurts or does not hurt)
- ◦ May not understand cause and effect (such as swallowing medicine to make pain go away)
- ◦ Views clothing and possessions as part of self and does not like having them removed
- ◦ May think illness or injury is punishment for bad behavior or thoughts
- ◦ Believes others see things from child's own viewpoint
- • Language milestones: Uses complete sentences, asks many questions, imitates adult conversation
- • Anatomic and physiologic considerations
- ◦ Ribs and sternum are pliable; more resistant to rib fractures than those of adults, although the force of the injury is readily transmitted to the delicate tissues of the lung and may result in a pulmonary contusion, hemothorax, or pneumothorax.
- ◦ Cannot sustain rapid respiratory rates for long periods due to immature intercostal muscles.
- ◦ Oxygen requirements are approximately twice those of adolescents and adults (6 to 8 mL/kg/min in a child; 3 to 4 mL/kg/min in an adult).
- ◦ Children have a proportionately smaller functional residual capacity,

and therefore proportionally smaller oxygen reserves. Hypoxia develops rapidly because of increased oxygen requirements and decreased oxygen reserves.

- The liver and spleen of a small child are lower in the abdomen and less protected by the rib cage.
- A young child's vertebral column may withstand traction and torsion without evidence of deformity while the spinal cord tears.

- Physical milestones
  - Runs well, marches, stands on one foot briefly, pedals tricycle, feeds self well, puts on shoes and socks, unbuttons and buttons (3 years).
  - Skips on one foot, cuts with scissors (not well), can wash and dry face, dress self except ties, standing broad jump, throws ball overhead, high motor drive (4 years).
  - Hops, skips, climbs, runs, dresses without help, good balance, skates, rides wagon and scooter, prints simple letters, handedness established, ties shoes (5 years) (Figure 2-6).
  - Frequent associated minor injuries.
- Social and emotional milestones
  - Enjoys being with others, likes to "help," responds to verbal guidance (3 years)

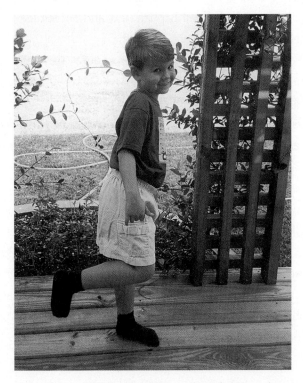

Figure 2-6   A 4-year-old child has sufficient balance to hop on one foot.

- ◦ Cooperative play, enjoys other children's company, highly social, may play loosely organized group games such as tag, duck-duck-goose (4 years)
- ◦ Organized, enjoys simple table games requiring turns and observing rules such as "school," feels pride in accomplishments (5 years)
- ◦ Accepts strangers, but slow to trust when ill or injured
- ◦ Modest about being undressed
- ◦ Likes to have control
- Common fears
  - ◦ Bodily injury and mutilation
  - ◦ Loss of control
  - ◦ The unknown and the dark
  - ◦ Being left alone
  - ◦ Being lost or abandoned
  - ◦ Adults that look or act mean
- Emergency care implications: Examine as for toddler plus
  - ◦ When possible, examine and treat the child in an upright position.
  - ◦ Explain procedures in brief, simple terms as they are performed.
  - ◦ Speak quietly in clear and simple language; avoid baby talk and frightening or misleading comments (e.g., shot, deaden, cut, germs, put to sleep) (see sidebar).
  - ◦ Allow the child to hold a transitional object or keep it in sight.
    - ▪ Tell the child what will happen next and encourage the child to help with his or her care.
    - ▪ Warn the child of a painful procedure just before carrying it out.
    - ▪ Offer the child treatment choices if possible.
    - ▪ Use an adhesive bandage after a procedure or when an injection has been given because the child may fear that "all of my blood will leak out" if a bandage is removed or not applied.
    - ▪ Respect the child's modesty.
    - ▪ Keep the child warm.
    - ▪ Allow caregiver to remain with the child whenever possible to help relieve the child's fear of separation from his or her caregiver.
    - ▪ Persistent irritability or inability to arouse patient may indicate physiologic distress.
    - ▪ Foreign body airway obstruction risk continues.

A child may feel vulnerable and out of control when lying down.

Give the child stickers or tokens for cooperation with procedures.

Selecting Nonthreatening Words or Phrases	
Words/Phrases to Avoid	**Suggested Substitutions**
Shot, bee sting, stick	Medicine under the skin
Organ	Special place in the body
Test	See how (specify body part) is working
Incision	Special opening
Edema	Puffiness
Stretcher, gurney	Rolling bed
Stool	Child's usual term
Dye	Special medicine
Pain	Hurt, discomfort, "owie," "boo-boo"
Deaden	Numb, make sleepy
Cut, fix	Make better
Take (as in "take your temperature" and "take your blood pressure")	See how warm you are Check your pressure; hug your arm
Put to sleep, anesthesia	Special sleep
Catheter	Tube
Monitor	TV screen
Electrodes	Stickers, ticklers
Specimen	Sample

From Wong DL, Hockenberry-Eaton M. *Wong's Essentials of Pediatric Nursing*, 6th ed. St. Louis: Mosby, 2001.

School-age Child (6 to 12 years)

- Cognitive milestones
  - Sees the world objectively and realistically
  - Understands concepts dealing with past and some future events
  - Masters reading, writing, and arithmetic
  - Engages in more flexible, relative thinking (a laceration may hurt a little or a lot)
  - Understands cause and effect and may be reasoned with (for example, understands that medicine will help pain go away)
  - May make up symptoms, but these will become inconsistent with distraction
  - Can reliably report where pain is located; quickly sees through falsehoods
  - Begins to understand death
- Language milestones: Uses language to communicate thoughts and learn what others are thinking
- Anatomic and physiologic considerations
  - Bones begin to lose flexibility around the age of 6 years, when the bony cortex begins to harden and thicken.
  - Lung volume increases to 200 mL by age 8.
  - In children younger than 13 years, penetrating injuries are likely to

be caused by accidental impalement on objects such as scissors or picket fences or by accidental discharge of a weapon.

- Physical milestones
  - Physical skills are well developed.
  - Better coordination reduces mishaps, but injuries due to risk-taking behavior increase (Figure 2-7).
- Social and emotional milestones
  - Has clear social skills
  - Can appreciate another's point of view; quickly senses shame, anger, frustration in adults
  - Usually modest about being undressed
  - Aware of bodily functions and internal organs
- Common fears
  - Fear of unknown setting
  - Separation from caregiver
  - Loss of control
  - Pain, loss of function
  - Bodily injury and mutilation
  - Failure to live up to the expectations of others
  - Rejection by peers
  - Death
  - Being unable to compete in school, sports, or play
  - Interruptions in daily routine

The growth spurt for girls can start as early as age $7^{1}/_{2}$ years and as late as age $11^{1}/_{2}$ years. The growth spurt for boys can start as early as age $10^{1}/_{2}$ years and as late as age 16.[5]

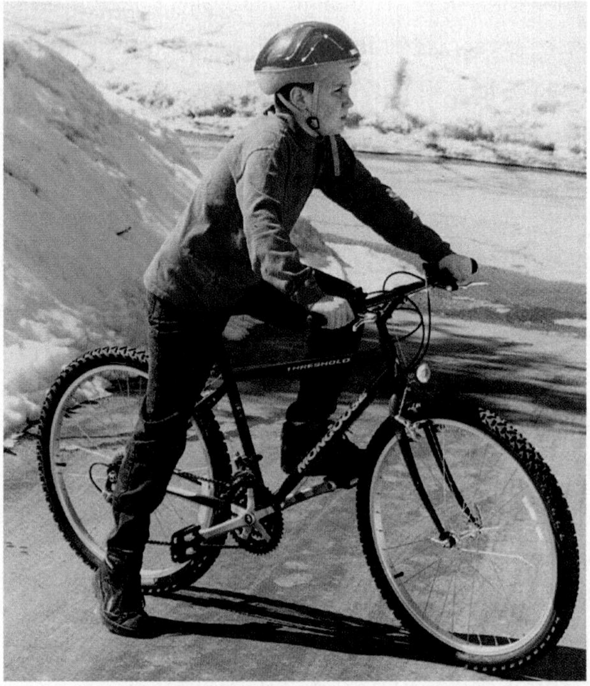

Figure 2-7   The school-aged child has good coordination, but injuries due to risk-taking behavior increase in this age group.

- Emergency care implications: Examine as for preschooler plus
  - Enlist the child's cooperation.
  - Introduce yourself to the child and approach him/her in a friendly, sympathetic manner.
  - Explain procedures before carrying them out.
  - Allow the child to see and touch samples of equipment that may be used in his or her care (e.g., medicine cup, cotton swab, tongue depressor).
  - Tell the child what will happen next and encourage the child to help with his or her care.
  - Warn the child of a painful procedure just before carrying it out.
  - Offer the child alternatives (e.g., "It is OK to yell, but don't move").
  - Make a contract with the child ("I promise to tell you everything I am going to do if you will help me by cooperating").
  - When speaking with the caregiver, include the child.
  - Include the child in discharge instructions.
  - Persistent irritability or inability to arouse patient may indicate physiologic distress.
  - Respect patient modesty.
  - Reassure patient of body integrity.
  - Address preoccupation about death when appropriate.

Honesty is particularly important when interacting with school-aged children.

Adolescent (13 to 18 years)

- Cognitive milestones
  - Engages in near-adult levels of abstract, objective, and rational thinking, but may have difficulty seeing adult perspectives
  - Has solid understanding of right and wrong; may be self-centered
  - Concerned about body image, scarring, and disfigurement
  - May be greatly influenced by opinions of peers
  - Capable of making up or misrepresenting physical or mental symptoms
  - Can reliably describe location of pain; can make decisions about care
- Language milestones: Language abilities approach adult levels, particularly in late adolescence
- Anatomic and physiologic considerations
  - Children grow at a faster rate during adolescence than at any other period except infancy.
  - Sebaceous glands increase sebum production in response to increased hormone levels. This gives the skin an oily appearance and predisposes the adolescent to acne.
  - By age 10, the size and flexibility of the airway matches that of adults.
  - Bone growth ends at age 20, when the epiphyses close.

- By 15 years of age, cardiac output is equal to that of an adult.
- Circulatory response to shock is similar to that of an adult.
- Breast tissue in females develops between 9 and 13 years of age. Mature adult breast tissue is achieved between 13 and 16 years of age.
- In children older than 13 years, 75% of penetrating trauma injuries are knife or handgun wounds inflicted by an assailant.[6]
- Physical milestones
  - Skills and coordination are similar to an adult's, but may lack adult strength and endurance in early adolescence.
  - Risk-taking or impulsive behavior may result in injuries or illness.
- Social and emotional milestones
  - Relates in direct, straightforward manner to adults who demonstrate respect
  - Appreciates being told the truth
  - Values privacy
  - Concerned about maintaining independence
  - Peer group is a major influence (Figure 2-8)
- Common fears
  - Being left out or socially isolated
  - Fear they will inherit parent's problems (e.g., alcoholism, mental illness)
  - Early and violent death
  - Loss of control
  - Altered body image
  - Separation from peer group
- Emergency care implications: Examine as for school-aged children, plus
  - Speak in a respectful, friendly manner, as if speaking to an adult.

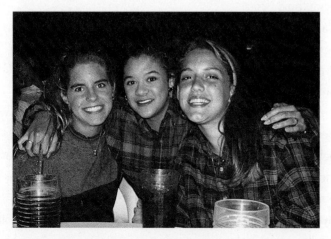

Figure 2-8   The peer group is a major influence in adolescent development.

- Obtain a history from the patient if possible.
- Respect independence; address the adolescent directly.
- Allow caregiver to be involved in examination if patient wishes.
- Explain things clearly and honestly; allow time for questions.
- Involve the patient in treatment whenever possible.
- Respect the patient's modesty.
- Address patient concerns of body integrity/disfigurement.
- Deal with the patient tactfully and fairly.
- Provide discharge instructions to the patient.
- Vital signs approach adult values.
- Consider the possibility of substance abuse, endangerment of self or others.

Case Study Resolution

This child's behavior is consistent with his age. Five-year-olds are very active and can hop, skip, climb, and run. When possible, examine a preschooler with his or her caregiver nearby. A 5-year-old will accept a stranger, but is slow to trust when ill or injured. If no obvious life-threatening injuries are present, begin your examination at his toes and work toward his head. Because a child of this age is modest about being undressed, keep him covered when possible and replace clothing promptly.

When talking with this child, expect him to answer in complete sentences and reliably explain where his pain is located (if present). If a procedure will hurt, be sure to warn the child just before the procedure.

References

1. Ludwig S, Loiselle J. Anatomy, growth, and development: impact on injury. In: Eichelberger MR, ed. *Pediatric trauma: prevention, acute care, and rehabilitation.* St. Louis, Mosby–Year Book, 1993, pp. 39–58.
2. Davis HW, Carrasco MM. Child abuse and neglect. In: Zitelli BJ, Davis HW, eds. *Atlas of pediatric physical diagnosis,* 4th ed. St. Louis: Mosby, 2002, pp. 153–224.
3. Jarvis C. *Pocket companion for physical examination and health assessment,* 2nd ed. Philadelphia: WB Saunders, 1996.
4. Meller JL, Shermeta DW. Falls in urban children: a problem revisited. *Am J Dis Child* 1987; 141:1271–1275.
5. Burke PJ. Developmental considerations. In: Kelly SJ, ed. *Pediatric emergency nursing,* 2nd ed. Norwalk, CT: Appleton & Lange, 1994, pp. 39–51.
6. Barkin RM, Marx JA. Abdominal trauma. In: Barkin RM, Rosen P, eds. *Emergency pediatrics: a guide to ambulatory care,* 5th ed. St. Louis: Mosby, 1999, pp. 476–487.

Chapter Quiz

1. The pediatric patient from birth to 1 month of age is called a(n):
    A) Newly born.
    B) Neonate.
    C) Infant.
    D) Toddler.

2. An infant is correctly defined as a pediatric patient:
    A) In the first minutes to hours following birth.
    B) From birth to 1 month of age.
    C) From 1 to 12 months of age.
    D) From 1 to 3 years of age.

3. Which of the following should be kept in mind when examining a 3-year-old?
    A) Remove clothing, examine, replace.
    B) Children of this age are unafraid of strangers.
    C) Toddlers prefer to be examined privately, away from the caregiver.
    D) Children of this age prefer direct eye contact with strangers.

4. Generally, an infant is responsive to his or her own name, gives and takes objects, and understands "no!" at age _____ .
    A) 1 to 3 months.
    B) 4 to 6 months.
    C) 7 to 9 months.
    D) 10 to 12 months.

5. At which age does a child begin to fear disfigurement?
    A) 1 to 3 years.
    B) 3 to 5 years.
    C) 6 to 12 years.
    D) 13 to 18 years.

6. Match each age group with the appropriate cognitive milestone.

_____ Preschooler (3 to 5 years).

_____ Infant (1 to 12 months) .

_____ Adolescent (13 to 18 years).

_____ Toddler (1 to 3 years).

_____ School-age child (6 to 12 years).

A) Says words, phrases, and simple sentences, understands simple directions, likes to look at books, short attention span, avoids simple hazards, can count to 10 but may get the numbers out of sequence.

B) Understands cause and effect and may be reasoned with; can reliably report where pain is located; quickly sees through falsehoods; begins to understand death.

C) Uses complete sentences, asks endless questions, learning to generalize, highly imaginative, dramatic, can classify objects by size, shape, and use; number skills are improving, long-term memory is expanding.

D) Looks, listens, smells, touches, and tastes to learn about the world.

E) Has a solid understanding of right and wrong; may be self-centered; concerned about body image, scarring, and disfigurement; may be greatly influenced by opinions of peers; capable of making up or misrepresenting physical or mental symptoms.

Chapter Quiz Answers

1. B. The pediatric patient from birth to 1 month of age is called a neonate.

2. C. An infant is correctly defined as a pediatric patient from birth to 12 months of age.

3. A. Toddlers are likely to resist examination and treatment and may scream, cry, or kick when touched. They do not like having their clothing removed so be sure to remove only the clothing necessary, examine the child, and replace the clothing as quickly as possible. Children of this age may be threatened by direct eye contact with strangers.

4. D. Generally, an infant 10 to 12 months of age is responsive to his or her own name, fears strangers, is curious, waves bye-bye, plays pat-a-cake, gives and takes objects, and understands "no!"

5. B. The 3 to 5 year old child fears pain, separation from his or her parents, and begins to fear disfigurement.

6. Matching exercise – cognitive milestones.
   (C) Preschooler (3 to 5 years).
   (D) Infant (1 to 12 months).
   (E) Adolescent (13 to 18 years).
   (A) Toddler (1 to 3 years).
   (B) School-age child (6 to 12 years).

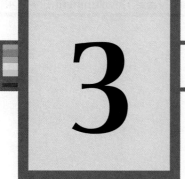

3 Patient Assessment

Case Study

Your patient is a 4-year-old boy with a fever. The boy clings to his father as Dad explains that the child has been sick with a fever for the past 2 days and has been crying frequently.

Using the Pediatric Assessment Triangle (PAT), your first impression of the child is that he is awake and aware of your presence. His respiratory rate is within normal limits for his age with no evidence of increased respiratory effort. Chest expansion appears symmetric. His nose is running and his skin appears flushed.

Based on the information provided, is this child "sick" or "not sick?" How should you proceed?

Objectives

1. Discuss the components of a pediatric assessment.
2. Describe techniques for successful assessment of infants and children.
3. Identify key anatomic and physiologic characteristics of infants and children and their implications.
4. Identify normal age-group–related vital signs.
5. Discuss the appropriate equipment used to obtain pediatric vital signs.
6. Identify the components of pediatric triage.

Initial Evaluation of the Acutely Ill or Injured Child

Scene Survey

- Hazards
  - Note any hazards or potential hazards and any visible mechanism or injury or illness (Figure 3-1)
  - Presence of pills, medicine bottles, or household chemicals may indicate a possible toxic ingestion
  - Injury and history that do not coincide with the mechanism of injury may indicate child abuse
- Relationships/interaction
  - Observe the interaction between the caregiver and the child and

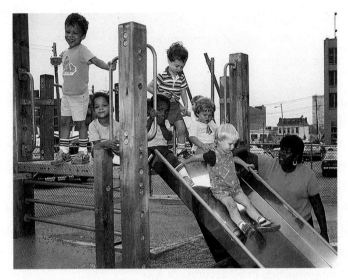

Figure 3-1   When evaluating the scene, note any hazards or potential hazards and any visible mechanism or injury or illness.

determine the appropriateness of their interaction. Does the interaction demonstrate concern, or is it angry or indifferent?

- Other important assessments that can be made during the scene survey include the following:
  - Orderliness, cleanliness, and safety of the home
  - General appearance of other children in the family
  - Presence of any medical devices used for the child (e.g., ventilator)
  - Indications of parental substance abuse. Parental substance abuse is associated with a more than twofold increase in the risk of exposure to childhood physical and sexual abuse.[1]
- Determine if additional resources are necessary including law enforcement, fire equipment, extrication equipment, special rescue services, additional medical personnel, or special transport services (aeromedical transport)

Pediatric Assessment: Components

The steps used to perform a pediatric assessment are described here as a linear process for clarity. In practice, some steps may be performed simultaneously, particularly if additional healthcare professionals are available to assist.

- Initial assessment
  - Pediatric Assessment triangle (PAT) (first impression)
  - Primary survey (ABCDE assessment)
  - Secondary survey
    - Vital signs

- Focused history
- Detailed physical examination
- Ongoing assessment

Pediatric Assessment Triangle (Figure 3-2)

- First impression/"across-the-room" assessment
  - Because approaching an ill or injured child can increase agitation, possibly worsening the child's condition, the PAT is performed **before** approaching or touching the child.
- Pause a short distance from the patient and, using your senses of sight and hearing (look and listen), quickly determine if a life-threatening problem exists that requires immediate intervention.
- Can be completed in 60 seconds or less.
- No equipment (cardiac monitor, blood pressure cuff, stethoscope) required.

The PAT and primary survey are used to quickly determine if a child is "sick" or "not sick." Remember that your patient's condition can change at any time. A patient who initially appears "not sick" may rapidly deteriorate and appear "sick." Reassess frequently.

- Establishes severity of illness or injury (sick [unstable] or not sick [stable])
- Identifies general category of physiologic abnormality (e.g., cardiopulmonary, neurologic, metabolic, toxicologic, trauma)
- Determines urgency of further assessment and intervention

Appearance

- Reflects the adequacy of oxygenation, ventilation, brain perfusion, homeostasis, and central nervous system function
- Assessment areas
  - **T**one (muscle tone)
  - **I**nteractivity/mental status
    - Level of responsiveness

Initial Assessment

TICLS (pronounced *tickles*) is a mnemonic used to recall the areas to be assessed related to the child's appearance.

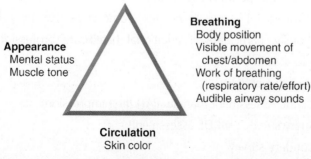

Figure 3-2   Pediatric Assessment Triangle.

- Interaction with caregiver
- Response to you or other healthcare professionals
  - **C**onsolability
  - **L**ook or gaze
  - **S**peech or cry
- Normal findings: Normal muscle tone, child responds to name (if older than 6 to 8 months), equal movement of all extremities, eyes open, normal speech or cry
- Abnormal findings
  - Agitation, marked irritability, reduced responsiveness, drooling (beyond infancy), limp or rigid muscle tone, inconsolable crying, failure to recognize caregiver, paradoxic irritability (irritable when held and lethargic when left alone; may be seen in infants and small children with neurologic infections).
  - If the child exhibits abnormal findings, proceed immediately to the primary survey.

(Work of) Breathing
- Reflects the adequacy of airway, oxygenation, and ventilation
- Assessment areas
  - Body position
  - Visible movement (chest/abdomen)
  - Respiratory rate
  - Respiratory effort
  - Audible airway sounds
- Normal findings: Quiet, nonlabored respirations; equal chest rise and fall, respiratory rate within normal range
- Abnormal findings
  - Abnormal body position (e.g., **sniffing position**, **tripod position**, **head bobbing**), **nasal flaring**, retractions, muffled or hoarse speech, **stridor**, **grunting**, **gasping**, **gurgling**, **wheezing**, respiratory rate outside normal range, accessory muscle use.
  - If the child exhibits abnormal findings, proceed immediately to the primary survey (Table 3-1).

Circulation
- Reflects the adequacy of cardiac output and perfusion of vital organs (i.e., core perfusion)
- Assessment areas: skin color
- Normal findings: color appears normal for child's ethnic group
- Abnormal findings
  - Pallor, mottling, cyanosis.
  - If the child exhibits abnormal findings, proceed immediately to the primary survey.

TABLE 3-1 *Abnormal Airway Sounds*

Gasping	Inhaling and exhaling with quick, difficult breaths
Grunting	Short, low-pitched sound heard at the end of exhalation that represents an attempt to generate positive end-expiratory pressure (PEEP) by exhaling against a closed glottis, prolonging the period of oxygen and carbon dioxide exchange across the alveolar-capillary membrane; a compensatory mechanism to help maintain patency of small airways and prevent atelectasis
Gurgling	Abnormal respiratory sound associated with collection of liquid or semisolid material in the patient's upper airway
Snoring	Noisy breathing through the mouth and nose during sleep, caused by air passing through a narrowed upper airway
Stridor	Harsh, high-pitched sound heard on inspiration associated with upper airway obstruction; frequently described as a high-pitched crowing or "seal-bark" sound
Wheezing	High-pitched "whistling" sounds produced by air moving through narrowed airway passages

Based on your first impression, decide if the child is sick (unstable) or not sick (stable).

- If the child's condition is urgent:
  - Proceed immediately with rapid assessment of airway, breathing, and circulation.
  - If a problem is identified, perform necessary interventions – "Treat as you find."
- If the child's condition is not urgent, proceed systematically:
  - Primary survey
  - Secondary survey
    - Vital signs
    - Focused history
    - Physical examination
  - Ongoing assessment

Primary Survey

The primary survey is also called the ABCDE assessment. During the primary survey, assessment and management occur simultaneously. The primary survey should be periodically repeated, particularly after any major intervention or when a change in the patient's condition is detected.

The primary survey focuses on basic life support (BLS) patient assessment and management. It usually requires less than 60 seconds to complete but may take longer if intervention is needed at any point.

- Systematic hands-on assessment
- Purpose: determine if life-threatening conditions exist
- Components: ABCDE
  - *A*irway and cervical spine protection
  - *B*reathing and ventilation

○ **C**irculation with bleeding control

○ **D**isability (mental status)

○ **E**xpose/environment

Airway and Cervical Spine Protection

- Assessment

  ○ Goals:

    ▪ Patent airway/absence of signs or symptoms of airway obstruction (e.g., stridor, dyspnea, hoarse voice)

    ▪ Able to handle oral secretions independently

    ▪ Patient speaks or makes appropriate sounds for age

  ○ Determine if the airway is patent, maintainable, or unmaintainable.

    ▪ Patent: able to be maintained independently

    ▪ Maintainable with positioning, suctioning

    ▪ Unmaintainable: requires assistance (e.g., tracheal intubation, cricothyrotomy, foreign body removal)

  ○ If cervical spine injury is suspected (by examination, history, or mechanism of injury), manually stabilize the head and neck in a neutral, in-line position or maintain spinal stabilization if already completed.

  ○ If the child is responsive and the airway is open (patent), move on to evaluation of the patient's breathing. If the child is responsive but cannot talk, cry, or cough forcefully, evaluate for possible airway obstruction.

  ○ If the child is unresponsive:

    ▪ Use manual airway maneuvers such as a head tilt–chin lift or jaw thrust without head tilt to open the airway (see Chapter 5). If trauma is suspected, use the jaw thrust without head tilt maneuver to open the airway.

    ▪ Assess the patient's airway

      • If the airway is patent (clear of debris and obstruction), move on to evaluation of the patient's breathing.

      • If the airway is not patent, assess for sounds of airway compromise (snoring, gurgling, or stridor). Gurgling is an indication for immediate suctioning.

      • Look in the mouth for blood, broken teeth, gastric contents, and foreign objects (e.g., loose teeth, gum, small toys). If present, position the patient to facilitate drainage and suction the mouth. If solid material is visualized, remove it with a gloved finger covered in gauze. If a foreign-body obstruction is suspected but not visualized, clear the obstruction by performing abdominal thrusts (if the patient is 1 year of age or older) or chest thrusts (if the patient is younger than 1 year of age).

The responsive child may have assumed a position to maximize his or her ability to maintain an open airway. Allow the child to maintain this position as you continue your assessment.

If blood, vomitus, or other secretions are visible, suction the oropharynx with a rigid (tonsil tip) suction catheter while manually opening the airway.

- Insert an airway adjunct (e.g., oropharyngeal [OPA] or naso-pharyngeal airway [NPA]) as needed to maintain a patent airway.
    - Use of an NPA is not recommended if trauma to the mid face is present or in cases of a known or suspected basilar skull fracture (see Chapter 9). If a basilar or cribriform plate fracture is present, the NPA may enter the cranial vault during insertion.
- Perform tracheal intubation if airway patency cannot be maintained by other means. Rapid sequence intubation (RSI) should be considered for those patients in whom intubation may otherwise be difficult due to combativeness, seizures, clenched teeth, or posturing (see Chapter 5).
  - Signs of distress may include the following:
    - Preferred posture (e.g., tripod position, holding head to maintain an open airway)
    - Drooling
    - Difficulty swallowing
    - Swelling of the lips and/or tissues of the mouth
    - Inadequate air movement
    - Obstruction by the tongue, blood, vomitus, foreign body
    - Abnormal airway sounds
- Interventions
  - Spinal stabilization as needed for trauma
  - Jaw thrust without head tilt
  - Head tilt–chin lift
  - Suction
  - Reposition
  - Removal of foreign body
  - Airway adjuncts (e.g., oropharyngeal airway, NPA)

> The head tilt–chin lift should *not* be used to open the airway if trauma is suspected.

Breathing and Ventilation

- Assessment
  - Goals:
    - Adequate gas exchange with no signs of hypoxia
      - Awake and alert
      - Pulse oximetry = oxygen saturation above 95%
      - Skin color normal; warm and dry
      - Respirations are spontaneous, unlabored, and at a normal rate for age
      - Chest expansion is equal bilaterally
      - Breath sounds are present, clear, and equal bilaterally
    - Absence of dyspnea, stridor, and signs of increased work of breathing (e.g., retractions, grunting, tracheal tugging, accessory muscle use, nasal flaring, head bobbing).

Evaluation of breathing should take no more than 10 seconds.

Look, listen, feel: inspect, auscultate, palpate.

Respiratory distress is increased work of breathing (respiratory effort).
Respiratory failure is a clinical condition in which there is inadequate blood oxygenation and/or ventilation to meet the metabolic demands of body tissues.

- Confirm that the child *is* breathing and note significant abnormalities in the work of breathing. If the patient is breathing, determine if breathing is adequate or inadequate. If breathing is adequate, move on to assessment of circulation.
  - Look
    - Assess the chest and abdomen for respiratory movement. Evaluate the depth (tidal volume) and symmetry of movement with each breath.
      - Tidal volume is the volume of air moved into or out of the lungs during a normal breath. Tidal volume can be indirectly evaluated by observing the rise and fall of the patient's chest and abdomen.
      - Minute volume is the amount of air moved in and out of the lungs in 1 minute and is determined by multiplying the tidal volume by the respiratory rate. Thus, a change in either the tidal volume *or* respiratory rate will affect minute volume.
    - Determine the respiratory rate.
      - The patient with breathing difficulty often has a respiratory rate outside the normal limits for his or her age (Table 3-2). Count the respiratory rate for 30 seconds and then double this figure to find the rate per minute.
      - **Tachypnea** is a rapid rate of breathing. It may be an abnormal finding because of a disease process or a compensatory response (and outside the normal resting respiratory rate ranges) secondary to excitement, anxiety, fever, and pain, among other causes. In the newly born, exposure to cold can increase the respiratory rate and may cause respiratory distress.
  - At any age, a respiratory rate greater than 60 per minute is abnormal.
  - As fatigue begins and hypoxia worsens, the child progresses to respiratory failure with slowing (and possible cessation) of the respiratory rate

TABLE 3-2 *Normal Respiratory Rates by Age*

Age	Breaths per Minute (At Rest)
Infant (1 to 12 mo)	30 to 60
Toddler (1 to 3 y)	24 to 40
Preschooler (4 to 5 y)	22 to 34
School-age (6 to 12 y)	18 to 30
Adolescent (13 to 18 y)	12 to 16

TABLE 3-3 *Signs of Respiratory Distress and Respiratory Failure*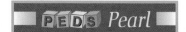

Respiratory Distress	Respiratory Failure
• Nasal flaring • Inspiratory retractions • Increased breathing rate (tachypnea) • Increased depth of breathing (hyperpnea) • Head-bobbing • Seesaw respirations (abdominal breathing) • Restlessness • Tachycardia • Grunting • Stridor	• Cyanosis • Diminished breath sounds • Decreased level of responsiveness or response to pain • Poor skeletal muscle tone • Inadequate respiratory rate, effort, or chest excursion • Tachycardia • Use of accessory muscles of respiration

- **Bradypnea** (abnormally slow rate of breathing) is an ominous sign in an acutely ill infant or child and may be caused by fatigue, hypothermia, or central nervous system depression, among other causes.
- Assess for the presence of respiratory distress/failure (Table 3-3). If respiratory distress is observed, *potential* respiratory failure is present.
  - Note signs of increased work of breathing (respiratory effort).
    - Anxious appearance, concentration on breathing
    - Use of accessory muscles: muscles of the neck, chest, and abdomen that become active during labored breathing
    - Leaning forward to inhale
    - Nasal flaring: widening of the nostrils on inhalation; an attempt to increase the size of the airway and increase the amount of available oxygen (Figure 3-3)
    - Retractions: sinking in of the soft tissues above the sternum (suprasternal) or clavicle (supraclavicular) or between (intercostal) or below (subcostal) the ribs during inhalation (Figures 3-4 and 3-5)
      - Indicate increased work of breathing.
      - In cases of severe obstruction, retractions may extend to the suprasternal notch and supraclavicular areas.
    - Seesaw (chest/abdominal) movement
      - Increased respiratory effort draws the chest in while thrusting the abdomen out.
      - Indicator of severe respiratory distress.
    - Note the rhythm of respirations (regular, irregular, periodic)

PEDS *Pearl*

Respirations in infants and children younger than 6 or 7 years are primarily abdominal (diaphragmatic) because the intercostal muscles of the chest wall are not well developed and fatigue easily from the work of breathing. Effective respiration may be jeopardized when diaphragmatic movement is compromised (e.g., gastric or abdominal distension) because the chest wall cannot compensate. As the child grows older, the chest muscles strengthen, and chest expansion becomes more noticeable.

The transition from abdominal (diaphragmatic) breathing to intercostal breathing begins between 2 and 4 years of age and is complete by 7 to 8 years of age.

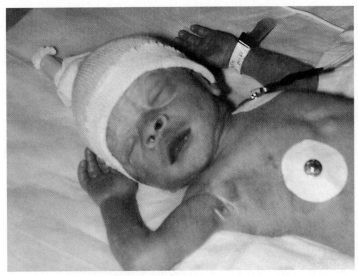

Figure 3-3   Nasal flaring. Widening of the nares may be seen in infants with respiratory distress.

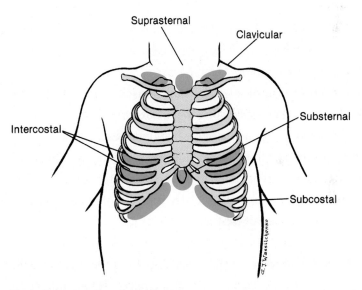

Figure 3-4   Location of retractions.

- ○ Prolonged inspiration suggests an upper airway obstruction.
  - ○ Prolonged expiration suggests a lower airway obstruction.
- ○ Listen
  - ■ Listen for air movement at the nose and mouth. Note if respirations are quiet, absent, or noisy (e.g., stridor, wheezing, snoring, crowing, gurgling). Wheezing may be heard throughout the lungs or, in the case of a foreign body obstruction, may be localized.
  - ■ Listen for the presence and quality of bilateral breath sounds and briefly listen to heart sounds.
    - • Breath sounds are normally quiet. Because the chest of a child is small and the chest wall is thin, breath sounds are easily

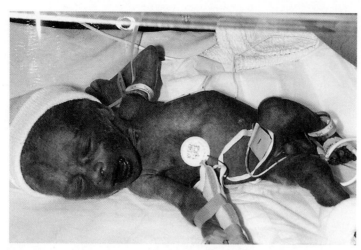

Figure 3-5   Retractions. The inward collapse of the lower anterior chest wall can be seen in this premature infant with respiratory distress syndrome.

transmitted from one side of the chest to the other. As a result, breath sounds may be heard despite the presence of a pneumothorax, hemothorax, or atelectasis. To minimize the possibility of sound transmission from one side of the chest to the other, listen along the midaxillary line (under each armpit) and in the midclavicular line under each clavicle (Figure 3-6). Alternate from side to side and compare your findings.

- Briefly listen to heart sounds to establish a baseline from which to compare (e.g., development of muffled heart sounds, a murmur, or rub).

○ Feel

■ Feel for air movement from the nose or mouth against your chin, face, or palm (Figure 3-7). Palpate the chest for tenderness, instability, and crepitation.

■ If the unresponsive patient is breathing adequately and there are no signs of trauma, place the patient in the recovery (lateral recumbent) position and administer supplemental oxygen (Figure 3-8).

■ If breathing is difficult and the rate is too slow or too fast, provide supplemental oxygen and, if necessary, positive-pressure ventilation.

■ If breathing is absent, insert an airway adjunct (if not previously done) and deliver two breaths with a pocket mask or bag-valve-mask with supplemental oxygen. Give each breath over 1 second. Ensure the patient's chest wall rises with each ventilation. Continue the primary survey.

The patient with inadequate breathing requires positive-pressure ventilation with 100% oxygen.

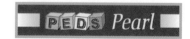

If the chest wall does not rise during positive-pressure ventilation, ventilation is inadequate or the airway is obstructed.

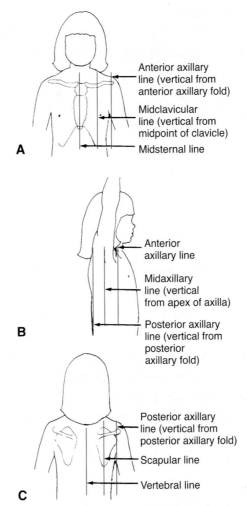

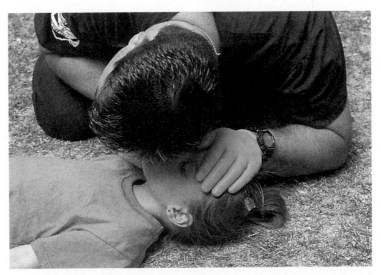

Figure 3-6   Landmarks of the chest. A, Anterior.
B, Right lateral. **C,** Posterior.

Figure 3-7   Feel for air movement from the nose or mouth against your chin, face, or palm.

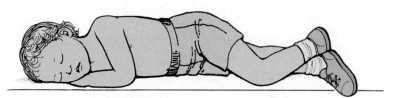

Figure 3-8   Recovery position.

- Interventions
  - Suction
  - Oxygen
  - Airway adjuncts
  - Positive-pressure ventilation

Circulation with Bleeding Control

- Goals   Assessment
  - Adequate cardiovascular function and tissue perfusion
    - Awake and alert
    - Central and peripheral pulses are strong and regular
    - Heart rate and blood pressure are within normal range for age
    - Skin color normal; warm and dry
    - Capillary refill time is less than 2 seconds (assess in children younger than 6 years)
    - Adequate oral intake and hydration
    - Adequate urine output for age and weight
  - Effective circulating fluid volume
    - No evidence of external bleeding
    - Vital signs within normal limits for age
    - Moist mucous membranes
    - Urine output of 1 to 2 mL/kg per hour
    - Hemoglobin and hematocrit values within normal range
    - Normal skin turgor
  - Normal core body temperature
- Control bleeding
  - Look for visible external hemorrhage. Control major bleeding, if present.
    - Apply direct pressure over the bleeding site.
    - Elevate the extremity (unless contraindicated).
    - Apply pressure over arterial pressure points.
    - Apply a pressure bandage.
  - Consider possible areas of major internal hemorrhage
    - Significant internal hemorrhage may occur in the chest, abdomen, pelvis, retroperitoneum, and femoral areas.
    - Pain or swelling in any of these areas may signal possible internal hemorrhage.

Hypotension often occurs well before the loss of central pulses.

- Compare the strength and quality of central and peripheral pulses
  - Palpation of pulses can be used to estimate heart rate, blood pressure, cardiac output, and systemic vascular resistance
  - Pulse quality reflects the adequacy of peripheral perfusion (Table 3-4)
    - A weak central pulse may indicate decompensated shock.
    - A peripheral pulse that is difficult to find, weak, or irregular suggests poor peripheral perfusion and may be a sign of shock or hemorrhage.
  - Determine if the patient's heart rate is within normal limits for the child's age. Normal heart rates by age are listed in Table 3-5.

Decreased skin perfusion is an early sign of shock.

- Evaluate skin color, temperature, moisture
  - Skin color: pink, pale, cyanotic, mottled
    - Pink = normal perfusion
      - The hands and feet are normally warm, dry, and pink.
      - A newborn often has acrocyanosis (cyanotic hands and feet, while the rest of the body is pink) (Figure 3-9).
    - Pale
      - May be observed in respiratory failure.
      - Cool, pale extremities are associated with decreased cardiac output, as seen in shock and hypothermia.

PEDS Pearl

The location for assessment of a central pulse varies according to the age of the child. In the newly born, assess the strength and quality of a central pulse by palpating the base of the umbilical cord between your thumb and index finger. In an infant and young child, assess the brachial or femoral pulse. Assess the carotid pulse in any child older than 1 year.

Assess a peripheral pulse while keeping one hand on the central pulse location. For example, if you are assessing a central pulse using the brachial artery, keep one hand on the brachial pulse and use your other hand to assess the peripheral (radial) pulse in the same extremity. Compare the strength and quality of the central and peripheral pulses. Although a peripheral pulse is not quite as strong as a central pulse, the rate and strength should be similar.

TABLE 3-4 *Grading of Pulses*

Description	Grade
Full, bounding, not obliterated with pressure	+4
Normal—easily palpated, not easily obliterated with pressure	+3
Difficult to palpate, obliterated with pressure	+2
Weak, thready, difficult to palpate	+1
Absent pulse	0

TABLE 3-5 *Normal Heart Rates by Age*

Age	Beats per Minute*
Infant (1 to 12 mo)	100 to 160
Toddler (1 to 3 y)	90 to 150
Preschooler (4 to 5 y)	80 to 140
School-age (6 to 12 y)	70 to 120
Adolescent (13 to 18 y)	60 to 100

*Pulse rates for a sleeping child may be 10% lower than the low rate listed in age group.

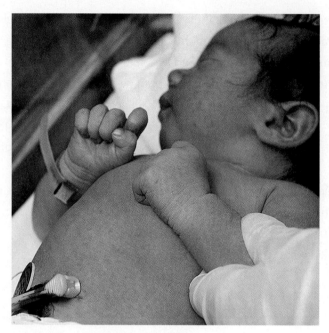

Figure 3-9   Acrocyanosis of the hands in a newborn.

- Blue (cyanosis)
  - Suggests hypoxemia or inadequate perfusion.
  - In dark skin, cyanosis may observed as ashen-gray lips and tongue.
- Mottled
  - Suggests decreased cardiac output, ischemia, hypoxia (Figure 3-10) but can be normal in an infant exposed to a cool environment.
- Skin temperature: hot, warm, cool
  - The skin surface is normally warm and equal bilaterally.
  - Use the dorsal surfaces of your hands and fingers to assess skin temperature.
  - As cardiac output decreases, coolness will begin in the hands and feet and ascend toward the trunk.
- Skin moisture: dry, moist, diaphoretic
  - The skin is normally dry with a minimum of perspiration.
  - Use the dorsal surfaces of your hands and fingers to assess the moisture of the skin.
- Skin **turgor**
  - To assess skin turgor (elasticity), grasp the skin on the abdomen between your thumb and index finger (Figure 3-11). Pull the skin taut and then release quickly. Observe the speed with which the skin returns to its original contour when released.

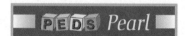

PEDS *Pearl*

Skin color is most reliably evaluated in the sclera, conjunctiva, nail beds, tongue, oral mucosa, palms, and soles.

A positive finding is more helpful than a negative one. Never assume a child is well hydrated on the basis of good skin turgor.

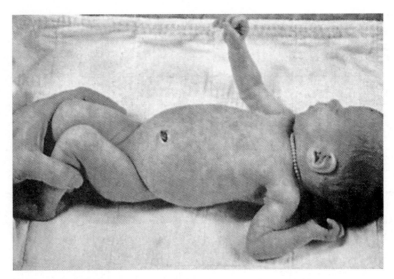

Figure 3-10   Mottling.

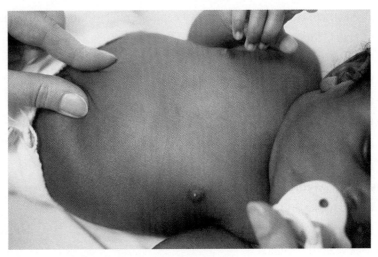

Figure 3-11   Assessing skin turgor in an infant.

- The skin should resume its shape immediately with no tenting or wrinkling. Good skin turgor indicates adequate hydration.
- Decreased skin turgor (a sign of dehydration and/or malnutrition) is present when the skin is released and it remains pinched (tented) and then slowly returns to its normal shape (Table 3-6).
- Evaluate capillary refill
  - To assess capillary refill, firmly press the skin over the warmest point on the child's body and release. Observe the time it takes for the blanched tissue to return to its original color.
    - If the ambient temperature is warm, color should return within 2 seconds.
    - Capillary refill time of 3 to 5 seconds is delayed and may indicate poor perfusion or exposure to cool ambient temperatures.

A positive finding is more helpful than a negative one. Never assume a child is well perfused on the basis of a good capillary refill time.

TABLE 3-6 *Evaluating Skin Turgor and Estimating Dehydration*

Elapsed Time for Skin to Return to Normal (Sec)	Approximate Degree of Dehydration
< 2	< 5% of child's body weight
2 to 3	5% to 8% of child's body weight
3 to 4	9% to 10% of child's body weight
> 4	> 10% of child's body weight

From Seidel HM, Ball JW, Dains JE, et al. *Mosby's guide to physical examination*, 5th ed. St. Louis: Mosby, 2003.

> **PEDs Pearl**
>
> If capillary refill is initially assessed in the hand or fingers and it is delayed, recheck it in a more central location, such as the chest.

- Capillary refill time longer than 5 seconds is markedly delayed and suggests shock (Figure 3-12).
  - Alternate sites for assessment of capillary refill include the forehead, chest, abdomen, or fleshy part of the palm.

Interventions

- Oxygen
- Position
- Chest compressions
- Bleeding control
- Fluid replacement
- Defibrillation

Disability (Mental Status)

Assessment

- Goal: Awake and alert
- Determine level of responsiveness using AVPU:
  - A = **A**lert
  - V = Responds to **v**erbal stimuli
  - P = Responds to **p**ainful stimuli
  - U = **U**nresponsive
- Another assessment tool that may be used is a version of the Glasgow Coma Scale (GCS) modified for pediatric use (Table 3-7). The pediatric GCS may be used to establish a baseline and for comparison in later, serial observations.
  - A GCS score that falls two points suggests significant deterioration. Urgent patient reassessment is required.
  - To avoid confusion with spinal reflexes, assess the patient's motor response by applying a stimulus above the neck.
- Question the parent/caregiver about the child's normal mood, activity level, attention span, and willingness and ability to cooperate.

Interventions

- Oxygen
- Ventilation

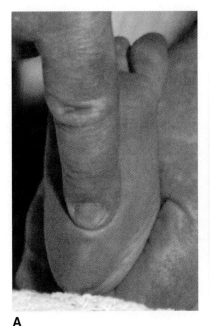
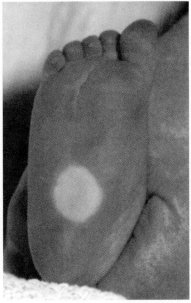
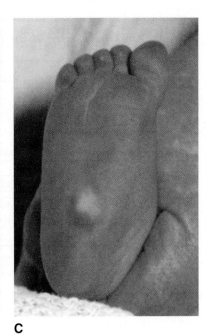

A   B   C

Figure 3-12 Capillary refill in a child in shock.

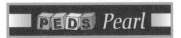

Maintaining appropriate temperature is particularly important in the pediatric patient because children have a large body surface area–to–weight ratio, providing a greater area for heat loss.

The Initial Assessment Algorithm is shown in Figure 3-14.

- Position
- Spinal stabilization

Expose/Environment
- Undress the patient
- Preserve body heat/maintain appropriate temperature
  - Respect modesty
  - Keep the child covered if possible and replace clothing promptly after examining each body area.

Secondary Survey

The secondary survey focuses on advanced life support (ALS) interventions and management.

- Obtain vital signs, attach pulse oximeter, electrocardiogram (ECG), and blood pressure monitor
- Obtain focused SAMPLE or CIAMPEDS history
- (Advanced) *A*irway
- *B*reathing
- *C*irculation
- *D*etailed (or focused) examination, differential diagnosis, diagnostic procedures
- *E*valuate interventions, pain management
- *F*acilitate family presence for invasive and resuscitative procedures

Vital Signs

See Tables 3-2 and 3-5 for normal values for respiratory rates and heart rates by age.

TABLE 3-7 *Adult, Child, and Infant Glasgow Coma Scale**

Glasgow Coma Scale	Adult/Child	Score	Infant
Eye opening	Spontaneous	4	Spontaneous
	To verbal	3	To verbal
	To pain	2	To pain
	No response	1	No response
Best Verbal response	Oriented	5	Coos, babbles
	Disoriented	4	Irritable cry
	Inappropriate words	3	Cries only to pain
	Incomprehensible sounds	2	Moans to pain
	No response	1	No response
Best Motor response	Obeys commands	6	Spontaneous
	Localizes pain	5	Withdraws from touch
	Withdraws from pain	4	Withdraws from pain
	Abnormal flexion (decorticate)	3	Abnormal flexion (decorticate)
	Abnormal extension (decerebrate)	2	Abnormal extension (decerebrate)
	No response	1	No response
	*Total = E + V + M	3 to 15	

- Temperature
  - Obtain the child's temperature by an appropriate route (e.g., oral, axillary, rectal, tympanic) considering the child's age and clinical condition (Figure 3-13).
  - Temperature varies with exercise, crying, stress, and clothing.
  - Common signs of increased body temperature include flushed face and skin, malaise, low energy level, increased respiratory and heart rates, and a "glassy look" to the eyes.
  - Infants and children may lose heat rapidly. Keep the child covered. It is particularly important to keep the head of an infant covered.
- Blood pressure
  - Blood pressure should be measured only after assessing pulse and respiration. Children often become agitated during this procedure, which increases their pulse and respiratory rate. To decrease the children's anxiety about blood pressure measurement, tell them you are going to give their arm "a hug."
  - Measure blood pressure in children older than 3 years. In children younger than 3 years, a strong central pulse is considered an acceptable sign of adequate blood pressure. Table 3-8 shows the lower limit of normal systolic blood pressure by age.
  - The blood pressure should be measured with a cuff, with the bladder completely encircling the extremity and the width covering one half to two thirds the length of the upper arm or upper leg.

Blood pressure is one of the *least* sensitive indicators of adequate circulation in children.

The cuff should be at heart level and the arm should be fully supported by the rescuer.

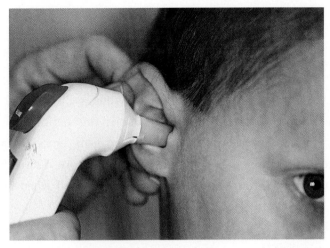

Figure 3-13 **Tympanic temperature assessment.** In a child older than 3 years, the pinna of the ear is pulled up and back to help straighten the ear canal for the infrared sensor to focus on the eardrum.

PEDS Pearl

To determine the *minimum* systolic blood pressure for a child 1 to 10 years of age, the following formula may be used: 70 + (2 × age in years).

TABLE 3-8 *Lower Limit of Normal Systolic Blood Pressure by Age*

Age	Lower Limit of Normal Systolic Blood Pressure
Term neonate (0 to 28 days)	> 60 mm Hg or strong central pulse
Infant (1 to 12 months)	> 70 mm Hg or strong central pulse
Child 1 to 10 years	> 70 + (2 × age in years)
Child ≥ 10 years	> 90 mm Hg

- Use of a cuff that is too large will result in a falsely low reading.
- Use of a cuff that is too small will result in a falsely high reading.
- Pulse pressure
  - **Pulse pressure** is the difference between the systolic and diastolic blood pressures.
  - Indicator of **stroke volume** (the amount of blood ejected by either ventricle during one contraction).
  - Narrowed pulse pressure is an indicator of circulatory compromise.
- Weight
  - Whenever possible, obtain a measured weight. If obtaining a measured weight is not possible, use a length-based measuring tape to estimate the child's weight if 35 kg or less, or ask the caregiver the child's last weight.
  - Pediatric weight formula
    - Weight in kg = 8 + (2 × age in years)
    - Use 3.0 kg for newborns
    - Use 7.0 kg for 6 month olds

- ◦ Weight conversion
  - ▪ Weight (lb) × 0.45 = Weight (kg)
  - ▪ Weight (kg) × 2.2 = Weight (lb)

Focused History

The history is often obtained simultaneously during the physical examination and while therapeutic interventions are performed. While performing the physical examination, ask the patient, family, bystanders, or others questions regarding the patient's history. SAMPLE is a mnemonic used to organize the information obtained when taking a patient history.

- **S**igns/symptoms: Assessment findings and history as they relate to the chief complaint.
  - ◦ When did it start/occur (time, sudden, gradual)? What was the child doing when it started/occurred?
  - ◦ How long did it last? Does it come and go? Is it still present?
  - ◦ Where is the problem? Describe character and severity if painful (use pain scale) (see Chapter 8).
  - ◦ Radiation? Aggravating or alleviating factors?
  - ◦ Previous history of same? If yes, what was the diagnosis?
- **A**llergies: To medications, food, environmental causes (e.g., pollen), and products (e.g., latex).
- **M**edications
  - ◦ Prescription and over-the-counter medications the child is currently taking.
  - ◦ Determine name of medication, dose, route, frequency, and indication for the medication.
- (Pertinent) **P**ast medical history
  - ◦ Is the child currently under a physician's care?
  - ◦ Serious childhood illnesses: age, complications
  - ◦ Hospitalizations: age, reason for admission, length of stay
  - ◦ Surgical procedures: age, reason for procedure, complications
  - ◦ Trauma/injuries and fractures/ingestions, burns: age, circumstances surrounding event, treatment, complications
  - ◦ Immunization status with regard to diphtheria, tetanus, pertussis, varicella, poliomyelitis, *Haemophilus influenza* type B, hepatitis B, rubeola, rubella, mumps, and so forth.
  - ◦ For infants and toddlers, obtain a birth history
    - ▪ Maternal age, gestational duration, prematurity, birth weight
    - ▪ Complications during pregnancy or delivery (e.g., cesarian delivery, forceps delivery)
    - ▪ Congenital anomalies
    - ▪ "Did the baby go home with you?"

- **L**ast oral intake
  - Time of last meal and fluid intake
  - Changes in eating pattern or fluid intake
  - For infants, determine if breast or bottle fed, if formula is used which type, feeding difficulties
- **E**vents leading to the illness or injury
  - Onset, duration, and precipitating factors
  - Associated factors such as toxic inhalants, drugs, alcohol
  - Injury scenario and mechanism of injury
  - Treatment given by caregiver

The Emergency Nurses Association (ENA) recommends use of the CIAMPEDS mnemonic.

- **C**hief complaint
  - Reason for the child's visit to the ED
  - Duration of complaint
- **I**mmunizations/Isolation
  - Evaluate scheduled immunizations for the child's age
  - Evaluate the child's exposure to communicable diseases (e.g., chickenpox, meningitis)
- **A**llergies: To medications, food, environmental causes (e.g., pollen), products (e.g., latex), and environment
- **M**edications
  - Prescription and over-the-counter medications the child is currently taking
    - Include herbal and dietary supplements
  - Determine name of medication, dose, route, frequency and indication for the medication
- **P**ast medical history
  - Child's health status including prior illnesses, injuries, hospitalizations, surgeries, and chronic physical and psychiatric illnesses
  - Use of alcohol, tobacco, drugs, or other substances of abuse
  - The neonate's history should include the prenatal and birth history including maternal complications during pregnancy or delivery, infant's gestational age and birth weight, number of days infant remained hospitalized after delivery
  - Date and description of last menstrual period
  - The history for sexually active patients should include type of birth control used, barrier protection, prior treatment for sexually transmitted diseases, pregnancies (gravida) and births, miscarriages, abortions, living children (para)
- **P**arent's/caregiver's impression of the child's condition
  - Identify the patient's primary caregiver

OPQRST is an acronym that may be used when evaluating pain.

- **O**nset: What were you doing when the pain started?
- **P**rovocation: What makes the pain better or worse? Coughing/deep breathing, anxiety/fear, treatment/procedure, movement/positioning, parent/caregiver not present?
- **Q**uality: What does the pain feel like (dull, sharp, pressure, burning, squeezing, stabbing, gnawing, shooting, throbbing)?
- **R**egion/Radiation: Where is the pain? Is the pain in one area or does it move?
- **S**everity: On a scale of 0 to 10, with 0 being the least and 10 being the worst, what number would you assign your pain or discomfort?
- **T**ime: How long ago did the problem/discomfort begin? Have you ever had this pain before? When? How long did it last?

- ◦ Consider cultural differences that may affect the caregiver's impressions
- ◦ Evaluate the caregiver's concerns and observations of the child's condition
- *E*vents surrounding illness/injury
  - ◦ Illness: Duration, including date of onset and sequence of symptoms; treatment provided before arrival at ED
  - ◦ Injury: Date/time of injury, mechanism of injury including use of restraints/protective devices, suspected injuries, prehospital vital signs and treatment, circumstances leading to the injury, witnessed or unwitnessed
- *D*iet/diapers
  - ◦ Time of last meal and fluid intake, changes in eating pattern or fluid intake
  - ◦ For infants, determine if breast or bottle fed, if formula is used which type, feeding difficulties
  - ◦ Special diet or dietary restrictions
  - ◦ Evaluation of child's urine and stool output
- (Associated) *S*ymptoms
  - ◦ Symptom identification and progression since onset of illness or injury

Physical Examination

The purpose of the physical examination in the secondary survey is to detect **non–life-threatening** conditions and provide care for those conditions/injuries. A detailed physical examination is presented here for completeness. A focused physical examination may be more appropriate, based on the patient's presentation and chief complaint.

- Inspect and palpate each of the major body areas for DCAP-BLS-TIC (*D*eformities, *C*ontusions, *A*brasions, *P*enetrations/punctures, *B*urns, *L*acerations, *S*welling/edema, *T*enderness, *I*nstability, *C*repitus).
- Auscultate breath and heart sounds.

Head/Face

- Scalp and skull
  - ◦ Inspect for DCAP-BLS
  - ◦ Palpate for DCAP-BLS-TIC, depressions, protrusions
  - ◦ In a child younger than 14 months, gently palpate the anterior and posterior fontanelles on the top of the head with the child in a sitting position (if no trauma is suspected).
    - ■ The posterior fontanelle normally closes by 2 months of age. In most infants, the anterior fontanelle closes between 7 and 14 months of age (Figure 3-15).
    - ■ A bulging anterior fontanelle may be due to crying, coughing,

The assessment procedure outlined here appears as a head-to-toes sequence; however, the sequence should be reversed (toes-to-head) in infants and young children. Infants and young children find it particularly threatening when strangers want to touch their faces. By beginning with the extremities and proceeding backward, you reduce the likelihood of frightening the child. Try to gain the child's trust as you proceed by being calm, friendly, and reassuring.

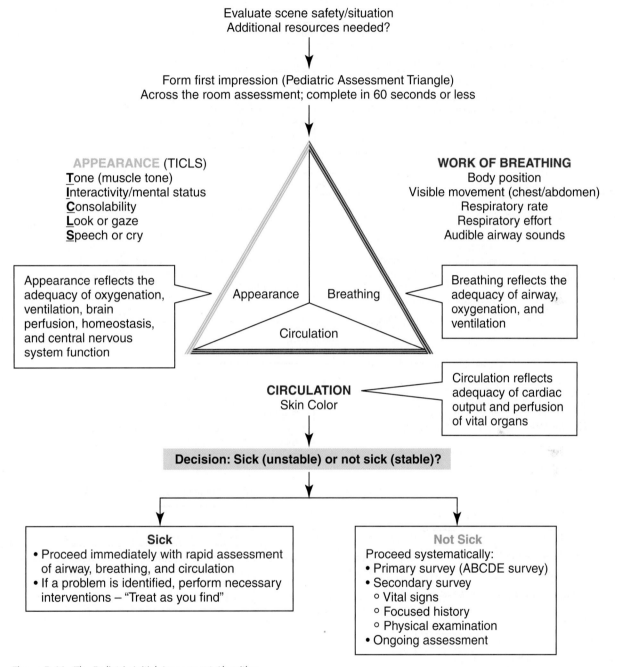

**PEDIATRIC INITIAL ASSESSMENT ALGORITHM
– FIRST IMPRESSION**

Evaluate scene safety/situation
Additional resources needed?

Form first impression (Pediatric Assessment Triangle)
Across the room assessment; complete in 60 seconds or less

APPEARANCE (TICLS)
Tone (muscle tone)
Interactivity/mental status
Consolability
Look or gaze
Speech or cry

WORK OF BREATHING
Body position
Visible movement (chest/abdomen)
Respiratory rate
Respiratory effort
Audible airway sounds

Appearance reflects the adequacy of oxygenation, ventilation, brain perfusion, homeostasis, and central nervous system function

Appearance   Breathing

Circulation

Breathing reflects the adequacy of airway, oxygenation, and ventilation

CIRCULATION
Skin Color

Circulation reflects adequacy of cardiac output and perfusion of vital organs

Decision: Sick (unstable) or not sick (stable)?

Sick
• Proceed immediately with rapid assessment of airway, breathing, and circulation
• If a problem is identified, perform necessary interventions – "Treat as you find"

Not Sick
Proceed systematically:
• Primary survey (ABCDE survey)
• Secondary survey
  ○ Vital signs
  ○ Focused history
  ○ Physical examination
• Ongoing assessment

Figure 3-14   The Pediatric Initial Assessment Algorithm..

vomiting, or increased intracranial pressure (ICP) due to a head injury, meningitis, or hydrocephalus. A depressed anterior fontanelle is seen in dehydrated or malnourished infants.

• Ears

  ◦ Inspect for DCAP-BLS, postauricular ecchymosis (Battle's sign), blood or clear fluid in the ears

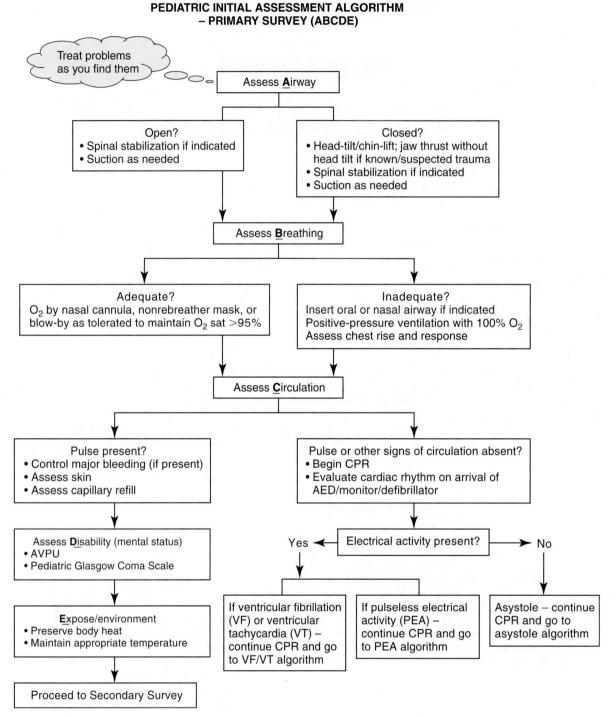

Figure 3-14, cont'd.

- ◦ Palpate for tenderness or pain
- • Face
  - ◦ Inspect for DCAP-BLS, singed facial hair, symmetry of facial expression
  - ◦ Palpate the orbital rims, zygoma, maxilla, mandible for DCAP-BLS-TIC, neurovascular impairment, muscle spasm, false motion or motor impairment

PEDIATRIC INITIAL ASSESSMENT ALGORITHM
– SECONDARY SURVEY (ABCDEF)

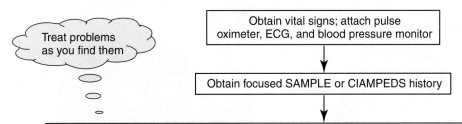

Treat problems as you find them

Obtain vital signs; attach pulse oximeter, ECG, and blood pressure monitor

Obtain focused SAMPLE or CIAMPEDS history

AIRWAY
• Reassess effectiveness of initial airway maneuvers and interventions
• Perform invasive airway management if needed

BREATHING
• Reassess ventilation
• If applicable, confirm tracheal tube placement (or other airway device) by at least two methods
• Provide positive-pressure ventilation (if applicable) and evaluate effectiveness of ventilations

CIRCULATION
• Establish vascular access / administer medications, if appropriate

DETAILED (OR FOCUSED) EXAMINATION, DIFFERENTIAL DIAGNOSIS, DIAGNOSTIC PROCEDURES
• If unresponsive or significant mechanism of injury, perform detailed (head-to-toes) physical exam. If responsive or no significant mechanism of injury, perform focused exam.
• Search for, find, and treat reversible causes
• Glucose check
• Laboratory and radiographic studies

EVALUATE interventions, pain management
FACILITATE family presence for invasive and resuscitative procedures

Perform an ongoing assessment
(Monitor and reassess)

• Reassess airway patency, oxygen saturation
• Reassess breathing effectiveness
• Reassess pulse rate and quality, perfusion status, cardiac rhythm
• Reassess capillary refill (if < 6 years)
• Reassess mental status and activity level
• Reassess and document vital signs
• Reevaluate emergency care interventions

Figure 3-14, cont'd.

To quickly assess the cranial nerves in a child who can follow commands, ask the child to close his or her eyes, open his or her eyes wide, follow a finger with his or her eyes, open his or her mouth, and stick out his or her tongue.

• Eyes
  ◦ Inspect for DCAP-BLS, foreign body, blood in the anterior chamber of the eye (hyphema) (Figure 3-16), presence of eyeglasses or contact lenses, periorbital ecchymosis (raccoon eyes) (Figure 3-17), color of sclera and conjunctiva, periorbital edema, pupils (size, shape, equality, reactivity to light), and eye movement (dysconjugate gaze, ocular muscle function).
  ◦ Determine Pediatric Coma Scale score or GCS score
• Nose
  ◦ Inspect for DCAP-BLS, blood or fluid from the nose, singed nasal hairs, nares for flaring

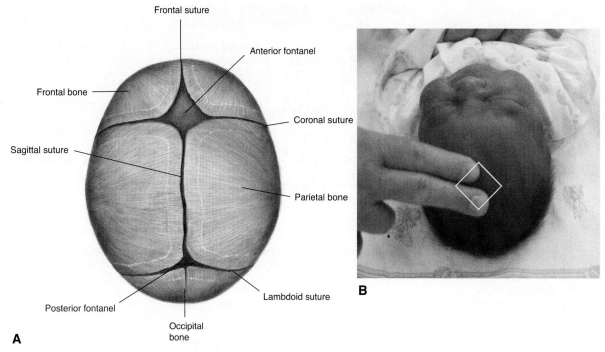

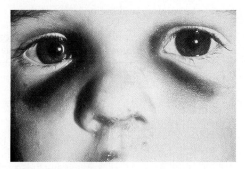

Figure 3-15 **A,** Location of sutures and fontanelles. **B,** Palpating the anterior fontanelle.

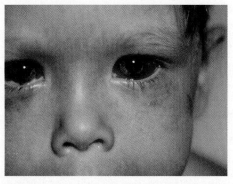

Figure 3-16 Blood in the anterior chamber of the eye (hyphema).

Figure 3-17 Raccoon eyes (periorbital ecchymosis).

- ◦ Palpate nasal bones
- • Mouth/throat/pharynx
  - ◦ Inspect for DCAP-BLS, blood, absent or broken teeth, gastric contents, foreign objects (e.g., loose teeth, gum, small toys), injured or swollen tongue, color of the mucous membranes of the mouth, note presence and character of fluids, vomitus, note sputum color, amount, and consistency
  - ◦ Listen for hoarseness, inability to talk
  - ◦ Note unusual odors (e.g., alcohol, feces, acetone, almonds)

Neck

- • Inspect for DCAP-BLS, neck veins (flat or distended), use of accessory muscles, and presence of a stoma or medical identification device. It is difficult to assess distended neck veins in infants and young children.

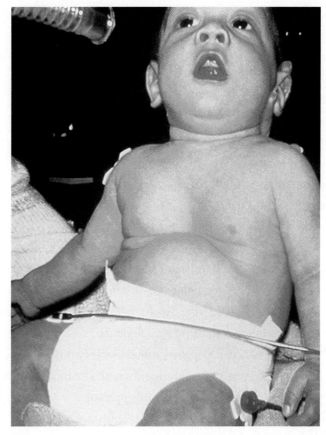

Figure 3-18 Inspect the chest and assess work of breathing, symmetry of movement, use of accessory muscles, and the presence of retractions.

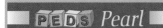 *Pearl*

If present, the following signs may help identify the nature and location of internal injuries:

- **Kehr's sign**: Left upper quadrant pain with radiation to the left shoulder suggests injury to the spleen or liver (pain occurs because of blood or bile irritating the diaphragm).
- **Cullen's sign**: A bluish discoloration around the umbilicus that may indicate intraabdominal or retroperitoneal hemorrhage.
- **Grey Turner's sign**: Bruising of the flanks that may indicate intraabdominal hemorrhage, often splenic in origin.

- Palpate for DCAP-BLS-TIC, subcutaneous emphysema, and tracheal position. To assess tracheal position, place your thumb and index finger on each side of the trachea and slide your fingers back and forth.

Chest

- Inspect: Work of breathing (Figure 3-18), symmetry of movement, use of accessory muscles, retractions; note abnormal breathing patterns, DCAP-BLS, vascular access devices
- Auscultate
  - Equality of breath sounds
  - Adventitious breath sounds (e.g., crackles, wheezes)
  - Heart sounds for rate, rhythm, murmurs, bruits, gallops, friction rub, muffled heart tones
- Palpate for DCAP-BLS-TIC, chest wall tenderness, symmetry of chest wall expansion, subcutaneous emphysema

Abdomen

- Inspect for DCAP-BLS, distention, scars from healed surgical incisions or penetrating wounds, feeding tubes, use of abdominal muscles during respiration, signs of injury, discoloration

- Auscultate to determine presence or absence of bowel sounds in all quadrants
- Palpate all four quadrants for DCAP-BLS, guarding or distention, rigidity, masses

Pelvis and Genitalia

- Inspect for DCAP-BLS
  - Discharge or drainage from the meatus
  - Priapism (spinal cord injury, sickle cell disease)
  - Scrotal bleeding or edema
- Palpate for DCAP-BLS-TIC
  - To assess the integrity of the pelvis:
    - First, gently palpate for point tenderness.
    - Next, place your hands on each iliac crest and press gently inward. If pain, crepitation, or instability is elicited, suspect a fracture of the pelvic ring. No further assessment is necessary if this assessment reveals positive findings.
    - If this assessment is negative, simultaneously push down on both iliac crests. Then place one hand on the pubic bone (over the symphysis pubis) and apply gentle pressure.
  - Assess strength and quality of femoral pulses.
  - In the hospital, assess anal sphincter tone.

Extremities

In an alert child, begin your assessment of the extremities by evaluating the lower extremities first. In an injured extremity, be sure to assess distal pulses and neurovascular integrity distal to the injury. Compare an injured extremity to an uninjured extremity and document your findings.

- Inspect for DCAP-BLS, vascular access devices, **purpura**, **petechiae** (Figures 3-19 and 3-20), presence of congenital anomalies (e.g., finger clubbing, club foot), abnormal extremity position, medical identification bracelet
- Palpate for DCAP-BLS-TIC
  - Assess skin temperature, moisture, and capillary refill in each extremity
  - Assess the strength and quality of pulses, motor function, and sensory function (PMS) in each extremity
    - If the child is alert, assess sensation by lightly touching the extremity and asking, "Do you feel me brushing your skin? Where?"
    - Assess motor function in an upper extremity in an alert patient by instructing the child to "Squeeze my fingers in your hand." To assess motor function in a lower extremity, instruct the child to "Push down on my fingers with your toes."

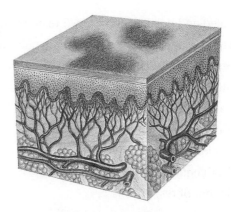

Purpura—red-purple nonblanch-able discoloration greater than 0.5cm diameter. Cause: Intravascular defects, infection

Figure 3-19 Purpuras are reddish-purple nonblanchable discolorations in the skin larger than 0.5 cm in diameter. Purpuras are produced by small bleeding vessels near the skin's surface.

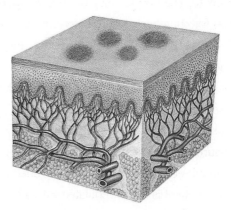

Petechiae—red-purple nonblanch-able discoloration less than 0.5 cm diameter Cause: Intravascular defects, infection

Figure 3-20 Petechiae are reddish-purple nonblanchable discolorations in the skin smaller than 0.5 cm in diameter.

If trauma is suspected, ensure manual in-line stabilization of the head and spine is maintained during the examination.

Ongoing Assessment

Posterior Body

- Inspect for DCAP-BLS, purpura, petechiae, rashes, edema
- Auscultate the posterior thorax
- Palpate the posterior trunk for DCAP-BLS

Purpose

- Reevaluate the patient's condition
- Assess the effectiveness of emergency care interventions provided
- Identify any missed injuries or conditions
- Observe subtle changes or trends in the patient's condition
- Alter emergency care interventions as needed

The ongoing assessment should be

- Performed on EVERY patient.
- Performed after ensuring completion of critical interventions.
- Performed after the detailed physical examination, if one is performed. (In some situations, the patient's condition may preclude performance of the detailed physical examination.)

- Repeated and documented every 5 minutes for an unstable patient.
- Repeated and documented every 15 minutes for a stable patient.

Components of the Ongoing Assessment

- Reassess airway patency, oxygen saturation
- Reassess breathing effectiveness
  - Rise and fall of the chest
  - Respiratory rate
  - Depth/equality of breathing
  - Rhythm of respirations
  - Signs of increased work of breathing (respiratory effort)
  - Breath sounds
- Reassess pulse rate and quality, perfusion status, cardiac rhythm
  - Look for changes in color of skin and mucous membranes
  - Feel for changes in skin temperature and moisture
  - Reassess capillary refill in infants and children younger than 6 years
  - Reassess mental status and activity level
- Reassess and document vital signs
- Reevaluate emergency care interventions
  - Ensure suction is readily available
  - If an OPA or NPA has been placed, ensure it is properly positioned
  - If the patient is being ventilated with a bag-valve device:
    - Ensure the device is connected to oxygen at 15 L per minute.
    - Reassess effectiveness of ventilation
      - Ensure adequate rise and fall of the chest.
      - Ensure adequate face-to-mask seal.
      - Evaluate lung compliance (resistance to ventilation). Increasing resistance suggests airway obstruction.
  - If oxygen is being delivered by nonrebreather mask:
    - Ensure the mask is connected to oxygen at 15 L per minute.
    - Ensure the reservoir bag is not pinched off and remains inflated.
    - Ensure the inhalation valve is not obstructed.
  - If oxygen is being delivered by nasal cannula:
    - Ensure the oxygen flow rate is set at no more than 6 L per minute.
    - Ensure the prongs are properly placed in the patient's nose.
  - Ensure open chest wounds have been properly sealed with an occlusive dressing.
  - Ensure bleeding is controlled. Assess and document the type and amount of drainage through dressings.
  - If intravenous (IV) fluids are administered, assess the IV site for patency. Document the type and amount of fluid administered.

○ If cardiopulmonary resuscitation (CPR) is performed, ensure pulses are produced with chest compressions.

○ Ensure the trauma patient's cervical spine is adequately stabilized.

○ Ensure injured extremities are effectively immobilized.

○ Ensure open wounds are properly dressed and bandaged.

Pediatric Triage in the Emergency Department

Goals of Triage

- Rapidly identify patients with life-threatening conditions
- Determine the most appropriate treatment area for patients presenting to the ED
- Optimize use of resources
- Decrease congestion in emergency treatment areas
- Provide ongoing assessment of patients
- Provide information to patients and families regarding services, expected care, and waiting times

Triage Guidelines

The triage interview is performed to gather enough information to make a clinical judgment regarding the patient's priority of care. Effective triage requires the use of sight, hearing, smell, and touch.

The ability to triage patients effectively and accurately is based on the following:

- The PAT
- Physical assessment findings
- The patient's pertinent medical history
- Appropriate use of guidelines and triage protocols
- Practical knowledge gained through experience and training

A 5-level triage classification system based on patient presentation and expected resource utilization has demonstrated reliability and is reviewed here.

Resuscitation (Critical)

A resuscitation condition is one that requires immediate medical attention and maximum use of resources. The patient presents with unstable vital functions with a high probability of mortality if immediate intervention is not begun to prevent further airway, respiratory, hemodynamic, and/or neurologic instability; a time delay would be harmful to the patient. Highest priority is given to conditions including the following:

- Apnea or severe respiratory distress
- Pale, diaphoretic, and lightheaded or weak
- Central cyanosis
- Unresponsive
- Pulseless
- Active seizure

An emergent condition is one that requires medical attention within 10 minutes and high resource utilization. The patient presents with threatened vital functions with a potential threat to life or limb. Highest priority is given to conditions including the following:

Emergent (High Risk)

- Altered mental status
- Unstable vital signs
- Vomiting with head injury
- Severe pain or distress
- Fever with signs of severe dehydration
- Moderate to severe respiratory distress
- Extremity injury with neurovascular compromise
- Fever with excessive drooling or difficulty swallowing
- Fever in an infant <6 months of age

Urgent (Moderate Risk)

An urgent condition is one that requires prompt treatment within 30 to 60 minutes. The patient presents with stable vital functions that are not likely to threaten life and requires medium resource utilization. The patient should be periodically reassessed (usually every 20 to 30 minutes) to ensure there is no deterioration in his or her condition.

- Infant fall >2 feet
- Foreign object ingested larger than a nickel
- Mild to moderate dehydration
- Mild to moderate respiratory distress
- Nonspecific chest pain
- Allergic reaction with hives >50% of body
- Abdominal pain with suspected abuse
- Moderate pain
- Nonpenetrating eye injury

Semi-Urgent (Low Risk)

A semi-urgent condition is one that may safely wait 1 to 2 hours to be evaluated without risk of morbidity or mortality. The patient presents with stable vital functions and has a low need for resource utilization. The patient's illness or injury has a low probability of progression to more serious disease or development of complications. The patient with a semi-urgent condition should be periodically reassessed (usually every 30 to 60 minutes) to ensure there is no deterioration in his or her condition.

- Simple laceration
- History of seizure (now awake and alert)
- Fever in a child 3 months to 3 years old
- Head trauma without symptoms

Non-Urgent (Low Risk)

A non-urgent condition is one that may safely wait 2 hours or more to be evaluated without risk of morbidity or mortality; the patient presents with stable vital functions and does not require resource utilization. The patient's illness or injury has a low probability of progression to more

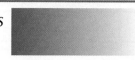

TABLE 3-9 *Triage Red Flags: Warning Signs of Serious Illness or Injury*

Airway	Apnea Choking Drooling Stridor
Breathing	Cyanosis Grunting Irregular respiratory pattern Respiratory rate above 60 breaths per minute Sternal retractions
Circulation	Decreased peripheral perfusion Decreased skin turgor Decreased tearing Dry tongue, mucous membranes Heart rate below 60 beats per minute Heart rate above 200 beats per minute Hypotension Hypothermia
Disability	Altered mental status Sunken or bulging fontanelle
Exposure/environment	Petechiae, purpura
Vital signs	Fever above 38.6° C (101° F) in an infant younger than 3 months Temperature above 40° C to 40.6° C (104° F to 105° F) at any age
History	Decreased urine output History of chronic illness Return emergency department visit within 24 hours Severe pain
Other	Sixth sense—a subjective feeling or intuition that a child is more seriously ill than objective data indicate

From Fredrickson JM. Triage. In: Kelly SJ, ed. *Pediatric emergency nursing*, 2nd ed. Norwalk, CT: Appleton & Lange, 1994.

serious disease or development of complications. The patient with a non-urgent condition should be periodically reassessed (usually every 60 to 120 minutes) to ensure there is no deterioration in his or her condition.

- Upper respiratory infection
- Fever in a child older than 36 months
- Impetigo
- Conjunctivitis
- Isolated soft-tissue injury
- Diaper rash
- Cold or flu
- Ear discomfort
- Sore throat
- Mild gastroenteritis
- Thrush

Case Study Resolution

Based on the information provided, this child is "not sick" (i.e., stable). Proceed systematically. Perform an initial assessment (i.e., primary survey), secondary survey (including vital signs, focused history, and detailed physical examination), and an ongoing assessment.

If the child appeared "sick" (unstable), you would proceed immediately with rapid assessment of airway, breathing, and circulation. If a problem were identified, you would perform necessary interventions ("treat as you find").

Reference

1. Walsh C, MacMillan HL, Jamieson E. The relationship between parental substance abuse and child maltreatment: findings from the Ontario Health Supplement. *Child Abuse Negl* 2003;27:1409–1425.

Chapter Quiz

1. The Pediatric Assessment Triangle (PAT):
   A) Is used to quickly determine if a child is "sick" or "not sick."
   B) Is a hands-on assessment of an infant or child.
   C) Is performed systematically from head-to-toes and requires the use of a stethoscope and blood pressure cuff.
   D) Should be repeated every fifteen to thirty minutes if the child appears very sick.

2. List the components of the Pediatric Assessment Triangle.

3. TICLS is a mnemonic used to recall the areas to be assessed related to a child's appearance. Explain the meaning of each of the letters of this mnemonic.
   T =
   I =
   C =
   L =
   S =

Questions 4–8 refer to the following patient situation.

A 2-year-old presents with shortness of breath. Mom states her son has had a three day history of a productive cough and runny nose. The child is holding a blanket and intently watching your movements while being held in his mother's arms. His respiratory rate appears to be within normal limits for his age with no evidence of increased work of breathing. Chest expansion appears equal and his skin is pink.

4. From the information provided, complete the following documentation regarding the Pediatric Assessment Triangle.
   Appearance:
   Breathing:
   Circulation:

5. Based on the information provided, is this child "sick" or "not sick?" How should you proceed?

6. To gain the child's cooperation you should:
   A) Introduce yourself and try to hold him.
   B) Sit down and listen attentively while speaking with the child's mother.
   C) Remove the child's clothing and inspect his airway with a pen light.
   D) Separate the mother and child and perform an initial assessment.

7. List the components of the Primary Survey.
   _____
   _____
   _____
   _____
   _____

8. A normal respiratory rate for a child of this age is _____ . A normal heart rate for a child of this age is _____ .

9. True or False: Respirations in a child younger than 8 years are primarily abdominal.

10. Match each abnormal respiratory sound with its description.

_____ Gasping

_____ Snoring

_____ Grunting

_____ Stridor

_____ Gurgling

A) Short, low-pitched sound heard at the end of exhalation; a compensatory mechanism to help maintain patency of small airways and prevent atelectasis.

B) Inhaling and exhaling with quick, difficult breaths.

C) Abnormal respiratory sound associated with collection of liquid or semi-solid material in the patient's upper airway.

D) Noisy breathing through the mouth and nose during sleep, caused by air passing through a narrowed upper airway.

E) Harsh, high-pitched sound heard on inspiration associated with upper airway obstruction.

11. Select the *incorrect* statement regarding assessment of blood pressure.

A) Use of a blood pressure cuff that is too large will result in a falsely low reading.

B) Blood pressure is one of the least sensitive indicators of adequate circulation in children.

C) Blood pressure should be measured only after assessing pulse and respiration.

D) To ensure an accurate patient assessment, it is essential to obtain serial blood pressure measurements in children younger than 3 years.

12. Match each of the acronyms/mnemonics listed with the primary reason for its use.

_____ OPQRST

_____ SAMPLE

_____ DCAP-BLS

_____ TICLS

_____ PAT

_____ ABCDE

A) Used to recall the areas to be assessed related to the child's appearance.

B) Used to recall what to look for when inspecting and palpating major body areas.

C) Used when evaluating pain.

D) Used to quickly determine if a child is "sick" or "not sick".

E) Used to recall the components of the Primary Survey.

F) Used to organize information obtained when taking a patient history.

13. Match each term with its description.

_____ Nasal flaring   _____ Tripod position

_____ Retractions   _____ Petechiae

_____ Head bobbing   _____ Purpura

_____ Sniffing position   _____ Stroke volume

_____ Pulse pressure

A) The child sits upright and leans forward with the chin slightly raised; in this position, the axes of the mouth, pharynx, and trachea are aligned, increasing airflow.

B) Reddish-purple nonblanchable discolorations in the skin less than 0.5 cm in diameter.

C) An indicator of increased work of breathing in infants; the head falls forward with exhalation and comes up with expansion of the chest on inhalation.

D) The difference between the systolic and diastolic blood pressure; an indicator of stroke volume.

E) Widening of the nostrils on inhalation; an attempt to increase the size of the airway and increase the amount of available oxygen.

F) The child sits upright and leans forward, supported by his or her arms, with the neck slightly extended, chin projected, and mouth open.

G) Sinking in of the soft tissues above the sternum or clavicle, or between or below the ribs during inhalation.

H) The amount of blood ejected by either ventricle during one contraction.

14. For each of the following conditions, indicate the appropriate triage classification.

_____ Respiratory arrest

_____ Active seizure

_____ Unresponsiveness

_____ Moderate respiratory distress

_____ Conjunctivitis

_____ Dehydration

_____ Ear discomfort

_____ Unstable vital signs

_____ Simple laceration

_____ Altered mental status

_____ Cold or flu

_____ Intubated patient

_____ Fever in an infant < 6 months of age

A) Resuscitation

B) Emergent

C) Urgent

D) Semi-Urgent

E) Non-Urgent

15. A 7-month-old infant has a two day history of poor feeding. Which of the following should be used to assess a central pulse in this infant?
    A) Carotid pulse.
    B) Femoral pulse.
    C) Radial pulse.
    D) Brachial pulse.

16. AVPU is an acronym used when describing a patient's level of responsiveness. Indicate the meaning of each of these letters.
    A =
    V =
    P =
    U =

17. The formula used to approximate the lower limit of systolic blood pressure in children 1 to 10 years of age is:
    A) $70 + (2 \times \text{age in years})$.
    B) Age in years x 2.2.
    C) $16 + \text{age in years}/4$.
    D) $2 \times 90/\text{age in years}$.

Chapter Quiz Answers

1. A. The PAT is used to 1) establish the severity of the child's illness or injury (sick or not sick), 2) identify the general category of physiologic abnormality (e.g., cardiopulmonary, neurologic, etc.), and 3) determine the urgency of further assessment and intervention. Because approaching an ill or injured child can increase agitation, possibly worsening the child's condition, the PAT is an "across the room" assessment that is performed before approaching or touching the child and can usually be completed in 60 seconds or less. No equipment is required.

2. The components of the Pediatric Assessment Triangle are 1) Appearance, 2) Breathing, and 3) Circulation.

3. TICLS is a mnemonic used to recall the areas to be assessed related to the child's appearance. TICLS stands for: Tone (muscle tone), Interactivity/mental status (e.g., level of responsiveness, interaction with parents/guardian, and response to you or other healthcare professionals), Consolability, Look or gaze, and Speech or cry.

4. Pediatric Assessment Triangle (first impression) findings:
   Appearance: Awake and alert, intently observing healthcare provider
   Breathing: Respiratory rate within normal limits for age, no evidence of increased respiratory effort, symmetrical chest expansion
   Circulation: Skin is pink

5. Based on the information provided, this patient is "not sick" (i.e., stable). Proceed systematically. Perform an initial assessment (i.e., primary survey), secondary survey (including vital signs, focused history, and detailed physical examination), and an ongoing assessment. If the child appeared "sick" (unstable), you would proceed immediately with rapid assessment of airway, breathing, and circulation. If a problem were identified, you would perform necessary interventions ("Treat as you find").

6. B. To gain the child's cooperation, sit down and listen attentively while speaking with the child's mother. Toddlers distrust strangers, are likely to resist examination and treatment, and do not like having their clothing removed. They fear pain, separation from their caregiver and separation from transitional objects (e.g., blanket, toy). Approach the child slowly and talk to him at eye level using simple words and phrases and a reassuring tone of voice. The child will understand your tone, even if he does not understand your words.

7. The Primary Survey is performed to determine if life-threatening conditions exist and consists of ABCDE: **A**irway and cervical spine protection, **B**reathing and ventilation, **C**irculation with hemorrhage control, **D**isability (neurologic status), and **E**xpose / environment.

8. A normal respiratory rate for a toddler (1 to 3 years of age) is 24 to 40 breaths/min. A normal heart rate for a child of this age is 90 to 150 beats/min.

9. True. Respirations in infants and children younger than 6 or 7 years are primarily abdominal (diaphragmatic) because the intercostal muscles of the chest wall are not well developed and fatigue easily from the work of breathing. The transition from abdominal breathing to intercostal breathing begins between 2 and 4 years of age and is complete by 7 to 8 years of age.

10. Matching exercise – abnormal respiratory sounds.
    (B) Gasping – Inhaling and exhaling with quick, difficult breaths.
    (D) Snoring – Noisy breathing through the mouth and nose during sleep, caused by air passing through a narrowed upper airway.
    (A) Grunting – Short, low-pitched sound heard at the end of exhalation; a compensatory mechanism to help maintain patency of small airways and prevent atelectasis.
    (E) Stridor – Harsh, high-pitched sound heard on inspiration associated with upper airway obstruction.
    (C) Gurgling – Abnormal respiratory sound associated with collection of liquid or semi-solid material in the patient's upper airway.

11. D. Use of a blood pressure cuff that is too large will result in a falsely low reading. Blood pressure is one of the least sensitive indicators of adequate circulation in children. Blood pressure should be measured only after assessing pulse and respiration. Children often become agitated during this procedure, which increases their pulse and respiratory rate. Measure blood pressure in children more than 3 years of age. In children less than 3 years of age, a strong central pulse is considered an acceptable sign of adequate blood pressure.

12. Matching exercise – acronyms and mnemonics.

    (C) OPQRST   (A) TICLS
    (F) SAMPLE   (D) PAT
    (B) DCAP-BLS   (E) ABCDE

13. Matching exercise – terminology.

    (E) Nasal flaring
    (G) Retractions
    (C) Head bobbing
    (A) Sniffing position
    (D) Pulse pressure
    (F) Tripod position
    (B) Petechiae
    (H) Stroke volume

14. Matching exercise – triage classification.

    _A__ Respiratory arrest
    _A__ Active seizure
    _A__ Unresponsiveness
    _B__ Moderate respiratory distress
    _E__ Conjunctivitis
    _C__ Dehydration
    _E__ Ear discomfort
    _B__ Unstable vital signs
    _D__ Simple laceration
    _B__ Altered mental status
    _E__ Cold or flu
    _A__ Intubated patient
    _B__ Fever in an infant < 6 months of age

15. D. The location for assessment of a central pulse varies according to the age of the child. In the newly born, assess the strength and quality of a central pulse by palpating the base of the umbilical cord between your thumb and index finger. In an infant and young child, assess the brachial or femoral pulse. Assess the carotid pulse in any child over 1 year.

16. A = <u>A</u>lert
    V = Responds to <u>v</u>erbal stimuli
    P = Responds to <u>p</u>ainful stimuli
    U = <u>U</u>nresponsive

17. A. The formula used to approximate the lower limit of systolic blood pressure in children 1 to 10 years of age is 70 + (2 x age in years).

Respiratory Distress and Respiratory Failure

4

Case Study

A 2-year-old boy is having difficulty breathing. His parents tell you the child has had a cold for the past 2 days. According to Mom, she picked the child up from daycare an hour ago because he was having difficulty breathing and noticed "a whistling sound when he breathes out." She recalls the child has had four or five similar breathing episodes during the past year, but none as severe as this one. Mom is unsure if the child has had a fever and says there is a family history of asthma. Both parents are smokers. The child has no allergies. The child's older brother had a cough and cold about 5 days ago, but he is fine now.

Using the Pediatric Assessment Triangle (PAT), your first impression reveals the child is awake and aware of your presence. His respiratory rate is faster than normal for his age. You observe moderate subcostal and supraclavicular retractions and hear expiratory wheezing. His skin color is pink.

Based on the information provided, is this child sick or not sick? What should you do next?

Objectives

1. Identify key anatomic and physiologic characteristics of infants and children and their implications in the patient with respiratory distress or respiratory failure.
2. Define respiratory distress, respiratory failure, and respiratory arrest.
3. Describe the physiologic progression of respiratory distress, failure, and arrest.
4. Discuss the assessment findings associated with respiratory distress and respiratory failure in infants and children.
5. Differentiate between upper airway obstruction and lower airway disease.
6. Describe the general approach to the treatment of children with upper airway obstruction or lower airway disease.

- The larynx of the pediatric airway is more anterior and superior in the neck.

- In a newborn, the larynx is located between C1 to C4. The epiglottis can pass behind the soft palate and lock into the nasopharynx. This creates two separate channels—one for air and one for food (i.e., the infant can breathe and eat at the same time). The connection between the epiglottis and soft palate is constant except during crying and disease. Oral respirations begin at 5 to 6 months.

- At age 7, the larynx level is at C3 to C5. At this point, the epiglottis no longer connects with the soft palate (i.e., the child does not have two separate channels for food and air).

- The larynx of the newborn and young child resembles a funnel with the narrowest portion being at the cricoid ring. This area creates a natural seal (a physiologic cuff) around a tracheal tube, making cuffed tubes unnecessary in children younger than 8 years.

- The trachea is smaller and shorter than that of an adult.

  - Movement of a tracheal tube may occur during changes in head position. The small, short trachea may result in intubation of the right mainstem bronchus or inadvertent extubation. Securing a tracheal tube before movement of an intubated infant or child is important to prevent tube displacement.

  - A small change in airway size results in a significant increase in resistance to air flow when edema or a foreign body is present. A marked increase in airway resistance can result in partial or complete airway obstruction (Figure 4-2).

- In infants and children, the diaphragm is the primary muscle of inspiration.

  - The diaphragm must generate significant negative intrathoracic pressure to expand the child's underdeveloped lungs.

  - The diaphragm is horizontal in infants and results in decreased contraction efficiency. (The diaphragm is oblique in adults.) Efficiency of the diaphragm increases with age. Because this is the main way for pediatric patients to breathe, any compromise is serious.

- The intercostal muscles are immature and fatigue easily from the work of breathing.

  - The intercostal muscles act more as rib stabilizers and not as efficient rib elevators.

  - Accessory muscles of respiration are quiet during normal breathing, but may be activated during periods of respiratory distress.

- Effective respiration may be jeopardized when diaphragmatic movement is compromised because the chest wall cannot compensate.

Blind finger sweeps are not performed in pediatric patients. Because the larynx is high in the neck, a blind finger sweep may push a foreign body into the larynx and obstruct the airway.

The narrowest portion of the upper airway of an infant and young child is at the level of the cricoid ring.

> The pediatric upper airway is susceptible to obstruction from foreign bodies, congenital anomalies, infection (e.g., croup, bacterial tracheitis), flexion or hyperextension, and soft-tissue swelling due to injury or inflammation. The lower airways are vulnerable to obstruction because of edema, mucus plugging, spasm, or a tumor.

Chest and Lungs

Use of the diaphragm leads to a characteristic "seesaw" or abdominal breathing pattern.

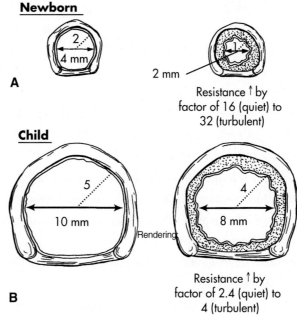

Newborn

Child

2 mm

Resistance ↑ by
factor of 16 (quiet) to
32 (turbulent)

Resistance ↑ by
factor of 2.4 (quiet) to
4 (turbulent)

Figure 4-2   **A**, A newborn's trachea is approximately 5 cm in length and approximately 4 mm in diameter. One millimeter of circumferential edema in a neonate's airway increases the resistance to air flow by a factor of 16 during quiet breathing and by a factor of 32 with turbulent airflow (e.g., crying, labored breathing). **B**, The trachea of a young adult is approximately 10 mm in diameter. One millimeter of circumferential edema in a young adult's airway increases the resistance to air flow by a factor of 2.4 during quiet breathing, and by a factor of 4 with turbulent airflow (e.g., crying, labored breathing).

> The compliant chest wall of an infant or young child should expand easily during positive-pressure ventilation. If the chest wall does not expand equally during positive-pressure ventilation, ventilation is inadequate or the airway may be obstructed.

- ○ Restraint for immobilization may impair chest wall movement.
- ○ Consider insertion of an orogastric or nasogastric tube if gastric distention is present and impairs ventilation.
- The chest wall of the infant and young child is pliable because it is composed of more cartilage than bone and the ribs are more horizontal.
- ○ Offers less protection to underlying organs.
- ○ Significant internal injury can be present without external signs.
- ○ Because of the flexibility of the ribs, children are more resistant to rib fractures than adults are, although the force of the injury is readily transmitted to the delicate tissues of the lung and may result in a pulmonary contusion, hemothorax, or pneumothorax.
- ○ Due to their pliability, the ribs may fail to support the lungs, leading to paradoxic movement during active inspiration, rather than lung expansion.
- ○ The thin chest wall allows for easily transmitted breath sounds. It is easy to miss a pneumothorax or misplaced tracheal tube because of transmitted breath sounds.

- Thoracic volume is small.
  - Children have fewer and smaller alveoli. Thus the potential area for gas exchange is less. Lung volume increases to 200 mL by age 8.
  - Fluids or air can more easily enter the interstitium (i.e., pneumo-thorax, pulmonary edema).
  - The oxygen requirements of infants and children are approximately twice those of adolescents and adults (6 to 8 mL/kg/min in a child; 3 to 4 mL/kg/min in an adult).
  - Children have a proportionately smaller functional residual capacity, and therefore proportionally smaller oxygen reserves. Hypoxia develops rapidly because of increased oxygen requirements and decreased oxygen reserves.
    - "Grunting" can help maintain functional residual capacity because it breaks the expiratory flow.
    - Grunting is not effective if there is reduced lung compliance (e.g., pneumonia, shock lung), impaired neurologic control (trauma, meningitis, drug effects), or an intubated trachea. Therefore the volume left in the lungs may not be enough to keep the alveoli open.

Respiratory Distress, Failure, and Arrest

Definitions

- **Respiratory distress** is increased work of breathing (respiratory effort).
- **Respiratory failure** is a clinical condition in which there is inadequate blood oxygenation and/or ventilation to meet the metabolic demands of body tissues.
- **Respiratory arrest** is the absence of breathing.

Respiratory Distress

Respiratory distress is characterized by the presence of increased respiratory effort, rate, and work of breathing.

Causes of Respiratory Distress in Children

Respiratory distress may result from a problem in the tracheobronchial tree, lungs, pleura, or chest wall.

- Asthma/reactive airway disease (RAD)
- Aspiration
- Foreign body
- Congenital heart disease
- Infection (e.g., pneumonia, croup, epiglottitis, bronchiolitis)
- Medication or toxin exposure
- Trauma

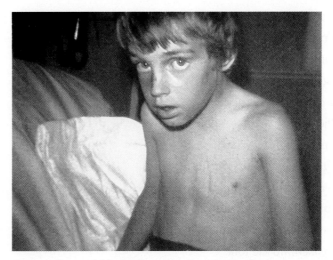

Figure 4-3   A child exhibiting signs of respiratory distress.

Signs of Respiratory Distress

- Alert, irritable, anxious, restless
- Stridor
- Grunting
- Gurgling
- Audible wheezing
- Respiratory rate faster than normal for age (tachypnea)
- Increased depth of breathing (hyperpnea)
- Intercostal retractions
- Head bobbing
- Seesaw respirations (abdominal breathing)
- Nasal flaring
- Neck muscle use
- Central cyanosis that resolves with oxygen administration
- Mild tachycardia

Respiratory Failure

- Respiratory failure is the most common cause of cardiopulmonary arrest in children. It is often preceded by respiratory distress in which the child's work of breathing is increased in an attempt to compensate for hypoxia.
- *Potential* respiratory failure is based on clinical observation of signs of respiratory distress.
- Failure to improve (or deterioration) after treatment for respiratory distress indicates respiratory failure.

Causes of Respiratory Failure in Children

- Infection (e.g., croup, epiglottitis, bronchiolitis, pneumonia)
- Foreign body
- Asthma/RAD

- Smoke inhalation
- Submersion syndrome
- Pneumothorax, hemothorax
- Congenital abnormalities
- Neuromuscular disease
- Medication or toxin exposure
- Trauma
- Congestive heart failure
- Metabolic disease with acidosis

Signs of Respiratory Failure

- Sleepy, intermittently combative, or agitated
- Decreased muscle tone
- Decreased level of responsiveness or response to pain
- Inadequate respiratory rate, effort, or chest excursion
- Tachypnea with periods of bradypnea; slowing to bradypnea/ agonal breathing

Signs of Respiratory Arrest: **Respiratory Arrest**

- Mottling; peripheral and central cyanosis
- Unresponsive to voice or touch
- Absent chest wall motion
- Absent respirations
- Weak to absent pulses
- Bradycardia or asystole
- Limp muscle tone

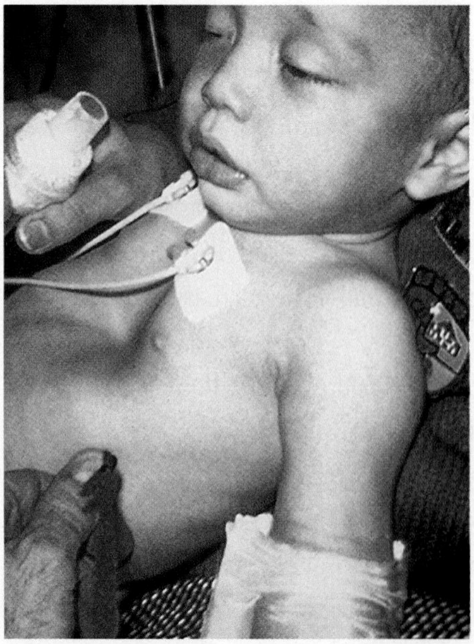

Figure 4-4   An infant exhibiting signs of respiratory failure.

Respiratory Assessment

Scene Safety

On arrival, ensure the scene is safe before proceeding with your assessment of the patient.

Initial Assessment

Remember, the PAT is your first impression of the patient. From a distance, evaluate the child's appearance, work of breathing, and circulation to determine the severity of the child's illness or injury (Table 4-1) and assist you in determining the urgency for care (Table 4-2).

If the child appears sick (unstable), proceed immediately with the primary survey and treat problems as you find them. If the child appears "not sick" (stable), complete the initial assessment. Perform a focused or detailed physical examination, based on the patient's presentation and chief complaint. Remember: Your patient's condition can change at any time. A patient that initially appears "not sick" may rapidly deteriorate and appear "sick." Reassess frequently.

Detailed initial assessment information and interventions were presented in Chapter 3 and are not repeated here. Additional history, signs and symptoms, and interventions specific to each disorder are listed.

TABLE 4-1 *First Impression of Respiratory Emergencies*

Assessment	Respiratory Distress	Respiratory Failure	Respiratory Arrest
Mental status	Alert, irritable, anxious, restless	Decreased level of responsiveness or response to pain	Unresponsive to voice or touch
Muscle tone	Able to maintain sitting position (children older than 4 mo)	Normal or decreased	Limp
Body position	May assume tripod position	May assume tripod position. May need support to maintain sitting position as he/she tires	Unable to maintain sitting position (infant older than 7 to 9 mo)
Respiratory rate	Faster than normal for age	Tachypnea with periods of bradypnea; slowing to bradypnea/agonal breathing	Absent
Respiratory effort	Intercostal retractions. Nasal flaring. Neck muscle use. Seesaw respirations	Inadequate respiratory effort or chest excursion	Absent
Audible airway sounds	Stridor, wheezing, gurgling	Stridor, wheezing, grunting, gasping	Absent
Skin color	Pink or pale; central cyanosis resolves with oxygen administration	Central cyanosis despite oxygen administration; mottling	Mottling; peripheral and central cyanosis

TABLE 4-2 *Immediate Interventions for Respiratory Emergencies based on the First Impression*

Emergency	Interventions
Respiratory distress	Approach promptly, but work at a moderate pace Permit the child to assume a position of comfort Correct hypoxia by giving oxygen without causing agitation Provide further interventions based on assessment findings
Respiratory failure	Move quickly Open the airway and suction if necessary Correct hypoxia by giving high-flow oxygen Begin assisted ventilation if the patient does not improve Provide further interventions on the basis of assessment findings
Respiratory arrest	Move quickly Immediately open the airway and suction if necessary Begin ventilating with 100% oxygen Reassess for return of spontaneous respiration Provide further interventions based on assessment findings

Modified from Foltin GL, Tunik MG, Cooper A, et al. *Teaching resource for instructors in prehospital pediatrics for paramedics.* New York: Center for Pediatric Emergency Medicine, 2002.

Focused History and Physical Examination

Focused History

In addition to the SAMPLE history, consider the following questions when obtaining a focused history for a condition affecting the respiratory system. This list will require modification on the basis of the patient's age and chief complaint.

- Is the child having any trouble breathing?
- When did it start/occur (time, sudden, gradual)? What was the child doing when it started/occurred?
- How long did it last? Does it come and go? Is it still present?
- Does the child have a cough? If yes, what does the cough sound like? When does it occur? Does he bring up any sputum when he coughs? What does the sputum look like?
- Previous history of a similar episode? If yes, what was the diagnosis?
- Does anything make the symptoms better or worse (e.g., cool air, tripod position, use of inhaler)?
- Allergies to medications, foods, pets, dust, perfume, pollen, or cigarette smoke? If yes, how does the child's allergy affect his or her breathing?
- History of asthma/RAD? Ever hospitalized or intubated for this condition?
- Medications: What are they (prescription, over-the-counter, recreational)? Last dose?

- Recent cold, flu, earache, pneumonia, other infection?
- Recent injuries/accidents (e.g., chest trauma, near-drowning)?
- Possibility of foreign body aspiration?
- History of trauma?
- Will the child drink? Has he or she been drooling?
- Has the child had a fever? For how long?
- Has the child's voice changed?
- Are siblings sick?
- Treatment given by caregiver?

Focused Physical Examination

A child presenting with a sudden onset of respiratory distress accompanied by fever, drooling, hoarseness, stridor, and tripod positioning may have a partial airway obstruction. Because agitation tends to worsen respiratory distress, keep the child as calm and as comfortable as possible, usually in the arms of the caregiver. Administer supplemental oxygen as discreetly as possible, usually via blow-by oxygen while the child is sitting on the caregiver's lap. Allow the child to assume a position of comfort and disturb the child as little as possible. Avoid procedures that may agitate the child until after the airway has been secured.

- Determine if the airway is patent, maintainable, or unmaintainable
  - Patent: able to be maintained independently
  - Maintainable with positioning, suctioning
  - Unmaintainable: requires assistance (e.g., tracheal intubation, cricothyrotomy, foreign body removal)
- Assess for signs of airway obstruction. Signs include absent breath sounds, tachypnea, intercostal retractions, stridor or drooling, choking, bradycardia, and/or cyanosis.
  - It is often helpful to put your stethoscope in your ears and look without listening. Many pediatric patients (particularly infants) sound terrible, but the sounds can be due to upper airway congestion. One can even feel transmitted sounds from the upper airway. Signs such as retractions, cyanosis, lethargy, nasal flaring, or similar signs are cause for concern (Table 4-3).
- Obtain a pulse oximeter reading (Figure 4-5)
- Adequate breathing requires a patent airway, an adequate tidal volume, and an acceptable respiratory rate (the rate is age dependent). Observe the chest wall for equal bilateral movement and time spent on inspiration and expiration.
- Tachycardia is commonly seen in the child with respiratory distress. Bradycardia is seen with severe hypoxemia and acidosis due to respiratory failure. Bradycardia in a child with respiratory failure is a warning of imminent cardiopulmonary arrest (Figure 4-6).

A quiet child is a sick child; a strong cry is a good cry.

For tachypnea without a distressed-looking patient, consider cardiac causes.

TABLE 4-3 *Signs of Increased Work of Breathing* 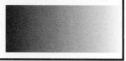	
Visible Signs (Look)	**Audible Signs (Listen)**
Anxious appearance, concentration on breathing	Stridor
Respiratory rate faster than normal for age	Wheezing
Use of accessory muscles	Crackles
Leaning forward to inhale	Grunting
Inspiratory retractions	Gurgling
Nasal flaring	Gasping
Head bobbing	
Seesaw (chest/abdominal) movement	

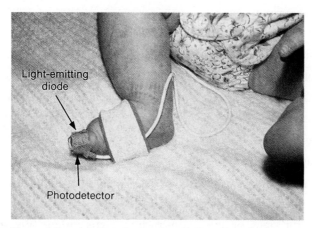

Figure 4-5   A pulse oximeter sensor is present on the great toe. The sensor is positioned with the light-emitting diode opposite the photodetector. The cord is secured to the foot with a self-adhering band to minimize movement of the sensor.

- Agitation and irritability may indicate hypoxemia. Lethargy and decreased responsiveness may signal severe hypoxemia and/or carbon dioxide retention.
- Expose the child as needed to complete your examination.

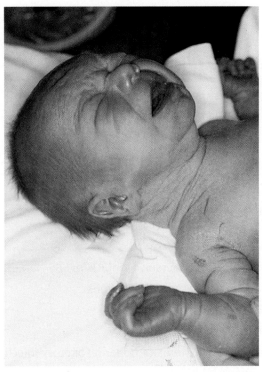

Figure 4-6   This ill infant exhibits cyanosis and poor skin perfusion.

Common Pediatric Upper Airway Emergencies

Croup

Description

Croup (laryngotracheobronchitis) is a respiratory infection that affects the upper respiratory tract. The area below the glottis is most commonly affected, resulting in swollen, inflamed mucosa with associated hoarseness, inspiratory stridor, and a barklike cough. The diagnosis is usually based on history and physical examination (Figure 4-7).

Etiology

Croup is caused by a respiratory virus. Parainfluenza type 1 is the most common cause, but it may also result from parainfluenza types 2 and 3, influenza A and B, adenovirus, respiratory syncytial virus (RSV), echovirus, rhinovirus, and mycoplasma (infrequently).

Epidemiology and Demographics

- Primarily affects children ages 6 months to 3 years; peaks at age 2 years
- The three parainfluenza viruses are observed most frequently in the fall. RSV has a midwinter peak and can be found in increasing numbers in the spring.

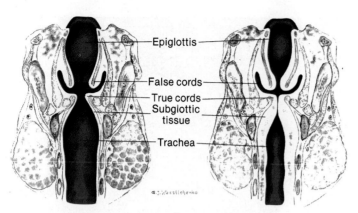

Figure 4-7   **A,** Normal larynx. **B,** Obstruction and narrowing resulting from edema of croup.

- Spread via person-to-person contact or by large droplets and contaminated nasopharyngeal secretions
- Incubation period: 2 to 4 days

History

- Typical history of symptoms of upper respiratory infection (URI) for 2 to 3 days, but may be spasmodic (usually wakes from a nap or sleep). Croup is usually worse at night or when the child is agitated.
- Obtain a thorough history to narrow diagnosis
  - Trauma
  - Cough or choking after playing with small toys

Physical Examination

- Vital signs: increased respiratory rate, increased heart rate, elevated temperature (usually less than 102.2° F)
- Loud stridor with hoarse voice and barky (seal-like) cough. Stridor becomes less as muscles fatigue.
- Nasal flaring
- Retractions

Croup Severity

- Mild croup: normal color, normal mental status, air entry with stridor audible only with stethoscope, no retractions
- Moderate croup: normal color, audible stridor, mild to moderate retractions, slightly diminished air entry in an anxious child (Figure 4-8)
- Severe croup: cyanosis, loud stridor, significant decrease in air entry, marked retractions in a highly anxious child

The croup score (Table 4-4) may be useful in determining the severity of airway obstruction. The croup score is based on a child's color, level of alertness, degree of stridor, air movement, and degree of retractions. Zero points are given if these findings are normal or not present. Up to five points are given for more severe symptoms. In general, a score of 3 necessitates hospitalization if unresponsive to therapy.

Croup is the most common infectious cause of acute upper airway obstruction in pediatrics, causing 90% of the cases.[1]

TABLE 4-4 *Westley Croup Score*

Criteria		Points
Retractions	None	0
	Mild	1
	Moderate	2
	Severe	3
Air entry	Normal	0
	Decreased but easily audible	1
	Severely decreased	2
Inspiratory stridor	None	0
	When agitated	1
	At rest, with stethoscope	2
	At rest, without stethoscope	4
Cyanosis	None	0
	With agitation	4
	At rest	5
Alertness/level of responsiveness	Alert	0
	Restless, anxious	2
	Altered mental status	5

Croup score 0-1, mild croup; croup score 2-7, moderate croup; croup score 8 or higher, severe croup.

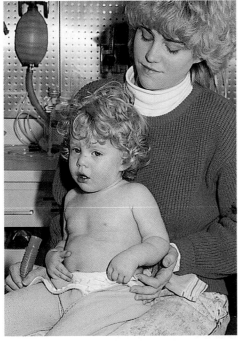

Figure 4-8   **Croup.** This toddler with moderate upper airway obstruction caused by croup had suprasternal and subcostal retractions. Her anxious expression was the result of mild hypoxia confirmed by pulse oximetry.

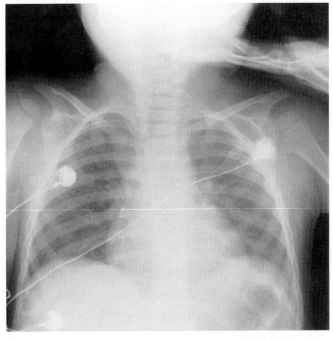

Figure 4-9   **Croup.** Radiograph of the airway of a patient with croup, showing typical subglottic narrowing ("steeple sign").

Acceptable Interventions

- Use personal protective equipment.
- Perform an initial assessment and obtain a focused history.
- Assist the child into a position of comfort, usually sitting up on the caregiver's lap.
- Maintaining an airway takes precedence over any other procedures. Ten percent of children require hospitalization and 3% require airway support.
- Avoid agitating the child. Keep the child as calm and as comfortable as possible, usually in the arms of the caregiver.
- Assess for foreign body airway obstruction (FBAO) (by history). Do not examine the oropharynx (may agitate the child and worsen respiratory distress).
- Initiate pulse oximetry, if available. Note: The use of pulse oximetry in croup can be inaccurate. This is because a large degree of upper airway obstruction is required to produce hypoxia in an otherwise previously healthy child.[2]
- If ventilation is adequate and the patient exhibits signs of respiratory distress, give high-concentration oxygen in a manner that does not agitate the child. Keep the oxygen saturation above 95%. If signs of respiratory failure or respiratory arrest are present, assist ventilation using a bag-valve-mask device with 100% oxygen.
- If the patient shows signs of respiratory failure or respiratory arrest, establish vascular access and administer normal saline at a rate sufficient to keep the vein open. In the field, do not delay transport to establish vascular access.
- In the child with mild croup, nebulized saline with no medication added may be used to provide a cool water vapor to help reduce inflammation and swelling.

Moderate to severe croup

- Give racemic epinephrine 0.05 mL/kg/dose (maximum dose is 0.5 mL) of 2.25% solution in 3 mL normal saline for inhalation, no more than every 1 to 2 hours or nebulized epinephrine 0.5 mL/kg of 1:1000 (1 mg/mL) in 3 mL normal saline (maximum dose is 2.5 mL for a child 4 years old, 5 mL for a child older than 4 years).[3]
  - The α-adrenergic effect of epinephrine is beneficial by reducing mucosal edema. Smooth-muscle relaxation due to β-adrenergic effects may benefit those children with croup who are also wheezing.[2]
  - Administer with supplemental oxygen.
  - Cardiac monitoring is **required** due to the tachycardic effect and potential for dysrhythmias.

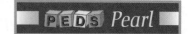

An upright lateral radiograph of the neck may be a useful aid in diagnosing croup, but should be reserved for the child in whom epiglottitis is *not* suspected. The radiograph may reveal laryngeal narrowing 5 to 10 mm below the vocal cords. This finding is referred to as the typical "steeple sign" associated with viral croup (Figure 4-9). However, the steeple sign may be absent in patients with croup, may be present in patients without croup as a normal variant, and may be present in patients with epiglottitis. In addition, the radiographs do not correlate well with disease severity.[5]

Cool, humidified air often helps alleviate the inflammation associated with croup.

A pulse oximeter provides information about oxygenation. It does not reflect the adequacy of ventilation.

Hold epinephrine administration for any heart rate above 200 beats per minute. Admit if more than one nebulization is required.

Drug Pearl: Epinephrine

- Epinephrine relaxes the smooth muscle of the bronchioles and reduces tissue swelling of related structures.
- Inhaled epinephrine may be used for the child with stridor at rest, in those with associated reduced air entry, and/or for those with retractions.
- Epinephrine can be used in the treatment of severe acute exacerbations of asthma if β_2-agonists (inhaled or parenteral) are not available. However, the possibility of adverse effects, particularly among hypoxic patients, is greater.
- In anaphylaxis, epinephrine is the bronchodilator of choice and is administered by subcutaneous or intramuscular injection.
- Adverse reactions include transient, moderate anxiety, apprehensiveness, restlessness, tremor, weakness, dizziness, sweating, palpitations, pallor, nausea and vomiting, and headache.

PEDS Pearl

- An episode of mild croup will usually break with humidification by cool-mist vaporizer, a steam bath in the bathroom (for 30 minutes or less at a time), or going into the cool, moist night air. Breathing cold freezer air can also be tried. Inspired air that is cooler than body temperature and less than 100% saturated with water vapor results in cooling of the mucosa, leading to vasoconstriction and lessened edema.
- Generally, sedatives should not be used in the child with croup because they can depress the respiratory drive and restlessness is used as one means of evaluating the severity of airway obstruction and the need for intubation. Opiates should not be used because they may depress respirations and dry secretions.

- The administration of nebulized epinephrine plays no role in the decision to admit or discharge the patient; therefore patient disposition should not be a consideration in the decision to provide this treatment.
- Consider dexamethasone 0.6 mg/kg (maximum dose 8 mg) intramuscular (IM) or by mouth (PO) as a single dose.[3] Some data show early treatment with dexamethasone may shorten the course and prevent the progression of croup to complete obstruction.
- Nebulized budesonide (2 mg) may also be tried.[2]
- The child with severe croup may progress to respiratory failure. If tracheal intubation is required, use a tracheal tube 0.5 to 1.0 mm smaller than that calculated for age because of the swelling and inflammation of the trachea at the subglottic level.

Unacceptable Interventions

- Failure to use personal protective equipment
- Failure to recognize signs of respiratory distress and the need for interventions
- Failure to allow the child to assume a position of comfort
- Failure to administer supplemental oxygen
- Failure to measure oxygen saturation
- Agitating the child with an intravenous (IV) start, placement of a face mask, blood pressure assessment, or medication administration unless the treatment is immediately lifesaving
- Failure to assist ventilation with a bag-valve-mask device and 100% oxygen if signs of respiratory failure or respiratory arrest are present

- Failure to reassess respiratory status after initiating assisted ventilations
- Performing tracheal intubation before treating respiratory failure with assisted ventilations via bag-valve-mask and 100% oxygen
- Failure to anticipate the potential need for tracheal intubation
- Performing tracheal intubation in a child who responds to less invasive interventions
- Failure to recognize signs of deterioration to respiratory failure or arrest and the need for more aggressive interventions
- If tracheal intubation is required, failure to confirm tracheal tube position using assessment and mechanical methods
- Failure to administer nebulized epinephrine or racemic epinephrine to a child with moderate to severe croup
- Failure to monitor the cardiac rhythm if signs of respiratory failure or respiratory arrest are present, or if racemic or nebulized epinephrine is administered
- Failure to use an accurate method for weight and medication dosage determination
- Medication errors
- Ordering a dangerous or inappropriate intervention
- Performing any technique resulting in potential harm to the patient

Epiglottitis

Description

Epiglottitis is a bacterial infection of the upper airway that may progress to complete airway obstruction and death within hours unless adequate treatment is provided (Figure 4-10). Diagnosis is often based on history and observation of the child from a distance.

Epiglottitis is more accurately called acute supraglottitis, because inflammation of the supraglottic structures can cause the symptoms of epiglottitis, without actually involving the epiglottis.

Etiology

In the past, *Haemophilus influenzae* type B (HiB) was the most commonly identified cause of acute epiglottitis. Due to the widespread use of the HiB vaccine in the United States, invasive disease due to HiB in pediatric patients has been reduced by 80% to 90%. *Streptococcus pyogenes, Streptococcus pneumoniae,* and *Staphylococcus aureus* now represent a larger proportion of pediatric cases of epiglottitis.

Epidemiology and Demographics

- Can occur at any age; typically affects children 3 to 7 years of age
- Decreased incidence in children because of widespread use of *H. influenzae* vaccine; increasing prevalence in adolescents and adults
- No seasonal preference

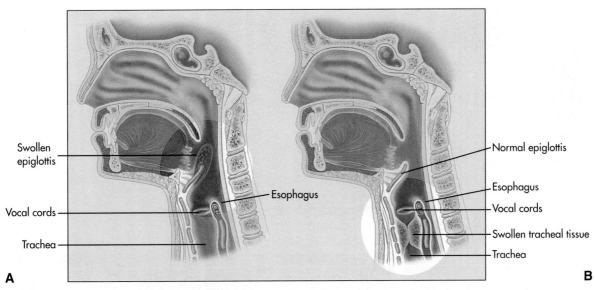

Figure 4-10   **A**, Acute epiglottitis. **B**, Laryngotracheobronchitis (croup).

The child's muffled voice may be referred to as "hot potato" voice because it sounds as if the child is talking with a hot potato in his or her mouth.

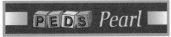

PEDS *Pearl*

Never force a child with respiratory distress to lie down. This may compromise the airway and cause immediate obstruction.

History

- Quiet wet stridor, a muffled voice, dysphagia, and a preference for sitting upright are characteristic of supraglottic disorders. Absence of a cough is an important diagnostic clue.
- Sudden onset of high fever.
- Typically, no other family members are ill with an acute upper respiratory illness.

Physical Examination

- Vital signs: increased respiratory rate, increased heart rate, elevated temperature, usually 102° F to 104° F
- Difficulty swallowing, sore throat, drooling
- Muffled voice
- Shallow breathing
- Prefers to sit up and lean forward (tripod position), with the mouth open (Figure 4-11)
- Stridor is a late finding and suggests near-complete airway obstruction
- Child appears acutely ill ("toxic")

Acceptable Interventions

Because an aggressive physical examination, attempt to visualize the epiglottis, laboratory tests, or IV placement can precipitate complete airway obstruction, these procedures should be deferred until the diagnosis of epiglottitis is confirmed and the airway is secured. Close observation and frequent reassessment is essential.

- Use personal protective equipment.

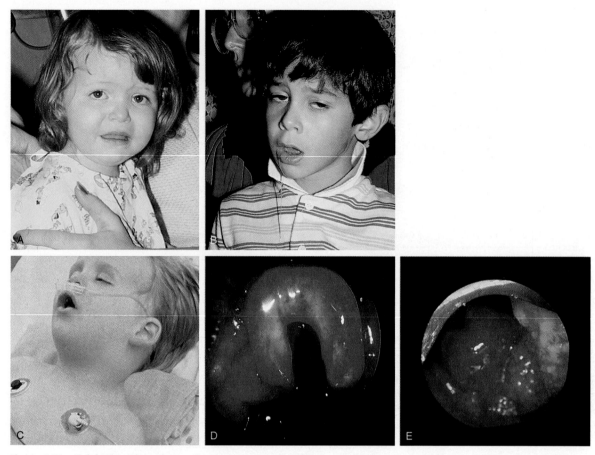

Figure 4-11   Epiglottitis. These three patients with acute epiglottitis demonstrate the varying degrees of distress that may be seen, depending on age and time of presentation. **A,** This 3-year-old seen a few hours after the onset of symptoms was anxious and still, but had no positional preference or drooling. **B,** This 5-year-old, who had been symptomatic for several hours, holds his neck extended with the head held forward, is mouth breathing and drooling, and shows signs of tiring. **C,** This 2-year-old was in severe distress and was too exhausted to hold his head up. **D** and **E,** In the operating room, the epiglottis was visualized and appears intensely red and swollen. It may retain its omega shape or resemble a cherry.

- Perform an initial assessment and obtain a focused history.
- Assist the child into a position of comfort, usually sitting up on the caregiver's lap.
- Avoid agitating the child. Keep the child as calm and as comfortable as possible, usually in the arms of the caregiver.
- Do not examine the oropharynx (may agitate the child and worsen respiratory distress).
- Initiate pulse oximetry, if available.
- If ventilation is adequate and the patient exhibits signs of respiratory distress, give high-concentration oxygen in a manner that does not agitate the child. Keep the oxygen saturation above 95%. If signs of respiratory failure or respiratory arrest are present, assist ventilation using a bag-valve-mask device with 100% oxygen. If total obstruction occurs, ventilate with high pressures.

- Do not administer anything by mouth.
- Management options[3]
  - If the child is unstable (unresponsive, cyanotic, bradycardic), the clinician most skilled in pediatric intubation should emergently intubate. Tracheal intubation should be performed using a tracheal tube 0.5 to 1 mm smaller than that calculated for age.
  - If the child is stable with a high suspicion of epiglottitis, the patient should be escorted with an epiglottitis team (e.g., senior pediatrician, anesthesiologist, and otolaryngologist) for endoscopy and intubation under general anesthesia.
  - If the child is stable with a moderate or low suspicion of epiglottitis, and no evidence of obstruction exists, some clinicians prefer to obtain a radiograph of the nasopharynx and upper airway before direct visualization of the pharynx.
    - A child with suspected epiglottitis should be accompanied by a clinician capable of intubating the patient and intubation equipment *at all times*, including the trip to and from the radiology department.
    - The radiograph may show swelling of the epiglottis, also known as the "thumb" sign, because it resembles the size and shape of the human thumb (Figure 4-12); however, in many patients the lateral neck film may not be diagnostic.[4]
- After the airway is secured, an IV should be established and fluid therapy begun. Blood cultures, cultures of the epiglottis and supraglottic surfaces, and other tests may be performed and antibiotic therapy started. The patient should be monitored in the intensive care unit (ICU).

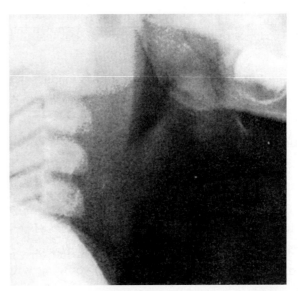

Figure 4-12   Epiglottitis. A lateral radiograph of the upper airway reveals a swollen epiglottis.

Unacceptable Interventions

- Failure to use personal protective equipment
- Failure to recognize signs of respiratory distress and the need for interventions
- Failure to allow the child to assume a position of comfort
- Failure to administer supplemental oxygen
- Failure to measure oxygen saturation
- Agitating the child with an IV start, placement of a face mask, blood pressure assessment, or medication administration unless the treatment is immediately lifesaving.
- Failure to assist ventilation with a bag-valve-mask device and 100% oxygen if signs of respiratory failure or respiratory arrest are present
- Failure to reassess respiratory status after initiating assisted ventilations
- Performing tracheal intubation before treating respiratory failure with assisted ventilations via bag-valve-mask and 100% oxygen
- Failure to anticipate the potential need for tracheal intubation
- Performing tracheal intubation in a child who responds to less invasive interventions
- Failure to recognize signs of deterioration to respiratory failure or arrest and the need for more aggressive interventions
- Failure to monitor the cardiac rhythm if signs of respiratory failure or respiratory arrest are present
- Failure to ensure a child with suspected epiglottitis is accompanied to and from the radiology department by a clinician capable of intubating the patient and with appropriate equipment.
- If tracheal intubation is required, failure to confirm tracheal tube position using assessment and mechanical methods
- Attempting a needle or surgical cricothyrotomy before attempting assisted ventilations via bag-valve-mask or tracheal tube and 100% oxygen
- Ordering a dangerous or inappropriate intervention
- Performing any technique resulting in potential harm to the patient

Bacterial Tracheitis

Description

Bacterial tracheitis (also called membranous tracheitis or pseudo-membranous croup) is an acute bacterial infection of the subglottic area of the upper airway that can cause a life-threatening airway obstruction. The diagnosis is based on evidence of bacterial upper airway disease, high fever, purulent airway secretions, and an absence of the classic findings of epiglottitis.

Etiology

Bacterial tracheitis most commonly involves infection with *S. aureus, H.*

influenzae, and *Corynebacterium diphtheriae,* but parainfluenza virus type 1, *Moraxella catarrhalis,* and anaerobic organisms have also been identified.

Epidemiology and Demographics

- Bacterial tracheitis occurs in the same age group as croup (children 6 months to 3 years), although older children have occasionally been affected.
- There are no clear gender differences in incidence or severity.
- Controversy exists as to whether bacterial tracheitis exists alone or whether it is a bacterial complication of a preexistent viral respiratory infection (such as croup).
- This life-threatening illness is now more common than epiglottitis.[5]
- Fifty percent of children with bacterial tracheitis have an associated pneumonia.

History

- The patient with bacterial tracheitis frequently has a several-day history of viral upper respiratory symptoms, such as fever, cough, and stridor, similar to croup. This may be followed by a rapid onset of high fever, respiratory distress, and a toxic appearance. Drooling is usually absent.
- Patients frequently have concurrent sites of infection, with pneumonia being the most common.
- Bacterial tracheitis is associated with swelling of the mucosa at the level of the cricoid cartilage that is complicated by copious thick, purulent secretions. The child may decompensate quickly due to airway obstruction from a purulent membrane that has loosened.

Physical Examination

Signs and symptoms are usually intermediate between epiglottitis and croup.

- Inspiratory stridor with or without expiratory stridor
- Barklike or brassy cough
- Hoarseness
- Variable degrees of respiratory distress: retractions, dyspnea, nasal flaring, cyanosis
- Sore throat (minimal)
- Dysphonia
- Typically, no drooling
- Worsening or abruptly occurring stridor or respiratory distress

Acceptable Interventions

The usual treatments for croup (e.g., mist, IV fluid, nebulized epinephrine) are ineffective for bacterial tracheitis. Close observation and frequent reassessment are essential. Toxic shock syndrome has been associated with tracheitis.

- Use personal protective equipment
- Perform an initial assessment and obtain a focused history.
- Assist the child into a position of comfort.
- Avoid agitating the child. Keep the child as calm and as comfortable as possible, usually in the arms of the caregiver.
- Initiate pulse oximetry, if available.

- If ventilation is adequate and the patient exhibits signs of respiratory distress, give high-concentration oxygen in a manner that does not agitate the child. Keep the oxygen saturation above 95%. If signs of respiratory failure or respiratory arrest are present, assist ventilation using a bag-valve-mask device with 100% oxygen.
- If required, tracheal intubation should be performed using a tracheal tube 0.5 to 1 mm smaller than that calculated for age because of the swelling and inflammation of the trachea at the subglottic level. Frequent suctioning is often necessary to maintain the patency of the tube.
- After the airway is secured, establish IV access and begin antibiotic therapy.

Unacceptable Interventions

- Failure to use personal protective equipment
- Failure to recognize signs of respiratory distress and the need for interventions
- Failure to allow the child to assume a position of comfort
- Failure to administer supplemental oxygen
- Failure to measure oxygen saturation
- Agitating the child with an IV start, placement of a face mask, blood pressure assessment, or medication administration unless the treatment is immediately lifesaving.
- Failure to assist ventilation with a bag-valve-mask device and 100% oxygen if signs of respiratory failure or respiratory arrest are present
- Failure to reassess respiratory status after initiating assisted ventilations
- Performing tracheal intubation before treating respiratory failure with assisted ventilations via bag-valve-mask and 100% oxygen
- Failure to anticipate the potential need for tracheal intubation
- Performing tracheal intubation in a child who responds to less invasive interventions
- Failure to recognize signs of deterioration to respiratory failure or arrest and the need for more aggressive interventions
- Failure to monitor the cardiac rhythm if signs of respiratory failure or respiratory arrest are present
- If tracheal intubation is required, failure to confirm tracheal tube position using assessment and mechanical methods
- If suctioning is required, failure to limit suctioning to 10 seconds or less per attempt
- Ordering a dangerous or inappropriate intervention
- Performing any technique resulting in potential harm to the patient

Foreign Body Airway Obstruction

Description

FBAO may be seen at any age, but children younger than 5 years of age are especially vulnerable. One third of aspirated objects are nuts, particularly peanuts. Laryngotracheal foreign bodies typically produce an acute obstruction. A foreign body in a bronchus may result in a more subtle presentation.

Etiology

- Common causes of foreign body aspiration in children include small foods such as nuts, raisins, sunflower seeds, popcorn, and improperly chewed pieces of meat, grapes, hot dogs, raw carrots, or sausages. Other items commonly found in the home that may cause FBAO include disc batteries, pins, rings, nails, buttons, coins, plastic or metal toy objects, and marbles (Figure 4-13).
  - Grapes, hot dogs, sausages, and balloons are more likely to cause tracheal obstruction and asphyxiation because they are round or smooth, or both.
  - Popular fruit-flavored gel snacks have been associated with an increased risk of aspiration in children.[6]
  - Hot dogs and bread are two of the most common causes of fatal aspiration.
- Because they absorb moisture, dried foods (such as beans and peas) may cause progressive airway obstruction.
- Peanut butter is particularly difficult to remove by coughing or with the use of instruments.

Epidemiology and Demographics

- Although an FBAO can occur in individuals of any age, it occurs most often in children younger than 5 years. Children younger than 3 years account for 73% of cases of FBAO.
- Children are at risk of FBAO because
  - They are inherently curious.
  - Infants and young children learn about their world by putting an object in their mouth.
  - They lack molar teeth, decreasing their ability to sufficiently chew food.
  - They tend to talk, laugh, and run while chewing.
  - Parents may have unrealistic expectations regarding what their child should be able to eat or do at a given age.
- More than 90% of pediatric deaths due to foreign body aspiration occur in children younger than 5 years; 65% of victims are infants.
- In adults, an FBAO most often occurs during eating. In infants and children, most episodes of choking occur during eating or play. Occasionally, poor supervision by adults or older siblings is a contributing factor.

Ages at highest risk of FBAO: 6 months to 5 years

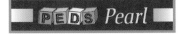

PEDS *Pearl*

"A positive history must never be ignored. A negative history may be misleading."[11] Suspect FBAO in any previously well, afebrile child with a sudden onset of respiratory distress and associated coughing, choking, stridor, or wheezing.

Children will eat, swallow, and place into any body cavity anything they can get hold of, even if it is "yucky" tasting or appearing. Never doubt that they could or would!

PEDS Pearl

A bronchial foreign body may produce obstruction from a variety of mechanisms, depending on its size. Most foreign bodies end up in the right mainstem bronchus because it is wider and originates at a less acute angle from the trachea.

- If the foreign body is only slightly smaller than the airway, air gets in during inspiration but no air escapes during expiration (check valve effect), resulting in air trapping (obstructive overinflation). In this situation, breath sounds are diminished over the affected area and localized wheezing may be noted on inspiration. If no air escapes on expiration, no wheezing occurs (Figure 4-14).
- If the foreign body is dislodged during exhalation but reimpacts on inhalation (ball valve effect), distal atelectasis results. Breath sounds are diminished over the affected area (Figure 4-15).
- If the foreign body is as large as the airway, inspired air is not permitted to pass the obstruction, resulting in distal atelectasis (stop valve effect). Breath sounds are diminished over the affected area (Figure 4-16).
- If the foreign body is much smaller than the airway, a partial obstruction to the inflow and outflow of air is produced (bypass valve effect). No change in breath sounds and no adventitial sounds occur if airflow is not impeded. If there is some decrease in airflow past the foreign body, localized wheezing and diminished breath sounds are noted over the affected area.

agitate the child. Keep the oxygen saturation above 95%. If signs of respiratory failure or respiratory arrest are present, assist ventilation using a bag-valve-mask device with 100% oxygen.

Unacceptable Interventions

- Failure to use personal protective equipment
- Failure to recognize signs of respiratory distress and the need for interventions
- Failure to correctly perform FBAO maneuvers, if indicated
- Failure to assist ventilation with a bag-valve-mask device and 100% oxygen if signs of respiratory failure or respiratory arrest are present
- Failure to reassess respiratory status after initiating assisted ventilations
- Failure to recognize signs of deterioration to respiratory failure or arrest and the need for more aggressive interventions
- Performing tracheal intubation in a child who responds to less invasive interventions
- Attempting a needle or surgical cricothyrotomy before attempting assisted ventilations via bag-valve-mask or tracheal tube and 100% oxygen
- Ordering a dangerous or inappropriate intervention
- Performing any technique resulting in potential harm to the patient

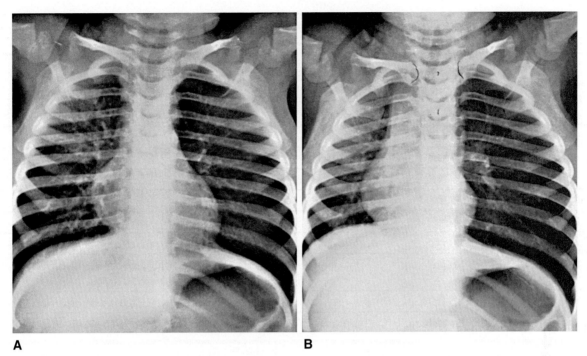

A   **B**

Figure 4-15   **A,** Normal inspiratory chest radiograph in a toddler with a peanut fragment in the left main bronchus. **B,** Expiratory radiograph of the same child showing the classic obstructive emphysema (air trapping) on the involved (left) side. Air leaves the normal right side, allowing the lung to deflate. The mediastinum shifts toward the unobstructed side.

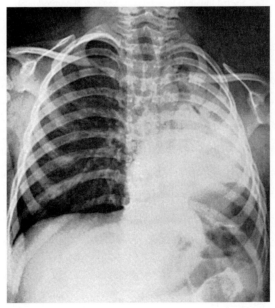

Figure 4-16   Obstructive atelectasis of the left lung caused by a foreign body lodged in the left mainstem bronchus. Notice that the heart is drawn completely into the left side of the chest.

TABLE 4-5 *Comparison of Upper Airway Emergencies*

	Croup	Epiglottitis	Bacterial Tracheitis	Foreign Body
Age	6 mo to 3 y	3 to 7 y	6 mo to 3 y	< 5 y most common
Cause	Viral	Bacterial	Bacterial	Food, toys, coins
Incidence	80%	8%	2%	2%
Seasonal preference	Late fall, early winter	None	None	None
Onset	Gradual	Sudden	Gradual	Sudden
Fever	Low	High	High	No
Appearance	Nontoxic	Toxic	Toxic	Varies depending on location
Posture	No preference	Upright, leaning forward, drooling	Upright	Varies depending on location
Sore throat	No	Yes	Minimal	Varies depending on location
Cry	Bark, stridor	Muffled	Bark, stridor	Varies depending on location

PEDIATRIC RESPIRATORY DISTRESS – UPPER AIRWAY ALGORITHM

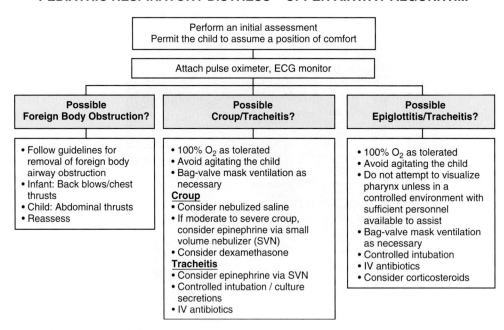

Common Pediatric Lower Airway Emergencies

Asthma/Reactive Airway Disease

Asthma is a reversible obstructive airway disease characterized by chronic inflammation, hyperreactive airways, and episodes of bronchospasm.

Wheezing occurs commonly in young children and has been associated with certain viral infections. Due to emotional, financial, and other implications involved with a diagnosis of asthma, some physicians have been reluctant to call these children "asthmatics." Therefore, they sometimes call the clinical presentation, "reactive airway disease," or RAD.[8]

Etiology

• Allergens trigger the release of immunoglobulin E (IgE), causing mast cell release of histamine and other inflammatory mediators. The resulting edema of the bronchial mucosa, bronchospasm, cellular infiltration, and mucus plugging vary in severity depending on the age of the child, the size and anatomy of the airways, the type of irritant that precipitates the obstruction, and the duration and severity of the asthma attack[9] (Figure 4-17).

   ○ The increased work of breathing caused by use of accessory muscles and increased obstruction to airflow results in increased oxygen consumption and cardiac output.

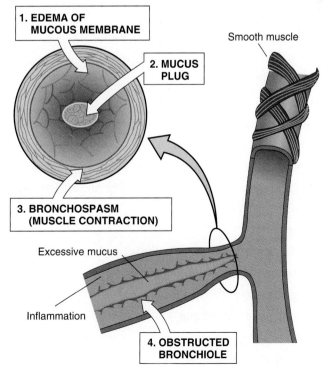

Figure 4-17   Asthma. Acute episode.

- This level of exertion is difficult for young children to maintain because of their small glycogen reserves and the likelihood that caloric intake is inadequate because of illness.
- In most children, both larger and smaller airways are obstructed. The obstruction results from hypertrophy of smooth muscle, inflammatory exudate, and mucus plugs. Ineffective ventilation results in hypoxemia, which stimulates hyperventilation with hypocapnia and respiratory alkalosis.
  - As the obstruction becomes more severe, there is air trapping, inadequate ventilation, more severe hypoxemia, and hypercapnia (hypoventilation) with respiratory acidosis. Respiratory failure is imminent.
- In 50% of asthmatics, there are two phases to an asthma episode: the early asthmatic response (EAR) and the late asthmatic response (LAR)[10] (Figure 4-18).
  - Mast cell activation and the resultant effects of mast cell mediators within the first 20 to 30 minutes are known as the EAR. The early phase is characterized by bronchospasm and increased mucus secretion. This phase usually resolves within 1 hour after the child is removed from the allergen.
  - The late phase typically develops 6 to 8 hours after the early phase and results from the recruitment of inflammatory cells by mediators released during the early phase. Symptoms during the late phase can be more severe than in the early phase. The late phase may last hours to days.

Epidemiology and Demographics

- Asthma is the most common pediatric chronic disease.
- Nearly 5 million children younger than 18 years have been diagnosed with asthma. Fifty percent to 80% of children develop symptoms by 5 years of age.
- Asthma is the third leading cause of hospitalization among children under the age of 15.
- The prevalence of asthma is greater in African Americans than in whites. The asthma prevalence in inner-city African American children may be 12% to 15%.
- Risk factors
  - Personal or family history of asthma or allergy
  - Exposure to passive cigarette smoke
  - Male gender (in early childhood)
  - Maternal history of asthma
  - Viral respiratory infection
  - Smaller airways in early life
  - Low birth weight

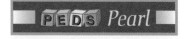

PEDS *Pearl*

- Wheezing is an unreliable sign when evaluating the degree of distress in an asthmatic patient. An absence of wheezing may represent severe obstruction. With improvement, wheezing may become more prominent.
- In infants, breathlessness sufficiently severe to prevent feeding is an important symptom of impending respiratory failure.

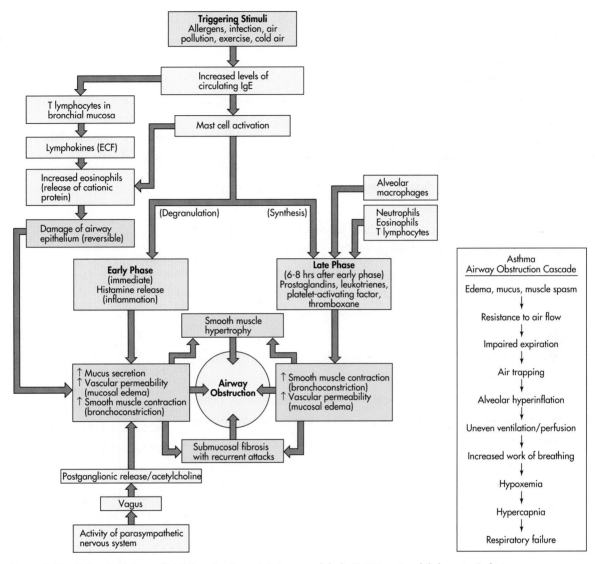

Figure 4-18   Pathophysiology of childhood asthma. *IgE,* Immunoglobulin E; *ECF,* eosinophil chemotactic factor.

History

- Recurrent respiratory symptoms (cough, wheeze, difficulty breathing, chest tightness) that are often worse at night
- Symptoms occur or worsen in the presence of exercise, viral infections, animals with fur or feathers, house dust mites, molds, smoke (tobacco, wood), pollen, changes in weather, strong emotional depression, airborne chemicals or dusts

Physical Examination

- Wheezing (most common symptom)
- Dry cough
- Chest tightness
- Shortness of breath with exertion
- Retractions

- Tachypnea
- Poor air entry
- Prolonged expiratory phase

Acceptable Interventions

Goals of treatment are to reverse bronchospasm, improve hypoxia, and correct dehydration

- Use personal protective equipment.
- Perform an initial assessment and obtain a focused history.
- Assist the child into a position of comfort.
- Initiate pulse oximetry, if available.
- If ventilation is adequate and the patient exhibits signs of respiratory distress, give high-concentration oxygen in a manner that does not agitate the child. Keep the oxygen saturation above 95%. If signs of respiratory failure or respiratory arrest are present, assist ventilation using a bag-valve-mask device with 100% oxygen.
- Place the child on a cardiac monitor.
- Obtain vascular access if the patient shows signs of severe respiratory distress, respiratory failure, or respiratory arrest.
- If the patient shows signs of respiratory distress or respiratory failure with clinical evidence of bronchospasm or a history of asthma:
  - Administer albuterol (Proventil, Ventolin), a rapid-acting β_2-agonist.
    - Give nebulized albuterol (0.5% solution) 0.15 mg/kg/dose up to 5 mg diluted in 2 to 3 mL of normal saline. The patient in severe distress may require albuterol nebulizations every 20 minutes for up to 1 hour. Repeated dosing produces incremental bronchodilation.
    - Severe airflow obstruction may benefit from continuous albuterol nebulization (0.6 to 1 mg/kg/hr). Watch for tachycardia and vomiting.
  - Evaluate the patient's response to the initial inhaled albuterol treatments.
    - Because PEF measurements require the child's cooperation in making a maximal expiratory effort (and coaching by a person trained in making these measurements), PEF measurements are used to assess the severity of an episode and the response to therapy in children older than 5 years.
    - The effort required to produce a PEF measurement is a full inspiration to total lung capacity followed by a short maximal exhalation in a standing position. PEF measurements should be compared with the patient's own previous best measurements.
  - Administer systemic glucocorticosteroids if no immediate response, if the patient recently took an oral glucocorticosteroid, or if the

Continue monitoring oxygen saturation until a clear response to therapy has occurred.

An infant or young child can become quickly dehydrated because of an increased respiratory rate and decreased oral intake. Be sure to assess fluid status and treat appropriately.

Although rapid-acting inhaled β_2-agonists are generally administered by nebulization, equivalent results can be achieved with a more rapid onset and fewer side effects using a metered-dose inhaler (MDI) with a spacer.[11] However, for some children, administration by nebulizer may be easier.

In children with asthma, peak expiratory flow (PEF) can be normal as airflow obstruction and gas trapping worsens. Therefore PEF can underestimate the degree of airflow obstruction.

TABLE 4-6 *Severity of Asthma Exacerbations**

	Mild	Moderate	Severe	Respiratory Arrest Imminent
Symptoms				
Breathless	Walking Can lie down	Talking Infant—softer shorter cry; difficulty feeding Prefers sitting	At rest Infant stops feeding Hunched forward	
Talks in	Sentences	Phrases	Words	
Alertness	May be agitated	Usually agitated	Usually agitated	Drowsy or confused
Signs				
Respiratory rate	Increased	Increased	Often > 30 breaths per minute	
Accessory muscles and suprasternal retractions	Usually not	Usually	Usually	Paradoxic thoracoabdominal movement
Wheeze	Moderate, often only end expiratory	Loud	Usually loud	Absence of wheeze
Pulse (beats per minute)	<100	100 to 120	>120	Bradycardia
Pulsus paradoxus	Absent < 10 mm Hg	May be present 10 to 25 mm Hg	Often present >25 mm Hg (adult) 20 to 40 mm Hg (child)	Absence suggests respiratory muscle fatigue
Functional Assessment				
PEF after initial bronchodilator % predicted or % personal best	Over 80%	Approximately 60% to 80%	<60% predicted or personal best (< 100 L/min adults) or response lasts < 2 h	
Pao_2 (on air) And/or $Paco_2$	Normal Test not usually necessary < 45 mm Hg	> 60 mm Hg < 45 mm Hg	< 60 mm Hg Possible cyanosis > 45 mm Hg: Possible respiratory failure	
$SaO2$% (on air)	> 95%	91% to 95%	< 90%	
	Hypercapnia (hypoventilation) develops more readily in young children than in adults and adolescents.			

Adapted from *Global strategy for asthma management and prevention*. National Institutes of Health, National Heart, Lung, and Blood Institute, Revised 2002. NIH Publication No 02-3659.

PEF, peak expiratory flow; Sao_2, oxygen saturation.

*Note: The presence of several parameters, but not necessarily all, indicates the general classification of the exacerbation.

Risk factors for death from asthma:	• Use of more than two metered-
• History of sudden severe exacerbations	dose inhaler (MDI) canisters of short-acting inhaled β_2-agonist per month
• Prior intubation for asthma	• Current use of oral corticosteroids
• Prior admission for asthma to an intensive care unit	or recent withdrawal from oral corticosteroids
• Two or more hospitalizations for asthma in the past year	• Serious psychiatric disease, including depression, or
• Three or more emergency care visits for asthma in the past year	psychosocial problems
• Hospitalization or emergency department visit for asthma in past month	• Difficulty perceiving airflow obstruction or its severity

episode is severe. The time to peak effect of systemic corticosteroids is at least 4 hours. The early use of steroids can shorten recovery time and reduce the need for hospitalization or shorten the hospital stay.

◦ Tracheal intubation may be necessary in the asthmatic patient with acute respiratory failure.

• If the patient is experiencing a moderate episode (PEF, 60% to 80% predicted/personal best; physical examination reveals moderate symptoms; accessory muscle use):

◦ Inhaled β_2-agonist and inhaled anticholinergic every 60 minutes

◦ Consider glucocorticosteroids

◦ Continue treatment for 1 to 3 hours, provided there is improvement

• If the patient is experiencing a severe episode (PEF less than 60% predicted/personal best, physical examination reveals severe symptoms at rest, chest retractions; history of high-risk patient; no improvement after initial treatment):

◦ Inhaled β_2-agonist and inhaled anticholinergic. Ipratropium bromide 0.25 to 0.5 mg nebulized with albuterol may be beneficial for moderate to severe exacerbations and may produce better bronchodilation than either drug alone.

◦ Systemic glucocorticosteroids.

◦ Consider subcutaneous, intramuscular, or IV β_2-agonist.

◦ Consider subcutaneous administration of a β_2-agonist if inhaled agents are not immediately available, if a child with severe respiratory distress and poor air exchange is not responding to inhaled albuterol, or if the patient is unable to cooperate with a nebulizer.

◦ Epinephrine 0.01 mL/kg subcutaneously (1:1000, maximum single dose 0.35 mL) or terbutaline 0.01 mg/kg subcutaneously (maximum single dose 0.4 mg) may be administered every 20 minutes up to three doses if necessary.

Many asthma medications (e.g., glucocorticosteroids, β_2-agonists, theophylline) are metabolized faster in children than in adults, and young children tend to metabolize drugs faster than older children.

Injectable β_2-agonists tend to produce more adverse effects (tachycardia, headache, tremor) than inhaled agents do.

Poor perception of the severity of asthma on the part of the patient and healthcare professional has been cited as a major factor causing delay in treatment and may contribute to increased severity and mortality from asthma exacerbations.[13]

Evaluate the asthma patient's ability to complete a sentence (age dependent) and the presence of cough, breathlessness, and chest tightness. Assess pulse rate, respiratory rate, breath sounds, use of accessory muscles, and presence of suprasternal retractions. Close monitoring is *essential*.

- ○ Consider IV methylxanthines (e.g., aminophylline, theophylline).
- ○ Consider magnesium sulfate 75 mg/kg IV (maximum 2 g) over 20 minutes every 6 hours. Monitor magnesium levels.
- Nonpharmacologic interventions
  - ○ Environmental control
  - ○ Irritant and allergen avoidance

Unacceptable Interventions

- Failure to use personal protective equipment
- Failure to recognize signs of respiratory distress and the need for interventions
- Failure to allow the child to assume a position of comfort
- Failure to administer supplemental oxygen
- Failure to measure oxygen saturation
- Failure to administer a bronchodilator for a child in respiratory distress with a history of asthma
- Failure to use an accurate method for weight and medication dosage determination
- Failure to monitor and correctly interpret the patient's electrocardiogram (ECG) rhythm
- Agitating the child with an IV start, placement of a face mask, blood pressure assessment, or medication administration unless the treatment is immediately lifesaving.
- Failure to assist ventilation with a bag–valve–mask device and 100% oxygen if signs of respiratory failure or respiratory arrest are present
- Failure to reassess respiratory status after initiating assisted ventilations

---

Drug Pearl
Albuterol (Proventil, Ventolin)

- Albuterol is a sympathomimetic bronchodilator that possesses a relatively selective specificity for β_2 (pulmonary) receptors and therefore is less likely to cause unwanted cardiovascular effects.
- Before administration, inquire about the medications the patient may have already taken. If the patient has been using an inhaler, ascertain the frequency and last application.
- The onset of action of inhaled bronchodilators is within 5 minutes. Their duration of action in severe asthma is unknown and may vary with the severity of the disease.
- Continuous cardiac monitoring is essential during bronchodilator administration because these medications may cause tachycardia and other dysrhythmias.
- After administration, reassess pulse and respiratory rate, oxygen saturation, and peak expiratory flow rate. Any deterioration may require prompt intervention.

- Performing tracheal intubation before treating respiratory failure with assisted ventilations via bag-valve-mask and 100% oxygen
- Failure to anticipate the potential need for tracheal intubation
- Performing tracheal intubation in a child who responds to less invasive interventions
- Failure to recognize signs of deterioration to respiratory failure or arrest and the need for more aggressive interventions
- Failure to monitor the cardiac rhythm if signs of respiratory failure or respiratory arrest are present
- If tracheal intubation is required, failure to confirm tracheal tube position using assessment and mechanical methods
- Failure to recognize signs of a tension pneumothorax
- Failure to perform needle decompression in a rapidly deteriorating patient with signs of a tension pneumothorax
- Medication errors
- Ordering a dangerous or inappropriate intervention
- Performing any technique resulting in potential harm to the patient

Respiratory Syncytial Virus/Bronchiolitis

Bronchiolitis is an inflammation of the smaller bronchioles caused by a virus and characterized by thick mucus. It occurs primarily in winter and early spring and is rare in children over 2 years of age. RSV is the primary cause of bronchiolitis and pneumonia in children younger than 1 year.

Etiology

- The cause of bronchiolitis is RSV in 45% to 75% of cases.
  - Parainfluenza viruses are the second most common cause.
  - Other agents that cause bronchiolitis include influenza virus, rhinovirus, adenovirus, and *Mycoplasma pneumoniae*.
- In bronchiolitis, airway obstruction is usually gradual and is caused by inflammation, secretions, and edema of varying degrees in the small bronchi and bronchioles. Areas of hyperinflation may exist with air trapping (Figure 4-19) due to partial obstruction or areas of atelectasis or nonaeration resulting from total obstruction.

  Inflammation and edema make the small air passages in infants particularly vulnerable to obstruction.

- RSV is highly contagious. The incubation period from exposure to first symptoms is about 4 days. The virus is shed in nasal secretions for varying periods, usually 5 to 12 days, although excretion of the virus for 3 weeks and longer has been documented.

  Hand washing and the use of disposable gloves and gowns are important.

  - RSV is spread from respiratory secretions through close contact with infected persons or contact with contaminated surfaces or objects. Infection can occur when infectious material contacts mucous membranes of the eyes, mouth, or nose, and possibly through the inhalation of droplets generated by a sneeze or cough.

PEDIATRIC ASTHMA ALGORITHM

• **Mild episode** = PEF > 80% predicted or personal best

• **Moderate episode** = PEF 60 to 80% predicted/personal best, physical exam reveals moderate symptoms, accessory muscle use

• **Severe episode** = < 60% predicted / personal best, physical exam reveals severe symptoms at rest, chest retractions; history of high-risk patient; no improvement after initial treatment

Perform an initial assessment

• Permit the child to assume a position of comfort
• Attach pulse oximeter and ECG monitor, assess peak expiratory flow (PEF) rate
• Administer oxygen; establish vascular access if the patient shows signs of severe respiratory distress, respiratory failure, or respiratory arrest

Initial Treatment*
• Inhaled rapid-acting β2-agonist, usually by nebulization, one dose every 20 minutes for 1 hour
• Systemic glucocorticosteroids if no immediate response, or if patient recently took oral glucocorticosteroid, or if episode is severe

• Assess clinical signs of respiratory distress including pulse and respiratory rate, oxygen saturation, and peak expiratory flow (PEF) rate. Any deterioration may require prompt intervention.

GOOD RESPONSE
• Response sustained 60 minutes after last treatment
• Physical exam normal
• PEF > 70%
• No distress
• O2 saturation > 95%

INCOMPLETE RESPONSE WITHIN 1 TO 2 HOURS
• History: high-risk patient
• Physical exam: mild to moderate symptoms
• PEF < 70%
• O2 saturation not improving

POOR RESPONSE WITHIN 1 HOUR
• History: high-risk patient
• Physical exam: severe symptoms, drowsiness, confusion
• PEF < 30%
• PCO2 > 45 mm Hg
• PO2 < 60 mm Hg

• Inhaled β2-agonist and inhaled anticholinergic every 60 minutes
• Consider glucocorticosteroids
• Continue treatment 1 to 3 hours, provided there is improvement

• Inhaled β2-agonist and inhaled anticholinergic
• Systemic glucocorticosteroid
• Consider SC, IM, or IV β2-agonist
• Consider IV methylxanthines
• Consider IV magnesium

Observe for at least one hour before discharge home

Admit to Hospital
• Inhaled β2-agonist ± inhaled anticholinergic
• Systemic glucocorticosteroid
• Oxygen
• Consider IV methylxanthines
• Monitor PEF, O2 saturation, pulse, theophylline

Admit to Intensive Care
• Inhaled β2-agonist + anticholinergic
• IV glucocorticosteroid
• Consider SC, IM, or IV β2-agonists
• Oxygen
• Consider IV methylxanthines
• Possible intubation and mechanical ventilation

*Note: Preferred treatments are inhaled β2-agonists in high doses and systemic glucocorticosteroids.
Adapted from *Global Strategy for Asthma Management and Prevention*. National Institutes Of Health, National Heart, Lung, and Blood Institute, Revised 2002. NIH Publication No 02-3659.

Drug Pearl
Ipratropium Bromide (Atrovent)

- Ipratropium bromide (Atrovent) blocks the contraction of bronchiolar smooth muscle and the increase in mucus secretion resulting from increased vagal (i.e., parasympathetic) activity.
- Anticholinergics produce preferential dilation of the larger central airways, in contrast to β-agonists, which affect the peripheral airways.
- Continuous cardiac monitoring is essential during bronchodilator administration because these medications may cause tachycardia and other dysrhythmias.
- Studies indicate that ipratropium use in combination with β-agonists is associated with lower hospitalization rates and greater improvement in peak expiratory flow.
- After administration, reassess pulse and respiratory rate, oxygen saturation, and peak expiratory flow rate.

Drug Pearl
Methylxanthines

- Methylxanthines (e.g., theophylline, aminophylline) produce bronchodilation, increase pulmonary blood flow, and strengthen diaphragmatic contractions (reduce diaphragm fatigue). In higher doses, methylxanthines increase heart rate (chronotropy) and force of contraction (inotropy).
- Methylxanthines treat asthma symptoms for longer periods than β₂-agonists (except salmeterol and formoterol) do.
- Methylxanthines have an equivalent bronchodilator effect to inhaled β₂-agonists, but because of increased side effects, methylxanthines should only be considered as an alternate therapy.
- Before administration, obtain a theophylline level if the child is currently receiving a theophylline preparation.
- Assess the patient's respiratory rate, tidal volume, breath sounds, heart rate, ECG, and blood pressure before, during, and after administration. Continuous ECG monitoring is essential during administration of methyl-xanthines. Watch closely for signs of cardiac irritability, particularly premature ventricular complexes (PVCs) and tachycardia.
- Hypotension may occur following rapid administration.

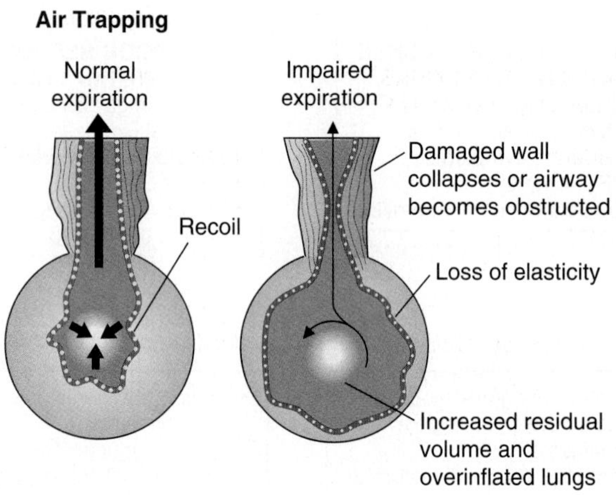

Air Trapping

Figure 4-19   Air trapping.

- In the healthcare setting, RSV is often spread from child to child on the hands of caregivers.
  - RSV in secretions can survive only a few hours on countertops, paper tissues, and cloth, and for half an hour on the skin. The virus is readily inactivated with soap and water and disinfectants.

Epidemiology and Demographics

- RSV occurs in yearly epidemics. In temperate climates, these epidemics occur each winter and last 4 to 5 months. In the Northern Hemisphere, epidemics usually peak in January, February, or March, but peaks have been recognized as early as December and as late as June.[12]
- Parainfluenza type 3 occurs primarily spring to fall, type 1 occurs in epidemics in the fall every other year, and type 2 occurs in the fall.
- RSV is most common in infants younger than 1 year.

- Fifty percent of all infants will be infected with RSV by the end of the first year of life. Infants 1 to 4 months old are at particular risk of severe infection and hospitalization.
- Almost all infants are infected by the virus by the end of their second winter, and half experience two infections during their first two winters.
- Risk factors for early-onset disease and subsequent hospitalization include low birth weight, prematurity, lower socioeconomic group, crowded living conditions, parental smoking, absence of breast feeding, chronic lung or cardiac conditions, and day care.

History

- URI with rhinorrhea and cough for several days
  - Low-grade fever common
  - Increasingly productive cough
  - Increasing respiratory distress
  - Caregiver often reports wheezing at home
- Otitis media common
- Contact with older siblings or children at day care who have viral respiratory symptoms
- Hypoxemia in severe cases
- Apnea may occur in former premature infants and infants younger than 4 months old
- Family history of asthma or allergies

Physical Examination

An RSV infection can affect any part of the respiratory tract.

- RSV begins with signs and symptoms limited to an upper respiratory tract infection, such as rhinorrhea and pharyngitis.
  - Within 1 to 3 days, a cough usually appears and may be accompanied by sneezing and a low-grade (below 101° F) fever.
  - Wheezing develops soon after the cough appears and may be detectable without a stethoscope. Auscultation often reveals diffuse rhonchi, fine rales or crackles, and wheezes. A chest radiograph at this stage is frequently normal.
  - Mild cases of RSV may not progress beyond this stage.
- If RSV progresses, coughing and wheezing increase and air hunger follows. These signs and symptoms are accompanied by an increased respiratory rate, intercostal and subcostal retractions, hyperexpansion of the chest, restlessness, and peripheral cyanosis.
- Signs of dehydration (e.g., sunken eyes, dry mucous membranes, sunken fontanelle, and fatigue) may be present due to decreased fluid intake and increased fluid losses from fever and tachypnea.
- Tachypnea and tachycardia are often present.
- Signs of severe, life-threatening illness include central cyanosis, tachypnea of more than 70 breaths per minute, listlessness, and apnea

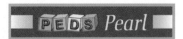

Because asthma and bronchiolitis present similarly, it may be difficult to distinguish between these conditions. Keep in mind that asthma rarely occurs before 1 year of age; bronchiolitis is more common in children of this age.

spells. At this stage, the chest may be greatly hyperexpanded and almost silent on auscultation because of poor air exchange.

Acceptable Interventions

- Use personal protective equipment
- Perform an initial assessment and obtain a focused history.
- Assist the child into a position of comfort, usually sitting up on the caregiver's lap.
- Avoid agitating the child. Keep the child as calm and as comfortable as possible, usually in the arms of the caregiver.
- Initiate pulse oximetry, if available.
- If ventilation is adequate and the patient exhibits signs of respiratory distress, give high-concentration oxygen in a manner that does not agitate the child. Keep the oxygen saturation above 95%. If signs of respiratory failure or respiratory arrest are present, assist ventilation using a bag-valve-mask device with 100% oxygen.
- Mild dehydration is often present. Fluid replacement is important; however, excessive fluid replacement may encourage interstitial edema formation. Close monitoring is essential.
- Use of bronchodilators is controversial.
  - Nebulized albuterol has been shown to produce a modest short-term improvement in clinical signs and symptoms, but has not shown improvement in the reduction of hospital admissions or in the length of hospital stay.
  - Nebulized epinephrine has been shown to improve clinical signs and symptoms, improve oxygenation, decrease the time spent in the emergency department, and reduce the rate of hospital admissions.
  - Although conflicting evidence regarding the efficacy of broncho-dilator therapy exists, current practice is to try a β_2-agonist such as albuterol (0.15 mg/kg per dose) and evaluate the patient's clinical response to the medication. If the patient responds favorably (an improvement is noted in retractions, respiratory rate, and wheezing), bronchodilator therapy is continued and the patient's response assessed every 5 to 10 minutes.

Unacceptable Interventions

- Failure to use personal protective equipment
- Failure to recognize signs of respiratory distress and the need for interventions
- Failure to allow the child to assume a position of comfort
- Failure to administer supplemental oxygen
- Failure to measure oxygen saturation
- Agitating the child with an IV start, placement of a face mask, blood

Oxygen administration and supportive care with fluid replacement are the mainstays of treatment.

Remember: Nebulized epinephrine may be more effective.

Drug Pearl
Drugs for RSV

Ribavirin, a broad-spectrum antiviral agent administered by aerosol, was approved for use by the U.S. Food and Drug Administration (FDA) in 1986. Treatment with ribavirin has been limited because of its high cost, lack of demonstrated benefit in decreasing the duration of hospitalization or mortality, and concern about potential toxic effects among exposed healthcare personnel.

RSV-IGIV (RespiGam) and palivizumab (Synagis) are two products approved by the FDA for the prevention of RSV infection in children younger than 2 years who have lung problems due to prematurity or bronchopulmonary dysplasia. Both products must be given in five monthly doses.

RSV-IGIV is an IV preparation of immunoglobulin G that provides neutralizing antibodies against specific strains of RSV. It is given on an inpatient or outpatient basis before or during the RSV epidemic season.

Palivizumab is administered intramuscularly. Palivizumab is preferred for most high-risk children because of its ease of administration (intramuscular), lack of interference with measles-mumps-rubella vaccine and varicella vaccine, and lack of complications associated with IV administration of human immune globulin products.

RSV-IGIV is contraindicated and palivizumab is not recommended for children with cyanotic congenital heart disease.

---

pressure assessment, or medication administration unless the treatment is immediately lifesaving.

- Failure to assist ventilation with a bag-valve-mask device and 100% oxygen if signs of respiratory failure or respiratory arrest are present
- Failure to reassess respiratory status after initiating assisted ventilations
- Failure to recognize signs of deterioration to respiratory failure or arrest and the need for more aggressive interventions
- Performing tracheal intubation before treating respiratory failure with assisted ventilations via bag-valve-mask and 100% oxygen
- Failure to anticipate the potential need for tracheal intubation
- Performing tracheal intubation in a child who responds to less invasive interventions
- Failure to monitor the cardiac rhythm if signs of respiratory failure or respiratory arrest are present, or if bronchodilators are administered
- If tracheal intubation is required, failure to confirm tracheal tube position using assessment and mechanical methods
- Failure to use an accurate method for weight and medication dosage determination
- Medication errors

- Ordering a dangerous or inappropriate intervention
- Performing any technique resulting in potential harm to the patient

Pneumonia is an inflammation and infection of the lower airway and lungs caused by a viral, bacterial, parasitic, or fungal organism. Pneumonia may occur as a primary infection or secondary to another illness or infection and is often classified by anatomic location (Figure 4-20):

- Lobar pneumonia: localized to one or more lobes of the lung
- Bronchopneumonia: inflammation around medium-sized airways, which causes patchy consolidation of parts of the lobes
- Interstitial pneumonia: inflammation of lung tissue between air sacs, usually generalized, often viral symptom

Etiology

- The organism responsible for pneumonia varies with the age of the child.
- The responsible organism is not definitively identified in 20% to 60% of pneumonia cases.
- The more common pathogens include:
  - Virus: RSV, parainfluenza, influenza, adenovirus
  - Bacteria: *S. pneumoniae, Streptococcus pyogenes, S. aureus, Streptococcus agalactiae,* HiB
  - *M. pneumoniae*

Pneumonia

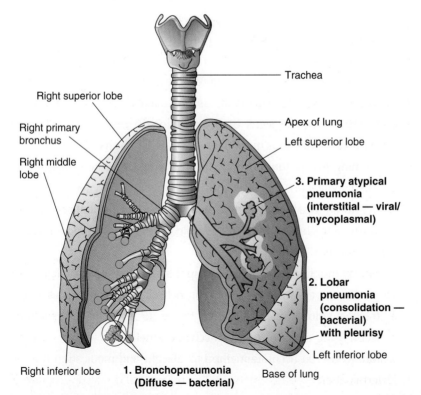

Figure 4-20   Types of pneumonia.

- *Chlamydia trachomatis, Chlamydia pneumoniae*
- *Mycobacteria tuberculosis*

Epidemiology and Demographics

- Although a virus is the cause of 60% to 90% of pneumonias, three fourths of all deaths from pneumonia result from bacterial infections.
- Pneumonia is most prevalent in the winter months.
- Children who are immunocompromised or who have underlying lung disease are at greater risk for significant pneumonia.

History

- Pneumonia is often preceded by symptoms of an URI.
- Signs and symptoms may include fever, malaise, anorexia, and chest pain.

Physical Examination

- Fever (less prominent in viral pneumonia, high in bacterial pneumonia)
- Chills
- Malaise
- Headache
- Lethargy
- Anorexia or poor feeding in infants
- Grunting
- Tachypnea
- Tachycardia
- Crackles may be present over affected lobes (other lobes normal) in lobar pneumonia; scattered crackles in bronchopneumonia; scattered crackles and wheezes in interstitial pneumonia
- Retractions
- Chest pain
- Apnea spells

Acceptable Interventions

- Use personal protective equipment
- Perform an initial assessment and obtain a focused history.
- Assist the child into a position of comfort, usually sitting up on the caregiver's lap.
- Avoid agitating the child. Keep the child as calm and as comfortable as possible, usually in the arms of the caregiver.
- Initiate pulse oximetry, if available.
- If ventilation is adequate and the patient exhibits signs of respiratory distress, give high-concentration oxygen in a manner that does not agitate the child. Keep the oxygen saturation above 95%. If signs of respiratory failure or respiratory arrest are present, assist ventilation using a bag-valve-mask device with 100% oxygen.
- Obtain vascular access for hydration or medication administration if necessary.

An infant or young child can become quickly dehydrated because of an increased respiratory rate and decreased oral intake. Be sure to assess fluid status and treat appropriately.

- Antibiotics may be used to treat bacterial pneumonia. Most viral pneumonias are treated symptomatically; however, specific antiviral therapy may be beneficial in certain situations.
- Antipyretics (e.g., acetaminophen) may be used to control fever.

Unacceptable Interventions

- Failure to use personal protective equipment
- Failure to recognize signs of respiratory distress and the need for interventions
- Failure to allow the child to assume a position of comfort
- Failure to administer supplemental oxygen
- Failure to measure oxygen saturation
- Agitating the child with an IV start, placement of a face mask, blood pressure assessment, or medication administration unless the treatment is immediately lifesaving.
- Failure to assist ventilation with a bag-valve-mask device and 100% oxygen if signs of respiratory failure or respiratory arrest are present
- Failure to reassess respiratory status after initiating assisted ventilations
- Performing tracheal intubation before treating respiratory failure with assisted ventilations via bag-valve-mask and 100% oxygen
- Failure to anticipate the potential need for tracheal intubation
- Performing tracheal intubation in a child who responds to less invasive interventions
- Failure to recognize signs of deterioration to respiratory failure or arrest and the need for more aggressive interventions
- Failure to monitor the cardiac rhythm if signs of respiratory failure or respiratory arrest are present
- If tracheal intubation is required, failure to confirm tracheal tube position using assessment and mechanical methods
- If suctioning is required, failure to limit suctioning to 10 seconds or less per attempt
- Ordering a dangerous or inappropriate intervention
- Performing any technique resulting in potential harm to the patient

Bronchopulmonary Dysplasia

Bronchopulmonary dysplasia (BPD) is a chronic lung disease that occurs most commonly in children who were born as premature infants with respiratory problems in the first few days after birth.

Etiology

Etiologic factors have not been proven. Prolonged treatment with positive-pressure ventilation and high oxygen concentrations are among those suggested.

Epidemiology and Demographics

- The most important risk factor for BPD is prematurity. Ninety percent of the infants who develop BPD are premature and weigh less than 1500 g (3.5 lb). The more premature the newborn is, the higher the risk for developing BPD.

- Approximately 5,000 to 10,000 new cases of BPD (20% to 30% of infants surviving respiratory distress syndrome) occur each year.
- Although BPD is most common in premature infants, it can occur in term infants who need mechanical ventilation and oxygen under pressure for problems such as neonatal pulmonary hypertension.
- Improved neonatal critical care now makes it possible for most infants weighing at least 500 g to survive. This increased survival of very-low-birth-weight infants is a major factor contributing to the increasing incidence of BPD.
- Complications associated with BPD include recurrent respiratory infections, increased airway resistance, trapping of air in the lungs, and exercise-induced bronchospasm.

History

- History of recent viral infection or exercise-induced bronchospasm
- Although the criteria differ among neonatologists, the diagnosis of BPD is usually based on the following:
  ◦ A history of lung injury in the first days after birth,
  ◦ A continuing need for supplemental oxygen at age 28 days, and
  ◦ Persistence of the clinical signs of respiratory difficulty beyond 28 days of age

Physical Examination

- Very low birth weight
- Tachypnea
- Tachycardia
- Increased work of breathing with retractions, nasal flaring, and grunting
- Poor weight gain
- Seesaw respirations
- Wheezing
- Arterial blood gases may reveal acidosis, hypercarbia, and hyperoxia
- Chest radiograph may reveal decreased lung volume, areas of atelectasis, and hyperinflation.

Acceptable Interventions

The treatment for BPD is primarily supportive.

- Use personal protective equipment
- Perform an initial assessment and obtain a focused history.
- Assist the child into a position of comfort, usually sitting up on the caregiver's lap.
- Avoid agitating the child. Keep the child as calm and as comfortable as possible, usually in the arms of the caregiver.

- Initiate pulse oximetry, if available. Hypoxia may occur because of a decrease in respiratory drive, alterations in pulmonary mechanics, excessive stimulation, and bronchospasm.
- If ventilation is adequate and the patient exhibits signs of respiratory distress, give high-concentration oxygen in a manner that does not agitate the child. Keep the oxygen saturation above 95%. If signs of respiratory failure or respiratory arrest are present, assist ventilation using a bag-valve-mask device with 100% oxygen.
- Bronchodilators may be used to improve airflow in the lungs.
- Corticosteroids may be used to reduce airway swelling and inflammation.
- Diuretics may be administered to decrease fluid accumulation in the lungs.
- Antibiotics may be administered to control infection.
- Chest physiotherapy is often used to assist the lungs in expelling mucus.

Mechanical ventilation and supplemental oxygen are provided to overcome respiratory failure and maintain blood oxygen levels.

Unacceptable Interventions
- Failure to use personal protective equipment
- Failure to recognize signs of respiratory distress and the need for interventions
- Failure to allow the child to assume a position of comfort
- Failure to administer supplemental oxygen
- Failure to measure oxygen saturation
- Agitating the child with an IV start, placement of a face mask, blood pressure assessment, or medication administration unless the treatment is immediately lifesaving.
- Failure to assist ventilation with a bag-valve-mask device and 100% oxygen if signs of respiratory failure or respiratory arrest are present
- Failure to reassess respiratory status after initiating assisted ventilations
- Performing tracheal intubation before treating respiratory failure with assisted ventilations via bag-valve-mask and 100% oxygen
- Failure to anticipate the potential need for tracheal intubation
- Performing tracheal intubation in a child who responds to less invasive interventions
- Failure to recognize signs of deterioration to respiratory failure or arrest and the need for more aggressive interventions
- Failure to monitor the cardiac rhythm if signs of respiratory failure or respiratory arrest are present
- If tracheal intubation is required, failure to confirm tracheal tube position using assessment and mechanical methods
- Failure to use an accurate method for weight and medication dosage determination
- If suctioning is required, failure to limit suctioning to 10 seconds or less per attempt

- Medication errors
- Ordering a dangerous or inappropriate intervention
- Performing any technique resulting in potential harm to the patient

Cystic Fibrosis

Cystic fibrosis (CF) is an inherited multisystem disease affecting approximately 30,000 children and adults in the United States. A defective gene causes the body to produce abnormally thick, sticky mucus that affects multiple organs, most commonly the lungs, pancreas, liver, and small intestine (Figure 4-21).

Etiology

- Patients with CF have an abnormality in the glands that produce or secrete sweat and mucus.
  - CF patients lose excessive amounts of salt when they sweat.
  - Inadequate water in mucous secretions ("sticky mucus") results in very thick mucus that accumulates in the intestines and lungs. The result is malnutrition, poor growth, frequent respiratory infections, and breathing difficulty.
- Although multiple organ systems are affected, progressive lung destruction (bronchiectasis) is the major cause of morbidity and mortality in those affected with CF.

Epidemiology and Demographics

- CF occurs in approximately one of every 3200 live white births (in one of every 3900 live births of all Americans).
  - CF occurs most often in whites whose ancestors came from northern Europe, although it affects all races and ethnic groups.

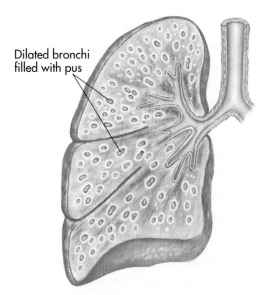

Dilated bronchi filled with pus

Figure 4-21   In cystic fibrosis, abnormally thick mucus may cause progressive clogging of the bronchi and bronchioles and subsequent pulmonary infections.

- ◦ Accordingly, it is less common in African Americans, Native Americans, and Asian Americans.
- About 1000 new cases of CF are diagnosed each year.
- More than 80% of patients are diagnosed by age 3 years; however, nearly 10% of newly diagnosed cases are age 18 or older.
- More than 10 million Americans are symptomless carriers of the defective CF gene. An individual must inherit two defective CF genes (one from each parent) to have CF. Each time two carriers conceive, there is a 25% chance that their child will have CF; a 50% chance that the child will be a carrier of the CF gene; and a 25% chance that the child will be a noncarrier.
- According to the CF Foundation's National Patient Registry, the median age of survival for a person with CF is 33.4 years.
- ◦ As more advances have been made in the treatment of CF, the number of adults with CF has steadily grown.
- ◦ Today, nearly 40% of the CF population is age 18 years and older. Adults, however, may experience additional health challenges including CF-related diabetes and osteoporosis.

History

- Some children with CF have symptoms at birth. Some are born with meconium ileus.
- CF most often presents in early childhood with persistent respiratory illness (50%), malnutrition and poor growth (40%), diarrhea (30%), or a combination of these.

In CF, the meconium can be too thick and sticky to pass and can completely block the intestines.

Physical Examination

- Respiratory system: nasal congestion, sinusitis, chronic cough, increased anterior-posterior diameter of the chest, use of accessory muscles for respiration, tachypnea, hemoptysis, cyanosis, wheezing
- Gastrointestinal system: poor weight gain, abdominal distention, diffuse tenderness; steatorrhea (fat in stools); rectal prolapse (protrusion of the rectum through the anus)
- Musculoskeletal system: digital clubbing from chronic hypoxia, thin extremities, muscle wasting, salty-tasting skin (usually noticed by the caregiver when kissing the child), profuse sweating in warm weather
- Other: increase in amount and thickness of secretions, frequent infections

Acceptable Interventions

- Use personal protective equipment.
- Perform an initial assessment and obtain a focused history.
- Assist the child into a position of comfort, usually sitting up on the caregiver's lap.
- Avoid agitating the child. Keep the child as calm and as comfortable as possible, usually in the arms of the caregiver.

Treatment is primarily directed at respiratory and nutritional support.

- Initiate pulse oximetry, if available.
- If ventilation is adequate and the patient exhibits signs of respiratory distress, give high-concentration oxygen in a manner that does not agitate the child. Keep the oxygen saturation above 95%. If signs of respiratory failure or respiratory arrest are present, assist ventilation using a bag-valve-mask device with 100% oxygen.
- Obtain vascular access for hydration or medication administration if necessary.
  - Because patients with CF have frequent infections, many will have an implanted central vascular access device in place.
- Decongestants and/or bronchodilators (before and after chest physiotherapy) are used to relieve bronchospasm, enable the removal of thick secretions, and improve airflow in the lungs.
- Mucolytics may be administered to alter the consistency of mucus (making it more fluid and easier to expectorate).
- Corticosteroids may be used to reduce airway swelling and inflammation.
- Antibiotics may be administered to control infection. More than one antibiotic is often necessary to treat suspected pathogens.
- Chest physiotherapy.
  - Chest percussion and vibration (to help loosen mucus from lungs)
  - Postural drainage (to help drain mucus from lungs)
- Pancreatic enzymes may be administered to help with digestion and treat pancreatic deficiency.
- Vitamins and other dietary supplements may be administered to add nutrients to the diet.

Ideally, chest physiotherapy should be performed two or three times daily.

Unacceptable Interventions
- Failure to use personal protective equipment
- Failure to recognize signs of respiratory distress and the need for interventions
- Failure to allow the child to assume a position of comfort
- Failure to administer supplemental oxygen
- Failure to measure oxygen saturation
- Agitating the child with an IV start, placement of a face mask, blood pressure assessment, or medication administration unless the treatment is immediately lifesaving.
- Failure to assist ventilation with a bag-valve-mask device and 100% oxygen if signs of respiratory failure or respiratory arrest are present
- Failure to reassess respiratory status after initiating assisted ventilations
- Performing tracheal intubation before treating respiratory failure with assisted ventilations via bag-valve-mask and 100% oxygen

PEDIATRIC RESPIRATORY DISTRESS – LOWER AIRWAY ALGORITHM

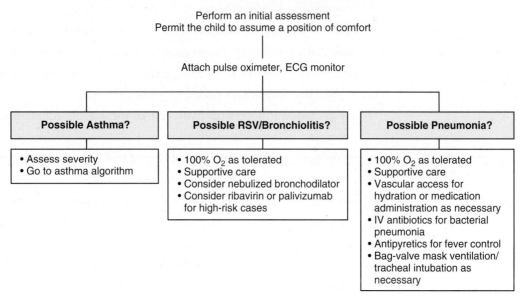

- Failure to anticipate the potential need for tracheal intubation
- Performing tracheal intubation in a child who responds to less invasive interventions
- Failure to recognize signs of deterioration to respiratory failure or arrest and the need for more aggressive interventions
- Failure to monitor the cardiac rhythm if signs of respiratory failure or respiratory arrest are present
- If tracheal intubation is required, failure to confirm tracheal tube position using assessment and mechanical methods
- Failure to use an accurate method for weight and medication dosage determination
- If suctioning is required, failure to limit suctioning to 10 seconds or less per attempt
- Medication errors
- Ordering a dangerous or inappropriate intervention
- Performing any technique resulting in potential harm to the patient

Case Study Resolution

This child is sick. His presentation is consistent with acute bronchospasm. Move quickly. Use personal protective equipment. Perform an initial assessment and obtain a focused history. Assist the child into a position of comfort. Initiate pulse oximetry (initial SpO_2 on room air was 84%). Correct hypoxia by giving high-flow oxygen in a manner that does not agitate the child (blow-by oxygen was administered while the child was seated in Mom's lap). Place the child on a cardiac monitor. Give nebulized albuterol and assess response. Begin assisted ventilation and establish vascular access if the child does not improve. Provide further interventions on the basis of assessment findings and the patient's response to therapy.

Web Resources

- www.vh.org/pediatric/provider/pediatrics/ElectricAirway/ElectricAirway.html (Electric Airway: Upper Airway Problems in Children)
- www.med.monash.edu.au/paediatrics/resources/asthma.html (Asthma: Monash University)
- www.kidshealth.org/parent/infections/bacterial_viral/bronchiolitis.html (Bronchiolitis: Kidshealth.org)

References

1. Scruggs K, Johnson MT, eds. Pediatric Treatment Guidelines. Laguna Hills, CA: Current Clinical Strategies Publishing 2004, 112.

2. Wright RB, Pomerantz WJ, Joseph W, et al. New approaches to respiratory infections in children: bronchiolitis and croup. *Emerg Med Clin North Am* 2002;20:93–114.

3. Soileau-Burke M. Emergency management. In: Gunn VL, Nechyba C, eds. *The Harriet Lane handbook: a manual for pediatric house officers,* 16th ed. Philadelphia: Mosby, 2002, pp. 10–11.

4. Barkin RM, Rosen P, eds. *Pulmonary disorders in emergency pediatrics: a guide to ambulatory care,* 5th ed. St. Louis: Mosby, 1999, pp. 786–788.

5. Roosevelt GE. Acute inflammatory upper airway obstruction. In: Behrman RE, Kliegman RM, Jenson HB, eds. *Nelson textbook of pediatrics,* 17th ed. Philadelphia: WB Saunders, 2004, pp. 1405–1409.

6. Oureshi S, Mink R. Aspiration of fruit gel snacks. *Pediatrics* 2003;111:687–689.

7. Holinger LD. Foreign bodies of the airway. In: Behrman RE, Kliegman RM, Jenson HB, eds. *Nelson textbook of pediatrics,* 17th ed. Philadelphia: WB Saunders, 2004, pp. 1410–1411.

8. Hopp RJ. Recurrent wheezing in infants and young children: a perspective. *J Asthma* 1999; 36:547–553.

9. Huether SE, McCance KL. *Alterations of pulmonary function in children in understanding pathophysiology,* 2nd ed. St. Louis: Mosby, 2000, pp. 775–788.

10. Moy JN. Asthma. In: Finberg L, Kleinman RE, eds. *Saunders manual of pediatric practice,* 2nd ed. Philadelphia: WB Saunders, 2002.

11. Cates CC, Bara A, Crilly JA, et al. Holding chambers versus nebulisers for beta-agonist treatment of acute asthma. *Cochrane Database Syst Rev* 2003;3:CD000052.

12. McIntosh K. Respiratory syncytial virus. In: Behrman RE, Kliegman RM, Jenson HB, eds. *Nelson textbook of pediatrics,* 16th ed. Philadelphia: WB Saunders, 2000, pp. 991–993.

13. Nowak RM, Pensler MI, Sarkar DD, et al. Comparison of peak expiratory flow and FEV1 admission criteria for acute bronchial asthma. *Ann Emerg Med* 1982;11:64–69.

Chapter Quiz

1. The most important risk factor for bronchopulmonary dysplasia is:
   A) Prematurity.
   B) Current use of oral corticosteroids.
   C) Serious psychiatric disease, including depression.
   D) Use of more than two metered-dose inhaler (MDI) canisters of short-acting inhaled β2-agonist per month.

2. Which of the following should be suspected in any previously well, afebrile child with a sudden onset of respiratory distress and associated coughing, choking, stridor, or wheezing?
   A) Asthma.
   B) Epiglottitis.
   C) Foreign body airway obstruction.
   D) Croup.

3. Epiglottitis most commonly occurs in children _____ . Croup most commonly occurs in children _____ .
   A) 6 months to 3 years of age; 2 to 5 years of age.
   B) 3 months to 6 years of age; 6 to 12 years of age.
   C) 2 to 5 years of age; 6 months to 3 years of age.
   D) 6 to 12 years of age; 3 months to 6 years of age.

Questions 4–6 pertain to the following patient situation.

An 8-month-old infant presents with a cough, clear nasal discharge, and difficulty breathing. Mom states the infant has had a cold for the past two days. She is concerned because his breathing is "different" today and he has been feeding poorly. You note the infant appears tired and limp in his mother's arms and his color is dusky. His respiratory rate is rapid and shallow. Nasal flaring and intercostal and subcostal retractions are visible.

4. From the information provided, complete the following documentation regarding the Pediatric Assessment Triangle.
   Appearance:
   Breathing:
   Circulation:

5. Your initial assessment reveals a patent airway. The infant's respiratory rate is 56/min. Auscultation of the chest reveals fine crackles and wheezes bilaterally. A brachial pulse is easily palpated at a rate of 148 beats/min. The skin is dusky and dry. Capillary refill is 2 to 3 seconds; temperature is 100.4° F. Based on the patient's age and clinical presentation, you suspect the patient has:
   A) Asthma
   B) Bronchiolitis
   C) Epiglottitis
   D) Pneumonia

6. Is this patient sick or not sick? Describe your approach to the initial management of this patient.

7 Which of the following types of medications is *not* routinely used in the treatment of broncho-pulmonary dysplasia?
   A) Corticosteroids.
   B) Bronchodilators.
   C) Diuretics.
   D) Beta-blockers.

8. Which of the following is an *early* sign of impending respiratory difficulty?
   A) Delayed capillary refill.
   B) An increase in heart rate.
   C) An increase in respiratory rate.
   D) A decrease in blood pressure.

9. The cough that accompanies croup is typically characterized as:
   A) A "whooping" sound.
   B) Barky (seal-like).
   C) Loose, productive.
   D) Brassy, dry.

10. Which of the following lists conditions that affect the upper airway?
   A) Bacterial tracheitis, epiglottitis, pneumonia
   B) Bronchiolitis, croup, asthma
   D) Asthma, bronchiolitis, pneumonia
   E) Croup, epiglottitis, bacterial tracheitis

Chapter Quiz Answers

1. A. The most important risk factor for bronchopulmonary dysplasia (BPD) is prematurity. Ninety percent of the infants who develop BPD are premature and weigh less than 1500 grams (3.5 pounds). The more premature the newborn is, the higher the risk for developing BPD.

2. C. Suspect a foreign body airway obstruction (FBAO) in any previously well, afebrile child with a sudden onset of respiratory distress and associated coughing, choking, stridor, or wheezing.

3. C. Epiglottitis most commonly occurs in children 2 to 5 years of age. Croup most commonly occurs in children 6 months to 3 years of age.

4. Pediatric Assessment Triangle (first impression) findings:
   Appearance: Awake but appears tired and limp
   Breathing: Respirations are rapid and shallow; increased work of breathing evident
   Circulation: Skin color is dusky; no evidence of bleeding

5. B. The patient's age and clinical presentation are consistent with bronchiolitis/respiratory syncytial virus (RSV). In bronchiolitis, airway obstruction is usually gradual and is caused by inflammation, secretions, and edema of varying degrees in the small bronchi and bronchioles. Inflammation and edema make the small air passages in infants particularly vulnerable to obstruction.

6. This infant is sick. Move quickly. Open the airway and suction if necessary. Correct hypoxia by giving high-flow oxygen. Begin assisted ventilation if the patient does not improve. Provide further interventions based on assessment findings.

7. D. Because beta-blockers impede bronchodilation, they are not routinely used in the management of bronchopulmonary dysplasia. Bronchodilators may be used to improve airflow in the lungs. Corticosteroids may be used to reduce airway swelling and inflammation. Diuretics may be administered to decrease fluid accumulation in the lungs. Antibiotics may be administered to control infection.

8. C. An increase in the respiratory rate (tachypnea) is an early sign of impending respiratory difficulty.

9. B. The cough that accompanies croup is typically described as barky or seal-like.

10. E. Croup, epiglottitis, and bacterial tracheitis are conditions that affect the upper airway. Pneumonia, asthma, and bronchiolitis are conditions that affect the lower airway.

Respiratory Interventions

5

Case Study

A 4-year-old girl has a fever and difficulty breathing. Mom states the child has had a cough and runny nose for the past 3 to 4 days, and the cough appears to be getting worse. Several family members have had symptoms of a cold recently. The child had a fever of 104° F yesterday that decreased to 101° F after she was given acetaminophen. Last night the child began breathing fast and her cough sounded "wet." The child's cough is productive for greenish-yellow sputum. Today she is "not acting right" and is having more difficulty breathing.

Using the Pediatric Assessment Triangle, your first impression reveals the child is awake, but is unconcerned about your presence. Her respiratory rate is faster than normal for her age and shallow, and her skin is pale. The Primary Survey reveals the child is slow to respond to your questions. Her airway is patent. Her respiratory rate is approximately 65 breaths per minute, shallow and labored. Capillary refill is 5 seconds and the extremities are cool in a warm environment. Peripheral pulses are weak and rapid. The skin is pale and dry.

Based on the information provided, is this child sick or not sick? What should you do next?

Objectives

1. Describe the head-tilt/chin-lift and jaw-thrust without head-tilt methods for opening the airway.
2. Describe the preferred method of opening the airway in cases of suspected cervical spine injury.
3. Describe the procedures used to relieve foreign body airway obstruction (FBAO) in infants and children.
4. Describe correct suctioning technique and complications associated with this procedure.
5. Discuss oxygen delivery systems used for infants and children.
6. Describe the oxygen liter flow per minute and estimated oxygen percentage delivered for a nasal cannula, simple face mask, partial nonrebreather mask, nonrebreather mask, and bag-valve-mask (BVM) device.
7. Describe the method of correct sizing, insertion technique, and

possible complications associated with insertion of the oropharyngeal airway (OPA) and nasopharyngeal airway (NPA).

8. Discuss appropriate ventilation devices for infants and children.

9. Discuss complications of improper use of ventilation devices with infants and children.

10. Discuss the indications for and use of cricoid pressure.

11. List the indications for gastric decompression for infants and children.

12. State the indications for tracheal intubation of infants and children.

13. Discuss appropriate tracheal intubation equipment for infants and children.

14. Identify complications of an improper tracheal intubation procedure in infants and children.

15. State the indications for rapid sequence intubation (RSI) of infants and children.

Airway Maneuvers

Overview

- In the unresponsive patient, a partial airway obstruction may occur if
  - The tongue falls back against the back of the throat due to a loss of muscle control (Figure 5-1)
  - The epiglottis acts as a flap to obstruct the airway at the level of the larynx
- If the patient is breathing, snoring respirations are a characteristic sign of airway obstruction due to displacement of the tongue. In the apneic patient, airway obstruction caused by the tongue may go undetected until ventilation is attempted.
- Ventilating an apneic patient with an airway obstruction is difficult. If the airway obstruction is due to the tongue, repositioning of the patient's head and jaw may be all that is needed to open the airway.

Head Tilt–Chin Lift

The head tilt–chin lift is the preferred technique for opening the airway of an unresponsive patient without suspected cervical spine injury.

- Indications
  - Unresponsive patient who does not have a mechanism for cervical spine injury
  - Unresponsive patient who is unable to protect his or her own airway
- Contraindications
  - Awake patient
  - Known or suspected cervical spine injury

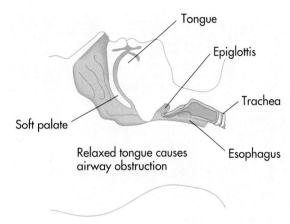

Figure 5-1 In the unresponsive patient, a partial airway obstruction may occur if the tongue falls back against the back of the throat due to a loss of muscle control.

- Advantages
  - No equipment required
  - Simple, noninvasive
- Disadvantages
  - Head tilt hazardous to patients with cervical spine injury
  - Does not protect the lower airway from aspiration
- Procedure
  - Place the patient in a supine position
  - Place the hand closest to the child's head on the forehead. Apply firm downward pressure with your palm to tilt the patient's head gently back into a neutral or slightly extended position (Figure 5-2).
  - Place the tips of the fingers of your other hand under the *bony* part of the patient's chin and gently lift the jaw upward and outward to open the airway.

> **PEDS** *Pearl*
>
> Hyperextension of the patient's neck or compression of the soft tissue under the patient's chin can obstruct the airway.

Jaw Thrust without Head Tilt Maneuver

Studies have shown that this maneuver does cause some movement of the cervical spine. If an assistant is available, ask him or her to maintain manual in-line stabilization to minimize movement of the head and neck when performing this maneuver.

The jaw thrust without head tilt maneuver is the preferred method of opening the airway when cervical spine injury is suspected.

- Indications
  - Unresponsive patient with possible cervical spine injury
  - Unable to protect own airway
- Contraindications
  - Awake patient
- Advantages
  - Noninvasive
  - Requires no special equipment
  - May be used with cervical collar in place
- Disadvantages
  - Difficult to maintain

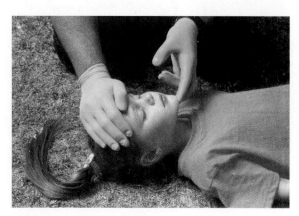

Figure 5-2   Head tilt–chin lift.

- ○ Requires second rescuer for BVM ventilation
- ○ Does not protect against aspiration
- Technique
  - ○ Place the patient in a supine position
  - ○ While stabilizing the patient's head in a neutral position, grasp the angles of the patient's lower jaw with both hands, one on each side, and displace the mandible forward (Figure 5-3).

Rescue Breathing

- Determine if the child is breathing (assess for up to 10 seconds).   **Assessment**
  - ○ LOOK for rise and fall of the chest and abdomen.
  - ○ LISTEN for exhaled air.
  - ○ FEEL for exhaled air.
- If the child is breathing, maintain a patent airway.
- If the child is not breathing:
  - ○ Remove any obvious airway obstruction.
  - ○ Begin rescue breathing while maintaining a patent airway with a chin lift or jaw thrust without head tilt.

- Rescue breathing should be performed with a mask equipped with a   **Rescue Breathing**
  one-way valve or similar device. Personal protective equipment should always be readily available, including masks with one-way valves for ventilating pediatric patients.
- Deliver two breaths (1 second per breath), pausing after the first breath.

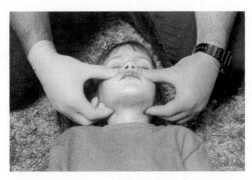

Figure 5-3   Jaw thrust without head tilt maneuver.

- Pausing allows the rescuer to take a breath to maximize oxygen content and minimize carbon dioxide (CO_2) concentration in delivered breaths. Failing to do so will result in rescue breaths low in oxygen and high in CO_2.
- Rapid rescue breathing may cause gastric distention.
- Excessive gastric distention may inhibit rescue breathing by elevating the diaphragm and reducing lung volume.
- The volume of air delivered should be sufficient to cause gentle chest rise. The airway is clear if air enters freely and the chest rises.
- If the child's chest does not rise during rescue breathing, ventilation is not effective.
  - If the chest does not rise, either the airway is obstructed or more volume or pressure is needed to provide effective ventilation.
  - A common cause of obstruction is improper positioning of the airway. Readjust the position of the head, ensure the mouth is open, and reattempt to ventilate.
- Suspect an FBAO if the chest fails to rise despite attempts to ventilate.

Relief of Foreign Body Airway Obstruction

FBAO should be suspected in infants and children with a *sudden* onset of respiratory distress associated with coughing, gagging, stridor, or wheezing.

Overview

The 2005 resuscitation guidelines refer to a "mild" airway obstruction as one in which the victim can cough and make some sounds.

- If the infant or child is conscious and maintaining his or her own airway *without* respiratory distress:
  - Do not interfere. Allow the child to continue his or her efforts to attempt to clear the foreign body.
  - Allow the child to assume a position of comfort and administer 100% oxygen as tolerated.

- ◦ Encourage the child to cough and provide emotional support.
- ◦ Removal of the foreign body by bronchoscopy or laryngoscopy should be attempted in a controlled environment.
- If the infant or child is conscious and maintaining his or her own airway but respiratory distress is present:
  - ◦ Do not interfere. Allow the child to continue his or her efforts to attempt to clear the foreign body.
  - ◦ Allow the child to assume a position of comfort and administer 100% oxygen as tolerated.
  - ◦ Encourage the child to cough and provide emotional support.
  - ◦ If the cough becomes ineffective and/or there is increasing respiratory difficulty accompanied by stridor, attempt to relieve the obstruction.

- Assess the infant. If the infant can cough or cry, watch him or her closely to ensure the object is expelled. If the infant is unable to cough or cry, provide care.
- Back blows
  - ◦ While supporting the infant's head and neck, place the infant face down over one arm (Figure 5-4).
  - ◦ Position the infant's head slightly lower than the rest of the body.
  - ◦ Using the heel of one hand, deliver up to five back blows forcefully between the infant's shoulder blades.
  - ◦ If the foreign body is not expelled, deliver chest thrusts.
- Chest thrusts
  - ◦ Support the infant's head and neck.
  - ◦ Position the infant between your hands and arms and turn the infant onto his or her back (Figure 5-5).
  - ◦ Imagine a line between the nipples. Place the flat part of your middle and ring fingers about one finger-width below this imaginary line. Deliver up to five quick downward chest thrusts.
  - ◦ Check the patient's mouth. If the foreign body is seen, remove it. **Do NOT perform a blind finger sweep!**
- Open the airway and attempt rescue breathing.
  - ◦ If rescue breathing does not cause the infant's chest to rise, reposition the head and reattempt rescue breathing.
  - ◦ If the chest does not rise (the airway remains obstructed), continue the sequence of up to five back blows, up to five chest thrusts, and breathing attempts until the object is dislodged (and expelled) and rescue breathing is successful, or the victim becomes unconscious.

Performance Guidelines for a Conscious Choking Infant

The 2005 resuscitation guidelines refer to a "severe" airway obstruction as one in which the victim cannot cough or make any sound.

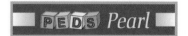
PEDS Pearl

Back blows are performed in an attempt to loosen the foreign body. Chest thrusts increase intrathoracic pressure, which may cause expulsion of the foreign body.

Do not sweep the mouth unless the foreign body is visible. Blind sweeps may push the foreign body into the glottic opening, resulting in complete obstruction.

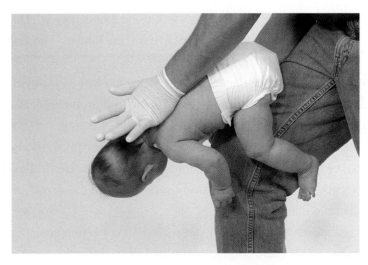

Figure 5-4   To clear a foreign body from a conscious infant's airway, deliver up to five back blows between the infant's shoulder blades using the heel of one hand.

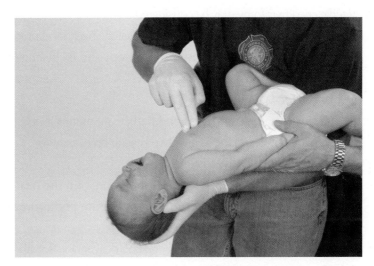

Figure 5-5   If back blows do not relieve the obstruction, deliver up to five chest thrusts about one finger's width below the nipple line.

Performance Guidelines for an Unconscious Choking Infant

- Place the infant in a supine position on a hard surface.
- Using a head tilt–chin lift (or jaw thrust without head tilt if trauma is suspected), open the airway.
  - Check the nose and mouth for secretions, emesis, a foreign body, and other obstructions. Suction fluids and particulate matter as necessary.

- If a foreign body is visible, remove it using a finger sweep. ***Do NOT perform a blind finger sweep!*** Remove the foreign body *only* if it is visualized.
- Attempt to ventilate the infant using a pocket mask or BVM device with 100% oxygen. If the chest does not rise, reposition the infant's head, reopen the airway, and try to ventilate again.
- If the chest does not rise, begin CPR. After 30 chest compressions, look into the mouth and remove the foreign body, if visualized. If the chest does not rise, reposition the patient's head, reopen the airway, and try again to ventilate.
- If basic airway maneuvers are not successful in clearing an obstructed airway:
  - Perform direct laryngoscopy and attempt to locate the obstruction. Remove the foreign body using pediatric Magill forceps if it is clearly visible. If removal is successful, reassess breathing and resume BVM ventilation.
  - If unsuccessful, attempt tracheal intubation and ventilate the patient.
  - If the infant cannot be intubated, attempt BVM ventilation.
  - Needle cricothyrotomy may be considered if complete airway obstruction exists and BVM ventilation is unsuccessful (check local protocol).
  - Removal of the foreign body by bronchoscopy should be attempted in a controlled environment.
- If the obstruction is removed:
  - Assess breathing. Suction fluids and particulate matter if necessary. If the infant is not breathing, give two rescue breaths.
  - Assess circulation and perfusion.
  - If there is no pulse or other signs of circulation, or if the heart rate is less than 60 beats per minute with signs of poor perfusion, begin chest compressions.
  - If breathing is absent but a pulse is present, deliver one breath every 3 to 5 seconds (12 to 20 breaths per minute) and monitor the infant's pulse.
  - If the infant is breathing (and breathing is effective), reassess frequently.
  - Assess mental status.
  - Expose as necessary to perform further assessments while maintaining the infant's body temperature.
  - Perform a focused history and detailed physical examination only if they will not interfere with lifesaving interventions.

PEDS Pearl

Positive-pressure ventilation can convert a complete airway obstruction to a partial one by pushing the foreign body into the lower airway, usually the right mainstem bronchus, allowing ventilation of the left lung (or part of the left lung).

Performance Guidelines for a Conscious Choking Child

- Assess the child's ability to speak or cough. Ask, "Are you choking?"
- If the child can cough or speak, watch the child closely to ensure the object is expelled.

The child may hold his or her neck with the thumb and fingers. This sign is the universal distress signal for a choking emergency.

- If the child cannot cough or speak, perform abdominal thrusts (Figure 5-6).
  - Stand behind the child and wrap your arms around the child's waist.
  - Abdominal thrusts should be delivered two finger's width above the navel. Make a fist with one hand. Place the fist thumb side in on the thrust site. Place your other hand on top of the fist. Perform a quick inward and upward thrust.
  - Continue performing abdominal thrusts until the foreign body is expelled or the child becomes unresponsive.

Performance Guidelines for an Unconscious Choking Child

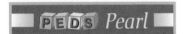

An infant or child with a partial airway obstruction and poor air exchange should be treated as if he or she has a complete airway obstruction.

- Confirm that the patient is unresponsive.
- Place the child in a supine position on a hard surface, being sure to protect the head, neck, and spine.
- Using a head tilt–chin lift (or jaw thrust without head tilt if trauma is suspected), open the airway.
  - Check the nose and mouth for secretions, emesis, a foreign body, and other obstructions. Suction fluids and particulate matter as necessary.
  - If a foreign body is visible, remove it using a finger sweep. **Do NOT perform a blind finger sweep!** Remove the foreign body only if it is visualized.

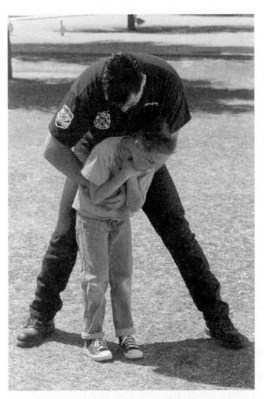

Figure 5-6   Clearing a foreign body airway obstruction—conscious child.

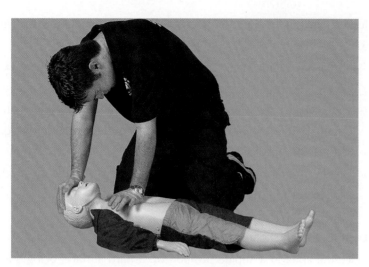

Figure 5-7   If the victim's chest does not rise, begin CPR.

- Attempt to ventilate the child using a BVM device with 100% oxygen. If the chest does not rise, reposition the child's head, reopen the airway, and try again to ventilate with the BVM.
- If the chest does not rise, begin CPR. After 30 chest compressions, look into the mouth and remove the foreign body, if visualized. If the chest does not rise, reposition the patient's head, reopen the airway, and try again to ventilate (Figure 5-7).
- If basic airway maneuvers are not successful in clearing an obstructed airway:
  - Perform direct laryngoscopy and attempt to locate the obstruction. Remove the foreign body using pediatric Magill forceps if it is clearly visible. If removal is successful, reassess breathing and resume BVM ventilation.
  - If unsuccessful, attempt tracheal intubation and ventilate the patient.
  - If the child cannot be intubated, attempt BVM ventilation.
  - Needle cricothyrotomy may be considered if complete airway obstruction exists and BVM ventilation is unsuccessful (check local protocol).
  - Removal of the foreign body by bronchoscopy should be attempted in a controlled environment.
- If the obstruction is removed:
  - Assess breathing. If the child is not breathing, give two rescue breaths.

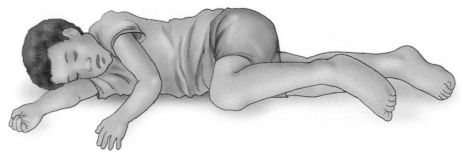

Figure 5-8   Recovery position.

PEDS *Pearl*

Many recovery positions have been used in the management of pediatric patients. The ideal position should enable maintenance of a patent airway, maintenance of cervical spine stability, minimize the risk for aspiration, limit pressure on bony prominences and peripheral nerves, allow visualization of the child's respiratory effort and appearance, and permit access to the patient for procedures.

- Assess circulation and perfusion.
  - If there is no pulse or other signs of circulation, or if the heart rate is less than 60 beats per minute with signs of poor perfusion, begin chest compressions.
  - If breathing is absent but a pulse is present, deliver one breath every 3 to 5 seconds (12 to 20 breaths per minute) and monitor the child's pulse.
- If the victim is breathing (and breathing is effective):
  - Turn the child to the side (recovery position) if trauma is not suspected (Figure 5-8).
  - Reassess the child frequently.
- Assess mental status.
- Expose as necessary to perform further assessments while maintaining the child's body temperature.
- Perform a focused history and detailed physical examination only if they will not interfere with lifesaving interventions.

Suctioning

Purpose of Suctioning
- Remove vomitus, saliva, blood, meconium (in newly born infants), and other secretions from the patient's airway
- Improve gas exchange
- Prevent atelectasis
- Obtain secretions for diagnosis

Suction Devices
- Bulb syringe (nasal aspirator)
  - A bulb syringe is most often used to remove secretions from the

nose and mouth of newborns and infants up to approximately 4 months of age, but can also be used to clear the airway of a child.

- Soft suction catheters
  - Also called "whistle-tip" or "French" catheters.
  - Long, narrow, flexible piece of plastic used to clear thin secretions from the mouth, trachea, nasopharynx, or tracheal tube.
  - A side opening is present at the proximal end of most catheters that is covered with the thumb to produce suction. (In some cases, suctioning is initiated when a button is pushed on the suction device itself.)
  - Can be inserted into the nares, mouth, through an OPA or NPA, or through a tracheal tube or tracheostomy tube.
- Rigid suction catheters
  - Also called "hard," "tonsil tip," or "Yankauer" suction catheters.
  - The rigid suction catheter is made of hard plastic and is angled to aid in the removal of thick secretions and particulate matter from the mouth and oropharynx.
  - A rigid suction catheter typically has one large and several small holes at the distal end through which particles may be suctioned.
  - Because of its size, the rigid suction catheter is not used to suction the nares, except externally.

Suctioning Technique

- Using personal protective equipment, preoxygenate the patient with 100% oxygen for at least 30 seconds before suctioning.
- Bulb syringe
  - Depress the rounded end of the bulb to remove air from the syringe (Figure 5-9).
  - Place the tip of the syringe snugly into one side of the nose (or mouth).
  - Release the bulb slowly; the bulb will operate as a vacuum to remove the secretions from the nose or mouth.

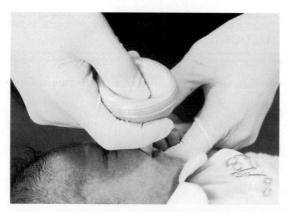

Figure 5-9   A bulb syringe may be used to suction the nose and mouth of newborns and infants.

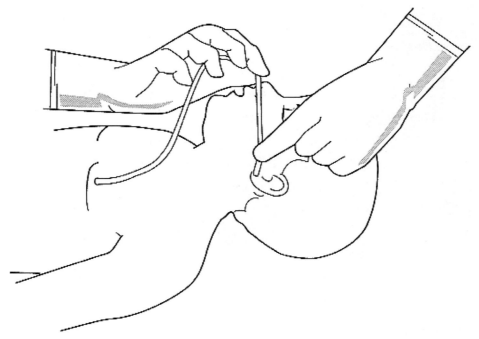

Figure 5-10   When using a soft suction catheter, estimate the depth to suction by holding the catheter next to the child's face and measuring from the tip of the nose to the ear lobe.

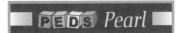 *Pearl*

Before suctioning, note the child's heart rate, oxygen saturation, and color. Monitor the child's heart rate and clinical appearance during suctioning. Bradycardia may result from stimulation of the posterior pharynx, larynx, or trachea. If bradycardia occurs or the child's clinical appearance deteriorates, interrupt suctioning and ventilate with high-concentration oxygen until the child's heart rate returns to normal.

- When the bulb is reinflated, remove the syringe and empty the contents.
- Soft suction catheter
  - Ensure the suction device is powered on and mechanical suction is present.
  - When preparing to suction to nose or mouth, measure the proper distance the catheter should be inserted by holding the catheter next to the child's face and measuring from the tip of the nose to the ear lobe (Figure 5-10). To estimate the correct catheter depth for tracheobronchial suctioning, measure from the nose (or mouth) to the ear and add the distance from the ear to the sternal notch.
  - Gently insert the catheter up to the measured distance **without** applying suction (Figure 5-11). Apply intermittent suction while withdrawing the catheter.
  - Before repeating the procedure, ventilate the patient with 100% oxygen for at least 30 seconds and rinse the suction catheter in sterile saline or water.
- Rigid suction catheter (Figure 5-12)
  - Ensure the suction device is powered on and mechanical suction is present.
  - **Without** applying suction, gently place the tip of the catheter in the child's mouth along one side of the mouth until it reaches the posterior pharynx

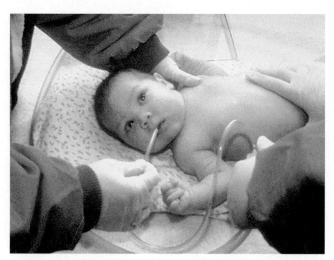

Figure 5-11 A soft suction catheter may be used to clear thin secretions from the mouth, trachea, nasopharynx, or tracheal tube.

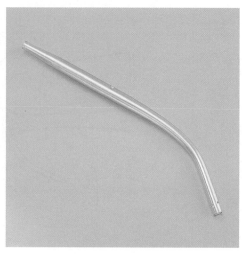

Figure 5-12 Rigid suction catheter.

○ Apply intermittent suction while withdrawing the catheter

○ Before repeating the procedure, ventilate the patient with 100% oxygen for at least 30 seconds and rinse the suction catheter in sterile saline or water.

- Hypoxia
- Dysrhythmias
- Increased intracranial pressure (ICP)
- Local edema
- Hemorrhage
- Tracheal ulceration
- Tracheal infection
- Bronchospasm
- Bradycardia and hypotension from stimulation of the posterior pharynx, larynx, or trachea
- Tachycardia may result from sympathetic stimulation.

Suctioning: Possible Complications

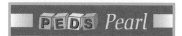

Insertion of a suction catheter and suctioning should take no longer than 10 seconds per attempt. When suctioning to remove material that completely obstructs the airway, more time may be necessary.

Airway Adjuncts

Description and Function

An OPA is a J-shaped plastic device designed for use in an unresponsive patient without a gag reflex (Figure 5-13). When correctly positioned, the OPA extends from the patient's lips to the pharynx. The flange of the device rests on the patient's lips or teeth. The distal tip lies between the base of the tongue and the back of the throat, preventing the tongue from occluding the airway. Air passes around and through the device.

Oropharyngeal Airway (Oral Airway)

An OPA does not protect the lower airway from aspiration.

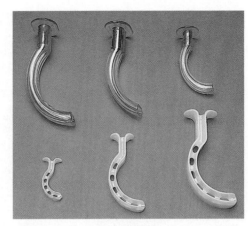

Figure 5-13   Oropharyngeal airways are available in a variety of sizes.

Indications

- To aid in maintaining an open airway in an unresponsive patient who is not intubated
- To aid in maintaining an open airway in an unresponsive patient with no gag reflex who is being ventilated with a BVM or other positive-pressure device
- May be used as a bite block after insertion of a tracheal tube or orogastric tube

Contraindications

- Patient with an intact gag reflex

Advantages

- Positions the tongue forward and away from the posterior pharynx
- Easily placed

Disadvantages

- Does not protect the lower airway from aspiration
- May produce vomiting if used in a responsive or semiresponsive patient with a gag reflex

Sizing

The size of the airway is based on the distance, in millimeters, from the flange to the distal tip.

- Available in many sizes varying in length and internal diameter (ID).
- Proper airway size is determined by holding the device against the side of the patient's face and selecting an airway that extends from the corner of the mouth to the angle of the jaw (Figure 5-14).

Insertion

An OPA should only be inserted by persons properly trained in their use.

Before inserting an OPA, use personal protective equipment, open the airway, and ensure the mouth and pharynx are clear of secretions, blood, and vomitus. After selecting an OPA of proper size, open the patient's mouth by applying thumb pressure on the chin.

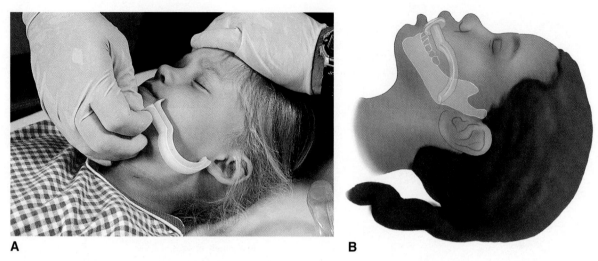

A   **B**

Figure 5-14   Proper airway size is determined by (**A**) holding the device against the side of the patient's face and selecting an airway that (**B**) extends from the corner of the mouth to the angle of the jaw.

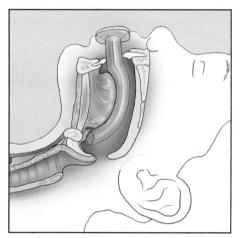

Figure 5-15   Place the oropharyngeal airway over the tongue down into the mouth until the flange of the airway rests against the patient's lips. When correctly positioned, the distal tip of the oropharyngeal airway lies between the base of the tongue and the back of the throat, preventing the tongue from occluding the airway.

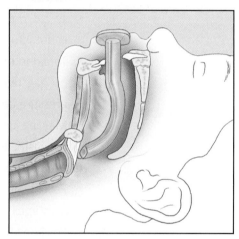

Figure 5-16   If an oropharyngeal airway is too long, it may press the epiglottis against the entrance of the larynx resulting in a complete airway obstruction.

Depress the tongue with a tongue blade and gently insert the OPA with the curve downward. Place the airway over the tongue down into the mouth until the flange of the airway rests against the patient's lips (Figure 5-15).

Special Considerations

- The OPA should only be used in an unresponsive patient. Use in responsive or semiresponsive patients may stimulate the gag reflex when the back of the tongue or posterior pharynx is touched, resulting in retching, vomiting, and/or laryngospasm.

- Use of an OPA does not eliminate the need for maintaining proper head position.

The preferred technique for OPA insertion in an infant or child requires the use of a tongue blade.

TABLE 5-1 *Selection of Appropriate Oropharyngeal Airway Size Based on Broselow Resuscitation Tape*		
Age	**Weight (kg)**	**Airway Size**
Newborn / small Infant (0 to 3 mo)	3 to 5	Newborn
Infant (3 to 6 mo)	6 to 7	Infant/small child
Infant (7 to 10 mo)	8 to 9	Infant/small child
Toddler (11 to 18 mo)	10 to 11	Small child
Small child (19 to 35 mo)	12 to 14	Child
Child (3 to 4 y)	15 to 18	Child
Child (5 to 6 y)	19 to 22	Child/small adult
Large child (7 to 9 y)	24 to 30	Child/small adult
Adult (10 to 12 y)	32 to 40	Medium adult

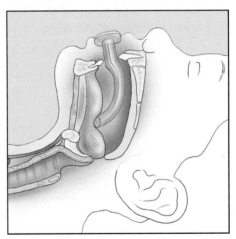

Figure 5-17 If an oropharyngeal airway is too short, the tongue may be pushed back into the pharynx resulting in an airway obstruction, or the airway may advance out of the mouth.

- An improperly positioned OPA may compromise the airway.
- If the airway is too long, it may press the epiglottis against the entrance of the larynx resulting in complete airway obstruction (Figure 5-16).
- If the airway is too short, the tongue may be pushed back into the pharynx resulting in an airway obstruction, or the airway may advance out of the mouth (Figure 5-17).

Nasopharyngeal Airway (Nasal Trumpet, Nasal Airway)

Description and Function

- Soft, uncuffed rubber or plastic tube designed to keep the tongue away from the posterior pharynx

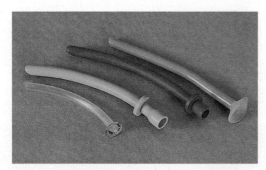

Figure 5-18 Nasopharyngeal airways are available in a variety of sizes.

- The device is placed in one nostril and advanced until the distal tip lies in the posterior pharynx just below the base of the tongue, while the proximal tip rests on the external nares.
- Available in many sizes varying in length and ID (Figure 5-18).

Indications

- To aid in maintaining an airway when use of an OPA is contraindicated or impossible (e.g., trismus, seizing patient, biting, clenched jaws or teeth)
- May be useful in patients requiring frequent suctioning (decreases tissue trauma, bleeding)
- Dental or oral trauma

Contraindications

- Patient intolerance
- Nasal obstruction
- Significant mid-face trauma
- Presence of cerebrospinal fluid drainage from the nose
- Moderate to severe head trauma
- Known or suspected basilar skull fracture

Advantages

- Provides a patent airway
- Reasonably well tolerated in the responsive patient
- Does not require the mouth to be open
- Less likely than an OPA to stimulate a gag reflex and cause vomiting

Disadvantages

- Improper technique may result in severe bleeding; resulting epistaxis may be difficult to control
- Does not protect the lower airway from aspiration
- Small internal size of an airway that will fit a child does not allow adequate air flow

Sizing

- Proper airway size is determined by holding the device against the side of the patient's face and selecting an airway that extends from the tip of the nose to the angle of the jaw or the tip of the ear (Figure 5-19).

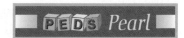
PEDS *Pearl*

Nasopharyngeal airways are not useful in infants and small children. The small internal size of an airway that will fit these patients does not allow adequate air flow.

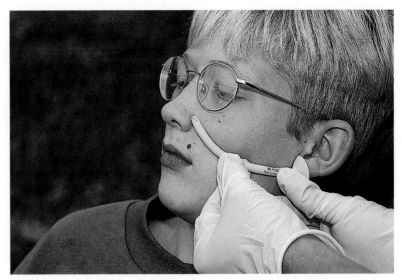

Figure 5-19   Sizing a nasopharyngeal airway.

- ◦ If the NPA is equipped with an adjustable flange, adjust the flange up or down as necessary to obtain the appropriate length.
- An NPA that is too long may stimulate the gag reflex or enter the esophagus, causing gastric distention and hypoventilation. One that is too short may not be inserted far enough to keep the tongue away from the posterior pharynx.

Insertion

An NPA should only be inserted by persons properly trained in their use.

- Before inserting an NPA, use personal protective equipment and open the airway.
- Lubricate the distal tip of the device liberally with a water-soluble lubricant to minimize resistance and decrease irritation to the nasal passage.
- After selecting an NPA of the proper size, hold the device at its flange end like a pencil and slowly insert it into the patient's nostril with the bevel pointing toward the nasal septum.

If blanching of the nostril is present after insertion of an NPA, the diameter of the device is too large. Remove the NPA, select a slightly smaller size, and reinsert.

- Advance the airway along the floor of the nostril, following the natural curvature of the nasal passage, until the flange rests against the outside of the nostril.
  - ◦ The nasal cavity is very vascular. During insertion, do not force the airway because it may cause abrasions or lacerations of the nasal mucosa and result in significant bleeding, increasing the risk of aspiration.
  - ◦ If resistance is encountered, a gentle back-and-forth rotation of the device between your fingers may ease insertion. If resistance continues, withdraw the NPA, reapply lubricant, and attempt insertion in the other nostril.
- When correctly positioned, the NPA extends from the patient's nose to

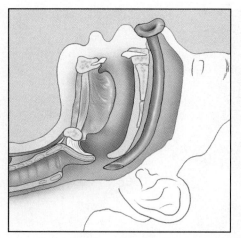

Figure 5-20   When correctly positioned, the nasopharyngeal airway extends from the patient's nose to the pharynx. The flange of the device rests against the outside of the nostril. The distal tip lies between the base of the tongue and the back of the throat, preventing the tongue from occluding the airway.

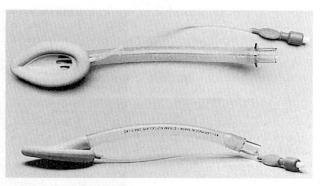

Figure 5-21   The laryngeal mask airway (LMA).

the pharynx. The flange of the device rests against the outside of the nostril and the distal tip lies between the base of the tongue and the back of the throat, preventing the tongue from occluding the airway. Air passes around and through the device (Figure 5-20).

Special Considerations

- The NPA does not protect the lower airway from aspiration.
- Use of the NPA does not eliminate the need for maintaining proper head position.
- Small-diameter NPAs can become easily obstructed with blood, mucus, vomitus, or the soft tissues of the pharynx.
- Suctioning may be necessary to keep the NPA open; however, suctioning through an NPA is difficult.
- Although most responsive and semiresponsive patients can tolerate an NPA, the gag reflex may be stimulated in sensitive patients, precipitating coughing, laryngospasm, or vomiting.

- An LMA is a device that functions intermediately between an OPA and a tracheal tube, and does not require direct visualization of the airway for insertion. The LMA is available in sizes for neonates, infants, young children, older children, and small, average, and large adults.
- The LMA consists of a tube fitted with an oval mask and an inflatable rim (Figure 5-21). The tube opens into the middle of the mask by means of vertical slits that prevent the tip of the epiglottis from falling back and blocking the lumen of the tube. The LMA is inserted through

Laryngeal Mask Airway

According to the 2005 resuscitation guidelines, there is insufficient evidence to recommend for or against the routine use of LMAs during cardiac arrest.

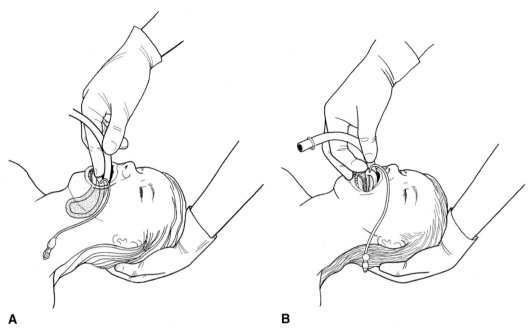

A   **B**

Figure 5-22 **A,** The laryngeal mask airway (LMA) is inserted through the mouth into the pharynx without visualization with the mask opening facing anteriorly. **B,** The LMA is advanced until resistance is felt, using the right index finger to maintain firm pressure on the device against the hard palate.

PEDS Pearl

The current LMA design does not provide a route for suctioning or delivering medications. There have been a few reports of administering medications through the LMA with contrasting results. In one cadaver study, epinephrine was successfully delivered to the lungs in "reasonable" amounts. However, in 100 anesthetized patients using a special cannula, medications were found in only 27% of the patients. Therefore administration of medications through an LMA is unreliable.

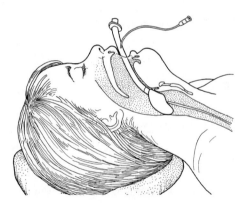

Figure 5-23 The laryngeal mask airway surrounds the larynx and forms a seal to permit ventilation.

the mouth into the pharynx without visualization. The LMA is advanced until resistance is felt, using the right index finger to maintain firm pressure on the device against the hard palate (Figure 5-22). The rim of the mask is then inflated to seal the mask around the larynx and the base of the tongue (Figure 5-23), and the LMA is connected to a ventilation device.

- The inflatable LMA mask does not ensure an airtight seal to protect the airway against gastric regurgitation. Leakage of the mask may allow aspiration of emesis and gastric distention may occur with misplacement.

The LMA should only be inserted by persons properly trained in the use of the device.

TABLE 5-2 *Airway Adjuncts*

Device	Indications	Sizing
Oropharyngeal airway (oral airway, OPA)	To aid in maintaining an open airway in an unresponsive patient who is not intubated To aid in maintaining an open airway in an unresponsive patient with no gag reflex that is being ventilated with a bag-valve-mask or other positive-pressure device May be used as a bite block after insertion of a tracheal tube or orogastric tube	Corner of mouth to the angle of the jaw
Nasopharyngeal airway (nasal airway, NPA)	To aid in maintaining an airway when use of an OPA is contraindicated or impossible (e.g., trismus, seizing patient, biting, clenched jaws or teeth) May be useful in patients requiring frequent suctioning Dental or oral trauma	From the tip of the nose to the angle of the jaw or the tip of the ear
Laryngeal mask airway (LMA)	Patient in whom intubation has been unsuccessful and ventilation is difficult Patient in whom airway management is necessary but healthcare provider is untrained in the technique of visualized orotracheal intubation Many elective surgical procedures	Because masks are available in several sizes, the LMA can be used in patients of all ages, from neonates to adults.

Oxygen Delivery Systems

The oxygen delivery systems described in this section may be used for the spontaneously breathing infant or child with effective ventilation (i.e., adequate chest movement and breath sounds). If spontaneous breathing is inadequate, assisted ventilation is required (discussed later in this chapter).

General Principles

- Administer high-concentration oxygen to any seriously ill or injured child with signs or symptoms of respiratory compromise, shock, or trauma.
- Humidified oxygen should be used when possible. Humidification helps prevent drying of the mucous membranes and loosens secretions.
- Cool-mist systems may produce hypothermia in the small child; heated humidification systems are preferred.

Indications for Oxygen Administration

- All cases of cardiopulmonary arrest
- Suspected hypoxemia of any cause

- Any condition of respiratory difficulty that may potentially lead to cardiopulmonary arrest

Types of Oxygen Delivery Systems

- Oxygen therapy is referred to as the fraction of inspired gas that is oxygen (FiO_2).
- Oxygen delivery systems are categorized as low-flow, high-flow, or enclosure systems.
    - A low-flow oxygen delivery system, such as a nasal cannula, provides oxygen at a flow rate that is less than the patient's maximum inspiratory flow. The inspired oxygen is diluted with room air and the FiO_2 that enters the patient's airway is affected by the relationships between oxygen flow, the patient's inspiratory flow, and the patient's breathing pattern.
    - A high-flow oxygen delivery system can provide a specific delivered oxygen concentration at flow rates that exceed the patient's inspiratory flow requirement so that the patient's breathing pattern and inspiratory flow do not affect the FiO_2.
    - Enclosure systems (such as an oxygen hood, closed incubator, or oxygen tent) provide a means of controlling oxygen concentration, temperature, and humidity.

Nasal Cannula (Nasal Prongs)

Secure the nasal cannula in place and then slowly start the oxygen flow to avoid frightening the child.

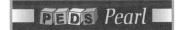

Because the lungs of a child are small in relationship to his or her metabolic needs, and a child has fewer and smaller alveoli than an adult, oxygen reserves can be rapidly depleted. Administer high-concentration oxygen to any child who exhibits signs of respiratory distress, failure, or arrest, or any time you are in doubt about the child's respiratory status.

Description and Function

A nasal cannula is a piece of plastic tubing with two soft prongs that project from the tubing. The prongs are inserted into the patient's nares, and the tubing secured to the patient's face (Figure 5-24). Oxygen flows from the cannula into the patient's nasopharynx, which acts as an anatomic reservoir.

- Low-flow oxygen delivery device used for the infant or child who requires only low levels of supplemental oxygen.
- Oxygen flow rate: 1 to 6 L/min.
- Concentration delivered: up to 50%.
- A high FiO_2 may result when the flow rate exceeds the patient's inspiratory flow and minute ventilation.

Advantages

- Easy to use
- Allows the patient to eat and drink
- Does not require humidification
- No rebreathing of expired air
- Does not interfere with patient assessment or impede patient communication with healthcare personnel

Disadvantages

- Can only be used in the spontaneously breathing patient

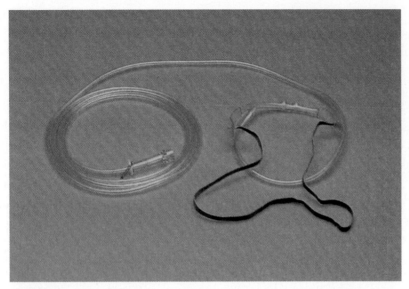

Figure 5-24   Nasal cannula.

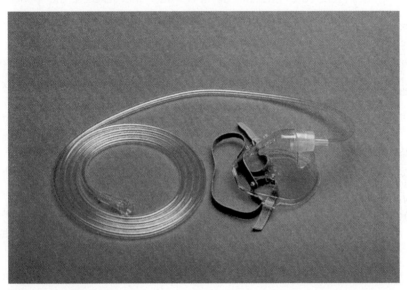

Figure 5-25   Simple face mask.

- Easily displaced
- Nasal passages must be patent
- Drying of mucosa
- May irritate nose
- May cause sinus pain

Description and Function

A simple face mask is a plastic reservoir designed to fit over the patient's nose and mouth. Small holes on each side of the mask allow the passage of inspired and expired air. Supplemental oxygen is delivered through a small-diameter tube connected to the base of the mask (Figure 5-25). The mask is secured in position by means of an elastic strap around the back

Simple Face Mask
(Standard Mask)

of the patient's head. The internal capacity of the mask produces a reservoir effect.

- Oxygen flow rate: 6 to 10 L/min.
- Concentration delivered: 35% to 60%.
- The patient's actual inspired oxygen concentration will vary because the amount of air that mixes with supplemental oxygen is dependent on the patient's inspiratory flow rate and breathing pattern.

Advantages

- Higher oxygen concentration delivered than by nasal cannula
- Patient accessibility

Disadvantages

- Can only be used with spontaneously breathing patients
- Not tolerated well by severely dyspneic patients (feeling of suffocation)
- FIO_2 varies with inspiratory flow rate
- Can be uncomfortable
- Dangerous for the child with poor airway control and at risk for emesis
- Difficult to hear the patient speaking when the device is in place
- Must be removed at meals
- Requires a tight face seal to prevent leakage of oxygen

Partial Rebreather (rebreathing) Mask

Description and Function

- The partial rebreather mask is similar to a simple oxygen mask but has an attached oxygen-collecting device (reservoir) at the base of the mask (Figure 5-26).
- Depending on the patient's respiratory pattern, oxygen flow rate, and the presence of a snug mask fit, oxygen concentrations of 50% to 60% can be delivered when an oxygen flow rate of 10 to 12 L/min is used.

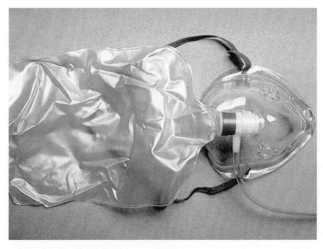

Figure 5-26 Partial rebreather mask.

- Fill the reservoir bag with oxygen before placing the mask on the patient.
- After placing the mask on the patient, adjust the flow rate so the bag does not completely deflate when the patient inhales.

Advantages

- Higher oxygen concentration delivered than by nasal cannula
- Patient accessibility

Disadvantages

- Same as for simple mask

Description and Function

- A nonrebreather mask is equipped with a one-way valve that separates the reservoir (bag) from the mask and directs exhaled air out through the side ports on the mask. This valve prevents the patient's exhaled air from returning to the reservoir bag (thus the name "nonrebreather"), ensuring a supply of 100% oxygen to the patient with minimal dilution from the entrainment of ambient air (Figure 5-27).
- Provides a higher inspired oxygen concentration than the nasal cannula, simple face mask, and partial rebreather mask
- Delivery device of choice when high concentrations of oxygen are needed in the spontaneously breathing patient because it can consistently deliver an inspired oxygen concentration of up to 95% at a flow of 10 to 15 L/min.
  - Fill the reservoir bag with oxygen before placing the mask on the patient
  - After placing the mask on the patient, adjust the flow rate so the bag does not completely deflate when the patient inhales.

Advantages

- Higher oxygen concentration delivered than by nasal cannula, simple face mask, and partial rebreather mask

Disadvantages

- Same as for simple mask

Nonrebreather (nonrebreathing) Mask

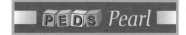

PEDS Pearl

When using a nonrebreather or partial rebreather mask, ensure that the bag does not collapse when the child inhales. Should the bag collapse, increase the oxygen flow rate in small increments until the bag remains inflated. The reservoir bag must remain at least two thirds full so that sufficient supplemental oxygen is available for each breath.

Description and Function

- Large, soft plastic bucket that fits loosely around the child's face and lower jaw (Figure 5-28)

Advantages

- Permits access to the face and nose for suctioning
- Can provide warmed or cooled humidified oxygen

Disadvantages

- Oxygen concentrations in excess of 40% cannot be reliably provided, even with an oxygen flow rate of 10 to 15 L/min

Face Tent (Face Shield)

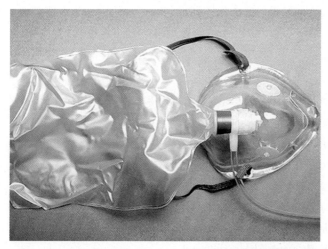

Figure 5-27   Nonrebreather mask.

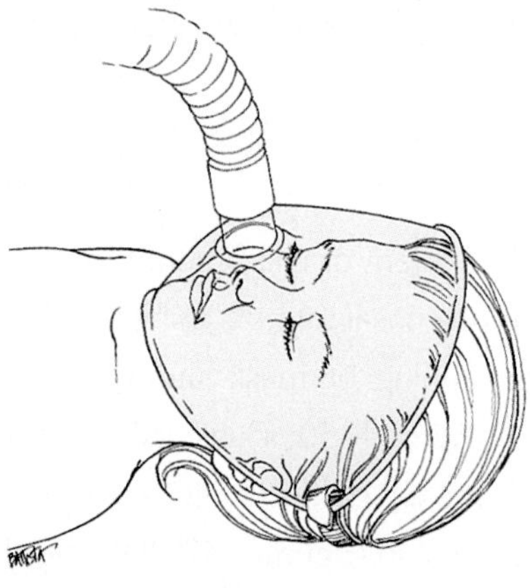

Figure 5-28   Face tent.

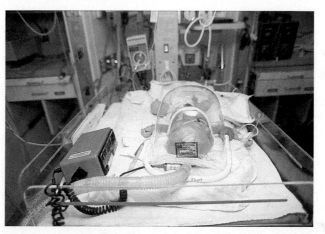

Figure 5-29   Oxygen administered to an infant by means of a plastic hood.

Oxygen Hood

Description and Function

- An oxygen hood is a clear plastic dome that encircles the child's head (Figure 5-29). The hood size should be adjusted to the patient's size.
- Used for neonates and infants smaller than 10 kg who will not tolerate a face mask
- Permits control of oxygen concentration, temperature, and humidity
- At 10 to 15 L/min, can deliver an inspired oxygen concentration of approximately 80% to 90%
- An oxygen flow rate of at least 10 L/min is required to flush accumulated CO_2 from inside the hood.

Advantages

- Oxygen concentration can be continuously monitored by means of a meter
- Permits access to the chest, trunk, and extremities for continued care

Disadvantages

- Generally not large enough to be used for children older than 1 year

- "Raining out" on the walls of the hood may obscure the patient's head from observation
- Noisy for the patient

When an infant or child cannot tolerate supplemental oxygen delivery by means of a nasal cannula or face mask, blow-by oxygen may be used. The oxygen tubing or mask should be directed near the child's nose and mouth (Figure 5-30). Consider attaching the oxygen tubing to a toy and encourage the child to hold the toy near the face or try placing the tubing in a paper cup (Figure 5-31), then ask the child to "drink from the cup."

In a recent study,[1] researchers sought to determine the FIO_2 actually administered to patients with blow-by oxygen delivery. Three different methods of oxygen delivery were studied: an infant resuscitator bag, a

Blow-by Oxygen Delivery

When possible, allow the child's caregiver to administer blow-by oxygen.

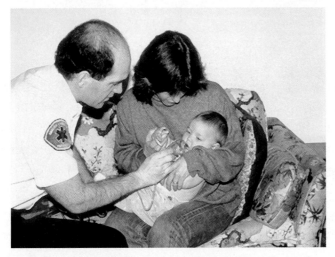

Figure 5-30   When an infant or child cannot tolerate supplemental oxygen delivery by means of a nasal cannula or face mask, blow-by oxygen may be used.

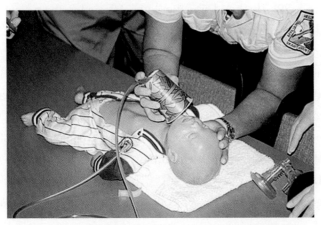

Figure 5-31   When administering blow-by oxygen, consider attaching the oxygen tubing to a toy and encourage the child to hold the toy near the face or try placing the tubing in a paper cup and then ask the child to "drink from the cup."

Device	Approximate Inspired Oxygen Concentration	Liter Flow (L/min)
Nasal cannula	Up to 50%	1 to 6
Simple face mask	35% to 60%	6 to 10
Partial rebreather mask	50% to 60%	10 to 12
Nonrebreather mask	60% to 95%	10 to 15
Face tent	35% to 40%	10 to 15
Oxygen hood	80% to 90%	10 to 15
Blow-by (via face mask)	30% to 40%	10

TABLE 5-3 *Oxygen Percentage Delivery by Device*

standard pediatric face mask, and oxygen tubing. Flow rates of 5 L/min and 10 L/min were used and the oxygen concentration was measured in 10% increments using an oxygen meter. Contour lines of oxygen concentration were constructed for each delivery method.

The researchers determined that the resuscitator bag was unsatisfactory because the flow-back valve may close and result in insignificant levels of oxygen delivery. Oxygen tubing gave a useable area too narrow for use with an active patient, with 30% oxygen concentration being available in an area with a width of only 18 cm. This is, however, a suitable method in short-term attended administration, either during feeding or in the situation of a neonatal resuscitation. At a flow rate of 10 L/min, the pediatric face mask delivered 30% oxygen to an area 35 cm wide × 32 cm from the top of the mask. At 10 L/min, 40% oxygen was delivered to an area 16 cm wide and 14 cm from the top of the mask.

Ventilation Devices

If the patient's respiratory efforts are inadequate, breathing may be assisted by forcing air into the lungs (i.e., delivering positive-pressure ventilation). Several methods may be used to deliver positive-pressure ventilation including mouth-to-mask ventilation and BVM ventilation. Regardless of the method used, effective positive-pressure ventilation requires the delivery of an adequate volume of air at an appropriate rate.

Cricoid Pressure (Sellick Maneuver)

Purpose

Positive-pressure ventilation, especially if performed rapidly, may cause gastric distention. The cricoid cartilage is the most inferior of the laryngeal cartilages and is the only completely cartilaginous ring in the larynx. Compression of the cricoid cartilage pushes the trachea posteriorly, compressing the esophagus against the cervical vertebrae (Figure 5-32). This helps minimize inflation of the stomach during ventilation, reducing the likelihood of vomiting and aspiration.

Technique

Cricoid pressure (also called the Sellick maneuver) is used only in unresponsive patients and is usually applied by an assistant during positive-pressure ventilation.

- Locate the cricoid cartilage.
- Apply pressure on the cricoid cartilage with the thumb and index or middle finger, just lateral to the midline. In an infant or young child, cricoid pressure is applied using only one finger (Figure 5-33).
- During tracheal intubation, do not release cricoid pressure until the tracheal tube is in the trachea, the cuff of the tube is inflated (if a cuffed tracheal tube is used), and proper position of the tube is verified.

Precautions

- If excessive pressure is applied, cricoid pressure can cause complete airway obstruction.
- If active regurgitation occurs while performing cricoid pressure, release cricoid pressure to avoid rupture of the stomach or esophagus.

Description and Function

- The device used for mouth-to-mask ventilation is commonly called a **pocket mask**, pocket face mask, or ventilation face mask.
- A ventilation face mask permits the rescuer to oxygenate and ventilate a patient. The device can be used with an NPA or OPA during spontaneous, assisted, or controlled ventilation.

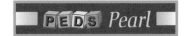

PEDs Pearl

Positive-airway pressure therapy refers to the application of higher than ambient airway pressures during inspiration and/or exhalation for the purpose of improving pulmonary and respiratory function. Positive pressure applied during *inspiration* is usually referred to as positive-pressure ventilation (PPV). Positive pressure applied during *exhalation* is usually referred to as positive end-expiratory pressure (PEEP).[7]

Mouth-to-Mask Ventilation

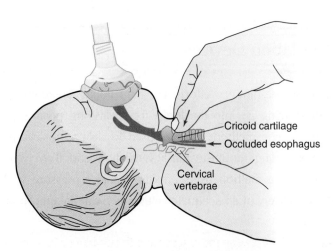

Cricoid cartilage
Occluded esophagus
Cervical vertebrae

Figure 5-32 Compression of the cricoid cartilage pushes the trachea posteriorly, compressing the esophagus against the cervical vertebrae.

Assisted ventilation using a bag-mask or mouth-to-mask device is indicated in the following scenarios:
- The patient is in severe respiratory failure or respiratory arrest.
- High-concentration oxygen does not improve the child's muscle tone, mental status, work of breathing, and respiratory rate.
- You are uncertain about the degree of respiratory compromise.

In the latter case, if the child does not resist assisted ventilation, you can safely assume that the child is sick enough to need it.[2]

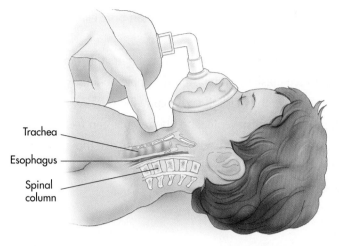

Trachea
Esophagus
Spinal column

Figure 5-33   In an infant or young child, cricoid pressure is applied using only one finger.

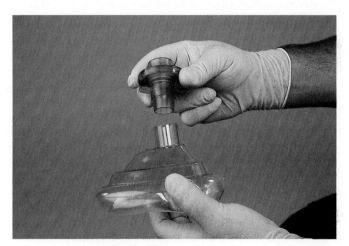

Figure 5-34   A pocket mask should be made of transparent material to allow evaluation of the patient's lip color and detection of blood, vomitus, or secretions and equipped with a one-way valve that diverts the patient's exhaled gas, reducing the risk of infection.

- Ventilation masks may be disposable or reusable. Some have an oxygen inlet on the mask, allowing delivery of supplemental oxygen; others do not.
- A ventilation mask should be made of transparent material to allow evaluation of the patient's lip color and detection of blood, vomitus, or secretions. It should be equipped with a one-way valve to divert the patient's exhaled air, reducing the risk of infection (Figure 5-34).

Advantages
- Aesthetically more acceptable than mouth-to-mouth ventilation.
- Easy to teach and learn.
- Physical barrier between the rescuer and the patient's nose, mouth, and secretions.
- Reduces the risk of exposure to infectious disease.

- Use of a one-way valve at the ventilation port eliminates exposure to patient's exhaled air.
- If the patient resumes spontaneous breathing, the mask can be used as a simple face mask by administering supplemental oxygen through the oxygen inlet on the mask (if so equipped).
- With mouth-to-mask ventilation, the rescuer can feel the **compliance** of the patient's lungs. Compliance refers to the resistance of the patient's lung tissue to ventilation.

Disadvantages

- Rescuer fatigue

Technique

- Using personal protective equipment, position yourself at the top of the supine patient's head. If needed, clear the patient's airway of secretions or vomitus. Open the patient's airway with a head tilt–chin lift or, if trauma is suspected, perform the jaw thrust without head tilt maneuver. If the patient is unresponsive, insert an OPA.
- Select a mask of appropriate size and place it on the patient's face.
  - Ventilation masks are available in a variety of sizes. The mask should have limited dead space and an inflatable rim and should provide a tight seal without pressure on the eyes. A mask of proper size should extend from the bridge of the nose to the crease of the chin (Figure 5-35).
  - Apply the narrow portion (apex) of the mask over the bridge of the patient's nose and stabilize it in place with your thumbs.
  - Lower the mask over the patient's face and mouth.
  - Use the remaining fingers of both hands to stabilize the wide end (base) of the mask over the groove between the lower lip and chin and maintain proper head position.
  - Ventilate the patient through the one-way valve on the top of the mask, and deliver each breath over 1 second (Figure 5-36). Stop ventilation when adequate chest rise is observed. Allow the patient to exhale between breaths.

Description and Function

- The BVM is the most common mechanical aid used to deliver positive-pressure ventilation in emergency care. A BVM may also be referred to as a bag-mask device or bag-mask resuscitator (when the mask is used), or a bag-valve device (when the mask is not used, i.e., when ventilating a patient with a tracheal tube in place).
- A BVM consists of a self-inflating bag; a nonrebreathing valve with an adapter that can be attached to a mask, tracheal tube, or other invasive airway device; and an oxygen inlet valve (Figure 5-37).

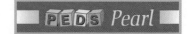
PEDs *Pearl*

Selection of a mask of proper size is essential to ensuring a good seal. If the mask is not properly positioned and a tight seal maintained, air will leak from between the mask and the patient's face, resulting in delivery of less tidal volume and lower oxygen concentrations to the patient.

If the patient is unresponsive and an assistant is available, cricoid pressure may be applied to reduce the risk of vomiting and aspiration.

Bag-Valve-Mask Ventilation

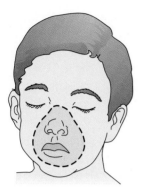

Figure 5-35 A proper-fitting mask should extend from the bridge of the nose to the crease of the chin.

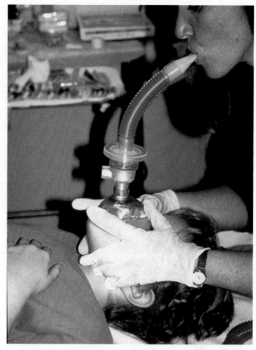

Figure 5-36 When using with a pocket mask, ventilate the patient through the one-way valve on the top of the mask, and deliver slow, steady breaths. Stop ventilation when adequate chest rise is observed.

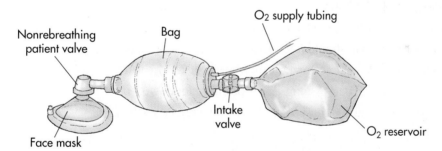

Nonrebreathing patient valve

Bag

O₂ supply tubing

Intake valve

O₂ reservoir

Face mask

Figure 5-37 Components of a bag-valve-mask device.

To disable a pop-off valve, depress the valve with a finger during ventilation or twist the pop-off valve into the closed position.

- The BVM used for resuscitation should have either no pop-off (pressure-release) valve or a pop-off valve that can be disabled during resuscitation (Figure 5-38). Pop-off valves were originally added to pediatric devices to guard against pulmonary hyperinflation and barotrauma. However, some situations require higher ventilatory pressure, such as near-drowning, cardiopulmonary resuscitation (CPR), pulmonary edema, asthma, partial upper airway obstruction, or initial resuscitation of the newly born. To effectively ventilate a patient in these situations, the ventilatory pressure needed may exceed the limits of the pop-off valve. Thus a pop-off valve may prevent generation of sufficient tidal volume to overcome the increase in airway resistance. Disabling the pop-off valve, or using a BVM with no pop-off valve, helps ensure delivery of adequate tidal volumes to the patient during resuscitation.

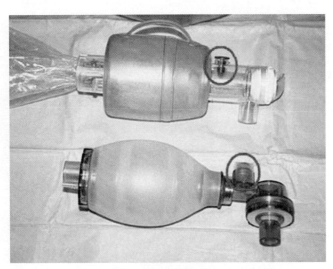

Figure 5-38   These bag-valve-mask devices have pop-off valves. If used for resuscitation, the pop-off valve should be disabled. This can be done by depressing the valve with a finger during ventilation or twisting the pop-off valve into the closed position.

- BVM devices are available in various sizes. It is important to select a device with sufficient volume for the patient's size:
  - At least 450 to 500 mL (pediatric bag) for full-term newly born infants, infants, and children
  - 1200 mL (adult bag) for larger children and adolescents
  - A 250-mL (neonatal) bag should not be used because this size does not provide sufficient volume for term newborns. A child can be ventilated with a larger bag as long as proper technique is used—squeeze the bag just until the chest begins to rise, then release the bag.

Oxygen Delivery
- A BVM used without supplemental oxygen will deliver 21% oxygen (room air) to the patient (Figure 5-39).
- A BVM should be connected to an oxygen source. Attach one end of a piece of oxygen connecting tubing to the oxygen inlet on the BVM and the other end to an oxygen regulator.
  - A pediatric BVM used with supplemental oxygen set at a flow rate of 10 L/min will deliver approximately 30% to 80% oxygen to the patient.
  - An adult BVM used with supplemental oxygen set at a flow rate of 15 L/min will deliver approximately 40% to 60% oxygen to the patient (Figure 5-40).
- An oxygen-collecting device (reservoir) should be attached to the BVM to consistently deliver high-concentration oxygen. The reservoir collects a volume of 100% oxygen equal to the capacity of the bag. After squeezing the bag, the bag reexpands, drawing in 100% oxygen from the reservoir into the bag.

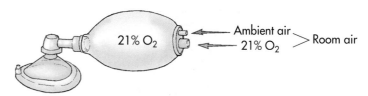

Figure 5-39   A bag-valve-mask used without supplemental oxygen will deliver 21% oxygen (room air) to the patient.

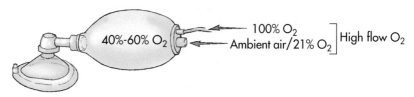

Figure 5-40   An adult bag-valve-mask used with supplemental oxygen set at a flow rate of 15 L/min will deliver approximately 40% to 60% oxygen to the patient.

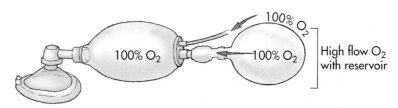

Figure 5-41   An adult BVM used with supplemental oxygen (set at a flow rate of 15 L/min) and an attached reservoir will deliver approximately 90% to 100% oxygen to the patient.

- A pediatric BVM used with supplemental oxygen (set at a flow rate of 10 to 15 L/min) and an attached reservoir will deliver approximately 60% to 95% oxygen to the patient.
- An adult BVM used with supplemental oxygen (set at a flow rate of 15 L/min) and an attached reservoir will deliver approximately 90% to 100% oxygen to the patient (Figure 5-41).

Advantages

- Provides a means for delivery of an oxygen-enriched mixture to the patient
- Conveys a sense of compliance of the patient's lungs to the BVM operator
- Provides a means for immediate ventilatory support
- Can be used with the spontaneously breathing patient as well as the apneic patient

Disadvantages

- The most frequent problem with the BVM is the inability to provide adequate ventilatory volumes. This is due to the difficulty in providing a leak-proof seal to the face while simultaneously maintaining an open airway.

PEDS *Pearl*

Gastric distention is a complication of positive-pressure ventilation that can lead to regurgitation and subsequent aspiration. Gastric distention also restricts movement of the diaphragm, impeding ventilation. Insertion of a gastric tube to alleviate gastric distention is recommended when the patient requires BVM ventilation (Figure 5-42).

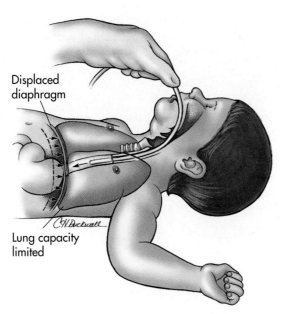

Displaced
diaphragm

Lung capacity
limited

Figure 5-42   Gastric distention, which interferes with
ventilation by causing pressure on the
diaphragm, can be relieved by placement of
an orogastric tube.

- Difficult to use by inexperienced operators
- Gastric distention

BVM Ventilation: Technique

- Using personal protective equipment, position yourself at the top of the supine patient's head.
- Select an appropriate bag for ventilation based on the patient's size.
  - The bag should have an oxygen reservoir.
  - Connect one end of the oxygen tubing to an oxygen source and the other end to an oxygen flow meter. Set the flow meter to the appropriate liter flow.
- Open the patient's airway using a head tilt–chin lift or, if trauma is suspected, perform the jaw thrust without head tilt maneuver. If needed, clear the patient's airway of secretions or vomitus.
- If the patient is unresponsive, insert an oral airway.
- Select a mask of appropriate size and place it on the patient's face. Apply the narrow portion (apex) of the mask over the bridge of the patient's nose and the wide end (base) of the mask over the groove between the lower lip and chin. If the mask has a large, round cuff surrounding a ventilation port, center the port over the mouth.
- One-handed technique ("E-C clamp")
  - Stabilize the mask in place with your thumb and index finger, creating a "C" (Figure 5-43).
  - With gentle pressure, push down on the mask to establish an adequate seal.

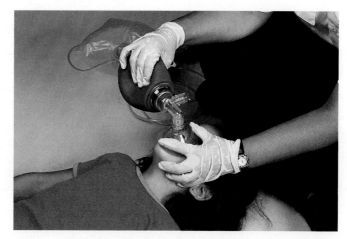

Figure 5-43   One-handed bag-valve-mask ventilation using the "E-C clamp" technique.

Avoid compressing the soft tissues of the face and neck and ensure that the mask does not compress the eyes.

If the patient is unresponsive and an assistant is available, cricoid pressure may be applied to reduce the risk of vomiting and aspiration.

- Place your third, fourth, and fifth fingers along the patient's jaw, forming an "**E**." Use these fingers to lift the jaw along the bony portion of the mandible.
- Connect the bag to the mask (if not already done) and ensure the bag is connected to oxygen.
- Squeeze the bag with your other hand (or with one hand and your arm or chest if necessary).
- Begin by delivering two ventilations, allowing 1 second per breath, while watching for chest rise.
  - If the chest rises, assess for the presence of a pulse. If a pulse is present, resume ventilation. If there is no pulse or other signs of circulation, or if the heart rate is less than 60 beats per minute with signs of poor perfusion, begin chest compressions.
  - If the chest does not rise, reassess the patient's head position, reposition the airway, and attempt to ventilate again.
- Ventilate with the correct tidal volume. Squeeze the bag gently. As soon as chest rise is visible, release the bag. Wait for the chest to fall before ventilating again.
- Ventilate at a rate of 12 to 20 breaths/minute (1 breath every 3 to 5 seconds).
- Two-handed technique
  - BVM ventilation is optimally a two-rescuer operation—one to hold the mask to the face (ensuring a good mask to face seal) and maintain an open airway, the other to compress the bag with two hands.
  - Ask an assistant to squeeze the bag with two hands until the patient's

TABLE 5-4 *Selection of Appropriate Resuscitation Bag and Oxygen Mask Size Based on Broselow Resuscitation Tape*

Age	Weight (kg)	Resuscitation Bag	Oxygen Mask
Newborn /small infant (0 to 3 mo)	3 to 5	Infant	Newborn
Infant (3 to 6 mo)	6 to 7	Child	Newborn
Infant (7 to 10 mo)	8 to 9	Child	Newborn/Pediatric
Toddler (11 to 18 mo)	10 to 11	Child	Pediatric
Small child (19 to 35 mo)	12 to 14	Child	Pediatric
Child (3 to 4 y)	15 to 18	Child	Pediatric
Child (5 to 6 y)	19 to 22	Child	Pediatric
Large child (7 to 9 y)	24 to 30	Child/adult	Adult
Adult (10 to 12 y)	32 to 40	Adult	Adult

chest begins to rise while you press the mask firmly against the patient's face with both hands and simultaneously maintain proper head position.

- Assess the effectiveness of ventilation
  - ◦ Ensure the mask forms an airtight seal on the patient's face.
  - ◦ Evaluate lung compliance (resistance to ventilation).
  - ◦ Observe the rise and fall of the patient's chest with each ventilation.
  - ◦ Assess for an improvement in the color of the patient's skin or mucous membranes.
  - ◦ Assess for an improvement in the patient's mental status, heart rate, perfusion, and blood pressure.
  - ◦ Auscultate for bilateral breath sounds.

Troubleshooting Bag-Valve-Mask Ventilation
- If the chest does not rise with BVM ventilation, ventilation is not effective—either the airway is obstructed or more volume or pressure is needed to provide effective ventilation.
  - ◦ A common problem when ventilating with a BVM device is placing the mask tightly on the face without performing an adequate maneuver to open the patient's airway. This results in an airway obstruction because of improper airway positioning. Readjust the patient's head position, ensure the mouth is open, and reattempt to ventilate.
- Inadequate tidal volume delivery may be the result of gastric distention, improper mask seal, or incomplete bag compression.
  - ◦ Gastric distention may cause regurgitation with a risk of subsequent aspiration. Gastric distention may also impair movement of the diaphragm, resulting in inadequate ventilation. Insert an orogastric or nasogastric tube to decompress the stomach.

Increasing resistance during positive-pressure ventilation suggests airway obstruction.

Bag-Valve-Mask Ventilation

The pressure and volume delivered by a bag-valve-mask device depends on the following:
- The set-point of the pop-off (pressure-release) valve, if present.
- How hard the bag is squeezed.
- Any leak present between the mask and the patient's face.

According to the 2005 resuscitation guidelines, an orogastric or nasogastric tube should be inserted *after* placement of an endotracheal (ET) tube. If a gastric tube is inserted before the ET tube, the gastric tube can interfere with the gastroesophageal sphincter and may result in vomiting.

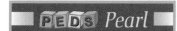

The pediatric patient ranges in size and weight from the newly born to 18 years of age. When considering pediatric equipment needed for resuscitation or for a procedure, plan to have a range of equipment sizes available to accommodate these variations in size and weight.

- ○ An inadequate mask seal may result in hypoxia or hypoventilation.
  - If air is escaping from under the mask, reposition your fingers and the mask.
  - If the leak persists:
    - Ask for assistance with the patient's airway.
    - Consider using another mask.
    - Use the two-handed technique.
- ○ Remember that in certain situations (e.g., severe asthma, cardio-pulmonary arrest), higher than normal inspiratory pressures may be required for adequate ventilation. Check to see if the BVM has a pop-off valve. If a pop-off valve is present, disable the valve and attempt to ventilate again.
- Reevaluate the effectiveness of bag compression.
  - ○ Check for obstruction.
  - ○ Lift the jaw.
  - ○ Suction the airway as needed.
- If the chest still does not rise, suspect an airway obstruction.

Tracheal Intubation

Tracheal intubation is an advanced airway procedure in which a tube is placed directly into the trachea. This procedure requires special training and frequent refresher training to maintain skill proficiency.

Description and Function

For prehospital professionals with short transport times, oxygenation and ventilation of the patient using a bag-valve-mask device is recommended instead of tracheal intubation because of the high incidence of misplaced and displaced tracheal tubes.

Tracheal intubation may be performed for a variety of reasons including the delivery of anesthesia, assisting a patient's breathing with positive-pressure ventilation, and protection of the patient's airway from aspiration.

Special equipment and supplies are required including a laryngoscope handle, laryngoscope blades, extra batteries, tracheal tubes of various sizes, a 10-mL syringe for inflation of the tracheal tube cuff (if present), a stylet, a BVM device with supplemental oxygen and a reservoir, suction equipment, a commercial tube holder or tape, water-soluble lubricant, a bite-block or OPA, and an end-tidal carbon dioxide ($ETCO_2$) detector and/or esophageal detector. Pulse oximetry and electrocardiogram (ECG) monitoring should be performed throughout this procedure.

- Laryngoscope
  - ○ A laryngoscope is an instrument that consists of a handle and blade used for examining the interior of the larynx, specifically visualization of the glottic opening (the space between the vocal cords).
  - ○ A standard laryngoscope is made of plastic or stainless steel. The laryngoscope handle contains the batteries for the light source.

- Attaches to a plastic or stainless steel blade that has a bulb located in the blade's distal tip. The point where the handle and the blade attach to make electrical contact is called the fitting.
- The bulb on the laryngoscope blade lights when the blade is attached to the laryngoscope handle and elevated to a right angle.
- Laryngoscope blades
  - There are two primary types of laryngoscope blades—straight and curved (Figure 5-44).
  - The straight blade is also referred to as the Miller, Wisconsin, or Flagg blade.
    - During orotracheal intubation, the tip of the straight blade is positioned under the epiglottis. When the laryngoscope handle is lifted anteriorly, the blade directly lifts the epiglottis out of the way to expose the glottic opening.
    - A straight blade should be used when intubating a child younger than 8 years. The straight blade is preferred because
      - The straight blade provides greater movement of the large tongue into the floor of the mouth and visualization of the glottic opening.
      - A curved blade may not adequately control and retract a child's longer, more pliable epiglottis to permit a clear view of the glottic opening.[2]
  - The curved blade is also called the MacIntosh blade.
    - It is inserted into the vallecula, the space (or "pocket") between the base of the tongue and the epiglottis.
    - When the laryngoscope handle is lifted anteriorly, the blade elevates the tongue and indirectly lifts the epiglottis, allowing visualization of the glottic opening.

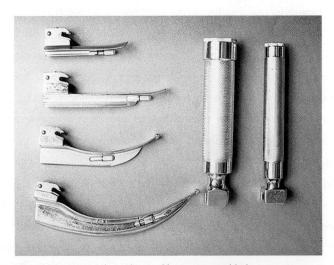

Figure 5-44   Straight and curved laryngoscope blades.

- Select the appropriate blade size with the laryngoscope blade held next to the patient's face.
    - Blades are available in a variety of sizes ranging from 0 to 4.
    - A blade of proper size should reach between the patient's lips and larynx.
    - If unsure of the correct size, it is usually best to select a blade that is too long, rather than too short.
- Tracheal tube
    - A tracheal tube is a curved tube that is open at both ends. A standard 15-mm connector is located at the proximal end for attachment of a device for delivery of positive-pressure ventilation.
    - The distal end of the tube is beveled to facilitate placement between the vocal cords.
    - The distal end may include a Murphy eye (a hole in the side wall of the tube). This helps prevent complete tube occlusion if the tracheal tube should become blocked.
    - Tracheal tubes are measured in millimeters (mm) by their ID and external diameter (OD). Centimeter markings on the tracheal tube are used as reference points.
        - Aids in placement of the tracheal tube.
        - Assists in detecting accidental displacement of the tube.
    - Some tracheal tubes have an inflatable balloon cuff that surrounds the distal tip of the tube. When the distal cuff is inflated, it contacts the wall of the trachea as it expands, sealing off the trachea from the remainder of the pharynx, reducing the risk of aspiration. The cuff is attached to a one-way valve through a side tube with a pilot balloon that is used to indicate if the cuff is inflated.
    - Tracheal tubes are available in lengths ranging from 12 to 32 cm. Internal tube diameters range from 2.5 to 4.5 mm (uncuffed) and 5.0 to 10.0 mm (cuffed).
- Stylet
    - A stylet is a flexible plastic-coated wire inserted into a tracheal tube used for molding and maintaining the shape of the tube during intubation. A stylet may be needed with smaller-sized tracheal tubes because of their thin structure.
    - If a stylet is used, be sure the stylet is free of kinks to allow easy removal after successful intubation. Some advocate lubrication of the stylet with a water-soluble lubricant before placement in the tracheal tube. This aids removal once the tube has been placed, avoiding accidental extubation. A petroleum-based lubricant should never be used because it may damage the tracheal tube and cause tracheal inflammation.

According to the 2005 resuscitation guidelines, cuffed ET tubes are as safe as uncuffed ET tubes in the in-hospital setting for infants beyond the newborn period and in children.

The length of a tracheal tube is directly related to its ID. The larger the ID, the longer the tube.

Cooling the tracheal tube (while still in its sterile container) until just before use may eliminate the need for a stylet.

- Isolates the airway
- Keeps the airway patent
- Reduces the risk of aspiration of gastric contents
- Ensures delivery of a high concentration of oxygen
- Permits suctioning of the trachea
- Provides a route for administration of some medications ("ALONE": atropine, lidocaine, oxygen, naloxone, epinephrine)
- Ensures delivery of a selected tidal volume to maintain lung inflation

- Considerable training and experience required
- Special equipment needed
- Bypasses physiologic function of upper airway (e.g., warming, filtering, humidifying of inhaled air)
- Requires direct visualization of vocal cords

Advantages

Disadvantages

Using personal protective equipment (at a minimum, use gloves, protective eyewear, and a mask), open the patient's airway with a head tilt–chin lift (or jaw thrust without head tilt if trauma is suspected).

1. Oxygenate and ventilate the patient.
   - Ask an assistant to preoxygenate the patient while you auscultate bilateral lung sounds to establish a baseline. Preoxygenation is particularly important in children because they have less oxygen reserve in their lungs and their metabolic oxygen consumption is proportionately greater than that in adults.
     ◦ If possible, avoid using a BVM for ventilation to reduce the risk of gastric distention and possible regurgitation. If the patient is breathing spontaneously and ventilations are adequate, deliver 100% oxygen by face mask.
     ◦ If ventilation by BVM is necessary, apply cricoid pressure. Cricoid pressure must be maintained until tracheal tube placement is confirmed. To avoid the possibility of esophageal rupture, release cricoid pressure if the patient actively vomits.
   - Place the patient on a cardiac monitor and attach the pulse oximeter.
2. Prepare the equipment.
   - While your assistant continues to preoxygenate the patient, assemble and prepare the equipment needed for intubation, including suction equipment.
   - Select the proper size blade and then assemble the laryngoscope. Attach the blade to the handle and check the blade for a "white, bright, light." After verifying the light is in working order, move the blade to its unlocked position to conserve battery life until the light is needed.

Technique

The 12 Steps of Pediatric Tracheal Intubation[2]
1. Oxygenate and ventilate the patient
2. Prepare the equipment
3. Position the patient
4. Provide suctioning and oxygenation
5. Open the patient's mouth
6. Control the patient's tongue
7. Control the patient's epiglottis
8. Locate landmarks for intubation
9. Insert the tracheal tube
10. Confirm correct placement
11. Secure the tube in place
12. Resume oxygenation and ventilation

The *minimum* equipment prerequisites that must be present to ensure a safe intubation can be remembered by the mnemonic "SALTT": Suction, Airway (oral), Laryngoscope, Tube and Tape (or Tube holder).

- Select the proper size tracheal tube.
  - If a cuffed tracheal tube is used, test the cuff for leaks. If there are no leaks, completely deflate the cuff. Refill the syringe with air and leave the syringe attached to the inflation valve on the tracheal tube.
  - Be sure to have at least two additional tracheal tube sizes available (one 0.5 mm smaller and one 0.5 mm larger than the selected size).

A petroleum-based lubricant should never be used because it may damage the tracheal tube and cause tracheal inflammation.

- If a stylet will be used, insert it into the tracheal tube, making sure that the end of the stylet is recessed at least 0.5 cm from the tip of the tracheal tube.
  - Bend the proximal end of the stylet over the tracheal tube to prevent it from sliding down into the tube. Lubricate the distal end of the tracheal tube with water-soluble lubricant.
  - Bend the tracheal tube and stylet into a gentle curve to help place the distal end of the tube into the glottic opening during intubation.

Do not place the patient's head in a sniffing position if trauma is suspected.

3. Position the patient.
  - To achieve direct visualization of the laryngeal opening, the three axes of the pharynx-glottis, glottis-trachea, and mouth-pharynx must be aligned. Proper positioning of the patient's head and neck will vary depending on the patient's age and clinical situation.
  - The smaller the child, the greater the proportion between the size of the cranium and midface and the greater the propensity of the posterior pharyngeal area to "buckle" as the relatively large occiput forces passive flexion of the cervical spine.[4]

In the sniffing position, hyperflexion occurs at C5 to C6 and hyperextension at C1 to C2.

  - In the absence of trauma, use the sniffing position to align the axes of the airway. In the sniffing position, the child looks as if he is putting his head forward to sniff a flower.
  - To achieve this position, elevate the child's head 3 to 4 inches (8 to 10 cm) and tilt it posteriorly. Do not hyperextend the neck, particularly when positioning infants and young children, who have a prominent occiput. Hyperextension may cause the tracheal rings to collapse and interfere with ventilation.
    - When placing an obese adolescent patient in the sniffing position, padding may need to be placed under the shoulders and head.
    - If trauma to the head, neck, or spine is suspected, do **not** place the patient in the sniffing position. Instead, use an assistant to keep the head and neck in a neutral, in-line position throughout the procedure.

4. Provide suctioning and oxygenation.

- If necessary, suction the patient's mouth and pharynx of secretions. After suctioning, ventilate the patient with high-concentration oxygen for at least 30 seconds.
- Stop ventilations and remove the ventilation face mask and OPA (if present). Do not exceed 30 seconds from ventilation to ventilation for each intubation attempt.
- Direct an assistant to apply cricoid pressure and maintain pressure until the airway is secured. If the patient begins to vomit, discontinue cricoid pressure until vomiting stops and the airway has been cleared.

5. Open the patient's mouth.
- Open the patient's mouth by applying thumb pressure on the chin. Alternatively, an unresponsive patient's mouth may be opened using the crossed-finger method.
  ◦ Cross the fingers and thumb of your nondominant hand.
  ◦ Press your thumb against the child's upper teeth and your fingers against the lower teeth and push them apart.

6. Control the patient's tongue.
- The flange and tip of the laryngoscope blade are used to control the tongue and epiglottis.
- Holding the laryngoscope in the left hand and with the tip of the blade pointing away from you, insert the blade into the right side of the patient's mouth, sweeping the tongue to the left.
  ◦ If the tongue is not pushed far enough to the left, your view of the glottic opening will be obscured.
  ◦ If the blade is initially placed in the middle of the tongue (instead of the right side of the mouth), the tongue will fold over the lateral edge of the blade and obscure your view of the glottic opening.
- The laryngoscope is held in the left hand because most laryngoscopes are designed for right-handed individuals. This allows the dominant (right) hand to be used for manipulation of the tracheal tube.
- Advance the laryngoscope blade slowly along the tongue until the distal end reaches the base of the tongue. Lift the laryngoscope to elevate the mandible without putting pressure on the front teeth and visualize the glottis. Do NOT use the patient's teeth or gums as a fulcrum. Do not allow the blade to touch the patient's teeth.

7. Control the patient's epiglottis.
- After visualizing the epiglottis, place the blade in the proper position.
- If you are using a straight blade, advance the tip under the epiglottis. If you are using a curved blade, advance the tip of the blade into the vallecula.

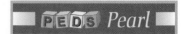
PEDs Pearl

If cervical spine injury is suspected, an assistant should manually maintain the head and neck in a neutral position throughout the intubation procedure. To maintain the cervical spine in a neutral position, it is often necessary to place padding under the child's torso. The padding should be firm, evenly shaped, and extend from the shoulders to the pelvis. For an infant or young child, the padding should be of appropriate thickness so that the child's shoulders are in horizontal alignment with the ear canal (see Chapter 9).

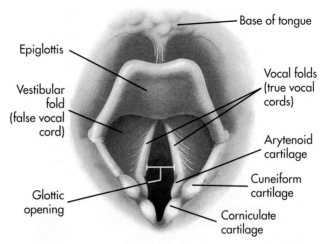

Figure 5-47   Landmarks for tracheal intubation.

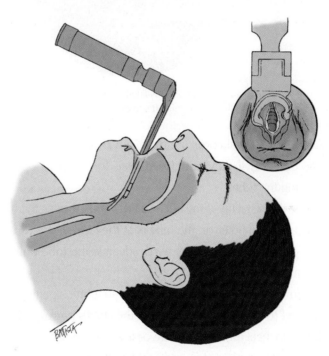

Figure 5-48   When the straight blade is lifted anteriorly, the blade directly lifts the epiglottis out of the way to expose the glottic opening.

8. Locate landmarks for intubation (Figure 5-47).
   - When the straight blade is lifted anteriorly, the blade directly lifts the epiglottis out of the way to expose the glottic opening (Figure 5-48).
   - When the curved blade is lifted anteriorly, the blade indirectly lifts the epiglottis to expose the glottic opening (Figure 5-49).
   - Visualize the vocal cords.
9. Insert the tracheal tube.
   - While holding the laryngoscope steady with your left hand, grasp the tracheal tube with your right hand and gently introduce it into the right corner of the patient's mouth.

Do not attempt to pass the tracheal tube through the channel in the laryngoscope blade. Doing so will obstruct your view of the glottic opening.

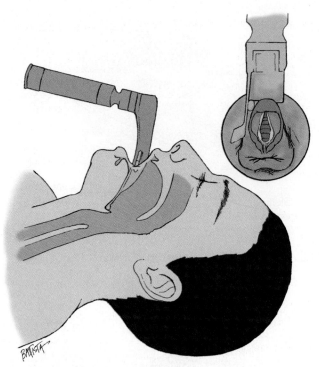

Figure 5-49   When the curved blade is lifted anteriorly, the blade indirectly lifts the epiglottis to expose the glottic opening.

- If the patient's vocal cords are open, advance the tube through the glottic opening. If they are closed, wait for them to open before advancing the tube.
- Visualize the distal tip of the tracheal tube and advance the tube until the vocal cord marker on the tube is at the level of the vocal cords.
  - If a cuffed tracheal tube is used, advance the tube until the cuff lies just beyond the vocal cords.
  - If you cannot advance the tube into the glottic opening, the tube may be too large to pass through the child's narrow cricoid ring.
  - If the tracheal tube is too large or if you were unable to visualize the glottic opening, stop and ventilate the patient using the BVM before trying again. Reposition the airway if necessary.
  - If the same problems are encountered during a second attempt, discontinue intubation attempts and resume BVM ventilation.
- While holding the tracheal tube firmly with your thumb and index finger against the child's lip or upper gum, remove the laryngoscope blade from the patient's mouth.
- While continuing to hold the tracheal tube in place, remove the stylet from the tracheal tube (if used).
- If a cuffed tracheal tube was used, inflate the distal cuff with air, and then disconnect the syringe from the inflation valve.
  - Check the pilot balloon on the tracheal tube to verify inflation.
- Detach the face mask from the BVM device. Attach the bag-valve-

PEDS *Pearl*

Viewing the vocal cords may be facilitated with the use of the BURP (*B*ackward, *U*pward, *R*ightward *P*ressure) technique. With this maneuver, the larynx is displaced in three specific directions (a) posteriorly against the cervical vertebrae, (b) superiorly as possible, and (c) slightly laterally to the right. This maneuver has been shown to improve visualization of the larynx more easily than simple back pressure on the larynx (cricoid pressure) because the back-up-right pressure moves the larynx back to the position from which it was displaced by a right-handed (held in the operator's left hand) laryngoscope.

mask device to the tracheal tube and ventilate the patient at an age-appropriate rate.

- If a cuffed tracheal tube was used, the distal cuff should be inflated just until the air leak heard during ventilation disappears.

10. Confirm correct placement.

- While holding the tube securely against the corner of the patient's mouth, use primary and secondary methods to confirm proper placement of a tracheal tube.

- **Primary** methods include clinical assessments.

- Visualize the passage of the tracheal tube between the vocal cords.
- Visualize symmetrical chest rise during positive-pressure ventilation.
- Confirm the absence of sounds over the epigastrium during positive-pressure ventilation.

  - After intubation, the presence of bubbling or gurgling sounds during auscultation of the epigastrium suggests the tube is incorrectly positioned in the esophagus. To correct this problem, deflate the tracheal tube cuff (if a cuffed tube was used), remove the tube, and preoxygenate before reattempting intubation.
  - Breath sounds may be heard over the stomach in infants but should not be louder than midaxillary sounds.

- Auscultate for bilateral breath sounds.

  - Auscultate for breath sounds in the second or third intercostal space in the anterior axillary line. Listen for two breaths on the right side of the chest, and then listen to the left side and compare.
  - If baseline breath sounds (i.e., breath sounds before intubation) were equal bilaterally, diminished breath sounds on the left side after intubation suggests that the tracheal tube has entered the right mainstem bronchus (Figure 5-50). To correct this problem, auscultate the left side of the chest while slowly withdrawing the tube until breath sounds are equal and chest expansion is symmetric.
  - If baseline breath sounds were equal bilaterally and are absent bilaterally after intubation, the tracheal tube is most likely in the esophagus. To correct this problem, deflate the tracheal tube cuff (if a cuffed tube was used), remove the tube, and preoxygenate before reattempting intubation.

- Absence of vocal sounds after placement of the tracheal tube
- Assess the child's skin color and heart rate. If poor skin color and bradycardia persist after intubation, consider the following possible causes:

  - The tracheal tube is too small, allowing air leaks.

Fogging or vapor condensation on the inside of the tracheal tube is **not** a reliable indicator of proper tube position.

If an uncuffed tracheal tube of appropriate size is used, a small air leak will be detectable during ventilation. If a significant air leak is detectable, the tube is too small and may need to be replaced. If no air leak is detectable, the tube is too large. A tube that is too large may result in excessive pressure at the cricoid cartilage and contribute to the development of laryngeal edema or stenosis. The tube may need to be replaced.

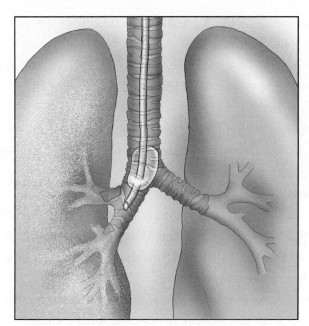

Figure 5-50   Right mainstem bronchus intubation with a cuffed tracheal tube.

- The tracheal tube cuff (if used) is underinflated.
- The pop-off valve on the bag-valve-mask device is not disabled.
- The bag-valve-mask device operator is not delivering an adequate volume for each breath.
- A pneumothorax is present.
- The tracheal tube is clogged or kinked.
- Esophageal intubation.
- Mainstem bronchus intubation.
- There is a leak (or other malfunction) in the bag-valve-mask device (mechanical failure).
- Disconnected oxygen source (mechanical failure).

- *Secondary* methods include the use of a mechanical device.
  - Monitor for changes in the color (colorimetric device) or number (digital device) on an $ETCO_2$ detector (discussed later in this chapter).
  - Verify tube placement with an EDD.
    - EDDs are simple, inexpensive, and easy to use. An EDD is used as an aid in determining if a tracheal tube is in the trachea or esophagus.
    - These devices operate under the principle that the esophagus is a collapsible tube and the trachea a rigid one.
    - The syringe-type EDD is connected to a tracheal tube with the plunger fully inserted into the barrel of the syringe. If the tracheal tube is in the trachea, the plunger can be easily withdrawn from the syringe barrel.

An esophageal detector device (EDD) may be used in children 5 years or older or those who weigh more than 20 kg.

Displaced tube (e.g., right mainstem or esophageal intubation): Reassess tube position
Obstructed tube (e.g., blood or secretions are obstructing air flow): Suction
Pneumothorax (tension): Needle thoracostomy
Equipment problem/failure: Check equipment and oxygen source

PEDS *Pearl*

Movement of the head and neck of an intubated infant or child can affect the placement of the tube. Reassess and confirm the position of the tube
• Immediately after tube insertion
• Whenever the patient is moved or repositioned
• Whenever a procedure is performed (e.g., suctioning, tracheal medication administration)
• When there is a change in the patient's clinical status
• During transport

• If the tracheal tube is in the esophagus, the walls of the esophagus will collapse when negative pressure is applied to the syringe, preventing air from being drawn out of the device.
■ The bulb-type EDD is compressed before it is connected to a tracheal tube (Figure 5-51). A vacuum is created as the pressure on the bulb is released.
  • If the tracheal tube is in the trachea, the bulb will refill easily when pressure is released, indicating proper tube placement. If the tracheal tube is in the esophagus, the bulb will remain collapsed, indicating improper tube placement.
■ Special considerations
  • Results may be misleading in patients with morbid obesity or status asthmaticus, in the presence of copious tracheal secretions, and in patients in late pregnancy.
  • The EDD appears to be unreliable in infants younger than 1 year.
  • If an EDD is used to confirm placement of a cuffed tracheal tube, do NOT inflate the cuff before using the esophageal detector. Inflating the cuff moves the distal end of the tracheal tube away from the walls of the esophagus. If the tube was inadvertently inserted into the esophagus, this movement will cause the detector bulb to reexpand, falsely suggesting that the tube was in the trachea.

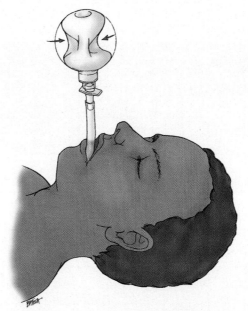

Figure 5-51 When using a bulb-type esophageal detector device, the bulb is compressed before it is connected to a tracheal tube.

○ On chest radiography, the tip of the tracheal tube should be positioned midway between the vocal cords and the carina.

11. Secure the tube in place.
- Secure the tracheal tube with a commercial tube holder or tape and provide ventilatory support with supplemental oxygen.
- After securing the tube, reassess to ensure the tracheal tube is in proper position.
- Record the tube depth at the patient's teeth.

12. Resume oxygenation and ventilation.

- Bleeding
- Laryngospasm
- Vocal cord damage
- Mucosal necrosis
- Barotrauma
- Aspiration
- Cuff leak
- Esophageal intubation
- Right mainstem intubation

Tracheal Intubation: Complications

TABLE 5-5 *Equipment Selection for Pediatric Tracheal Intubation Based on Broselow Resuscitation Tape*

Age	Weight (kg)	Blade Size	Blade Type	Tracheal Tube Size (mm)	Tracheal Tube Cuff	Tracheal Tube Length (cm at lip)	Stylet (F)
Newborn /small infant (0 to 3 mo)	3 to 5	0 to 1	Straight	2.5 to 3.5*	Uncuffed	10 to 10.5	6
Infant (3 to 6 mo)	6 to 7	1	Straight	3.5	Uncuffed	10 to 10.5	6
Infant (7 to 10 mo)	8 to 9	1	Straight	3.5 to 4.0	Uncuffed	10.5 to 12	6
Toddler (11 to 18 mo)	10 to 11	1	Straight	4.0	Uncuffed	11 to 12	6
Small child (19 to 35 mo)	12 to 14	2	Straight	4.5	Uncuffed	12.5 to 13.5	6
Child (3 to 4 y)	15 to 18	2	Straight or curved	5.0	Uncuffed	14 to 15	6
Child (5 to 6 y)	19 to 22	2	Straight or curved	5.5	Uncuffed	15.5 to 16.5	14
Large child (7 to 9 y)	24 to 30	2 to 3	Straight or curved	6.0	Cuffed	17 to 18	14
Adult (10 to 12 y)	32 to 40	3	Straight or curved	6.5	Cuffed	18.5 to 19.5	14

*Use 2.5 for premature infant. Use 3.0 to 3.5 for term infant.

- Occlusion caused by patient biting the tube or secretions
- Laryngeal or tracheal edema
- Tube occlusion
- Hypoxia due to prolonged or unsuccessful intubation
- Dysrhythmias
- Trauma to the lips, teeth, tongue or soft tissues of the oropharynx
- Increased intracranial pressure

Devices to Monitor Respiratory Function

Pulse Oximetry:
Description

When using a pulse oximeter, check that the pulse rate according to the oximeter is consistent with that obtained by palpation to ensure an accurate measurement. Be aware that tissue injury may occur at the measuring site because of probe misuse (e.g., pressure sores from prolonged application).

- **Pulse oximetry** (SpO_2) is a noninvasive method of monitoring the percentage of hemoglobin (Hb) that is saturated with oxygen by using selected wavelengths of light. A pulse oximeter consists of a probe that is placed over thin tissue with reasonably good blood flow (such as a finger, toe, or ear lobe) and connected to a computerized unit. The unit displays the percentage of Hb saturated with oxygen and provides an audible signal for each heartbeat, a calculated heart rate, and in some models, a graphic display of the blood flow past the probe.
- The probe consists of two light–emitting diodes (LEDs) and a photo detector. One LED transmits red light and the other transmits infrared light. Both lights flash through the blood onto the photo detector.
- Hb absorbs red and infrared light waves differently when it is bound with oxygen (oxyhemoglobin) than when it is not (deoxygenated or reduced Hb). Oxyhemoglobin absorbs more infrared light and allows more red light to pass through the blood. Deoxygenated Hb absorbs more red light and allows more infrared light to pass through. From this ratio, the pulse oximeter calculates Hb saturation. This calculation is called the saturation of peripheral oxygen or SpO_2.
- A pulse oximeter is an adjunct to, not a replacement for, vigilant patient assessment. It is essential to correlate your assessment findings with pulse oximeter readings to determine appropriate treatment interventions for your patient.
  - A pulse oximeter reading of 95% to 100% suggests adequate peripheral arterial oxygenation.
  - A reading between 91% and 95% suggests mild hypoxia.
  - A reading lower than 91% suggests severe hypoxia.

Indications

Continuous monitoring of oxygen saturation by means of pulse oximetry is considered the standard of care in any circumstance in which detection of hypoxemia is important. However, in critical situations, do not delay lifesaving interventions to initiate pulse oximetry.

Pulse oximetry should be used in the following scenarios:

- For infants and children exhibiting abnormal findings involving the work of breathing, respiratory rate, or mental status
- For infants and children with a history of respiratory difficulty or chronic pulmonary disease, such as asthma
- During and after delivery of supplemental oxygen
- During and after tracheal intubation
- During transport of a sick or injured child

- Pulse oximetry does not provide information about hypocapnia, hypercapnia, or acid-base disturbances.
- A pulse oximeter reading may be misleading in the following circumstances:
  - Presence of abnormal Hb (methemoglobin [congenital or due to drug exposure], carboxyhemoglobin [carbon monoxide poisoning], fetal Hb)
  - Presence of intravenous (IV) dyes (e.g., methylene blue, indocyanine green)
  - Sickle cell disease
  - Low peripheral perfusion states (e.g., severe hypotension, hypothermia, use of vasoconstrictive drugs, cardiac failure, some cardiac dysrhythmias)
  - Increased venous pulsations
  - Excessive ambient light on sensor probe
  - Patient movement, shivering
  - Patient use of nail polish

Because pulsatile blood flow is necessary for a pulse oximeter to work, it may provide inaccurate results in a child with poor peripheral perfusion. Pulse oximetry may also be inaccurate in children with chronic hypoxemia (e.g., cyanotic heart disease, pulmonary hypertension).

Limitations

A pulse oximeter measures oxygen saturation, but does not measure CO_2. Therefore a pulse oximeter does not measure the effectiveness of ventilation.

- **Capnography:** Continuous analysis and recording of CO_2 concentrations in respiratory gases.
- **Capnometry:** Measurement of CO_2 concentrations without a continuous written record or waveform.
- **Capnometer:** Device used to measure the concentration of CO_2 at the end of exhalation.
- **End-tidal CO_2 (ETCO$_2$) detector:** Capnometer that provides a noninvasive estimate of alveolar ventilation, the concentration of exhaled CO_2 from the lungs, and arterial CO_2 content

Exhaled or End-Tidal Carbon Dioxide (ETCO$_2$) Monitoring: Terminology

- Verification of tracheal tube placement
  - Because the air in the esophagus normally has very low levels of CO_2, capnometry is considered a rapid method of preventing unrecognized esophageal intubation.

Indications

An $ETCO_2$ detector can accurately confirm tracheal placement of a tracheal tube in children with spontaneous circulation who weigh more than 2 kg.

Types of Devices

Use a pediatric $ETCO_2$ detector for patients weighing 2 to 15 kg. Use an adult $ETCO_2$ detector if the patient weighs more than 15 kg.

PEDS Pearl

Ventilate the patient at least six times before evaluating tracheal tube placement using an end-tidal CO_2 detector. This will quickly wash out any retained CO_2 in the stomach and esophagus after BVM ventilation. CO_2 detected after this procedure can then be assumed to come from the trachea.

During CPR, a positive test suggests that the tracheal tube is in the airway; but a negative result (suggesting esophageal placement) requires an alternate means of confirming the position of the tube (e.g., esophageal detector), because end-tidal CO_2 may be very low during CPR.

○ Capnography should not be used as the *only* means of assessing tracheal tube placement.
* Assessment of progressive respiratory failure in the nonintubated patient
* Assessment of conscious sedation safety
* Evaluation of mechanical ventilation

* $ETCO_2$ detectors are available as electronic monitors or disposable colorimetric devices. The $ETCO_2$ detector is placed between a tracheal tube and a ventilation device.
* The presence of CO_2 (evidenced by a color change on the colorimetric device or number/light on the electronic monitor) suggests placement of the tube in the trachea. In a patient with a pulse, a lack of CO_2 (no color change on colorimetric detector or indicator on the electronic monitor) during exhalation suggests tube placement in the esophagus.
* Disposable colorimetric devices provide CO_2 readings by chemical reaction on pH-sensitive litmus paper housed in the detector.
  ○ The paper in the $ETCO_2$ detector changes according to the amount of CO_2 detected.
    ▪ In a patient with a pulse, a lack of color change during exhalation suggests esophageal tube placement.
    ▪ In a pulseless patient, possible reasons for a lack of color change include hypoperfusion, inadequate CPR, improper tube placement, or the patient is not viable.
  ○ If there is a small amount of CO_2 detected, the color will change slightly from its original color.
    ▪ The tube may be in the correct position, but the patient may not be ventilating or perfusing adequately (e.g., shock, cardiopulmonary arrest).
    ▪ The tube may be in the esophagus and the CO_2 detector is reading CO_2 retained in the esophagus from BVM ventilation, ingestion of a carbonated beverage, or alcohol.
  ○ If a normal amount of CO_2 is detected during exhalation, the color will change noticeably from its original color (i.e., confirms tracheal placement of the tube).
  ○ Colorimetric capnography is susceptible to inaccurate results due to exposure of the paper to medications, the environment, patient secretions (e.g., vomitus), and the age of the paper.

Rapid Sequence Intubation

RSI is the use of medications to sedate and paralyze a patient to rapidly achieve tracheal intubation. In addition to sedatives and paralytics, other medications may be used to minimize or prevent the physiologic responses of intubation such as the cough reflex, gag reflex, cardiac dysrhythmias, increased ICP, pain, hypoxia, hypertension, and increased ocular pressure.

Rapid Sequence Intubation: Description

- Excessive work of breathing, which may lead to fatigue and respiratory failure
- Loss of protective airway reflexes (e.g., cough, gag)
- Combative patients requiring airway control
- Uncontrolled seizure activity (to provide airway control)
- Functional or anatomic airway obstruction
- Head trauma and Glasgow Coma Scale score less than 8
- Severe asthma
- Inadequate central nervous system control of ventilation
- Need for high peak inspiratory pressure or positive-end expiratory pressure to maintain effective alveolar gas exchange
- To permit sedation for diagnostic studies while ensuring airway protection and control of secretions

Rapid Sequence Intubation: Indications

1. **Prepare** (zero minus 10 minutes)
   - Obtain a SAMPLE medical history and perform a focused physical examination
   - Assemble age-appropriate equipment. Alternative airways should be readily available to assist in the management of a difficult airway such as LMAs, needle cricothyrotomy equipment, and surgical cricothyrotomy equipment.
   - Apply the cardiac monitor and pulse oximeter.
   - Assemble personnel. If available, assign an assistant to perform cricoid pressure. If cervical spine injury is suspected, assign another assistant to manually stabilize the neck in a neutral position. Assign another assistant to monitor the patient's heart rate, ECG rhythm, blood pressure, and pulse oximeter readings.
   - Establish an IV. Assemble and draw up all medications that will be used during the procedure.
2. **Preoxygenate** (zero minus 5 minutes) with 100% oxygen for 3 minutes.
3. **Premedicate** (zero minus 3 minutes)

The initial medications administered during RSI are used to minimize the

Rapid Sequence Intubation: Procedure

Ensure all equipment is in working order.

The Seven P's of RSI

- **P**reparation (zero minus 10 minutes)
- **P**reoxygenate (zero minus 5 minutes)
- **P**remedicate (zero minus 3 minutes)
- **P**aralysis with sedation (zero)
- **P**rotect the airway (zero plus 15 seconds)
- **P**ass the tube and proof of placement (zero plus 45 seconds)
- **P**ostintubation management (zero plus 60 seconds)

"I SOAP ME" is a memory aid that can help you recall the equipment and medications required for rapid sequence intubation.
- **I**V: Ensure a secure IV is in place.
- **S**uction: Connect, power on, verify it is in working order.
- **O**xygen: Ensure patient is adequately ventilated and preoxygenated.
- **A**irway equipment: Laryngoscope with various blade sizes, stylet, tracheal tube for body length and age. tubes 0.5 mm larger and smaller, tape or a commercial tube holder, oropharyngeal and nasal airways, nasogastric tube, Magill forceps, and alternative airways.
- **P**harmacologic agents: Decide what medications will be used, calculate correct doses, and draw up.
- **M**onitoring equipment: ECG monitor, pulse oximeter, capnometer, and blood pressure equipment.
- **E**ndotracheal versus esophageal detection method for confirmation of tube position.

physiologic responses sometimes associated with intubation. These medications are referred to "adjunctive medications" or "adjunctive agents."

- Atropine or glycopyrrolate
  - Atropine is given to decrease airway secretions and minimize the bradycardia that may result from vagal stimulation during intubation.
    - Atropine administration should be standard for all children younger than 1 year, children who are bradycardic, children younger than 5 years who are to receive succinylcholine, and adolescents who receive a second dose of succinylcholine. Ketamine increases secretions. Atropine is suggested if ketamine is administered.
  - Glycopyrrolate (Robinul)
    - Like atropine, glycopyrrolate is an anticholinergic
    - Used for the same indications as atropine
- Lidocaine
  - Give lidocaine for head injury or increased ICP
  - Lidocaine diminishes the cough and gag reflexes, and may diminish the rise in ICP associated with intubation
  - If indicated, administer 2 to 5 minutes before the RSI procedure.

4. Paralyze and sedate (zero)

- Agents used for sedation during RSI include barbiturates, benzodiazepines, opiates, nonbarbiturate sedatives, and dissociative agents. Select an appropriate sedative on the basis of the patient's age, clinical condition, and the effects of the medication being considered for administration. Select a sedative that lasts as long as or longer than the paralytic agent to be administered or be prepared to

For maximum effect at the time of intubation, atropine should be given at least 1 to 2 minutes before the procedure.

Paralysis without sedation has been described as comparable to being buried alive. The patient should ***never*** be awake while paralyzed.

administer additional sedation. Administer the sedative *before* the paralytic agent.

- Administer a paralytic agent. ***Once a paralytic has been administered, you assume complete responsibility for maintaining an adequate airway and ventilations***.
  - Fasciculations are muscle twitches. A defasciculation agent is a medication that is given to inhibit muscle twitching.
  - Administration of a defasciculating dose (one tenth of the paralyzing dose) of a nondepolarizing paralytic agent (e.g., vecuronium, pancuronium) is recommended for children 5 years of age and older if succinylcholine is the paralytic agent selected for use.

5. **Protect** the airway (zero plus 15 seconds)
- To reduce the risk of aspiration, apply cricoid pressure when the patient becomes unresponsive.
- Position the patient for intubation.

6. **Pass the tube and proof** of placement (zero plus 45 seconds)
- Relaxation of the mandible and decreased resistance to manual ventilation indicates that the patient is ready to be intubated.
- If intubation is unsuccessful, maintain cricoid pressure and ventilate the patient with a BVM. After the patient is reoxygenated, either attempt another intubation or use an alternative airway technique.
- Confirm tube placement.
- Release cricoid pressure.

7. **Postintubation** management (zero plus 60 seconds)
- Verify the tracheal tube is positioned at the correct depth (centimeters at the lips should be three times the tracheal tube diameter).
- Secure the tube in place with tape or a commercial tracheal tube holder.
- Begin mechanical ventilation.
- Reassess the patient's vital signs, including pulse oximetry and $ETCO_2$ readings.
- Administer additional medications as necessary (e.g., sedatives, long-lasting muscle relaxants).
- Obtain a chest radiograph to confirm correct tube placement.

Absolute Contraindications
- Patients in whom alternative airway control (i.e., cricothyrotomy) would be difficult or impossible due to anatomy or massive neck swelling
- Patients who would be difficult or impossible to intubate after paralysis
- Operator unfamiliarity with the medications used for the RSI procedure

Relative Contraindications
The risk of complications must be weighed against the benefit of obtaining airway control.

Rapid Sequence Intubation: Contraindications

Before initiating RSI, the individual performing the procedure must be trained, appropriately credentialed, and prepared to perform a cricothyrotomy in the event of a failed airway.

- Severely increased ICP
- Known hypersensitivity to the medications used for the procedure
- Known unstable cervical spine injury or fracture

Rapid Sequence Intubation: Complications

- Prolonged apnea
- Bradycardia
- Fasciculations
- Death due to anoxia in a patient who cannot be intubated or ventilated
- Hypotension (secondary to sedative administration)
- Hyperkalemia (adverse effect associated with succinylcholine)
- Increased intragastric pressure
- Malignant hyperthermia

TABLE 5-6 *Medications Used During Rapid Sequence Intubation*

	Dosage (Intravenous)	Onset	Duration
Adjunctive Medications			
Atropine	0.01 to 0.02 mg/kg; minimum 0.1 mg, maximum 1.0 mg	2 to 3 min	> 30 min
Glycopyrrolate	0.005 to 0.01 mg/kg (maximum 0.2 mg)	60 sec	> 30 min
Lidocaine	1 to 2 mg/kg	2 to 5 min	> 30 min
Sedatives			
Etomidate	0.2 to 0.6 mg/kg (child >10 yrs)	30 to 45 sec	10 to 20 min
Fentanyl	2 to 4 mcg/kg	Almost immediate	30 to 90 min
Ketamine	1 to 2 mg/kg	30 to 60 sec	5 to 20 min
Midazolam	6 mo to 5 yrs: 0.05–0.1 mg/kg; total dose up to 0.6 mg/kg 6–12 yrs: 0.025–0.5 mg/kg; total dose up to 0.4 mg/kg 12–16 yrs: 0.3–0.35 mg/kg; total dose up to 0.6 mg/kg	2 to 3 min	20 to 30 min
Propofol	2.5–3.5 mg/kg (3 to 16 years of age)	10 to 30 sec	3 to 5 min
Thiopental	2 to 4 mg/kg	10 to 40 sec	10 to 20 min
Paralytics			
Pancuronium	0.1 to 0.2 mg/kg	1 to 2 min	45 to 90 min
Rocuronium	0.6 to 1.2 mg/kg	30 to 60 sec	30 to 60 min
Succinylcholine	2 mg/kg for infants/small children; 1 mg/kg older children/adolescents	30 to 60 sec	3 to 12 min
Vecuronium	0.08–0.10 mg/kg	1 to 2 min	30 to 90 min

TABLE 5-7 *Sedative Options During Rapid Sequence Intubation for Common Clinical Situations*

Clinical Condition	Blood Pressure	Adjunctive Agent	Sedative
Status asthmaticus	N/A	Atropine*	Ketamine *OR* midazolam
Head injury or increased intracranial pressure	Normal	Lidocaine	Etomidate *OR* thiopental *OR* midazolam
	Decreased	Lidocaine	Etomidate *OR* thiopental (low dose) *OR* midazolam
Status epilepticus	N/A		Thiopental *OR* midazolam *OR* propofol[†]
Shock	Mild	Atropine (if ketamine used)	Etomidate (low dose) *OR* ketamine *OR* midazolam (low dose)
	Severe	Atropine (if ketamine used)	Etomidate (low dose) *OR* ketamine *OR* none
No head injury or increased intracranial pressure	Normal	Atropine (if ketamine used)	Etomidate *OR* thiopental *OR* midazolam *OR* ketamine *OR* propofol
	Decreased	Atropine (if ketamine used)	Etomidate *OR* midazolam (low dose) *OR* ketamine

N/A, not applicable.
*Atropine administration should be standard for all children younger than 1 year, children who are bradycardic, children younger than 5 years who are to receive succinylcholine, and adolescents who receive a second dose of succinylcholine. Atropine is suggested if ketamine is used.
[†]Use with caution in critically ill or injured children.

Needle Cricothyrotomy

Description

- Needle cricothyrotomy (also called percutaneous cricothyrotomy) is a method of providing ventilation by insertion of a large-bore, over-the-needle catheter into the cricothyroid membrane. This procedure may be indicated in cases of upper airway obstruction that *cannot be relieved by less invasive methods* such as head positioning, suctioning, foreign body airway maneuvers, BVM ventilation, and tracheal intubation.
- Needle cricothyrotomy may be extremely difficult to perform in infants and young children because of the mobility of the larynx and trachea and the softness of the laryngeal cartilage in these patients, making palpation of the landmarks for the procedure difficult and collapse of the upper airway with labored breathing more likely.[5] This procedure requires special training and frequent refresher training to maintain skill proficiency.

Indications

- Conditions in which intubation is difficult or impossible
- Craniofacial abnormalities

- Congenital laryngeal anomalies
- Excessive oropharyngeal hemorrhage
- Massive traumatic or congenital deformities
- Complete upper airway obstruction
- Laryngeal fracture
- Pharyngeal/laryngeal burns
- Subglottic stenosis
- Respiratory arrest or near arrest in patients who cannot be tracheally intubated
- Cervical spine fracture with respiratory compromise in patients who cannot be tracheally intubated

Contraindications
- Unavailable or inadequate equipment

Advantages
- Allows rapid entrance to the airway for temporary oxygenation and ventilation

Disadvantages
- Does not allow for efficient elimination of CO_2
- Invasive procedure
- Requires skilled rescuers to perform with frequent retraining

Equipment Needed
- Personal protective equipment
- Oxygen source
- Suction equipment
- Antiseptic solution
- Bag-valve-mask device (size appropriate for patient)
- 14-gauge (or larger) over-the-needle catheter
- 3-mL syringe
- Adapter from the top of a 3.0-mm tracheal tube
- Tape or commercial tube holder

Procedure
- Place the patient in a supine position.
- Identify landmarks (Figure 5-52). Palpate the cricothyroid membrane between the thyroid and cricoid cartilages.
- Cleanse the site. Attach a 3-mL syringe to a 14-gauge (or larger) over-the-needle catheter.
- Stabilize the cricoid and thyroid cartilage between the thumb and finger of one hand. Using the over-the-needle catheter, carefully puncture the skin in the midline, directly over the cricothyroid membrane (Figure 5-53).
- Direct the needle and catheter toward the feet at a 45-degree angle. Carefully insert the needle and catheter through the cricothyroid membrane, maintaining negative pressure (pulling back) on the syringe

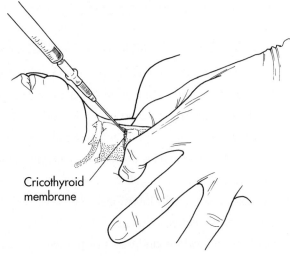

Figure 5-53   Stabilize the cricoid and thyroid cartilage between the thumb and finger of one hand. Using the over-the-needle catheter, carefully puncture the skin in the midline, directly over the cricothyroid membrane. Direct the needle and catheter toward the feet at a 45-degree angle.

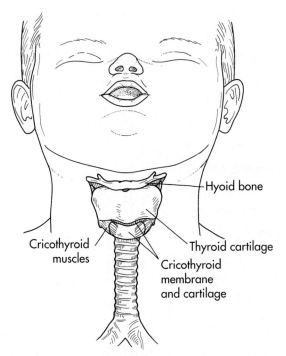

Cricothyroid membrane

Figure 5-52   Anatomic landmarks for cricothyroidotomy.

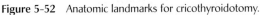

as the needle is advanced. A return of air signifies entry into the tracheal lumen.

- Advance the catheter over the needle, being careful to avoid the posterior tracheal wall, until the catheter hub is flush with the skin. Hold the catheter hub in place to prevent displacement.
- Withdraw the needle carefully, advancing the catheter downward into position in the trachea.
- Attach the hub of the IV catheter to a 3.0-mm pediatric tracheal tube adapter and ventilate with 100% oxygen using a bag-valve-mask device. (Alternatively, attach the barrel of a 3-mL syringe to the IV catheter and an 8-mm tracheal tube adapter to the syringe barrel.)
- Monitor carefully for chest rise and auscultate for adequate ventilation. Assess $ETCO_2$, pulse oximetry, ECG, and vital signs.
- Secure the catheter in place.

Complications

- Bleeding
- Infection
- Hematoma
- Hypoxemia
- Catheter dislodgement
- Subcutaneous and/or mediastinal emphysema
- Inadequate ventilation resulting in hypoxia and death

Surgical Cricothyrotomy

Description

- A surgical cricothyrotomy is the creation of an opening into the crico-thyroid membrane with a scalpel to allow rapid entrance to the airway for temporary oxygenation and ventilation. This procedure may be indicated in cases of upper airway obstruction that *cannot be relieved by less invasive methods* such as head positioning, suctioning, foreign body airway maneuvers, BVM ventilation, and tracheal intubation.
- Because surgical cricothyrotomy may be difficult to perform in infants and young children because of the difficulty in palpating and identifying the important landmarks of the neck, and because of the small diameter of the cricoid cartilage, the procedure is not recommended in children under the age of 10.[6] This procedure requires special training and frequent refresher training to maintain skill proficiency.

Indications

Surgical cricothyrotomy is rarely indicated for the infant or young child. If the procedure is necessary, it should be performed by the most experienced person available, preferably an experienced surgeon.

- Conditions in which intubation is difficult or impossible
- Craniofacial abnormalities
- Congenital laryngeal anomalies
- Excessive oropharyngeal hemorrhage
- Massive traumatic or congenital deformities
- Complete upper airway obstruction
- Laryngeal fracture
- Pharyngeal/laryngeal burns
- Subglottic stenosis
- Respiratory arrest or near arrest in patients who cannot be tracheally intubated
- Cervical spine fracture with respiratory compromise in patients who cannot be tracheally intubated

Contraindications

- Children younger than 10 years
- Adequate nonsurgical airway
- Unavailable or inadequate equipment
- Bleeding diatheses

Advantages

- Allows rapid entrance to the airway for temporary oxygenation and ventilation

Disadvantages

- Invasive procedure
- Requires skilled rescuers to perform with frequent retraining

Equipment Needed

- Personal protective equipment
- Oxygen source
- Suction equipment
- Antiseptic solution
- Bag-valve-mask device (size appropriate for patient)
- Scalpel
- Tracheal tube or tracheostomy tube
- Tape or commercial tube holder

Procedure

The most prominent structures in the anterior neck of the infant or child are the hyoid bone and the cricoid cartilage.

In an older child, a horizontal incision may be made directly through the skin, muscle, and cricothyroid membrane if landmarks are obvious.

To reduce the possibility of subglottic stenosis and voice change secondary to the procedure, it has been suggested that a cricothyrotomy be converted to a tracheostomy when the infant or child is stabilized.

- Place the patient in a supine position. If not contraindicated, extend the neck to expose landmarks.
- Identify landmarks (hyoid bone, thyroid cartilage, cricoid cartilage, cricothyroid membrane). Palpate the hyoid bone high in the neck. Next, locate the thyroid cartilage and then the cricoid cartilage. Identify the cricothyroid membrane between the thyroid and cricoid cartilages.
- Cleanse the site. Use a local anesthetic if the patient is conscious and if time permits.
- Stabilize the larynx between the finger and thumb of one hand. Make a vertical incision over the thyroid and cricoid cartilages.
- Expose the cricothyroid membrane (Figure 5-54). Make a horizontal incision through the cricothyroid membrane into the airway and listen/feel for air flow.
- Insert a tracheostomy or tracheal tube of appropriate size through the cricothyroid membrane, directing the tube caudally into the lower trachea.
- Connect the tracheostomy (or tracheal) tube to a bag-valve-mask device and ventilate the patient with 100% oxygen.
- Monitor carefully for chest rise and auscultate for adequate ventilation. Assess ETCO$_2$, pulse oximetry, ECG, and vital signs.
- Secure the tube to prevent dislodgement.

Complications

- Asphyxia
- Aspiration (blood)
- Creation of a false passage into the tissues
- Mediastinal emphysema
- Hemorrhage or hematoma formation
- Vocal cord paralysis
- Hoarseness
- Laceration of the trachea/esophagus
- Subglottic stenosis
- Tube dislodgement

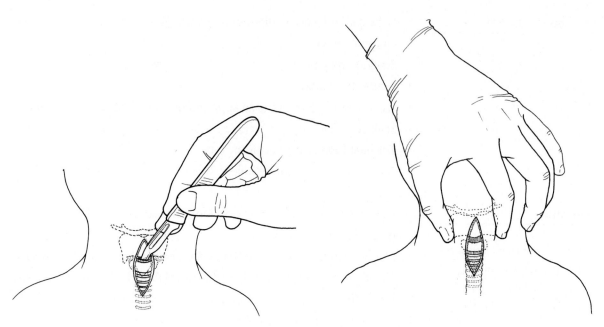

Figure 5-54   Identify the hyoid bone, thyroid cartilage, cricoid cartilage, and cricothyroid membrane. Stabilize the larynx between the finger and thumb of one hand. Make a vertical incision over the thyroid and cricoid cartilages. Expose the cricothyroid membrane. In an older child, a horizontal incision may be made directly through the skin, muscle, and cricothyroid membrane if landmarks are obvious.

Needle Thoracostomy

Needle thoracostomy (also called needle decompression) is the insertion of an over-the-needle catheter into the chest to relieve a tension pneumothorax. The procedure converts a tension pneumothorax to a simple, open pneumothorax.

Description

Suspected tension pneumothorax as evidenced by:

Indications

- Progressively worsening dyspnea
- Tachypnea
- Tachycardia
- Poor ventilation despite an open airway
- Restlessness and agitation
- Increased airway resistance when ventilating patient (poor bag compliance)
- Hyperresonance to percussion on the affected side
- Diminished or absent breath sounds on the affected side
- Decreased level of responsiveness
- Hypotension
- Tracheal deviation away from side of injury (may or may not be present)

- Distended neck veins (may not be present if hypovolemia is present or hypotension is severe)
- Cyanosis

Contraindications

There are no contraindications to this procedure if the patient's clinical presentation, history, and physical findings suggest the presence of a tension pneumothorax.

Equipment Needed

- Personal protective equipment
- Oxygen source
- Antiseptic solution
- 18-gauge, over-the-needle catheter for children younger than 8 years
- 14-gauge, over-the-needle catheter for children 8 years of age and older
- One-way valve (e.g., Heimlich valve)

Procedure

- Place the patient in a supine position and elevate the child's arm behind the head. Restrain as needed.
- Identify landmark: The second intercostal space at the midclavicular line.
- Cleanse the site. Use a local anesthetic if the patient is conscious and if time permits.
- Holding an over-the-needle catheter at a 90-degree angle to the chest wall, insert the needle through the skin.
  - Use an 18-gauge, over-the-needle catheter for children younger than 8 years.
  - Use a 14-gauge, over-the-needle catheter for children 8 years of age and older.
- Slowly advance the needle over the superior border of the rib until the pleural space is entered. Entry into the pleural space is evidenced by one or more of the following:
  - A "popping" sound or "giving way" sensation
  - A sudden rush of air
  - Ability to aspirate air into a syringe (if used)

Definitive treatment of a tension pneumothorax requires insertion of a chest tube, after which the needle thoracostomy catheter may be removed.

- Remove the needle from the catheter, leaving the catheter in place.
- Connect the catheter to a one-way valve (e.g., Heimlich valve) (An improvised one-way valve may be constructed from the finger of a surgical glove.)
- Secure the catheter and valve to the patient's chest wall to prevent dislodgement.
- Assess the patient's response to the procedure by evaluating respiratory status, breath sounds, jugular veins, tracheal position, and vital signs.

• Pneumothorax   **Complications**
• Pleural infection
• Laceration of the lung
• Laceration of the intercostal vessel(s) with resultant hemorrhage

Case Study Resolution

This child is sick. The presence of a high fever, productive cough, and tachypnea suggests pneumonia with signs of respiratory failure. Move quickly. Use personal protective equipment. Initiate pulse oximetry (initial SpO_2 on room air was 83%). Correct hypoxia by giving high-flow oxygen in a manner that does not agitate the child (SpO_2 on a nonrebreather mask was 87%). Place the child on a cardiac monitor and establish vascular access. Provide further interventions based on assessment findings. (Note: This child had decreased breath sounds in the right middle and lower lobes. Lower lobe consolidation was observed on her chest radiograph. She was preoxygenated, RSI was performed, and IV antibiotics were started.)

Web Resource

• www.storysmith.net/Articles/Rapid%20Sequence%20Intubation%20lecture%20notes.pdf (Rapid Sequence Intubation in Emergency Medicine)

References

1. Davies P, Cheng D, Fox A, et al. The efficacy of noncontact oxygen delivery methods. *Pediatrics* 2002;110:964–967.

2. Foltin GL, Tunik MG, Cooper A, et al. *Teaching resource for instructors in prehospital pediatrics for paramedics.* New York: Center for Pediatric Emergency Medicine, 2002.

3. King BR, Baker MD, Braitman LE, et al. Endotracheal tube selection in children: a comparison of four methods. *Ann Emerg Med* 1993;22:530–534.

4. McSwain NE, Frame S, Salomone JP, eds. *Special considerations in trauma of the child,* 5th ed. St. Louis: Mosby, 2003.

5. Bower CM. The surgical airway. In: Dieckmann RA, Fiser DH, Selbst SM, eds. *Illustrated textbook of pediatric emergency & critical care procedures,* St. Louis: Mosby–Year Book, 1997.

6. Gerardi MG. Evaluation and management of the multiple trauma patient. In: Strange GR, Ahrens WR, Lelyveld S, et al, eds. *Pediatric emergency medicine: a comprehensive study guide,* 2nd ed. New York: McGraw-Hill, 2002.

7. Shapiro BA, Peruzzi WT. Respiratory care. In: Miller RD, ed. *Anesthesia,* 5th ed., Philadelphia: Churchill Livingstone, 2000.

Chapter Quiz

1. Which of the following is NOT a desirable feature of a bag-valve-mask device?
   A) A clear mask.
   B) A compressible, self-refilling bag.
   C) Availability in adult and pediatric sizes.
   D) Pop-off (pressure release) valve.

2. A 3-year-old child weighing 15 kilograms requires tracheal intubation.
   A) What type of blade should be used?
   B) What size laryngoscope blade should be used?
   C) What size tracheal tube should be used?
   D) Should you use a cuffed or uncuffed tracheal tube for this child?
   E) When the tracheal tube has been inserted to the proper depth, what is the cm marking that should appear at the patient's lips?

3. A six-year-old child in cardiopulmonary arrest has been intubated. Which of the following would indicate inadvertent esophageal intubation?
   A) Subcutaneous emphysema
   B) External jugular vein distention
   C) Gurgling sounds heard over the epigastrium
   D) Breath sounds present on only one side of the chest

4. Why is the cricoid cartilage used to minimize gastric distention during positive pressure ventilation?
   A) The cricoid cartilage is wider than the thyroid cartilage.
   B) The thyroid cartilage is not completely developed in infants and children.
   C) The cricoid cartilage is the only completely cartilaginous ring in the larynx.
   D) The thyroid cartilage is more difficult to palpate than the cricoid cartilage.

5. Stridor is:
   A) A high-pitched "whistling" sound produced by air moving through narrowed airway passages.
   B) A harsh, high-pitched sound heard on inspiration associated with upper airway obstruction.
   C) Abnormally rapid breathing.
   D) An abnormal respiratory sound associated with collection of liquid or semi-solid material in the patient's upper airway.

6. Tracheal intubation:
   A) Is contraindicated in an unresponsive patient.
   B) Eliminates the risk of aspiration of gastric contents.
   C) Should be performed in less than 60 seconds.
   D) Should be preceded by efforts to ventilate by another method.

7. The maximum length of time for suctioning an infant or child is:
   A) 5 seconds.
   B) 10 seconds.
   C) 15 seconds.
   D) 30 seconds.

8. Which of the following is the most useful for removing thick secretions and particulate matter from the pharynx?
   A) Oropharyngeal airway.
   B) Rigid plastic suction catheter.
   C) Flexible plastic suction catheter.
   D) Nonrebreather mask.

9. Under optimum conditions, a partial rebreather mask can deliver an oxygen concentration of _____ at a flow rate of 10 to 15 L/min.
   A) Up to 50%
   B) 25 to 45%
   C) 50 to 60%
   D) 60 to 95%

10. List five potential complications of tracheal intubation.
    1. _____
    2. _____
    3. _____
    4. _____
    5. _____

11. When intubating a patient with a curved blade, the tip of the blade should be placed:
    A) In the vallecula.
    B) In the glottic opening.
    C) Under the epiglottis.
    D) Under the thyroid cartilage.

12. A 6-year-old child has been intubated and a colorimetric $ETCO_2$ detector is being used as a secondary method of confirming proper placement of the tracheal tube. A pulse is present. Select the INCORRECT statement regarding the use of colorimetric capnography.
    A) Disposable colorimetric devices provide CO_2 readings by chemical reaction on pH–sensitive litmus paper housed in the detector.
    B) If a normal amount of CO_2 is detected, the color will change noticeably from its original color (i.e., confirms tracheal placement of the tube.
    C) The paper in the devices is unaffected by exposure to secretions, medications, or the environment.
    D) A small amount of CO_2 may be detected if the tube is in the correct position but the patient is not ventilating or perfusing adequately.

Questions 13–23 refer to the following patient situation.

A 7-year-old girl is having difficulty breathing. You find the child sitting upright and leaning forward, supported by her arms, with her mouth open. Although she is aware of your presence, she appears unconcerned. You note the child has nasal flaring, suprasternal retractions, and is using her intercostal muscles to breathe. You hear loud wheezes without the use of a stethoscope. Her skin color is pale. A family member states the child has a history of asthma. A neighbor visited their home about an hour ago and showed them a kitten she had acquired, not realizing that the patient is allergic to cats.

13. From the information provided, complete the following documentation regarding the Pediatric Assessment Triangle.
    Appearance:
    Breathing:
    Circulation:

14. Your initial assessment reveals labored respirations at a rate of 38/min. Auscultation reveals absent breath sounds bilaterally in the bases, and diminished breath sounds throughout the remaining lung fields. Her heart rate is 140 beats/min and blood pressure is 94/62. Her skin is pale, but warm and dry. Capillary refill is < 2 seconds. Speech is limited to 2 to 3 words. Is this patient sick or not sick? Describe your approach to the initial management of this patient.

15. What is the normal resting respiratory rate for a 7-year-old child? What is the normal resting heart rate for a 7-year-old child?

16. This child's appearance and assessment findings are consistent with:
    A) Respiratory distress.
    B) Respiratory failure.
    C) Respiratory arrest.
    D) Cardiopulmonary arrest.

17. The patient is now unresponsive. You have two other advanced life support personnel to assist you. Emergency equipment is immediately available. How will you open the patient's airway?

18. The patient's airway is now open. How should you proceed?

19. The patient's airway is clear. How should you proceed?

20. The patient is apneic. How will you determine the proper size oropharyngeal airway (OPA) for this child?

21. An oropharyngeal airway has been inserted. The patient remains apneic. A pulse is present at 70 beats/min. A bag-valve-mask is available to provide positive pressure ventilation. What size mask should be used for this child?

22. What size resuscitation bag should be used to ventilate this child? At what rate/minute should ventilations be delivered?

23. Which of the following types of medications are often used in the treatment of asthma?
    A) Bronchodilators, diuretics.
    B) Beta-blockers, methylxanthines.
    C) Corticosteroids, bronchodilators.
    D) Diuretics, beta-blockers.

24. Under optimum conditions, blow-by oxygen administered by means of a face mask can deliver an oxygen concentration of _____ at a flow rate of 10 L/min.
    A) 25 to 45%
    B) 35 to 40%
    C) 50 to 60%
    D) 60 to 95%

25. In the case of a suspected foreign body airway obstruction (FBAO) in an infant or child, reposition the airway and perform a blind finger sweep to remove the foreign body.
    A) True
    B) False

Chapter Quiz Answers

1. D. The BVM used for resuscitation should have either no pop-off (pressure-release) valve or a pop-off valve that can be disabled during resuscitation. Some resuscitation situations require higher than normal ventilatory pressure, such as near-drowning, CPR, pulmonary edema, asthma, partial upper airway obstruction, or initial resuscitation of the newly born. To effectively ventilate a patient in these situations, the ventilatory pressure needed may exceed the limits of the pop-off valve. Thus, a pop-off valve may prevent generation of sufficient tidal volume to overcome the increase in airway resistance.

2. Tracheal intubation of a 3-year-old, 15 kg child:
   A) A straight or curved blade may be used.
   B) A size 2 laryngoscope blade should be used.
   C) A 5.0 mm tracheal tube should be used. Be sure to have a 4.5 mm and 5.5 mm immediately available.
   D) Use an uncuffed tracheal tube for this child.
   E) When the tracheal tube has been inserted to the proper depth, the 14 to 15 cm marking should appear at the patient's lips

3. C. After intubation, the presence of bubbling or gurgling sounds during auscultation of the epigastrium suggests the tube is incorrectly positioned in the esophagus. To correct this problem, deflate the tracheal tube cuff (if a cuffed tube was used), remove the tube, and preoxygenate before reattempting intubation.

4. C. The cricoid cartilage is the most inferior of the laryngeal cartilages and is the only completely cartilaginous ring in the larynx. Compression of the cricoid cartilage pushes the trachea posteriorly, compressing the esophagus against the cervical vertebrae. This helps minimize inflation of the stomach during ventilation, reducing the likelihood of vomiting and aspiration.

5. B. Stridor is a harsh, high-pitched sound heard on inspiration associated with upper airway obstruction. Wheezes are high-pitched "whistling" sounds produced by air moving through narrowed airway passages. Tachypnea is abnormally rapid breathing. Gurgling is abnormal respiratory sound associated with collection of liquid or semi-solid material in the patient's upper airway.

6. D. Tracheal intubation should be preceded by attempts to ventilate by another method. Tracheal intubation reduces, but does not eliminate, the risk of aspiration of gastric contents. When attempted, tracheal intubation should be performed in less than 30 seconds.

7. B. Insertion of a suction catheter and suctioning should take no longer than 10 seconds per attempt. When suctioning to remove material that completely obstructs the airway, more time may be necessary.

8. B. A rigid (also called a "hard," "tonsil tip," or "Yankauer") suction catheter is made of hard plastic and is angled to aid in the removal of thick secretions and particulate matter from the mouth and oropharynx.

9. C. A partial rebreather mask can deliver an oxygen concentration of 50 to 60% at a flow rate of 10 to 15 L/min.

10. Complications of tracheal intubation include bleeding, laryngospasm, vocal cord damage, mucosal necrosis, barotrauma, aspiration, cuff leak, esophageal intubation, right mainstem intubation, occlusion caused by patient biting the tube or secretions, laryngeal or tracheal edema, tube occlusion, hypoxia due to prolonged or unsuccessful intubation, dysrhythmias; trauma to the lips, teeth, tongue, or soft tissues of the oropharynx; increased intracranial pressure.

11. A. When intubating a patient with a curved blade, the tip of the blade should be placed in the vallecula.

12. C. Disposable colorimetric devices provide CO_2 readings by chemical reaction on pH-sensitive litmus paper housed in the detector. The paper in the $ETCO_2$ detector changes according to the amount of CO_2 detected. In a patient with a pulse, a lack of color change during exhalation suggests esophageal tube placement. If there is a small amount of CO_2 detected, the color will change slightly from its original color. Possible causes for this finding: 1) the tube may be in the correct position, but the patient may not be ventilating or perfusing adequately (e.g., shock, cardiopulmonary arrest) or 2) the tube may be in the esophagus and the CO_2 detector is reading CO_2 retained in the esophagus from bag-valve-mask ventilation, or ingestion of a carbonated beverage or alcohol. If a normal amount of CO_2 is detected during exhalation, the color will change noticeably from its original color (i.e., confirms tracheal placement of the tube). Colorimetric capnography is susceptible to inaccurate results due to exposure of the paper to medications, the environment, patient secretions (e.g., vomitus), and the age of the paper.

13. Pediatric Assessment Triangle
    A)   Appearance: Awake, seated in tripod position; unconcerned about your presence
    B)   Breathing: Spontaneous breathing; increased respiratory effort evident
    C)   Circulation: Pale skin color; no evidence of bleeding

14. This child is sick. Move quickly. Open the airway and suction if necessary. Correct hypoxia by giving high-flow oxygen. Begin assisted ventilation if the patient does not improve. Provide further interventions based on assessment findings.

15. The normal respiratory rate for a 7-year-old is 18 to 30 breaths/min. This patient's respiratory rate is elevated for her age. The normal heart rate for a 7-year-old is 70 to 120 beats/min. This patient's heart rate is elevated for her age.

16. B. This child's appearance and assessment findings are consistent with respiratory failure.

17. Open the child's airway with a head-tilt–chin-lift.

18. Assess for sounds of airway compromise (snoring, gurgling, stridor) and look in the mouth for blood, gastric contents, foreign objects, etc.

19. Look, listen, and feel for breathing

20. Proper airway size is determined by holding the device against the side of the patient's face and selecting an airway that extends from the corner of the mouth to the angle of the jaw.

21. An adult mask should be used for this child.

22. A child or adult resuscitation bag may be used. Deliver one ventilation every 3 to 5 seconds (12 to 20/minute).

23. C. Because beta-blockers impede bronchodilation, they are not routinely used in the management of asthma. Bronchodilators are used to improve airflow in the lungs. Corticosteroids are used to reduce airway swelling and inflammation. Methylxanthines (e.g., theophylline) may be used as an alternative therapy.

24. B. Under optimum conditions, blow-by oxygen administered by means of a face mask can deliver an oxygen concentration of 35 to 40% at a flow rate of 10 L/min.

25. B. Blind finger sweeps should not be performed in an infant or child. Blind sweeps may push the foreign body into the glottic opening, resulting in complete obstruction.

6 Cardiovascular Emergencies

Case Study

Your patient is a 4-year-old boy who has a swollen left foot, inspiratory stridor, and hives on his face, chest, back, and extremities. Mom says the boy had been outside playing with a friend and came into the house complaining that a bug bit him in the foot. Your first impression reveals an anxious child who is laboring to breathe. Inspiratory stridor is audible. The child has no allergies, but his older sister has an allergy to penicillin.

Is this child sick or not sick? What should you do next?

Objectives

1. Define the following terms: *afterload, preload, cardiac output, stroke volume,* and *shock.*
2. List assessment findings consistent with circulatory compromise.
3. Discuss the common causes of shock in infants and children.
4. Describe the clinical classifications of shock.
5. Describe the assessment findings that indicate shock in infants and children.
6. Differentiate between compensated and decompensated shock.
7. Describe the initial management of hypovolemic, cardiogenic, distributive (septic, anaphylactic, neurogenic), and obstructive shock in infants and children.
8. Describe assessment findings that indicate cardiopulmonary failure or arrest in children.
9. Discuss the primary etiologies of cardiopulmonary arrest in infants and children.
10. Identify the major classifications of pediatric cardiac dysrhythmias.
11. Identify four essential questions to ask in the initial emergency management of a pediatric patient with a dysrhythmia.
12. Recognize the following dysrhythmias: bradycardia, sinus tachycardia, supraventricular tachycardia (SVT), ventricular tachycardia

(VT), ventricular fibrillation (VF), and asystole.

13. Differentiate sinus tachycardia from SVT and SVT from VT.

14. Recognize a "sick" (unstable) and "not sick" (stable) infant or child with a cardiac dysrhythmia.

15. Discuss the dysrhythmias associated with pediatric cardiopulmonary failure or arrest.

16. Discuss the management of cardiac dysrhythmias in infants and children.

17. Discuss the pharmacology of medications used during shock, symptomatic bradycardia, stable and unstable tachycardia, and cardiopulmonary arrest.

18. Given a patient situation, formulate a management plan (including assessment, airway management, cardiopulmonary resuscitation [CPR], pharmacologic, and electrical interventions where applicable) for a patient in shock, or presenting with symptomatic bradycardia, stable or unstable tachycardia, or cardiopulmonary arrest.

19. Discuss the etiology, pathophysiology, assessment findings, and emergency management of syncope.

20. Describe the causes of chest pain in children.

21. Describe common congenital heart defects.

Cardiovascular System: Anatomic and Physiologic Considerations

Review of the Cardiovascular System

Heart

- The heart is divided into four cavities or chambers but functions as a two-sided pump (Figure 6-1).
  - The right side of the heart is a low-pressure system that pumps venous blood to the lungs.
  - The left side is a high-pressure system that pumps arterial blood to the systemic circulation.

Pulmonary Circulation

- The right atrium receives blood low in oxygen and high in carbon dioxide from the superior and inferior vena cava and the coronary sinus.
- Blood flows from the right atrium through the tricuspid valve into the right ventricle. When the right ventricle contracts, the tricuspid valve closes.
- The right ventricle expels the blood through the pulmonic valve into the pulmonary trunk.
- The pulmonary trunk divides into a right and left pulmonary artery,

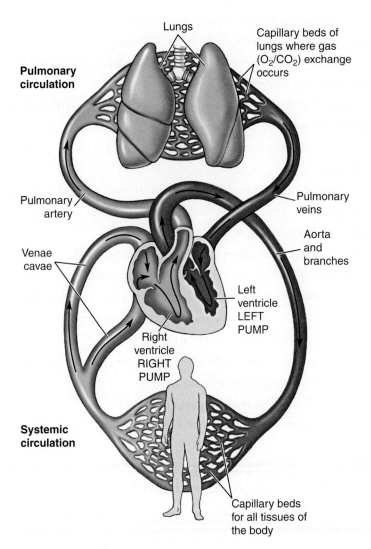

Figure 6-1   The right side of the heart (*blue*) is a low-pressure system that pumps venous blood to the lungs. The left side (*red*) is a high-pressure system that pumps arterial blood to the systemic circulation.

each of which carries blood to one lung (pulmonary circulation) (Figure 6-2).

Systemic Circulation

- Blood flows through the pulmonary arteries to the lungs, where oxygen and carbon dioxide are exchanged in the pulmonary capillaries, to the pulmonary veins.

- The left atrium receives oxygenated blood from the lungs via the four pulmonary veins (two from the right lung and two from the left lung).

- Blood flows from the left atrium through the mitral (bicuspid) valve into the left ventricle. When the left ventricle contracts, the mitral valve closes.

- Blood leaves the left ventricle through the aortic valve to the aorta and its branches and is distributed throughout the body (systemic circulation).

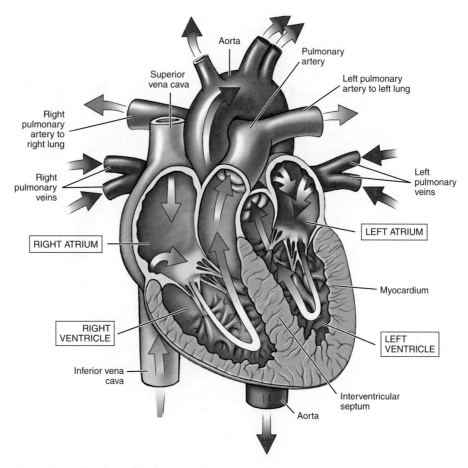

Figure 6-2   Chambers of the heart and the large vessels.

- Blood from the tissues of the head and neck is emptied into the superior vena cava. Blood from the lower body is emptied into the inferior vena cava. The superior and inferior vena cavae carry their contents into the right atrium.

Coronary Arteries

- Blood is supplied to the tissues of the heart during diastole by the first two branches of the aorta, the right and left coronary arteries.
- The openings to these vessels are just beyond the cusps of the aortic semilunar valve.

Blood Vessels

Arteries are conductance vessels.

- Arteries
  - Primary function of the large arteries is to conduct blood from the heart to the arterioles (Figure 6-3).
  - All arteries, except the pulmonary arteries, carry oxygen-rich blood.
  - Designed to carry blood under high pressure.
  - Arteries consist of three layers.
    - Outer layer = tunica adventitia
      - Consists of flexible fibrous connective tissue
      - Helps hold the vessel open

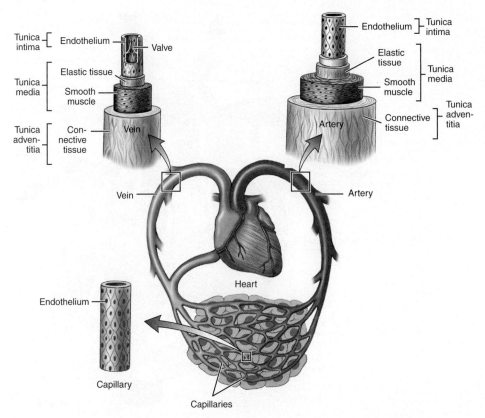

Figure 6-3   Blood vessel wall layers. With the exception of the capillaries, blood vessels contain three layers. Veins also contain valves that help direct the flow of blood back to the heart. The capillary wall consists of a single layer of cells (epithelium).

- ○ Middle layer = tunica media
  - Consists of smooth muscle tissue and elastic connective tissue.
  - This layer, encircled by smooth muscle and innervated by fibers of the autonomic nervous system (ANS), allows constriction and dilation of the vessel. Smooth muscle cells function to maintain vascular tone and regulate local blood flow depending on metabolic requirements.
- ○ Innermost layer = tunica intima
  - Made up of endothelium that lines the vascular system.
  - Endothelium is a single layer of cells in direct contact with the blood.

- Arterioles
  - ○ Arterioles are the smallest branches of the arteries.
  - ○ Arterioles connect arteries and capillaries. Precapillary sphincters are present where the arterioles and capillaries meet. These sphincters contract and relax to control blood flow throughout the capillaries.
  - ○ Arterioles are composed almost exclusively of smooth muscle.
    - The presence of smooth muscle in the vessel walls allows the vessel to alter its diameter, thereby controlling the amount of blood flow to specific tissues.

PEDs Pearl

Infants and children are capable of more effective vasoconstriction than adults are. As a result, a previously healthy infant or child is able to maintain a normal blood pressure and organ perfusion for a longer time in the presence of shock.

Arterioles are resistance vessels.

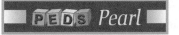

- Altering the diameter of the arterioles also affects the resistance to the flow of blood.
  - A dilated (widened) vessel offers less resistance to blood flow.
  - A constricted (narrowed) vessel offers more resistance to blood flow.
- Capillaries

Capillaries are exchange vessels.

  - Capillaries are the smallest and most numerous of the blood vessels.
  - Connect arterioles and venules.
  - The capillary wall consists of a single layer of cells (endothelium) with holes (pores) through which fluid, oxygen, carbon dioxide, electrolytes, glucose and other nutrients, and wastes are exchanged between the blood and tissues.
- Venules
  - Venules are the smallest branches of veins.
  - Venules connect capillaries and veins. Postcapillary sphincters are present where the venules and capillaries meet. Postcapillary sphincters contract and relax to control blood flow to body tissues.
  - Venules are designed to carry blood under low pressure.
  - The wall of a venule is slightly thicker than the wall of a capillary. The thickness of the wall increases as the venules join to form larger veins.
- Veins

Veins are capacitance (storage) vessels.

  - Veins carry deoxygenated (oxygen-poor) blood from the body to the right side of the heart. All veins, except the pulmonary veins, carry deoxygenated blood.
  - The walls of veins are thinner than arteries.
  - Because a high percentage (approximately 70%) of the blood is located in the veins at any one time, veins are called capacitance vessels.
  - Venous blood flow depends on skeletal muscle action, respiratory movements, and gravity. Valves in the larger veins of the extremities and neck are arranged to allow blood flow in one direction, toward the heart.

Cardiac Cycle
- The **cardiac cycle** refers to a repetitive pumping process that includes all of the events associated with the flow of blood through the heart. The cycle has two phases for each heart chamber—systole and diastole.
- **Systole** is the period during which the chamber is contracting and blood is being ejected. Systole includes contraction of both atrial and ventricular muscle.
  - When the left ventricle contracts, a wave of blood is sent through the arteries causing the arteries to expand and recoil. A **pulse** is the

regular expansion and recoil of an artery caused by the movement of blood from the heart as it contracts. A pulse can be felt anywhere an artery simultaneously passes near the skin surface and over a bone.

- ◦ Central pulses are located close to the heart. Peripheral pulses are located farther from the heart.
- ◦ Pulse sites that are normally readily palpable in the healthy infant or child include the carotid, axillary, brachial, radial, femoral, dorsalis pedis, and posterior tibial.

- **Diastole** is the period of relaxation during which the chamber is filling. Diastole includes relaxation of both atrial and ventricular muscle (Figure 6-4).
- During the cardiac cycle, the pressure within each chamber of the heart rises in systole and falls in diastole.
- The heart's valves ensure that blood flows in the proper direction. Blood flows from one heart chamber to another if the pressure in the chamber is more than that in the next.
- These pressure relationships depend on the careful timing of contractions. The heart's conduction system provides the necessary timing of events between atrial and ventricular systole.

Perfusion

- **Perfusion** is the circulation of blood through an organ or a part of the body. Perfusion delivers oxygen and other nutrients to the cells of all organ systems and removes waste products.
- **Hypoperfusion** (shock) is the inadequate circulation of blood through an organ or a part of the body.

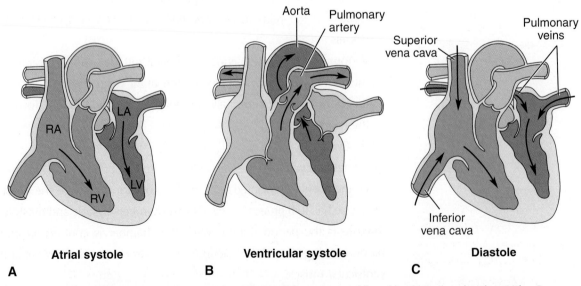

Atrial systole   **Ventricular systole**   **Diastole**

A   B   C

Figure 6-4   **Stages of the cardiac cycle. A,** Atrial systole. The atria contract and force blood into the relaxed ventricles. **B,** Ventricular systole. The ventricles contract, forcing blood into the pulmonary artery and aorta. **C,** Diastole. Both atria and ventricles are relaxed and fill with blood.

Heart Rate

- The heart is innervated by both the sympathetic and parasympathetic divisions of the ANS.
- The sympathetic division mobilizes the body, allowing the body to function under stress ("fight or flight" response).
- The parasympathetic division is responsible for the conservation and restoration of body resources ("feed and breed" response).

Venous Return

- The heart functions as a pump to propel blood through the systemic and pulmonary circulations. As the heart chambers fill with blood, the heart muscle is stretched.
- The most important factor determining the amount of blood pumped by the heart is the amount of blood flowing into it from the systemic circulation (**venous return**).

Cardiac Output

Cardiac output = stroke volume × heart rate (CO = SV × HR).

- **Cardiac output** (CO) is the amount of blood pumped into the aorta each minute by the heart. It is calculated as the SV (amount of blood ejected from a ventricle with each heartbeat) times the HR and is expressed in liters per minute. Adequate CO is necessary to maintain oxygenation and perfusion of body tissues.
- Normal CO
  - Neonates: 200 mL/kg per minute
  - Infants and children: 150 mL/kg per minute
  - Adolescents: 100 mL/kg per minute
- Changes in HR *or* SV can affect CO.
  - ↑ SV or HR → ↑ CO
  - ↓ SV or HR → ↓ CO
- Tachycardia is the initial compensatory response to the demand for increased CO.
  - Tachycardia shortens the length of time spent in diastole.
  - The coronary arteries are perfused during diastole. If the length of diastole is shortened (as in prolonged tachycardias), there is less time for adequate ventricular filling and coronary artery perfusion.
  - This may result in decreased SV, decreased CO, and myocardial ischemia.

Blood Pressure

- **Blood pressure** is the force exerted by the blood on the inner walls of the blood vessels.
  - Systolic blood pressure is the pressure exerted against the walls of the large arteries at the peak of ventricular contraction.
  - Diastolic blood pressure is the pressure exerted against the walls of the large arteries during ventricular relaxation.

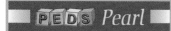

Because of the immaturity of sympathetic innervation to the ventricles, infants and children have a relatively fixed stroke volume and are therefore dependent on an adequate heart rate to maintain adequate cardiac output.

An early sign of impending shock is a slight increase in diastolic pressure without a change in the systolic pressure (i.e., narrowed pulse pressure).

- **Vascular resistance** is the amount of opposition that the blood vessels give to the flow of blood.
  - Resistance is affected by the diameter and length of the blood vessel, blood viscosity, and the tone of the vessel. The most significant changes in resistance are caused by the arterioles (Figure 6-5).
  - Even at rest, vascular tone is maintained by constant input from the sympathetic division of the ANS. This results in partial vasoconstriction throughout the body to ensure continued circulation of blood.
- Blood pressure is equal to CO times peripheral vascular resistance.
  - Blood pressure is affected by any condition that increases peripheral resistance or CO.
  - Thus an increase in either CO or peripheral resistance will result in an increase in blood pressure. Conversely, a decrease in either will result in a decrease in blood pressure.

Tone is a term that may be used when referring to the normal state of balanced tension in body tissues.

Effect of Resistance on Pressure

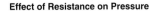
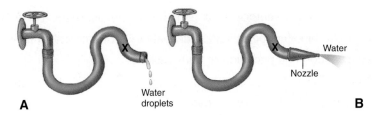

Effect of Resistance on Blood Pressure

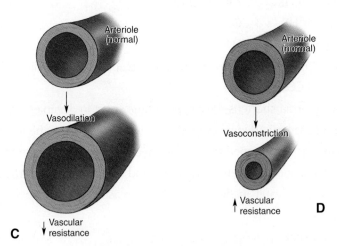

Figure 6-5   **The effect of resistance on pressure. A,** Water flows in large droplets from a wide hose. **B,** If a nozzle is applied to the hose, pressure within the hose increases (point x) as evidenced by the squirting water. Arterioles can function like nozzles. **C,** The nozzle is wide open (vasodilation), offering little resistance to flow. Pressure within the vessel decreases as the vessel dilates. **D,** Pressure within the vessel increases as the nozzle is tightened (vasoconstriction) and the resistance to flow increases.

Stroke Volume

- SV is determined by the following:
  - The degree of ventricular filling during diastole (preload)
  - The resistance against which the ventricle must pump (afterload)
  - The contractile state of the myocardium.

Preload

Fluid administration increases preload.

- **Preload** is the force exerted on the walls of the ventricles at the end of diastole.
- Preload in the right heart depends on venous return to the heart from the systemic circulation.
- Preload in the left heart depends on venous return from the pulmonary system.
  - The volume of blood returning to the heart influences preload.
  - Frank-Starling mechanism
    - The greater the preload, the more the ventricles are stretched.
    - To a point, as the greater the stretch of the ventricular fibers, the greater the contractile force.
  - More blood returning to the right atrium increases preload; less blood returning decreases preload.

Afterload

Afterload can be increased by giving vasopressors and can be decreased by giving vasodilators.

- **Afterload** is the pressure or resistance against which the ventricles must pump to eject blood.
- Afterload is influenced by arterial blood pressure, arterial distensibility (ability to become stretched), and arterial resistance.
  - The less the resistance (lower afterload), the more easily blood can be ejected. Increased afterload (increased resistance) results in increased cardiac workload.
  - Vasoconstriction $\rightarrow$ ↑ resistance $\rightarrow$ ↑ afterload $\rightarrow$ ↓ SV

Cardiovascular Assessment

Scene Safety

On arrival, ensure the scene is safe before proceeding with your assessment of the patient.

Initial Assessment

- From a distance, use the Pediatric Assessment Triangle to form your first impression of the patient. Evaluate the child's appearance, work of breathing, and circulation to determine the severity of the child's illness or injury (Table 6-1) and assist you in determining the urgency for care (Table 6-2).
- If the child appears sick (unstable), proceed immediately with the primary survey and treat problems as you find them.

TABLE 6-1 First Impression of Cardiovascular Emergencies

Assessment	Imminent Cardiopulmonary Failure	Cardiopulmonary Failure	Cardiopulmonary Arrest
Mental status	Alert, irritable, anxious, restless	Sleepy, intermittently combative, or agitated	Unresponsive to voice or touch
Muscle tone	Able to maintain sitting position (children older than 4 months)	Normal or decreased	Limp
Body position	May assume tripod position	May assume tripod position May need support to maintain sitting position as he/she tires	Unable to maintain sitting position (children older than 4 months)
Respiratory rate	Faster than normal for age	Tachypnea with periods of bradypnea; slowing to bradypnea/agonal breathing	Absent
Respiratory effort	Intercostal retractions Nasal flaring Neck muscle use Seesaw respirations	Nasal flaring Increased respiratory effort at sternal notch Marked use of accessory muscles Retractions, head bobbing Inadequate chest excursion See-saw respirations	Absent
Audible airway sounds	Stridor, wheezing, gurgling	Stridor, wheezing, grunting, gasping	Absent
Skin color	Pink or pale; central cyanosis resolves with oxygen administration	Central cyanosis despite oxygen administration; mottling	Mottling; peripheral and central cyanosis

- If the child appears "not sick" (stable), complete the initial assessment.
- Perform a focused or detailed physical examination based on the patient's presentation and chief complaint.
- Remember: Your patient's condition can change at any time. A patient who initially appears "not sick" may rapidly deteriorate and appear "sick." Reassess frequently.

Focused History

In addition to the SAMPLE history, consider the following questions when obtaining a focused history for a condition affecting the cardiovascular system. This list will require modification on the basis of the patient's age and chief complaint.

Shock

- History of trauma?
- Recent vomiting or diarrhea? Number of diaper changes or trips to the bathroom? Will the child drink?

Focused History and Physical Examination

	Interventions
Imminent cardiopulmonary failure	Approach promptly, but work at a moderate pace Permit the child to assume a position of comfort Correct hypoxia by giving oxygen without causing agitation Provide further interventions based on assessment findings
Cardiopulmonary failure	Move quickly Open the airway and suction if necessary Correct hypoxia by giving high-flow oxygen Begin assisted ventilation if the patient does not improve Provide further interventions based on assessment findings
Cardiopulmonary arrest	Move quickly Immediately open the airway and suction if necessary Use positioning or adjuncts as necessary Provide assisted ventilation with high-concentration oxygen Perform chest compressions as necessary Apply the cardiac monitor and determine the cardiac rhythm Perform endotracheal intubation if assisted ventilation is ineffective or if the airway cannot otherwise be maintained Administer fluids, medications, or defibrillation as indicated Reassess for return of spontaneous respiration and circulation Provide further interventions based on assessment findings

TABLE 6-2 *Immediate Interventions for Cardiovascular Emergencies based on the First Impression*

- Has the child had a fever? For how long?
- Associated symptoms (e.g., change in mental status, shortness of breath, feeling faint, dizziness)?
- History of severe asthma or allergic reactions? Previous treatment?
- Previous hospitalization for allergic reaction?
- Possible bite/sting or ingestion of nuts, shellfish, eggs? New medication?

Dysrhythmias

- When did it start/occur (time, sudden, gradual)? What was the child doing when it started/occurred?
- How long did it last? Does it come and go? Is it still present?
- Does anything make the symptoms better or worse (e.g., change in position, rest)?
- Associated symptoms (e.g., palpitations, change in mental status, shortness of breath, feeling faint, dizziness)?
- Previous hospitalization for heart-related problem?

Chest pain

- When did it start/occur (time, sudden, gradual)? What was the child doing when it started/occurred?

- Quality (e.g., crushing, tight, stabbing, burning, squeezing)?
- How long did it last? Does it come and go? Is it still present?
- Where is the problem? Describe the character and severity if pain is present (use pain scale) (see Chapter 8).
- Associated symptoms (e.g., shortness of breath, feeling faint, dizziness)?
- Previous history of a similar episode? If yes, what was the diagnosis?
- Does anything make the symptoms better or worse? (e.g., change in position)

Congestive heart failure

- When did it start/occur (time, sudden, gradual)?
- When was the child last well (i.e., without current symptoms)?
- History of CHD?
- Poor feeding? Recent weight gain? Decrease in activity?
- Does anything make the symptoms better or worse (e.g., lying down worsens symptoms)?

Focused Physical Examination

Assessment of adequate cardiovascular function includes the following objective measurements and clinical parameters:

- Compare the strength and quality of central and peripheral pulses.
  - Pulse quality reflects the adequacy of peripheral perfusion.
    - A weak central pulse may indicate decompensated shock.
    - A peripheral pulse that is difficult to find, weak, or irregular suggests poor peripheral perfusion and may be a sign of shock or hemorrhage.
  - HR is influenced by the child's age, size, and level of activity. A very slow or rapid rate may indicate or may be the cause of cardiovascular compromise. Normal HRs by age are listed in Table 6-3.
  - In an adult, a tachycardia is defined as a HR above 100 beats per minute. Because an infant or child's HR can transiently increase

TABLE 6-3 Normal Heart Rates by Age

Age	Beats per Minute*
Infant (1 to 12 mo)	100 to 160
Toddler (1 to 3 y)	90 to 150
Preschooler (4 to 5 y)	80 to 140
School-age (6 to 12 y)	70 to 120
Adolescent (13 to 18 y)	60 to 100

*Pulse rates for a sleeping child may be 10% lower than the low rate listed in age group.

- Hypovolemic shock may also be caused by a loss of plasma, fluids, and electrolytes or by endocrine disorders.
  - Plasma loss: burns, third spacing (e.g. pancreatitis, peritonitis)
  - Fluid and electrolyte loss: renal disorder, excessive sweating (e.g., cystic fibrosis), diarrhea, vomiting, dehydration
  - Endocrine: diabetes mellitus, diabetes insipidus, hypothyroidism, adrenal insufficiency
- Circulating blood volume
  - The average circulating blood volume is 80 mL/kg. Average circulating blood volumes by age are listed in Table 6-5.
  - In a healthy child, a loss of 10% to 15% of the circulating blood volume is usually well tolerated and easily compensated (Table 6-6).

Assessment Findings

- Compensated shock
  - Increased HR
  - Peripheral vasoconstriction: skin mottling, delayed capillary refill, cool extremities
  - Normal blood pressure
  - Narrowed pulse pressure
  - Normal or minimally impaired mental status
  - Decreased urine output
- Decompensated shock
  - Hypotension
  - Significant tachycardia
  - Markedly delayed capillary refill
  - Altered mental status: irritability, lethargy
  - Minimal urine output
  - Weak central pulses
  - Pale, mottled, mild peripheral cyanosis

A child may be in shock despite a normal blood pressure.

PEDS *Pearl*

The circulating blood volume is proportionately larger in infants and children than in adults; however, their *total* blood volume is smaller than in adults. As a result, a small volume loss can result in hemodynamic compromise. To understand this important point, consider a 2-year-old as our example. Using the pediatric weight formula, 8 + (2 × age in years), the child's weight is approximately 12 kg. Using a value of 70 mL/kg as the normal circulating blood volume for a child this age, her estimated blood volume is 840 mL. A volume loss of only 250 mL (approximately 30% of the circulating blood volume) is significant and likely to produce signs and symptoms of decompensated shock in this child.

TABLE 6-5 *Average Circulating Blood Volume By Age*

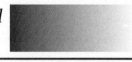

Age	Normal Blood Volume (Average)
Preterm infant	90 to 105 mL/kg
Term newborn	85 mL/kg
Infant older than 1 mo to 11 mo	75 mL/kg
Beyond 1 year	67 to 75 mL/kg
Adult	55 to 75 mL/kg

From: Barkin RM, Rosen P. *Emergency pediatrics: a guide to ambulatory care,* 5th ed. St. Louis: Mosby, 1999, p. 39.

TABLE 6-6 *Response to Fluid and Blood Loss in the Pediatric Patient*

	Class I	Class II	Class III	Class IV
Stage of shock	–	Compensated	Decompensated	Irreversible
% Blood volume loss	Up to 15%	15% to 30%	30% to 45%	More than 45%
Mental status	Slightly anxious	Mildly anxious; restless	Altered; lethargic; apathetic; decreased pain response	Extremely lethargic; unresponsive
Muscle tone	Normal	Normal	Normal to decreased	Limp
Respiratory rate/effort	Normal	Mild tachypnea	Moderate tachypnea	Severe tachypnea to agonal (preterminal event)
Skin color (extremities)	Pink	Pale, mottled	Pale, mottled, mild peripheral cyanosis	Pale, mottled, central and peripheral cyanosis
Skin turgor	Normal	Poor; sunken eyes and fontanelles in infant/young child	Poor; sunken eyes and fontanelles in infant/young child	Tenting
Skin temperature	Cool	Cool	Cool to cold	Cold
Capillary refill	Normal	Poor (more than 2 sec)	Delayed (more than 3 sec)	Prolonged (more than 5 sec)
Heart rate	Usually normal if gradual volume loss; increased if sudden loss of volume	Mild tachycardia	Significant tachycardia; possible dysrhythmias; peripheral pulse weak, thready, or may be absent	Marked tachycardia to bradycardia (preterminal event)
Blood pressure	Normal	Lower range of normal	Decreased	Severe hypotension
Pulse pressure	Normal or increased	Narrowed	Decreased	Decreased
Urine output	Normal; concentrated	Decreased	Minimal	Minimal to absent

Acceptable Interventions

- Use personal protective equipment.
- Perform an initial assessment and obtain a focused history. Obtain a history as soon as possible from the parent or caregiver to assist in identifying the etiology of shock.
- If trauma is suspected, maintain cervical spine stabilization and open the airway with a jaw thrust without head tilt maneuver, if necessary.
- Administer high-concentration oxygen; ensure effective ventilation and oxygenation. Apply a pulse oximeter. Maintain oxygen saturation at above 95%.

- If a pulse or other signs of circulation are absent, or if the HR is less than 60 beats per minute with signs of poor perfusion, begin chest compressions.
- Attach cardiac monitor. Identify the rhythm.

Ongoing assessment is crucial. Use mental status, blood pressure, HR, peripheral perfusion, capillary refill, and urine output to guide volume replacement.

- Obtain vascular access.
  - If immediate vascular access is needed, attempt intravenous (IV) access with two large peripheral IV lines. If unsuccessful, attempt intraosseous (IO) access.
  - Venous access may be difficult to obtain in an infant or child in shock. When shock is present, the most readily available vascular access site is preferred. Peripheral or central venous access is sufficient for fluid resuscitation in most patients.
  - If immediate vascular access is needed and reliable venous access cannot be rapidly achieved, establish IO access. If decompensated shock is present, *immediate* IO access is appropriate.
  - If CPR is in progress, attempt vascular access by the route most readily available that will not require interruption of CPR.

Large volumes of dextrose-containing solutions should not be given because hyperglycemia results, inducing osmotic diuresis.

- Volume resuscitation
  - Type and cross emergently if the child has severe trauma and life-threatening blood loss. Consider giving O-negative blood without crossmatch. Although type-specific crossmatched blood is preferred, O-negative blood may be used under urgent conditions. Order a consult with the trauma service as soon as possible.
  - Administer a bolus of 20 mL/kg of isotonic crystalloid solution (normal saline [NS] or lactated Ringer's [LR]) over 5 to 20 minutes. Assess response (i.e., mental status, capillary refill, HR, respiratory effort, blood pressure).
  - If there is no improvement, give another 20 mL/kg NS or LR fluid bolus and insert a urinary catheter. Assess response.

If blood is administered, it should be warmed before transfusion; otherwise, rapid administration may result in significant hypothermia.

  - If the child continues to demonstrate signs of inadequate perfusion:
    - Give a third 20-mL/kg fluid bolus of NS or LR **OR** give packed red blood cells and a 10-mL/kg fluid bolus of NS.
    - Repeat every 20 to 30 minutes as needed **OR** give a 20-mL/kg IV bolus of whole blood.
    - Repeat every 20 to 30 minutes as needed until systemic perfusion improves.

If severe and prolonged, hypoglycemia may cause brain damage.

- Check glucose. Some children in shock are hypoglycemic because of rapidly depleted carbohydrate stores. If the serum glucose is below 60 mg/dL, administer dextrose IV.
- Maintain normal body temperature.
- Insert a urinary catheter. Urine output is a sensitive measure of perfusion status and adequacy of therapy.

- Obtain appropriate laboratory studies.
  - ◦ Arterial blood gas. If the arterial pH is below 7.20 despite adequate ventilation, correction with sodium bicarbonate (1 mEq/kg) is usually indicated.
  - ◦ Electrolytes, glucose, complete blood count (CBC) with differential, coagulation studies
- Consider the use of vasopressors if poor perfusion persists despite adequate ventilation, oxygenation, and volume expansion.

Unacceptable Interventions

- Failure to use personal protective equipment
- If trauma is suspected, failure to maintain cervical spine stabilization
- If trauma is suspected, failure to open the airway with a jaw thrust without head tilt maneuver
- Failure to administer supplemental oxygen
- Failure to measure oxygen saturation
- Failure to assist ventilation with a bag-valve-mask device and 100% oxygen if signs of inadequate ventilation are present
- Failure to reassess respiratory status after initiating assisted ventilations
- Failure to rapidly establish vascular access
- Extended attempts to establish IV access in a child with decompensated shock when IO access could be established quickly
- Failure to administer a fluid bolus of 20 mL/kg in a child with signs of decompensated shock
- Failure to administer a fluid bolus of appropriate volume in less than 20 minutes
- Failure to assess serum glucose level
- Failure to administer dextrose for documented hypoglycemia
- Failure to use an accurate method for weight and medication dosage determination
- Administration of hypotonic or glucose-containing solutions for volume resuscitation
- Administration of a colloid solution as the initial fluid for volume resuscitation
- Administering vasopressors or boluses of a nonisotonic fluid in a patient with signs of adequate perfusion
- Failure to begin CPR if a pulse is absent or less than 60 beats per minute with signs of hypoperfusion
- Performing tracheal intubation before treating inadequate ventilation with assisted ventilations via bag-valve-mask and 100% oxygen
- Failure to anticipate the potential need for tracheal intubation
- Performing tracheal intubation in a child who responds to less invasive interventions

- If tracheal intubation is required, failure to confirm tracheal tube position using assessment (primary) and mechanical (secondary) methods
- Treating associated injuries (if present) before stabilization of the airway, oxygenation, and circulation
- Ordering a dangerous or inappropriate intervention
- Performing any technique resulting in potential harm to the patient

Cardiogenic Shock

Etiology

Inadequate pump

- Cardiogenic shock occurs because of impaired cardiac muscle function that leads to decreased CO (Figure 6-7).
- Cardiogenic shock may occur as a primary event in patients who have congenital heart disease (CHD) or may occur as a complication of shock of any cause.
  - Cardiomyopathy (CM): myocarditis, ischemia, hypoxia, hypoglycemia, acidosis
  - Myocardial dysfunction after cardiac surgery
  - Myocardial trauma
  - Congestive heart failure (CHF)
  - Hypothermia
  - Drug intoxication
  - Severe electrolyte or acid-base imbalances
  - Severe CHD
  - Hemodynamically significant cardiac dysrhythmias

Signs and symptoms are usually the result of decreased CO.

- Assessment findings
  - Compensated shock: anxiety, pale skin, cool extremities; diapho-

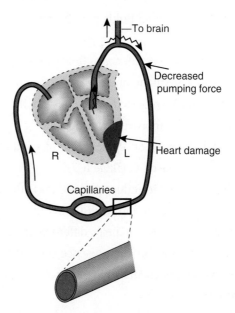

Figure 6-7   Cardiogenic shock.

resis, normal or delayed capillary refill; weak, thready peripheral pulses; mild tachycardia, jugular venous distention (indicating right ventricular failure), narrowed pulse pressure (rise in diastolic pressure with normal systolic blood pressure), mild basilar crackles, normal or mild decrease in urine output, orthopnea

- ○ Decompensated shock: lethargy; pale, mottled, or cyanotic skin; diaphoresis, markedly delayed capillary refill; weak, thready central pulses; peripheral pulses may be absent; hypotension, tachypnea with decreased tidal volume, increasing pulmonary congestion and crackles, oliguria

Acceptable Interventions

- Use personal protective equipment.
- Perform an initial assessment and obtain a focused history. Obtain a history as soon as possible from the parent or caregiver to assist in identifying the etiology of shock.
- Administer high-concentration oxygen; ensure effective ventilation and oxygenation. Apply a pulse oximeter. Maintain oxygen saturation at above 95%.
- If a pulse or other signs of circulation are absent, or if the HR is below 60 beats per minute with signs of poor perfusion, begin chest compressions.
- Attach cardiac monitor. Identify the rhythm.
- Obtain vascular access. If IV access cannot be rapidly established, place an IO needle.
- Check glucose and electrolyte levels. If the serum glucose is less than 60 mg/dL, administer dextrose IV.
- Give a small IV/IO fluid bolus of isotonic crystalloid solution (5 to 10 mL/kg of LR or NS). The fluid bolus may be repeated on the basis of the child's response.
  - ○ Repeat the primary survey after *each* fluid bolus. Monitor closely for increased work of breathing and the development of crackles.
  - ○ The fluid bolus may be repeated on the basis of the child's response. If the child fails to improve, consider giving an inotrope (e.g., dopamine, dobutamine, or epinephrine) to improve myocardial contractility and increase CO (Table 6-7).
- Vasodilators may be used to reduce preload and afterload.
- Treat dysrhythmias if present and contributing to shock.
- Obtain a chest radiograph to help differentiate cardiogenic from noncardiogenic shock, identify the presence of a pulmonary infection, cardiomegaly, pulmonary edema, or evolving acute respiratory distress syndrome (ARDS).
- Obtain a 12-lead electrocardiogram and cardiology consult.

Jugular venous distention (JVD) is difficult to assess in infants and young children.

The treatment of cardiogenic shock is generally based on increasing contractility, altering preload and afterload, and controlling dysrhythmias if they are present and contributing to shock.

Unacceptable Interventions

- Failure to use personal protective equipment
- Failure to administer supplemental oxygen
- Failure to measure oxygen saturation
- Failure to assist ventilation with a bag-valve-mask device and 100% oxygen if signs of inadequate ventilation are present
- Failure to reassess respiratory status after initiating assisted ventilations
- Failure to rapidly establish vascular access
- Extended attempts to establish IV access in a child with decompensated shock when IO access could be established quickly
- Failure to rapidly administer a 5 to 10 mL/kg of LR or NS fluid bolus to a child with signs of decompensated shock
- Failure to repeat the primary survey after each fluid bolus
- Failure to assess serum glucose level
- Failure to administer dextrose for documented hypoglycemia
- Failure to use an accurate method for weight and medication dosage determination
- Failure to consider addition of inotropes, vasopressors, or vasodilators if perfusion does not improve with fluid administration
- Failure to begin CPR if a pulse is absent or less than 60 beats per minute with signs of hypoperfusion
- Performing tracheal intubation before treating inadequate ventilation with assisted ventilations via bag-valve-mask and 100% oxygen
- Failure to anticipate the potential need for tracheal intubation
- Performing tracheal intubation in a child who responds to less invasive interventions

TABLE 6-7 *Medications Used for Cardiopulmonary Resuscitation*

	Positive Inotrope	Positive Chronotrope	Direct Pressor	Indirect Pressor	Vasodilator
Dopamine	++	+	±	++	++*
Dobutamine	++	±	–	–	+
Epinephrine	+++	+++	+++	–	–
Isoproterenol	+++	+++	–	–	+++
Norepinephrine	+++	+++	+++	–	–

From Krug SE. Chapter title. In: Behrman RE, Kliegman RM, eds. *The acutely ill or injured child in Nelson essentials of pediatrics,* 4th ed. Philadelphia: WB Saunders, 2002.
*Primarily splanchnic and renal in low doses (3 to 5 mcg/kg/min).

- If tracheal intubation is required, failure to confirm tracheal tube position using assessment (primary) and mechanical (secondary) methods
- Ordering a dangerous or inappropriate intervention
- Performing any technique resulting in potential harm to the patient

Distributive Shock

- In distributive shock, a relative hypovolemia occurs when vasodilation increases the size of the vascular space and the available blood volume must fill a greater space (container problem; increased vascular space) (Figure 6-8). This results in an altered distribution of the blood volume (relative hypovolemia) rather than actual volume loss (absolute hypovolemia).
- Distributive shock may be caused by a severe infection (septic shock), severe allergic reaction (anaphylactic shock), spinal cord injury (neurogenic shock), or certain overdoses (e.g., sedatives, narcotics).

Septic Shock

Terminology/Etiology

- **Bacteremia** is the presence of viable bacteria in the blood.
- **Systemic inflammatory response syndrome** (SIRS) is a response to infection manifested by derangement in two or more of the following: temperature, HR, respiratory rate, and white blood cell count.
- **Sepsis** is the systemic response to an infection.

Vessel/container problem; increased vascular space

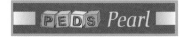

Signs and symptoms of distributive shock that are unusual in the presence of hypovolemic shock include warm, flushed skin (especially in dependent areas), and, in neurogenic shock, a normal or slow pulse rate (relative bradycardia).

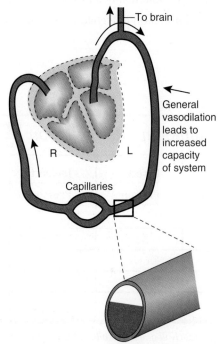

Neurogenic or Vascular Shock

To brain

General vasodilation leads to increased capacity of system

R   L

Capillaries

Figure 6-8   Distributive shock.

○ **Septicemia** refers to multiplication of bacteria in the bloodstream, resulting in an overwhelming infection.

○ Common sites of bacterial infection include the kidneys (upper urinary tract infection), liver or the gall bladder, bowel (usually seen with peritonitis), skin (cellulitis), and the lungs (bacterial pneumonia).

○ Septicemia may exist for some time before septic shock develops.

○ Risk factors for sepsis include extremes of age, a compromised immune system, malnourishment, and chronic antibiotic or steroid use.

• **Severe sepsis** is sepsis associated with organ dysfunction, hypoperfusion, or hypotension. Hypoperfusion and perfusion abnormalities may include, but are not limited to, lactic acidosis, oliguria, or an acute alteration in mental status.

• **Septic shock** is sepsis with hypotension, despite adequate fluid resuscitation, with the presence of perfusion abnormalities that may include, but are not limited to, lactic acidosis, oliguria, or an acute alteration in mental status. Patients who are on inotropic or vasopressor agents may not be hypotensive at the time that perfusion abnormalities are measured.

○ Fever, tachycardia, and vasodilation are common in children with benign infections.

  ▪ Septic shock should be suspected when a child with this inflammatory triad experiences a change in mental status evidenced by inconsolable irritability, lack of interaction with parents, or inability to be aroused.

○ Septic shock occurs in two clinical stages.

  ▪ The early (hyperdynamic) phase is characterized by peripheral vasodilation (warm shock) due to endotoxins that prevent catecholamine-induced vasoconstriction.

  ▪ The late (hypodynamic or decompensated) phase is characterized by cool extremities (cold shock) and resembles hypovolemic shock.

  ▪ Hypotension is not necessary for the clinical diagnosis of septic shock; however, its presence in a child with clinical suspicion of infection is confirmatory.[3]

Assessment Findings

• Early (hyperdynamic) phase (increased CO)

  ○ Warm, dry, flushed skin

  ○ Blood pressure may be normal or possible widened pulse pressure

  ○ Bounding peripheral pulses

  ○ Brisk capillary refill

  ○ Tachycardia

  ○ Tachypnea

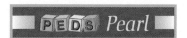

PEDS Pearl

If you observe a change in mental status in a febrile child (inconsolable, inability to recognize parents, unarousable), *immediately* consider the possibility of septic shock.

- Late (hypodynamic/decompensated) phase
  - Mottled, cool extremities
  - Diminished or absent peripheral pulses
  - Altered mental status
  - Tachycardia
  - Delayed capillary refill
  - Decreased urine output

Late septic shock is usually indistinguishable from other types of shock.

Acceptable Interventions

- Use personal protective equipment.
- Perform an initial assessment and obtain a focused history. Obtain a history as soon as possible from the parent or caregiver to assist in identifying the etiology of shock.
- Administer high-concentration oxygen; ensure effective ventilation and oxygenation. Apply a pulse oximeter. Maintain oxygen saturation at above 95%.
- If a pulse or other signs of circulation are absent, or if the HR is less than 60 beats per minute with signs of poor perfusion, begin chest compressions.
- Attach cardiac monitor. Identify the rhythm.
- Obtain vascular access. If IV access cannot be rapidly established, place an IO needle.
  - Rapidly give a 20-mL/kg isotonic crystalloid solution (NS or LR) fluid bolus.
  - If perfusion does not improve, repeat fluid boluses and reassess response, repeating the primary survey after *each* fluid bolus. Monitor closely for increased work of breathing and the development of crackles.
  - Therapeutic endpoints include objective measures such as urine output above 1 mL/kg per hour, normal mental status, normal blood pressure and pulse, and capillary refill less than 2 seconds.
- Check glucose and electrolyte levels. If the serum glucose is less than 60 mg/dL, administer dextrose IV.
- If septic shock lasts more than 1 hour despite aggressive fluid resuscitation[3]
  - Establish central venous access.
  - Establish arterial monitoring.
  - Dopamine is recommended as the first-line vasopressor for fluid resistant septic shock. Begin the infusion at 5 mcg/kg per minute. Continue administration of IV fluid boluses during the dopamine infusion.
  - If unresponsive to dopamine administration
    - Give epinephrine 0.1 to 0.5 mcg/kg per minute IV infusion for cold shock

Increased work of breathing, hypoventilation, and altered mental status are indications for intubation.

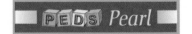

PEDS Pearl

Management of septic shock requires aggressive fluid administration. The patient in decompensated septic shock may require significant quantities of fluid. For example, some patients have required 100 to 200 mL/kg in the first few hours of resuscitation. Carefully monitor the patient for crackles and increased work of breathing during rapid fluid administration.

PEDS Pearl

The choice of IV solution used in septic shock is controversial. Crystalloid administration may result in pulmonary edema by lowering intravascular oncotic pressure and encouraging capillary leakage. Administration of a colloid solution may better maintain oncotic pressure, but may eventually leak into the interstitium due to the loss of vascular integrity. To restore adequate perfusion in septic shock, resuscitation may require the use of both crystalloid and colloid solutions.

- Give norepinephrine 0.03 to 1.5 mcg/kg per minute IV infusion for warm shock
- Administer IV antibiotics. Obtain cultures of blood or any other body fluid suspicious of being infected before administering antibiotics.
- The role of steroids in septic shock is controversial.

Unacceptable Interventions

- Failure to use personal protective equipment
- Failure to administer supplemental oxygen
- Failure to measure oxygen saturation
- Failure to assist ventilation with a bag-valve-mask device and 100% oxygen if signs of inadequate ventilation are present
- Failure to reassess respiratory status after initiating assisted ventilations
- Failure to rapidly establish vascular access
- Extended attempts to establish IV access in a child with decompensated shock when IO access could be established quickly
- Failure to administer a rapid fluid bolus of 20 mL/kg in a child with signs of decompensated shock
- Failure to repeat the primary survey after each fluid bolus
- Failure to assess serum glucose level
- Failure to administer dextrose for documented hypoglycemia
- Failure to use an accurate method for weight and medication dosage determination
- Administration of hypotonic or glucose-containing solutions for volume resuscitation
- Administration of a colloid solution as the initial fluid for volume resuscitation
- Administering vasopressors or boluses of a nonisotonic fluid in a patient with signs of adequate perfusion
- Failure to begin CPR if a pulse is absent or less than 60 beats per minute with signs of hypoperfusion
- Performing tracheal intubation before treating inadequate ventilation with assisted ventilations via bag-valve-mask and 100% oxygen
- Failure to anticipate the potential need for tracheal intubation
- Performing tracheal intubation in a child who responds to less invasive interventions
- If tracheal intubation is required, failure to confirm tracheal tube position using assessment (primary) and mechanical (secondary) methods
- Ordering a dangerous or inappropriate intervention
- Performing any technique resulting in potential harm to the patient

Anaphylactic Shock

Etiology

- Anaphylaxis or anaphylactic shock occurs when the body is exposed to a substance that produces a severe allergic reaction that usually occurs within minutes of the exposure. Common causes include insect stings, medications (e.g., penicillin, sulfa), and some foods (e.g., shellfish, nuts, strawberries).

- Type I hypersensitivity occurs when an individual is exposed to a specific allergen and develops IgE antibodies. These antibodies attach to mast cells in specific body locations, creating sensitized mast cells. On reexposure to the same allergen, histamine and other chemical mediators are released.

- These substances cause widespread arterial and venous vasodilation and increase capillary permeability (Figure 6-9).
  - Intravascular fluid leaks into the interstitial space resulting in a decrease in intravascular volume (relative hypovolemia).
  - Increased blood vessel permeability causes swelling that is noticeable in the mucous membranes of the larynx (stridor), trachea, and bronchial tree, increasing the potential for complete airway obstruction due to severe edema.
  - The decrease in intravascular volume results in decreased cardiac preload and exacerbates hypotension.

Assessment Findings

- Stridor, wheezing, coughing, hoarseness, intercostal and suprasternal retractions
- Tachycardia, hypotension, dysrhythmias
- Vomiting, diarrhea
- Anxiety, restlessness
- Facial swelling and angioedema
- Urticaria (hives)
- Abdominal pain, cramping
- Pruritus (itching)

Acceptable Interventions

- Use personal protective equipment.
- Perform an initial assessment and obtain a focused history.
- Remove/discontinue the causative agent.
- Administer high-concentration oxygen; ensure effective ventilation and oxygenation. Apply a pulse oximeter. Maintain oxygen saturation at above 95%.
- If a pulse or other signs of circulation are absent, or if the HR is less than 60 beats per minute with signs of poor perfusion, begin chest compressions.
- Attach cardiac monitor. Identify the rhythm.
- Give epinephrine 0.01 mg/kg (0.01 mL/kg) of 1:1000 intramuscular (IM) or subcutaneous (SC) solution. Maximum single dose 0.5 mg.[4] May be

---

Drug Pearl
Diphenhydramine (Benadryl)

- Diphenhydramine is an antihistamine/histamine-1 (H_1) receptor antagonist.
- Histamine is released from mast cells following exposure to an antigen to which the body has been previously sensitized. When released into the circulation following an allergic reaction, histamine acts on two different receptors: H_1 and H_2. Stimulation of H_1 receptors causes bronchoconstriction and contraction of the gut. Stimulation of H_2 receptors causes peripheral vasodilation and secretion of gastric acids.
- In anaphylaxis, diphenhydramine is used in conjunction with epinephrine and steroids. Epinephrine causes bronchodilation by stimulating β_2-adrenergic receptors. Diphenhydramine blocks cellular histamine response, but does not prevent histamine release.

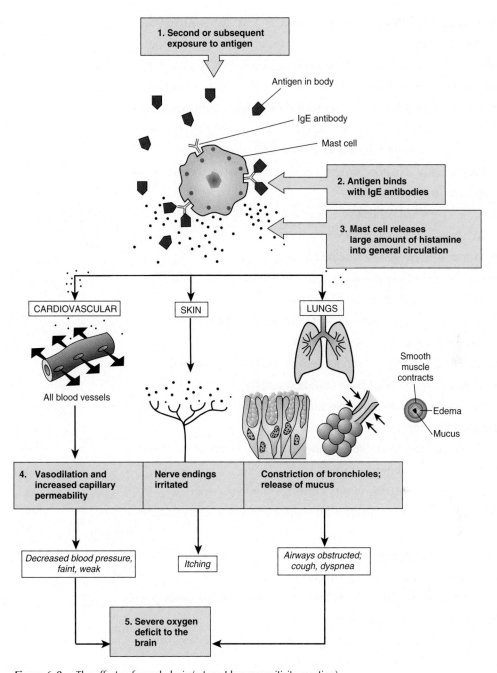

1. Second or subsequent exposure to antigen

Antigen in body

IgE antibody

Mast cell

2. Antigen binds with IgE antibodies

3. Mast cell releases large amount of histamine into general circulation

CARDIOVASCULAR

SKIN

LUNGS

Smooth muscle contracts

All blood vessels

Edema

Mucus

4. Vasodilation and increased capillary permeability

Nerve endings irritated

Constriction of bronchioles; release of mucus

Decreased blood pressure, faint, weak

Itching

Airways obstructed; cough, dyspnea

5. Severe oxygen deficit to the brain

Figure 6-9   The effects of anaphylaxis (a type I hypersensitivity reaction).

administered every 15 minutes up to three doses if necessary while attempting IV access.

- Obtain vascular access. If IV access cannot be rapidly established, place an IO needle.
  - Rapidly give a 20-mL/kg isotonic crystalloid solution (NS or LR) fluid bolus.
  - If perfusion does not improve, repeat one or two fluid boluses and reassess response, repeating the primary survey after *each* fluid bolus. Monitor closely for increased work of breathing and the development of crackles.

- Check glucose level. If the serum glucose is less than 60 mg/dL, administer dextrose IV.
- Consider inhaled bronchodilator therapy (e.g., albuterol).
- Administer other medications to help stop the inflammatory reaction.
  - Consider diphenhydramine 1.0 mg/kg IM or IV. Maximum dosage is 50 mg.
  - Consider methylprednisolone 1 to 2 mg/kg IV.
- Give epinephrine IV infusion for signs of decompensated shock.

Unacceptable Interventions

- Failure to use personal protective equipment
- Failure to administer supplemental oxygen
- Failure to measure oxygen saturation
- Failure to assist ventilation with a bag-valve-mask device and 100% oxygen if signs of inadequate ventilation are present
- Failure to reassess respiratory status after initiating assisted ventilations
- Failure to rapidly establish vascular access
- Extended attempts to establish IV access in a child with decompensated shock when IO access could be established quickly
- Failure to rapidly administer a rapid fluid bolus of 20 mL/kg in a child with signs of decompensated shock
- Failure to repeat the primary survey after each fluid bolus
- Failure to assess serum glucose level
- Failure to administer dextrose for documented hypoglycemia
- Failure to use an accurate method for weight and medication dosage determination
- Administering vasopressors or boluses of a nonisotonic fluid in a patient with signs of adequate perfusion
- Failure to begin CPR if a pulse is absent or less than 60 beats per minute with signs of hypoperfusion
- Performing tracheal intubation before treating inadequate ventilation with assisted ventilations via bag-valve-mask and 100% oxygen
- Failure to anticipate the potential need for tracheal intubation
- Performing tracheal intubation in a child who responds to less invasive interventions
- If tracheal intubation is required, failure to confirm tracheal tube position using assessment (primary) and mechanical (secondary) methods
- Ordering a dangerous or inappropriate intervention
- Performing any technique resulting in potential harm to the patient

Neurogenic Shock

Etiology

- Neurogenic shock is caused by a severe injury to the head or spinal cord (e.g., brainstem injuries, complete transection of the spinal cord)

In this type of shock, there is a disruption in the ability of the sympathetic nervous system to control vessel dilation and constriction.

that results in a loss of sympathetic vascular tone below the level of the spinal cord injury.

- The loss of peripheral vascular tone results in widespread vasodilation below the level of the injury → ↓ venous return → ↓ SV → ↓ CO → ↓ tissue perfusion
  - The total blood volume remains the same, but vessel capacity is increased (relative hypovolemia).
  - Normally, a decrease in blood pressure is accompanied by a compensatory increase in HR. In neurogenic shock, the patient does not become tachycardic because sympathetic activity is disrupted.
- Situations in which spinal cord damage may occur include high-speed motor vehicle crashes in which the child is a pedestrian, an unrestrained or improperly restrained passenger, falls from extreme heights, and diving accidents.

Assessment Findings

Widespread vasodilation may result in a loss of body heat. Be aware of possible hypothermia.

- Skin is warm and dry.
  - Immediately after the injury, the skin appears flushed due to vasodilation. Blood eventually pools, leaving the uppermost skin surfaces pale.
  - If neurogenic shock occurs with hypovolemia, the extremities often become cool.
  - Sweating does not occur below the level of the injury.
- HR within normal limits or bradycardic.
- Hypotension.
- Wide pulse pressure.
- Respiratory rate/effort and breathing pattern may be affected depending on the location of the injury.
  - Abdominal breathing may result if a high cord injury disrupts the intercostal nerves that control rib movement.
  - If the phrenic nerve is affected, breathing may be shallow, labored, and (possibly) irregular.

Acceptable Interventions

- Use personal protective equipment.
- Perform an initial assessment and obtain a focused history.
- If trauma is suspected, maintain cervical spine stabilization and open the airway with a jaw thrust without head tilt maneuver, if necessary.
- Administer high-concentration oxygen; ensure effective ventilation and oxygenation. Apply a pulse oximeter. Maintain oxygen saturation at above 95%.
- If a pulse or other signs of circulation are absent, or if the HR is less than 60 beats per minute with signs of poor perfusion, begin chest compressions.

- Attach cardiac monitor. Identify the rhythm.
- Obtain vascular access. If IV access cannot be rapidly established, place an IO needle.
  - Rapidly give a 20-mL/kg isotonic crystalloid solution (NS or LR) fluid bolus.
  - If perfusion does not improve, repeat fluid boluses and reassess response, repeating the primary survey after *each* fluid bolus. Monitor closely for increased work of breathing and the development of crackles.
  - Repeat every 20 to 30 minutes as needed until systemic perfusion improves.
- Check glucose. If the serum glucose is less than 60 mg/dL, administer dextrose IV.
- Maintain normal body temperature.
- Insert a urinary catheter. Urine output is a sensitive measure of perfusion status and adequacy of therapy.
- Consider the use of vasopressors if poor perfusion persists despite adequate ventilation, oxygenation, and volume expansion.

Unacceptable Interventions

- Failure to use personal protective equipment
- If trauma is suspected, failure to maintain cervical spine stabilization
- If trauma is suspected, failure to open the airway with a jaw thrust without head tilt maneuver
- Failure to administer supplemental oxygen
- Failure to measure oxygen saturation
- Failure to assist ventilation with a bag-valve-mask device and 100% oxygen if signs of inadequate ventilation are present
- Failure to reassess respiratory status after initiating assisted ventilations
- Failure to rapidly administer a rapid fluid bolus of 20 mL/kg in a child with signs of decompensated shock
- Failure to repeat the primary survey after each fluid bolus
- Failure to assess serum glucose level
- Failure to administer dextrose for documented hypoglycemia
- Failure to use an accurate method for weight and medication dosage determination
- Administering vasopressors or boluses of a nonisotonic fluid in a patient with signs of adequate perfusion
- Failure to begin CPR if a pulse is absent or less than 60 beats per minute with signs of hypoperfusion
- Performing tracheal intubation before treating inadequate ventilation with assisted ventilations via bag-valve-mask and 100% oxygen
- Failure to anticipate the potential need for tracheal intubation

- Performing tracheal intubation in a child who responds to less invasive interventions
- If tracheal intubation is required, failure to confirm tracheal tube position using assessment (primary) and mechanical (secondary) methods
- Treating associated injuries (if present), before stabilization of the airway, oxygenation, and circulation
- Ordering a dangerous or inappropriate intervention
- Performing any technique resulting in potential harm to the patient

Obstructive Shock

Shock that develops from cardiac tamponade, tension pneumothorax, or a massive pulmonary embolism is called obstructive shock because the common pathophysiology in these conditions is obstruction to blood flow from the heart.

Etiology

Ventricular outflow problem

- Tension pneumothorax
  - A tension pneumothorax can result from blunt or penetrating chest trauma, barotrauma secondary to positive-pressure ventilation (especially when using high amounts of positive end-expiratory pressure [PEEP]), as a complication of central venous catheter placement (usually subclavian or internal jugular), or when a chest tube is clamped or becomes blocked after insertion.
  - In a tension pneumothorax, air enters on inspiration but cannot escape. Intrathoracic pressure increases, the lung collapses, and air under pressure shifts the mediastinum away from the midline, toward the unaffected side. As intrathoracic pressure increases, the vena cava becomes kinked, decreasing venous return and altering CO (Figure 6-10).

In children, cardiac tamponade is more common in boys than in girls, with a male-to-female ratio of 7:3.

- Cardiac tamponade
  - The pericardial sac normally contains less than 1 mL/kg of fluid. In cardiac tamponade, excessive fluid accumulates in the pericardial sac, resulting in reduced ventricular filling, a decrease in SV, and a subsequent decrease in CO (Figure 6-11).
  - The right side of the heart is affected first, causing increased pressure in the systemic veins. If fluid accumulates rapidly in the pericardial sac, distended neck veins are often visible. If fluid accumulates slowly, a large amount of fluid can build up before signs appear because the pericardium adapts and stretches to accommodate the increased volume, without any significant effect on diastolic filling of the heart.
  - Excess fluid accumulation may occur from pericarditis, postcardiac surgery, after trauma, connective tissue diseases, radiation therapy, and as a complication of central venous catheters.

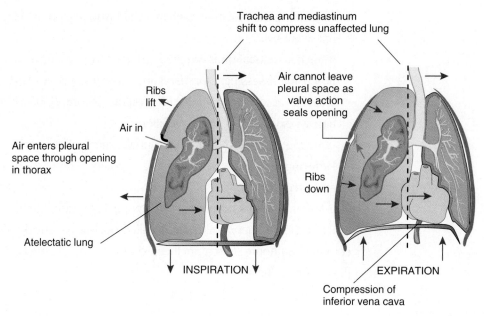

Figure 6-10   Tension pneumothorax.

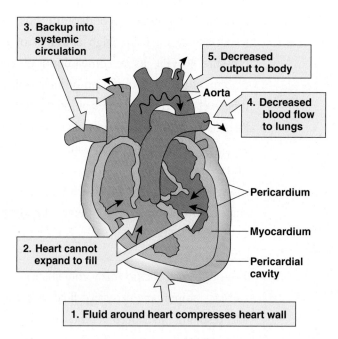

Figure 6-11   Effects of pericardial tamponade.

Assessment Findings

- Tension pneumothorax
  - Early
    - Dyspnea
    - Anxiety
    - Tachypnea
    - Tachycardia
    - Hyperresonance of the chest wall on the affected side
    - Diminished or absent breath sounds on the affected side

Cardiac tamponade and tension pneumothorax present with clear lung sounds; however, lung sounds are unequal in a tension pneumothorax.

- ◦ Late
  - Decreased level of responsiveness
  - Tracheal deviation toward the unaffected side
  - Hypotension
  - Distention of neck veins (may not be present if hypovolemic or in cases of severe hypotension)
  - Cyanosis
- Cardiac tamponade
  - ◦ Beck's triad: increased jugular venous pressure, hypotension, muffled heart sounds
  - ◦ Dyspnea
  - ◦ Anxiety, restlessness
  - ◦ Cold extremities
  - ◦ Pale, mottled, or cyanotic skin
  - ◦ Tachycardia
  - ◦ Weak or absent peripheral pulses
  - ◦ Narrowed pulse pressure
  - ◦ Pulsus paradoxus (i.e., a drop in blood pressure of 10 mm Hg or more during inspiration)

Acceptable Interventions

Management of obstructive shock depends on the cause.

- Use personal protective equipment.
- Perform an initial assessment and obtain a focused history. Obtain a history as soon as possible from the parent or caregiver to assist in identifying the etiology of shock.
- If trauma is suspected, maintain cervical spine stabilization and open the airway with a jaw thrust without head tilt maneuver, if necessary
- Administer high-concentration oxygen; ensure effective ventilation and oxygenation. Apply a pulse oximeter. Maintain oxygen saturation at above 95%.
- If a pulse or other signs of circulation are absent, or if the HR is less than 60 beats per minute with signs of poor perfusion, begin chest compressions.
- Attach cardiac monitor. Identify the rhythm.
- Obtain vascular access. If immediate vascular access is needed, attempt IV access. If unsuccessful, attempt IO access.
  - ◦ Administer a bolus of 20 mL/kg of isotonic crystalloid solution (NS or LR) over 5 to 20 minutes. Assess response (i.e., mental status, capillary refill, HR, respiratory effort, blood pressure).
  - ◦ If the child continues to demonstrate signs of inadequate perfusion, give a third 20-mL/kg fluid bolus of NS or LR. Repeat every 20 to 30 minutes as needed until systemic perfusion improves.
- Management of tension pneumothorax

- Perform needle decompression of the affected side. Reassess.
- After needle decompression, insert a thoracostomy tube. Reassess.
- Obtain a chest radiograph to assess for lung reexpansion and evaluate thoracostomy tube position.
- Management of cardiac tamponade
  - Volume expansion with isotonic crystalloid solution as necessary to maintain an adequate circulating blood volume
  - Administration of an inotropic drug such as dobutamine may be useful because it does not increase systemic vascular resistance while increasing CO.
  - Pericardiocentesis is the definitive treatment for cardiac tamponade.
- Check glucose. If the serum glucose is less than 60 mg/dL, administer dextrose IV.
- Maintain normal body temperature.
- Obtain appropriate laboratory studies.
- Insert a urinary catheter if necessary.

Unacceptable Interventions

- Failure to use personal protective equipment
- If trauma is suspected, failure to maintain cervical spine stabilization
- If trauma is suspected, failure to open the airway with a jaw thrust without head tilt maneuver
- Failure to administer supplemental oxygen
- Failure to measure oxygen saturation
- Failure to assist ventilation with a bag-valve-mask device and 100% oxygen if signs of inadequate ventilation are present
- Failure to reassess respiratory status after initiating assisted ventilations
- Failure to decompress a tension pneumothorax
- Failure to rapidly establish vascular access
- Extended attempts to establish IV access in a child with decompensated shock when IO access could be established quickly
- Failure to rapidly administer a rapid fluid bolus of 20 mL/kg in a child with signs of decompensated shock
- Failure to repeat the primary survey after each fluid bolus
- Failure to assess serum glucose level
- Failure to administer dextrose for documented hypoglycemia
- Failure to use an accurate method for weight and medication dosage determination
- Administration of hypotonic or glucose-containing solutions for volume resuscitation
- Administration of a colloid solution as the initial fluid for volume resuscitation

- Administering vasopressors or boluses of a nonisotonic fluid in a patient with signs of adequate perfusion
- Failure to begin CPR if a pulse is absent or less than 60 beats per minute with signs of hypoperfusion
- Performing tracheal intubation before treating inadequate ventilation with assisted ventilations via bag-valve-mask and 100% oxygen
- Failure to anticipate the potential need for tracheal intubation
- Performing tracheal intubation in a child who responds to less invasive interventions
- If tracheal intubation is required, failure to confirm tracheal tube position using assessment (primary) and mechanical (secondary) methods
- Treating associated injuries (if present) before stabilization of the airway, oxygenation, and circulation
- Ordering a dangerous or inappropriate intervention
- Performing any technique resulting in potential harm to the patient

PEDIATRIC SHOCK ALGORITHM

Perform an Initial Assessment (see Initial Assessment algorithm)

If **no** signs of congestive heart failure are present:

- Give a bolus of 20 mL/kg of isotonic crystalloid solution (NS or LR) IV/IO
  as rapidly as needed (< 20 minutes) to maintain circulating blood volume.
- Check glucose. Treat if < 60 mg/dL.
- Maintain normal body temperature
- Correct electrolyte and acid-base disturbances

Assess response (i.e., mental status, capillary refill, heart rate, respiratory effort, blood pressure).

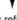

If inadequate response:

Hypovolemic	**Hypovolemic Shock – Nontraumatic:** Administer 1 or 2 additional fluid boluses as indicated. Reassess. Consider vasopressors if poor perfusion persists despite adequate ventilation, oxygenation, and volume expansion. **Hemorrhagic Shock:** Administer 1 or 2 additional fluid boluses as indicated and reassess; administer packed red blood cells if available at 10 mL/kg. Type and cross emergently if the child has severe trauma and life-threatening blood loss. Consider giving O-negative blood without crossmatch. Order a consult with Trauma Service as soon as possible.
Cardiogenic	• Consider giving a small IV/IO fluid bolus of isotonic crystalloid solution (5 to 10 mL/kg of LR or NS). Repeat the primary survey after *each* fluid bolus. The fluid bolus may be repeated based on the child's response. If the child fails to improve, consider giving an inotrope (e.g., dopamine, dobutamine, or epinephrine) to improve myocardial contractility and increase cardiac output. • Treat dysrhythmias if present and contributing to shock. Consult cardiologist for additional orders.
Distributive	**Anaphylaxis** • Remove/discontinue the causative agent. Give epinephrine 0.01 mg/kg (0.01 mL/kg) 1:1000 solution IM. Maximum single dose 0.5 mg. Repeat in 15 min if needed. • Give 1 or 2 additional fluid boluses as indicated. Reassess. Consider inhaled bronchodilator (albuterol), diphenhydramine 1.0 mg/kg IM or IV, methylprednisolone 1 to 2 mg/kg IV • Give epinephrine IV infusion for signs of decompensated shock **Septic** • Administer 1 or 2 additional fluid boluses as indicated. Reassess. • Administer a vasopressor by IV infusion for signs of decompensated shock. • Give IV antibiotics. **Neurogenic** • Administer 1 or 2 additional fluid boluses as indicated. Reassess.
Obstructive	Tension pneumothorax • Perform needle decompression followed by chest tube insertion. Reassess. Cardiac tamponade • Administer 1 or 2 additional fluid boluses as indicated. Reassess. • Pericardiocentesis is the definitive treatment for cardiac tamponade.

Cardiopulmonary Failure

Cardiopulmonary failure is a clinical condition identified by deficits in oxygenation, ventilation, and perfusion. Respiratory failure associated with decompensated shock leads to inadequate oxygenation, ventilation, and perfusion, resulting in cardiopulmonary failure. Without prompt recognition and management, cardiopulmonary failure will deteriorate to cardiopulmonary arrest.

Signs of Cardiopulmonary Failure

- Bradypnea with irregular, ineffective respirations
- Decreasing work of breathing (tiring)
- Delayed capillary refill time (longer than 5 seconds)
- Bradycardia
- Weak central pulses and absent peripheral pulses
- Cool extremities
- Mottled or cyanotic skin
- Diminished level of responsiveness

Cardiopulmonary Arrest

Cardiac arrest is the cessation of cardiac mechanical activity, confirmed by the absence of a detectable pulse, unresponsiveness, and apnea or agonal, gasping respirations. In adults, sudden nontraumatic cardiopulmonary arrests are usually the result of underlying cardiac disease. In children, cardiopulmonary arrest is usually the result of respiratory failure or shock that progresses to cardiopulmonary failure with profound hypoxemia and acidosis, and eventually cardiopulmonary arrest. The cause of cardiopulmonary arrest in the pediatric patient also varies with age, the underlying health of the child, and the location of the event (Table 6-8).

Rhythm Disturbances

ECG monitoring is an important aspect of pediatric emergency care and is indicated for any pediatric patient who shows signs of significant illness or injury. ECG monitoring may be used to assess the patient's HR, evaluate the effects of disease or injury on heart function, evaluate the response to medications, or to obtain a baseline recording before, during, and after a medical procedure. Although disorders of HR and rhythm are

- A **lead** is a record of electrical activity between two electrodes. A lead has a negative (−) and positive (+) electrode (pole).
  - Moving the lead selector on the ECG machine allows us to make any of the electrodes positive or negative. The position of the positive electrode on the body determines the portion of the heart "seen" by each lead.
  - Each lead senses the magnitude and direction of the electrical forces caused by the spread of waves of depolarization and repolarization throughout the heart. A 12-lead ECG views the surfaces of the left ventricle from 12 different angles. Lead II is most commonly used for ECG monitoring.
- Electrodes are applied at specific locations on the patient's chest wall and extremities in combinations of two, three, four, or five to view the heart's electrical activity from different angles and planes.
  - One end of a monitoring cable is attached to the electrode and the other end to an ECG machine.
  - When applying electrodes for ECG monitoring
    - Be sure the conductive gel in the center of the electrode is not dry.
    - Snap or connect the ECG/lead wires to the electrodes before applying them to the patient.
    - Place two of three electrodes on the shoulders or lateral chest, avoiding bony prominences. Place the third electrode on the lower abdomen or upper thigh (Figure 6-13).

Placing the electrodes in this manner ensures that chest compressions and paddle placement for defibrillation will not be hindered if these procedures are required.

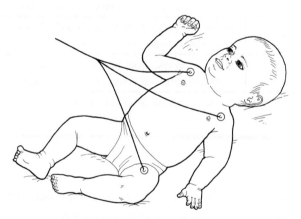

Figure 6-13   Electrode placement for electrocardiogram monitoring.

ECG Paper

- ECG paper is graph paper made up of small and large boxes. The smallest boxes are 1 mm wide and 1 mm high.
- The horizontal axis of the paper corresponds with time. Time is stated in seconds (Figure 6-14). ECG paper normally records at a constant speed of 25 mm per second; thus, each horizontal unit (1-mm box) represents 0.04 sec (25 mm per second × 0.04 sec = 1 mm)

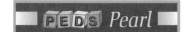

When viewing a rhythm strip, keep the following terms in mind:

- Waveform: movement away from the baseline in either a positive or a negative direction
- Segment: a line between waveforms; named by the waveform that precedes or follows it
- Interval: a waveform and a segment
- Complex: several waveforms

- There are five small boxes in each large box on the paper. A large box represents 0.20 second; five large boxes, each consisting of five small boxes, represent 1 second; 15 large boxes equal an interval of 3 seconds; 30 large boxes represent 6 seconds.
- The vertical axis of the paper represents voltage or amplitude of the ECG waveforms or deflections. The size or amplitude of a waveform is measured in millivolts or millimeters.

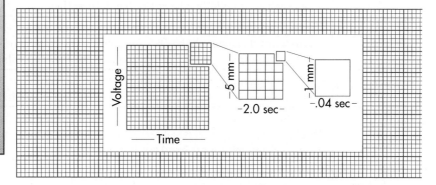

Figure 6-14 ECG paper. The horizontal axis represents time. The vertical axis represents amplitude or voltage.

Waveforms

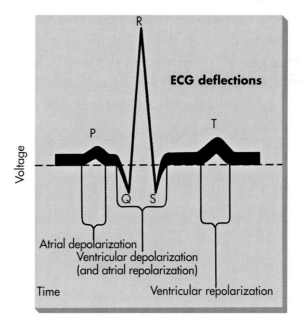

Figure 6-15 Electrocardiogram deflections: P, QRS, and T.

Artifact

Accurate ECG rhythm recognition requires a tracing in which the waveforms and intervals are free of distortion. Distortion of an ECG tracing by electrical activity that is noncardiac in origin is called **artifact**. Because artifact can mimic various cardiac dysrhythmias, including VF, it is *essential* to evaluate the patient before initiating any medical intervention.

TABLE 6-10 *Waveforms, Segments, Intervals, and Complexes*

P wave	First wave in the cardiac cycle Represents atrial depolarization and the spread of the electrical impulse throughout the right and left atria
PR interval	Measured from the point where the P wave leaves the baseline to the beginning of the QRS complex A normal PR interval indicates the electrical impulse was conducted normally through the atria, atrioventricular node, bundle of His, bundle branches, and Purkinje fibers
QRS complex	The QRS complex consists of the Q wave, R wave, and S wave. One or even two of the three waveforms that make up the QRS complex may not always be present Represents the spread of the electrical impulse through the ventricles (ventricular depolarization)
ST segment	Portion of the electrocardiogram tracing between the end of the QRS complex and the T wave Represents early part of repolarization of the right and left ventricles
T wave	Represents ventricular repolarization Absolute refractory period is still present during the beginning of the T wave; at peak of T wave, relative refractory period has begun
QT interval	Represents total ventricular activity—the time from ventricular depolarization (activation) to repolarization (recovery) Duration varies according to age, gender, and heart rate

Artifact may be due to loose electrodes (Figure 6-16), broken ECG cables or broken wires, muscle tremor (Figure 6-17), patient movement, external chest compressions, and 60-cycle interference. Proper preparation of the patient's skin and evaluation of the monitoring equipment (electrodes, wires) before use can minimize the problems associated with artifact.

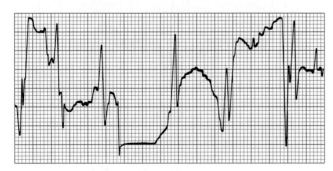

Figure 6-16 Artifact caused by a loose electrode.

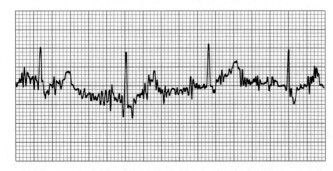

Figure 6-17 Artifact caused by muscle tremors.

Analyzing a Rhythm Strip

Determine if the rate is normal for age, too fast, too slow, or absent.

- Assess the rate.
  - The values used to define a tachycardia (above 100 beats per minute) and a bradycardia (less than 60 beats per minute) in an adult are not the same as those in the pediatric patient.
  - In infants and children, a tachycardia is present if the HR is faster than the upper limit of normal for the patient's age. A bradycardia is present when the HR is slower than the lower limit of normal.

Determine if the QRS is narrow or wide.

- Assess the width of the QRS complex.
  - The duration of the QRS complex is short in an infant and increases with age.
  - If the QRS measures 0.08 second (two small boxes) or less, the QRS is "narrow," and is presumed to be supraventricular in origin.
  - If the QRS is more than 0.08 second in duration, the QRS is "wide" and presumed to be ventricular in origin until proven otherwise.

Determine if the rhythm is regular or irregular.

- Assess rhythm/regularity
  - To determine if the ventricular rhythm is regular or irregular, measure the distance between two consecutive R-R intervals and compare that distance with the other R-R intervals.
  - To determine if the atrial rhythm is regular or irregular, measure the distance between two consecutive P-P intervals and compare that distance with the other P-P intervals.

Sick (unstable) or not sick (stable)?

- Evaluate the rhythm's clinical significance. How is the patient tolerating the rate and rhythm?
  - Stable: The infant or child is asymptomatic (i.e., normal blood pressure, mental status, and respiratory status).
  - Unstable: Decreased responsiveness, hypotension, or respiratory failure. Chest pain due to ischemia may be present in the older child and adolescent.

Rhythm Recognition

Pediatric dysrhythmias may be transient or permanent; congenital (in a structurally normal or abnormal heart) or acquired (rheumatic fever,

---

PEDS Pearl

The initial emergency management of pediatric dysrhythmias requires a response to four important questions:

1. Is a pulse (and other signs of circulation) present?
2. Is the rate within normal limits for age, too fast, too slow, or absent?
3. Is the QRS wide (ventricular in origin) or narrow (supraventricular in origin)?
4. Is the patient sick (unstable) or not sick (stable)?

myocarditis); caused by a toxin (diphtheria), cocaine, or theophylline; caused by proarrhythmic or antidysrhythmic medications; or a consequence of surgical correction of CHD.[5]

Sinus Rhythm

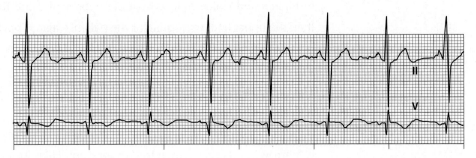

Figure 6-18   Sinus rhythm.

TABLE 6-11 *Characteristics of Sinus Rhythm*	
Rate	Within normal limits for age
Rhythm	Regular
P waves	Uniform in appearance, positive (upright) in lead II, one precedes each QRS complex
PR interval	Within normal limits for age and constant from beat to beat
QRS duration	0.08 sec or less

Sinus Arrhythmia

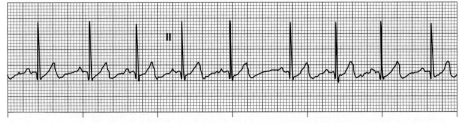

Figure 6-19   Sinus arrhythmia. This rhythm strip is from a 6-year-old girl complaining of abdominal pain. Note the irregular rhythm. The heart rate increases with inspiration (R-R intervals shorten) and decreases with expiration (R-R intervals lengthen).

TABLE 6-12 *Characteristics of Sinus Arrhythmia*	
Rate	Usually within normal limits for age
Rhythm	Irregular, phasic with respiration
P waves	Uniform in appearance, positive (upright) in lead II, one precedes each QRS complex
PR interval	Within normal limits for age and constant from beat to beat
QRS duration	0.08 sec or less
Clinical significance	Normal phenomenon that occurs with respiration and changes in intrathoracic pressure. Heart rate increases with inspiration (R-R intervals shorten) and decreases with expiration (R-R intervals lengthen). Commonly observed in infants and children.

Tachydysrhythmias: Too Fast Rhythms

In infants and children, a tachycardia is present if the HR is faster than the upper limit of normal for the patient's age. A tachycardia may represent either a normal compensatory response to the need for increased CO or oxygen delivery or an unstable dysrhythmia.

Three types of tachycardia are generally seen in children: sinus tachycardia, SVT, and VT with a pulse. Sinus tachycardia is the most common of these rhythms. As its name implies, SVT originates above the ventricles, while VT arises from within the ventricles, below the bifurcation of the bundle of His. SVT and VT can produce ventricular rates so rapid that ventricular filling time is reduced, SV decreases, and CO falls. Tachydysrhythmias seen in adults such as atrial flutter, ectopic atrial tachycardia, and junctional tachycardia are rare in children unless primary cardiac disease is present.

Sinus Tachycardia

Sinus tachycardia (Figure 6-20) is a normal compensatory response to the need for increased CO or oxygen delivery. In sinus tachycardia, the HR is usually less than 220 beats per minute in infants or 180 beats per minute in children. Onset of the rhythm occurs gradually. The ECG shows a

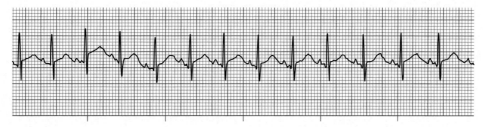

Figure 6-20   Sinus tachycardia.

TABLE 6-13 *Characteristics of Sinus Tachycardia*	
Rate	Faster than the upper limit of normal for age; rate usually less than 220 beats/min in infants and less than 180 beats/min in children
Rhythm	Regular
P waves	Uniform in appearance, positive (upright) in lead II, one precedes each QRS complex
PR interval	Within normal limits for age and constant from beat to beat
QRS duration	0.08 sec or less
Cause	Anxiety, fear, fever, crying, hypovolemia, hypoxemia, pain, congestive heart failure, respiratory distress, toxins/poisonings/drugs, myocardial disease
Clinical significance	Compensatory response to the body's need for increased cardiac output or oxygen delivery. Increased myocardial workload is usually well tolerated by the infant or child with a healthy heart.
Treatment	Identify and treat the underlying cause

regular, narrow QRS complex rhythm that often varies in response to activity or stimulation. P waves are present before each QRS complex. The history given typically explains the rapid HR (i.e., pain, fever, volume loss due to trauma, vomiting, or diarrhea).

Patient management includes treatment of the underlying cause that precipitated the rhythm (e.g., administering medications to relieve pain, administration of fluids to correct hypovolemia due to diarrhea). Electrical therapy and antidysrhythmics are not used in the treatment of sinus tachycardia.

Supraventricular Tachycardia

SVT (Figures 6-21 and 6-22) is the most common tachydysrhythmia that necessitates treatment in the pediatric patient. The most frequent age of presentation is in the first 3 months of life, with secondary peaks occurring at 8 to 10 years of age and again during adolescence.[6] No heart disease is found in about one-half of patients. Wolff-Parkinson-White (WPW) syndrome is present in 10% to 20% of cases and is evident only after conversion to sinus rhythm.[7]

Unlike sinus tachycardia, SVT is not a normal compensatory response to physiologic stress. In SVT, the HR is usually more than 220 beats per minute in infants or 180 beats per minute in children. Onset of the rhythm occurs abruptly. The ECG shows a regular, narrow QRS complex rhythm that does not vary in response to activity or stimulation. P waves are often indiscernible due to the rapid rate and may be lost in the T wave of the preceding beat. If P waves are visible, they differ in appearance from P

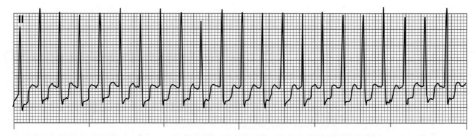

Figure 6-21   Supraventricular tachycardia (SVT) in a child complaining of chest pain.

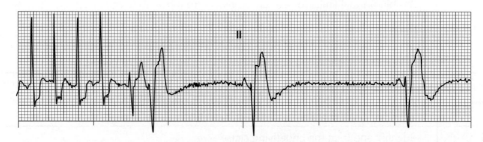

Figure 6-22   The same child as shown in Figure 6-21 after administration of one IV dose of adenosine.

TABLE 6-14 *Characteristics of Supraventricular Tachycardia*	
Rate	240 ± 40 beats/min; may be as high as 300 beats/min in infants
Rhythm	Regular
P waves	Often indiscernible due to rapid rate; may be lost in the T wave of the preceding beat. If P waves are visible, they differ in appearance from P waves that originate in the sinoatrial node and there is a one-to-one relationship to the QRS.
PR interval	Usually not measurable because P waves are not visible
QRS duration	0.08 sec or less unless an intraventricular conduction delay exists
Cause	Most often due to a reentrant mechanism that involves the atrioventricular junction or an accessory pathway
Clinical significance	Onset and termination of the rhythm are often abrupt (paroxysmal); tachydysrhythmias may result in decreased cardiac output (↑ heart rate → ↓ ventricular filling time → ↓ stroke volume → ↓ cardiac output)
Treatment	Vagal maneuvers, antidysrhythmics, or synchronized cardioversion depending on the stability of the patient; see tachycardia algorithm

Infants with SVT often present with heart failure because the tachycardia goes unrecognized for a long time.

waves that originate in the sinoatrial (SA) node. In the absence of known CHD, the history obtained is usually nonspecific (i.e., the history does not explain the rapid HR).

Rapid ventricular rates may be associated with lightheadedness, syncope, dyspnea, weakness, nervousness, and complaints of palpitations, chest pain, or pressure in the older child. Signs of shock may be evident depending on the duration and rate of the tachycardia, and the presence of primary cardiac disease. A child with normal cardiovascular function may tolerate a rapid ventricular rate for several hours before signs of CHF or shock will develop. Infants may tolerate the rapid ventricular rate associated with SVT for hours or days before developing signs of poor CO, CHF, and cardiogenic shock.

Vagal maneuvers (see Chapter 7) are used to slow conduction through the atrioventricular (AV) node, resulting in slowing of the HR. Success rates with vagal maneuvers vary and depend on the presence of underlying conditions in the patient, the patient's age, and level of cooperation.

> ### Drug Pearl
> ### *Adenosine*
>
> - Adenosine is found naturally in all body cells and is rapidly metabolized in the blood vessels. Adenosine slows the rate of the SA node, slows conduction time through the AV node, can interrupt reentry pathways that involve the AV node, and can restore sinus rhythm in SVT.
> - Reentry circuits are the underlying mechanism for most episodes of SVT in infants and children. Adenosine acts at specific receptors to cause a temporary block of conduction through the AV node, interrupting these reentry circuits.
> - Adenosine has a half-life of less than 10 seconds. It has an onset of action of 10 to 40 seconds and duration of 1 to 2 minutes. Because of its short half-life, and to enhance delivery of the drug to its site of action in the heart, select the injection port on the IV tubing that is nearest the patient and administer the drug using a two-syringe technique. Prepare one syringe with the drug, and the other with a NS flush of at least 5 mL. Insert both syringes into the injection port in the IV tubing. Administer the drug medication IV or IO as rapidly as possible (i.e., over a period of seconds) and *immediately* follow with the saline flush.
> - Adenosine may cause facial flushing because the drug is a mild cutaneous vasodilator and may cause coughing, dyspnea, and bronchospasm because it is a mild bronchoconstrictor.

TABLE 6-15 *Differentiation of Sinus Tachycardia and Supraventricular Tachycardia*

	Sinus Tachycardia	**Supraventricular Tachycardia**
Rate	Usually less than 220 beats/min in infants and less than 180 beats/min in children	Usually 220 beats/min or more in infants and 180 beats/min or more in children
Ventricular rate and regularity	Varies with activity/stimulation	Constant with activity/stimulation
Onset and termination	Gradual	Abrupt
P waves	Visible; normal appearance	Often indiscernible; if visible, differ in appearance from sinoatrial node P waves
History	History given explains rapid heart rate; pain, fever, volume loss due to trauma, vomiting, or diarrhea	In the absence of known congenital heart disease, history is usually nonspecific (i.e., history given does not explain rapid heart rate)
Physical examination	May be consistent with volume loss (blood, diarrhea, vomiting), possible fever, clear lungs, liver of normal size	Signs of poor perfusion including diminished peripheral pulses, delayed capillary refill, pallor, increased work of breathing, possible crackles, enlarged liver

Ventricular Tachycardia

VT is a serious cardiac dysrhythmia that originates in the ventricles (Figure 6-23). Because the rhythm originates below the AV junction, the ventricles may be depolarized without receiving the additional 10% to 30% of ventricular filling produced by atrial contraction. The inadequate ventricular filling and rapid ventricular rate associated with this rhythm result in decreased SV and CO.

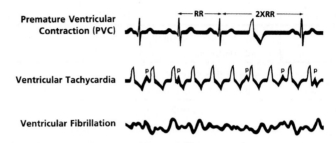

Figure 6-23   Examples of dysrhythmias originating in the ventricles.

Order a bedside glucose and toxicology screen for any child that presents with unexplained VT.

VT is uncommon in infants and children unless an underlying cardiovascular disorder exists. This dysrhythmia may be seen in children who have had open-heart surgical repair for tetralogy of Fallot (TOF) or other anomalies or who have a CM, myocarditis, or myocardial tumor. VT may occur in an infant or child with a preexisting conduction abnormality such as long QT syndrome (see sidebar), and may be seen in the end stages of acidosis, hypoxemia, hypovolemia, or hypothermia. Secondary causes of VT include electrolyte imbalance (as seen in hyperkalemia or hypomagnesemia) and ingestion of certain toxins (such as tricyclic antidepressants).

When the QRS complexes of VT are of the same shape and amplitude, the rhythm is termed *monomorphic VT* (Figure 6-24). When the QRS complexes of VT vary in shape and amplitude, the rhythm is termed *polymorphic VT* (Figure 6-25).

Polymorphic Ventricular Tachycardia

Polymorphic VT (Figure 6-25) is a rapid ventricular dysrhythmia with beat-to-beat changes in the shape and amplitude of the QRS complexes. Polymorphic VT associated with a long QT interval is called torsades de pointes (TdP). Polymorphic VT associated with a normal QT interval is simply called polymorphic VT.

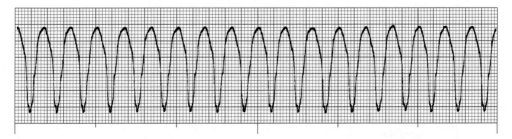

Figure 6-24   Monomorphic ventricular tachycardia.

TABLE 6-16 *Characteristics of Monomorphic Ventricular Tachycardia*

Rate	120 to 250 beats/min
Rhythm	Essentially regular
P waves	Usually not seen; if present, they have no set relationship to the QRS complexes appearing between them at a rate different from that of the ventricular tachycardia
PR interval	None
QRS duration	Greater than 0.08 sec; may be difficult to differentiate between the QRS and T wave
Cause	May be caused by acute hypoxemia, acidosis, electrolyte imbalance, reactions to medications, toxins/poisons/drugs, myocarditis
Clinical significance	Slower rates may be well tolerated. Rapid rates often result in decreased ventricular filling time and decreased cardiac output; may degenerate into ventricular fibrillation
Treatment	If no pulse, defibrillation. Pulse present: Antidysrhythmics or synchronized cardioversion depending on the stability of the patient; see tachycardia algorithm

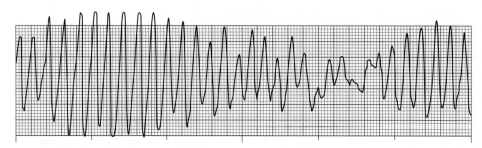

Figure 6-25   Polymorphic ventricular tachycardia.

TABLE 6-17 *Characteristics of Polymorphic Ventricular Tachycardia*

Rate	150 to 300 beats/min, typically 200 to 250 beats/min
Rhythm	May be regular or irregular
P waves	None
PR interval	None
QRS duration	Greater than 0.08 sec; gradual alteration in amplitude and direction of the QRS complexes
Causes	May be precipitated by slow heart rates; associated with medications or electrolyte disturbances that prolong the QT interval; a prolonged QT interval may be congenital or acquired; lengthening of the QT interval may be the only warning sign suggesting impending torsades de pointes
Clinical significance	Symptoms are usually related to the decreased cardiac output that occurs because of the fast ventricular rate; signs of shock are often present; patient may experience a syncopal episode or seizures; may occasionally terminate spontaneously and recur after several seconds or minutes; may deteriorate to ventricular fibrillation
Treatment	If no pulse, defibrillation. Pulse present: Magnesium sulfate is drug of choice; see tachycardia algorithm

Drug Pearl
Procainamide

- Procainamide is used for both atrial and ventricular dysrhythmias because it suppresses automaticity in the atria and ventricles and depresses conduction velocity within the conduction system.
- During administration, carefully monitor the patient's ECG and blood pressure. Observe the ECG closely for increasing PR and QT intervals, widening of the QRS complex, heart block, and/or onset of Torsades de Pointes. If the QRS widens to above 50% of its original width or hypotension occurs, stop the infusion.
- Procainamide should not be used in patients with a prolonged QRS duration or QT interval because of the potential for heart block or in patients with preexisting QT prolongation/TdP.
- Procainamide should not be used with other medications that prolong the QT interval (e.g., amiodarone).

Drug Pearl
Amiodarone

- Amiodarone directly depresses the automaticity of the SA and AV nodes, slows conduction through the AV node and in the accessory pathway of patients with WPW syndrome, inhibits α- and β-adrenergic receptors, and possesses both vagolytic and calcium-channel blocking properties. Because of these properties, amiodarone is used for a wide range of both atrial and ventricular dysrhythmias in adults and children.
- Amiodarone prolongs the PR, QRS, and QT intervals and has an additive effect with other medications that prolong the QT interval (e.g., procainamide, phenothiazines, some tricyclic antidepressants, thiazide diuretics, sotalol). Although prolongation of the QRS duration and QT interval may be beneficial in some patients, it may also increase the risk for TdP (a type of polymorphic VT associated with a long QT interval).
- Hypotension, bradycardia, and AV block are side effects of amiodarone administration. Slow the infusion rate or discontinue if seen.

Drug Pearl
Lidocaine

- Lidocaine depresses spontaneous ventricular depolarization but does not affect SA or AV node depolarization and is used in the treatment of ventricular dysrhythmias (e.g., VT, VF).
- If a lidocaine IV bolus was administered and resulted in conversion of the dysrhythmia, begin a lidocaine IV maintenance infusion. If there is a delay of more than 15 minutes between the initial dose of lidocaine and the start of the infusion, consider giving a second bolus of 0.5 to 1 mg/kg to reestablish a therapeutic level.
- Lidocaine toxicity may be seen in patients with persistently poor cardiac output and hepatic failure. Signs and symptoms of lidocaine toxicity are primarily central nervous system–related, including drowsiness, disorientation, muscle twitching, or seizures. The IV maintenance infusion rate should be decreased if reduced lidocaine clearance is expected or suspected (e.g., CHF, liver impairment). In these situations, the infusion rate should not exceed 20 mcg/kg per minute.
- To prepare a lidocaine infusion: 60 × body weight in kilograms = the number of milligrams of lidocaine to be added to an IV solution with a total volume of 100 mL (60 × kg = mg). Then: 1 mL per hour = 10 mcg/kg per minute. 2 mL per hour = 20 mcg/kg per minute, and so forth.
- Serum levels of lidocaine can be increased by drugs that reduce blood flow to the liver (β-blockers) and cimetidine (Tagamet). Concurrent administration with procainamide may result in additive central nervous system effects.

Acceptable Interventions: Tachycardia with Adequate Perfusion

- Use personal protective equipment.
- Perform an initial assessment and obtain a focused history.
- If the child is stable (i.e., normal blood pressure for age, alert with palpable distal pulses, and normal respiratory status)
  - Administer high-concentration oxygen; ensure effective ventilation and oxygenation. Apply a pulse oximeter. Maintain oxygen saturation at above 95%.
  - Attach a cardiac monitor and identify the rhythm.
  - Establish vascular access.
- If the rhythm is SVT
  - Ensure the patient's history does not indicate causes of *sinus* tachycardia (i.e., dehydration, fever)
  - Consider vagal maneuvers
    - Obtain a 12-lead ECG before and after a vagal maneuver and monitor the ECG continuously during the maneuver.
    - Vagal maneuvers are used to slow conduction through the AV node, resulting in slowing of the HR. Success rates with vagal maneuvers vary and depend on the presence of underlying conditions in the patient, the patient's age and level of cooperation.
  - If the rhythm persists, give adenosine IV.
    - Initial dose: adenosine 0.1 mg/kg rapid IV bolus. Follow immediately with a rapid normal saline IV flush of at least 5 mL. Reassess.
    - Second dose: If there is no response, give adenosine 0.2 mg/kg IV to a maximum individual dose of 12 mg, using the same technique. Reassess.
    - Once the patient has been converted to sinus rhythm, a longer acting medication should be selected for maintenance therapy.
- If the rhythm is VT
  - Consult a pediatric cardiologist.
  - Obtain a 12-lead ECG.
  - Obtain a focused history, including family history for ventricular dysrhythmias or sudden death.
  - Consider drug or metabolic causes of the VT, especially in a child without a known predisposing cause for the dysrhythmia
  - If the rhythm is monomorphic VT, give **one** of the following:
    - Amiodarone 5 mg/kg IV/IO over 20 to 60 minutes
    - Procainamide 15 mg/kg IV/IO over 30 to 60 minutes
- Identify and treat possible reversible causes of the dysrhythmia
  - Hypoxemia: give oxygen
  - Hypovolemia: replace volume

PEDS Pearl

SVT with abnormal (aberrant) conduction through the bundle branches produces a wide QRS complex. Differentiation of SVT with abnormal conduction (also called wide-QRS SVT) from VT is often difficult. Wide-QRS SVT is relatively uncommon, occurring in less than 10% of children with SVT.

Since almost all wide-QRS tachycardias are VT, any wide-QRS tachycardia in an infant or child should be presumed to be ventricular in origin and treated as VT.

In stable patients with SVT, adenosine is the drug of choice because of its rapid onset of action and minimal effects on cardiac contractility.

Amiodarone and procainamide should not be administered together because both prolong the QT interval.

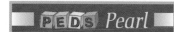

Be sure to obtain ECG tracings before, during, and after interventions for any patient experiencing a cardiac dysrhythmia.

- Hyperthermia: use simple cooling techniques
- Hyperkalemia/hypokalemia and metabolic disorders: correct electrolyte and acid–base disturbances
- Tamponade: pericardiocentesis
- Tension pneumothorax: needle decompression
- Toxins/poisons/drugs: antidote/specific therapy
- Thromboembolism
- Pain: ensure effective pain control

Unacceptable Interventions: Tachycardia with Adequate Perfusion

- Failure to use personal protective equipment
- Failure to adequately assess the patient
- Inability to quickly determine if the child is sick or not sick (i.e., unstable or stable)
- Failure to administer supplemental oxygen
- Failure to correctly identify the ECG rhythm
- Failure to establish vascular access
- Failure to use an accurate method for weight and medication dosage determination
- Administration of verapamil to an infant
- Failure to administer adenosine rapidly IV bolus
- Medication errors
- Attempting cardioversion or defibrillation for an infant or child in SVT or VT with signs of adequate perfusion
- Failure to correctly differentiate sinus tachycardia from SVT
- Ordering a dangerous or inappropriate intervention
- Performing any technique resulting in potential harm to the patient

Acceptable Interventions: Tachycardia with Inadequate Perfusion

Do not delay cardioversion to establish vascular access if the child is unresponsive or hypotensive.

- Use personal protective equipment.
- Perform an initial assessment and obtain a focused history.
- If the child is unstable ("sick") (i.e., increased work of breathing with altered mental status, hypotension, or CHF with diminished peripheral perfusion), immediate treatment with electrical or chemical (i.e., use of medications) cardioversion is warranted (see Tachycardia Algorithm).
- Administer high-concentration oxygen; ensure effective ventilation and oxygenation. Apply a pulse oximeter. Maintain oxygen saturation at above 95%.
- Attach a cardiac monitor and identify the rhythm.
- If the rhythm is SVT
  - If vascular access is already available, adenosine may be administered

before electrical cardioversion, but do not delay cardioversion if establishment of vascular access (IV or IO) will take more than 20 to 30 seconds to accomplish.

- If vascular access is immediately available, give adenosine 0.1 mg/kg rapidly IV or IO, immediately followed by a rapid normal saline IV flush of at least 5 mL. If there is no response, give adenosine 0.2 mg/kg IV/IO to a maximum individual dose of 12 mg, using the same technique.
- If vascular access has not been established, or if the child fails to respond to adenosine, perform synchronized cardioversion.
  - Begin with 0.5 to 1 J/kg.
  - If cardioversion does not terminate the dysrhythmia, increase the energy level to 2 J/kg.
- If the rhythm is VT
  - Perform synchronized cardioversion.
  - Begin with 0.5 to 1 J/kg.
  - If cardioversion does not terminate the dysrhythmia, increase the energy level to 2 J/kg.
- Establish vascular access.
- Identify and treat possible reversible causes of the dysrhythmia

> If the child is responsive, consider sedation and analgesia before performing cardioversion.

Unacceptable Interventions: Tachycardia with Inadequate Perfusion

- Failure to use personal protective equipment
- Failure to adequately assess the patient
- Inability to quickly determine if the child is sick or not sick (i.e., unstable or stable)
- Failure to administer supplemental oxygen
- Failure to assist ventilation with a bag-valve-mask device and 100% oxygen if signs of inadequate ventilation are present
- Failure to reassess respiratory status after initiating assisted ventilations
- Failure to correctly identify the ECG rhythm
- Failure to establish vascular access
- Extended attempts to establish IV access in a child with decompensated shock when IO access could be established quickly
- Failure to use an accurate method for weight and medication dosage determination
- Administration of calcium channel blockers (e.g., verapamil, diltiazem) or β-blockers to a sick (unstable) infant or child (due to negative inotropic effects) in SVT or VT
- Medication errors
- Attempting synchronized cardioversion or defibrillation for an infant or child in SVT or VT and signs of adequate perfusion

PEDIATRIC TACHYCARDIA ALGORITHM

Assess ABCs, ensure effective oxygenation and ventilation
Attach pulse oximeter and monitor/defibrillator
If pulseless, begin CPR - go to pulseless algorithm

Narrow-QRS (0.08 sec or less)
Probable sinus tachycardia or
supraventricular tachycardia (SVT)

Algorithm assumes
serious signs and
symptoms persist.

R H Y T H M

Probable Sinus Tachycardia:
*History explains rapid rate
*Gradual rhythm onset
*P waves present/normal
*Ventricular rate/regularity varies
with activity/stimulation
*Variable R to R interval with
constant PR interval
*Rate usually <220 beats/min
in infant and <180 beats/min
in child

R H Y T H M

Probable SVT:
*History does not explain rapid rate
*P waves absent/abnormal
*Rhythm onset - abrupt
*Ventricular rate/regularity constant
with activity/stimulation
*Abrupt rate changes
*Rate usually 220 beats/min
or more in infant and 180 beats/min
or more in child

Identify and treat underlying
cause

S T A B L E

Obtain 12-lead ECG, consult
pediatric cardiologist
Try vagal maneuvers
Start IV, identify/treat causes
Give adenosine IV
If rhythm persists, consider
amiodarone or procainamide

U N S T A B L E

Consider vagal maneuvers
If IV/IO in place,
consider adenosine
Sedate if possible, then
synchronized cardioversion with
0.5 to 1.0 J/kg;
2 J/kg if rhythm persists

Wide-QRS (>0.08 sec)
Probable ventricular tachycardia

S T A B L E

Obtain 12-lead ECG, consult
pediatric cardiologist
Start IV, identify/treat causes
Give amiodarone slowly IV

U N S T A B L E

If IV/IO in place, consider
adenosine
Sedate if possible, then
synchronized cardioversion
with 0.5 to 1.0 J/kg;
2 J/kg if rhythm persists
Consider amiodarone or
procainamide
before third shock

C O N S I D E R C A U S E S

*Hypoxemia - give oxygen
*Hypovolemia - replace volume
*Hypothermia - use simple
warming techniques
*Hyper-/hypokalemia and
metabolic disorders - correct
electrolyte and acid-base
disturbances
*Tamponade - pericardiocentesis
*Tension pneumothorax - needle
decompression
*Toxins/poisons/drugs - antidote/
specific therapy
*Thromboembolism
*Pain - ensure effective pain
control

D R U G S

Adenosine IV/IO: 0.1 mg/kg rapid IV bolus (maximum first dose 6 mg); if no
effect, may double and repeat dose once (max second dose 12 mg)
Amiodarone 5 mg/kg IV over 20 to 60 min*
Procainamide 15 mg/kg IV over 30 to 60 min*
*Do not routinely give amiodarone and procainamide together

- Delay cardioversion to establish vascular access
- Failure to correctly differentiate sinus tachycardia from SVT
- Failure to press the sync control after delivery of an initial synchronized shock in order to deliver additional synchronized shocks (does not apply to all defibrillator models)
- Failure to deliver the correct energy level(s) for the specific dysrhythmia
- Failure to identify and treat potentially reversible causes of the dysrhythmia
- Failure to anticipate the potential need for tracheal intubation
- Performing tracheal intubation in a child who responds to less invasive interventions
- If tracheal intubation is required, failure to confirm tracheal tube position using assessment and mechanical methods
- Ordering a dangerous or inappropriate intervention
- Performing any technique resulting in potential harm to the patient

Bradydysrhythmias: Too Slow Rhythms

In infants and children, a bradycardia is present if the HR is slower than the lower limit of normal for the patient's age. Bradycardias can be classified as either primary or secondary. A **primary bradycardia** is usually caused by structural heart disease. An infant or child with structural cardiac disease may develop bradycardia because of AV block or sinus node dysfunction. Physical examination of these children may reveal a midline sternal scar and they may have an implanted pacemaker to treat the bradycardia.

A **secondary bradycardia** is a slow HR due to a noncardiac cause. Causes of secondary bradycardias include increased vagal (parasympathetic) tone (vomiting, increased intracranial pressure, vagal maneuvers, suctioning, or tracheal intubation procedure), hypothermia, hyperkalemia, and ingestion of medications such as calcium channel blockers (verapamil, diltiazem), digoxin, and β-blockers (propranolol).

Remember that $CO = SV \times HR$. Therefore a decrease in either SV or HR may result in a decrease in CO. A bradycardia can produce significant symptoms unless SV increases to compensate for the decrease in HR. Unless corrected promptly, decreasing CO will eventually produce hemodynamic compromise.

Sinus Bradycardia

Atrioventricular Blocks

AV blocks are divided into three main types: first-, second-, and third-degree AV block (Figure 6-27). The clinical significance of an AV block depends on the degree (severity) of the block, the rate of the escape pacemaker (junctional vs. ventricular), and the patient's response to that ventricular rate.

In the pediatric patient, most slow rhythms occur secondary to hypoxia and acidosis.

Long QT Syndrome

Long QT syndrome (LQTS) is an abnormality of the heart's electrical system. The mechanical function of the heart is entirely normal. The electrical problem is thought to be due to defects in cardiac ion channels that affect repolarization. These electrical defects predispose affected persons to TdP that leads to a sudden loss of consciousness (syncope) and may result in sudden cardiac death.

LQTS may be acquired or inherited. The acquired form of LQTS is more common and usually caused by medications that prolong the QT interval. Inherited LQTS is caused by mutations of genes that encode the cardiac ion channels and is estimated to be present in one in 7000 persons in the United States. Inherited LQTS may cause as many as 3000 unexpected deaths in children and young adults per year.[13] Inherited LQTS is sometimes, but not always, associated with deafness. LQTS occurs in all races and ethnic groups, although the relative frequency in each group is not yet known because no systematic screening of different groups has been attempted.[13]

About one third of individuals with LQTS never exhibit symptoms. A lack of symptoms does not exclude an individual or family from having LQTS. Symptoms of LQTS include syncope or sudden death, typically occurring during physical activity or emotional upset. The syncopal episodes are often misdiagnosed as the common faint (vasovagal event) or a seizure. Actual seizures are uncommon in LQTS, but epilepsy is one of the common errors in diagnosis.

Cases in which LQTS should be considered include a sudden loss of consciousness during physical exertion or during emotional excitement, sudden and unexplained loss of consciousness during childhood and teenage years, a family history of unexplained syncope, any young person who has an unexplained cardiac arrest and epilepsy in children. Common triggers of LQTS include swimming, running, startle (e.g., an alarm clock, a loud horn, a ringing phone), anger, crying, test taking, or other stressful situations.

The diagnosis of LQTS is commonly suspected or made from the ECG. β-Blockers are frequently used in the management of patients with LQTS and are effective in about 90% of affected patients. New information regarding the genetics of the syndrome suggests that a subset of patients might be treated with other medications, either instead of or in addition to β-blockers.

- First-degree AV block
  - In first-degree AV block, all impulses from the SA node are conducted, but the impulses are delayed before they are conducted to the ventricles.
  - This delay in AV conduction results in a PR interval that is longer than normal, but constant.

- Second-degree AV block

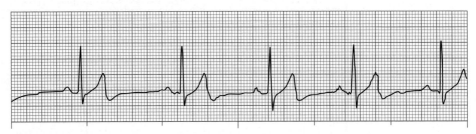

Figure 6-26 Sinus bradycardia.

TABLE 6-18 *Characteristics of Sinus Bradycardia*	
Rate	Slower than the lower range of normal for age
Rhythm	Essentially regular
P waves	Uniform in appearance, positive (upright) in lead II, one precedes each QRS complex
PR interval	Within normal limits for age and constant from beat to beat
QRS duration	0.08 sec or less
Cause	Hypoxemia, acidosis, increased vagal tone (e.g., suctioning, tracheal intubation)
Clinical significance	May be normal in conditioned adolescent athletes and in some children during sleep. In other patients, decreased cardiac output may occur because of slow rate, despite normal stroke volume
Treatment	Search for treatable cause. Ensure good oxygenation and ventilation. Begin chest compressions if the heart rate is below 60 beats/min in an infant or child with poor systemic perfusion despite oxygenation and ventilation. Establish vascular access. Epinephrine, atropine, possible pacing. See bradycardia algorithm

- In second-degree AV block, some impulses are not conducted to the ventricles.
- In second-degree AV block type I (also known as Wenckebach or Mobitz type I), P waves appear at regular intervals, but the PR interval progressively lengthens until a P wave is not conducted.
- In second-degree AV block type II (also known as Mobitz type II), P waves appear at regular intervals, and the PR interval is constant before each conducted QRS. However, impulses are periodically blocked—appearing on the ECG as a P wave with no QRS after it (dropped beat). This type of AV block may progress to third-degree AV block without warning.
- Third-degree AV block
  - In third-degree AV block (also known as complete heart block), the atria and ventricles beat independently of each other because impulses generated by the SA node are blocked before reaching the ventricles.

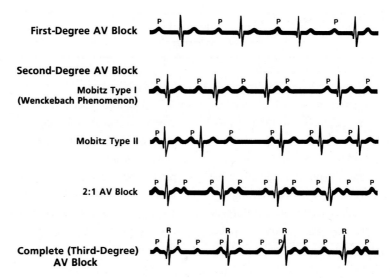

Figure 6-27 Examples of atrioventricular blocks.

Drug Pearl
Epinephrine

- Epinephrine is a direct-acting endogenous catecholamine with moderate β_2-(bronchodilation) and potent α- (vasoconstriction) and β_1- ($\rightarrow$ heart rate, $\rightarrow$ force of contraction) adrenergic properties.
- Although epinephrine's β_1 effects increase myocardial oxygen consumption, it is generally well tolerated in the pediatric patient.
- In cardiac arrest, epinephrine produces beneficial effects primarily because of its α-adrenergic stimulating effects: $\uparrow$ peripheral vascular resistance (vasoconstriction) $\rightarrow \uparrow$ diastolic pressure $\rightarrow \uparrow$ myocardial and cerebral blood flow during CPR.

- A secondary pacemaker (either junctional or ventricular) stimulates the ventricles; therefore, the QRS may be narrow or wide depending on the location of the escape pacemaker and the condition of the intraventricular conduction system.

Acceptable Interventions: Symptomatic Bradycardia

Interventions for a slow rhythm are unnecessary if the patient is asymptomatic. For example, adolescent athletes at rest or children who are sleeping may demonstrate no symptoms with a slow HR. If an infant or child is symptomatic because of a bradycardia, initial interventions focus on assessment of the airway and ventilation rather than administration of epinephrine, atropine, or other drugs because problems with adequate oxygenation and ventilation are more common in children than cardiac causes of bradycardia (see Bradycardia Algorithm).

Drug Pearl
Atropine

- Atropine enhances AV conduction and increases heart rate (positive chronotropic effect) by accelerating the SA node discharge rate and blocking the vagus nerve. Atropine has little or no effect on the force of contraction (inotropic effect).
- Anticholinesterase poisonings may require large doses of atropine.
- Epinephrine is the drug of choice if bradycardia is due to hypoxia and oxygenation and ventilation do not correct the bradycardia. Give atropine before epinephrine if the bradycardia is due to increased vagal tone or if AV block is present.
- Do not give atropine slowly or in smaller than recommended doses (0.1 mg) because paradoxic slowing of the heart rate can occur. Paradoxic slowing may last 2 minutes.

Drug Pearl
Dopamine

- Dopamine is an endogenous catecholamine with dose-related actions (there is some "overlap" of effects). At low doses (0.5 to 5 mcg/kg per minute), dopamine acts on dopaminergic receptors that are located mainly in mesenteric, renal, and coronary vessels, causing vasodilation. At moderate doses (5 to 10 mcg/kg per minute), dopamine stimulates the β_1-adrenergic receptors on the myocardium increasing myocardial contractility and stroke volume, thereby increasing cardiac output. At high doses (10 to 20 mcg/kg per minute), dopamine acts on vascular α-adrenergic receptors, producing systemic vasoconstriction. Because of the extreme variation in dosages required to activate receptor sites in patients, it is impossible to predict the infusion rate required for an individual patient.
- To prepare a dopamine infusion: $6 \times$ body weight in kilograms = the number of milligrams of dopamine to be added to an IV solution for a total volume of 100 mL ($6 \times$ kg = mg). Then: 1 mL per hour = 1 mcg/kg per minute, 2 mL per hour = 2 mcg/kg per minute, and so forth.

- Use personal protective equipment.
- Perform an initial assessment and obtain a focused history.
- If the child is unstable ("sick") (i.e., increased work of breathing with altered mental status, hypotension, or CHF with diminished peripheral perfusion) immediate intervention is necessary.
- Administer high-concentration oxygen; ensure effective ventilation and oxygenation. Apply a pulse oximeter. Maintain oxygen saturation at above 95%.
- Attach a cardiac monitor and identify the rhythm.
- If the HR is less than 60 beats per minute and accompanied by abnormal skin color, a decreased level of responsiveness, capillary refill above 2 seconds, or hypotension despite adequate oxygenation and ventilation, perform chest compressions.
- Establish vascular access.
- Identify and treat possible reversible causes of the dysrhythmia
- Give epinephrine
  - IV/IO: 0.01 mg/kg (1:10,000; 0.1 mL/kg), may repeat every 3 to 5 minutes
  - Endotracheal tube: 0.1 mg/kg (1:1000; 0.1 mL/kg), max 10 mg
- Give atropine before epinephrine if the bradycardia is due to suspected increased vagal tone, any type of AV block, or myocarditis
- Consider pacing

Unacceptable Interventions: Symptomatic Bradycardia

- Failure to use personal protective equipment
- Failure to adequately assess the patient
- Inability to quickly determine if the child is sick or not sick (i.e., unstable or stable)
- Treating an asymptomatic bradycardia
- Failure to administer supplemental oxygen
- Failure to assist ventilation with a bag-valve-mask device and 100% oxygen if signs of inadequate ventilation are present
- Failure to reassess respiratory status after initiating assisted ventilations
- Failure to correctly identify the ECG rhythm
- Failure to perform chest compressions if the HR is less than 60 beats per minute and accompanied by signs of inadequate perfusion despite adequate oxygenation and ventilation
- Failure to establish vascular access
- Extended attempts to establish IV access in a child with decompensated shock when IO access could be established quickly
- Failure to administer epinephrine for a symptomatic bradycardia unresponsive to basic life support interventions
- Failure to use an accurate method for weight and medication dosage determination
- Medication errors
- Attempting transcutaneous pacing for an infant or child with signs of adequate perfusion
- Failure to correctly perform transcutaneous pacing
- Failure to anticipate the potential need for tracheal intubation
- Performing tracheal intubation in a child who responds to less invasive interventions
- If tracheal intubation is required, failure to confirm tracheal tube position using assessment and mechanical methods
- Ordering a dangerous or inappropriate intervention
- Performing any technique resulting in potential harm to the patient

Absent/Pulseless Rhythms

In cardiopulmonary arrest, central pulses and the work of breathing are absent and the patient is unresponsive. Absent/pulseless rhythms include the following:

- Pulseless VT, in which the ECG displays a wide QRS complex at a rate faster than 120 beats per minute
- VF, in which irregular chaotic deflections that vary in shape and amplitude are observed on the ECG, but there is no coordinated ventricular contraction
- Asystole, in which no cardiac electrical activity is present

SYMPTOMATIC BRADYCARDIA ALGORITHM

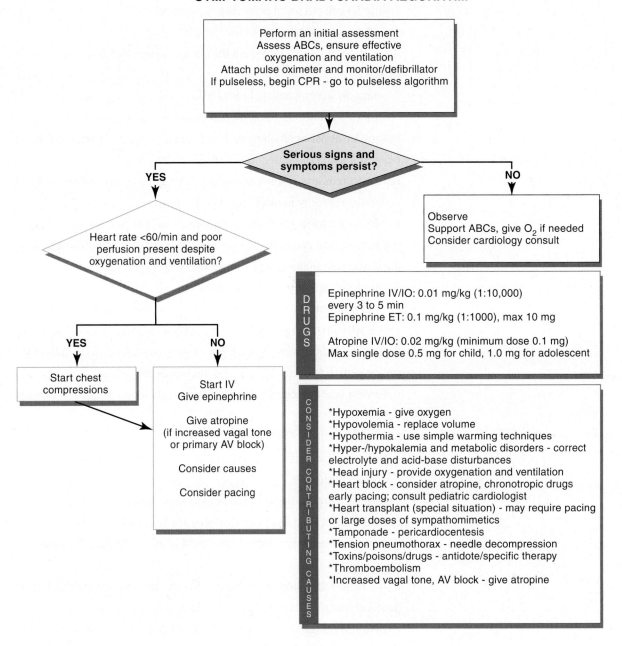

- Pulseless electrical activity (PEA), in which electrical activity is visible on the ECG but central pulses are absent

Ventricular Fibrillation

VF is a chaotic rhythm that originates in the ventricles. In VF, there is no organized depolarization of the ventricles. The ventricular myocardium quivers and, as a result, there is no effective myocardial contraction and no pulse. The resulting rhythm is irregularly irregular with chaotic deflections that vary in shape and amplitude. No normal-looking waveforms are visible.

Defibrillation and CPR are the most effective treatments for pulseless VT and VF.

VT and VF are uncommon in children. When these rhythms are seen, it usually signifies serious myocardial pathology or dysfunction due to CHD, cardiomyopathies, or an acute inflammatory injury to the heart (e.g., myocarditis) or due to a reversible cause including drug toxicity (e.g., recreational drugs, tricyclic antidepressants, digoxin overdose), metabolic causes (e.g., hyperkalemia, hypermagnesemia, hypocalcemia, or hypoglycemia), or hypothermia.

Commotio cordis (VF due to a blunt, nonpenetrating blow to the chest, most commonly from a baseball) is an underappreciated cause of sudden cardiac death in young patients. It most frequently occurs in males at a

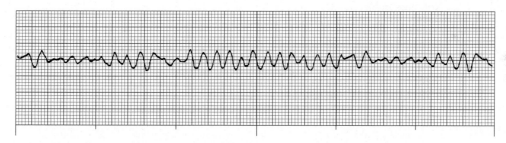

Figure 6-28 Ventricular fibrillation (VF). The patient in VF is unresponsive, apneic, and pulseless.

TABLE 6-19 *Characteristics of Ventricular Fibrillation*

Rate	Cannot be determined because there are no discernible waves or complexes to measure
Rhythm	Rapid and chaotic with no pattern or regularity
P waves	Not discernible
PR interval	Not discernible
QRS duration	Not discernible
Causes	Severe hypoxia and/or poor perfusion, electrolyte imbalance, hypothermia, toxins/poisons/drugs (e.g., digitalis, tricyclic antidepressants)
Significance	Terminal rhythm
Treatment	Confirm the patient is apneic and pulseless (check leads). Begin ventilation, oxygenation, and chest compressions until a defibrillator is available. See cardiac arrest algorithm

mean age of 14. Although once thought rare, an increasing number of these events have been reported. Prompt CPR and early defibrillation are associated with a favorable outcome.[8-10]

Asystole (Cardiac Standstill)

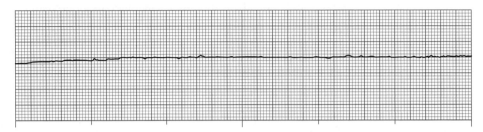

Figure 6-29 Asystole.

TABLE 6-20 Characteristics of Asystole

Rate	Ventricular usually not discernible but atrial activity may be observed ("P wave" asystole)
Rhythm	Ventricular not discernible, atrial may be discernible
P waves	Usually not discernible
PR interval	Not measurable
QRS duration	Absent
Causes	Hypoxia, hypokalemia, hyperkalemia, hypothermia, acidosis, toxins/poisons, respiratory failure, traumatic cardiac arrest (among other causes). Ventricular asystole may occur temporarily after termination of a tachydysrhythmia following medication administration, defibrillation, or synchronized cardioversion
Clinical significance	Absence of cardiac output; terminal rhythm. Patient is unresponsive, apneic, and pulseless.
Treatment	See cardiac arrest algorithm

Pulseless Electrical Activity

PEA is a clinical situation, not a specific dysrhythmia. PEA exists when organized electrical activity (other than VT) is observed on the cardiac monitor, but the patient is pulseless (Figure 6-30).

Many conditions may cause PEA. The mnemonic "4 H's and 4 T's" (see box) can be used to memorize the possible causes of PEA. PEA has a poor prognosis unless the underlying cause can be rapidly identified and appropriately managed.

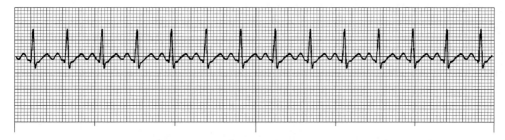

Figure 6-30 Pulseless electrical activity: organized electrical activity without a palpable pulse.

Causes of Pulseless Electrical Activity: Four H's and Four T's	
Hypovolemia	Tamponade, cardiac
Hypoxemia	Tension pneumothorax
Hypothermia	Thrombosis: lungs (massive pulmonary embolism)
Hyperkalemia	Tablets/toxins: drug overdose

Acceptable Interventions: Absent/Pulseless Rhythms

- Use personal protective equipment.
- Perform an initial assessment.
- Ensure effective oxygenation and ventilation.
- Perform CPR, attach monitor/defibrillator and identify the rhythm.
- If the rhythm is PEA or asystole
  - Confirm rhythm in a second lead (if the rhythm is asystole)
  - Establish vascular access without interrupting chest compressions
  - Give epinephrine every 3-5 minutes as long as the patient does not have a pulse
  - IV/IO: 0.01 mg/kg (1:10,000; 0.1 mL/kg), follow with saline flush
  - Endotracheal tube: 0.1 mg/kg (1:1000; 0.1 mL/kg), max 10 mg
  - Attempt to identify and treat possible reversible causes of the arrest
  - Consider placement of an advanced airway, confirm tube position with primary and secondary techniques
  - Reassess tube position, electrode position and contact, effectiveness of CPR, equipment in use is functioning properly, confirm appropriate interventions, consider alternative medications and special resuscitation circumstances
- If the rhythm is pulseless VT or VF
  - Turn off the oxygen flow (oxygen flow over the patient's torso during electrical therapy increases the risk of spark/fire). If the area is clear, shock once with 2 J/kg of equivalent biphasic energy.
  - Immediately resume CPR, starting with chest compressions. Start an IV and give epinephrine. Give epinephrine every 3 to 5 minutes as long as the patient does not have a pulse.

- Epinephrine IV/IO: 0.01 mg/kg (1:10,000; 0.1 mL/kg), follow with saline flush
- Epinephrine endotracheal tube: 0.1 mg/kg (1:1000; 0.1 mL/kg), max 10 mg
- After 5 cycles of CPR (about 2 minutes), recheck the rhythm. If pulseless VT/VF is present, turn off the oxygen flow, clear the patient, and shock using 4 J/kg (or equivalent biphasic energy). Immediately resume CPR, starting with chest compressions. Consider giving an antiarrhythmic. Given amiodarone (or lidocaine if amiodarone is not available). Consider magnesium sulfate if the rhythm is torsades. Consider placement of an advanced airway and possible causes of the arrest.
- Amiodarone 5 mg/kg IV/IO rapid bolus, follow with saline flush
- Lidocaine 1 mg/kg IV/IO bolus, follow with saline flush
- Magnesium sulfate 25 to 50 mg/kg IV/IO; maximum 2 g; follow with saline flush
- After 5 cycles of CPR (about 2 minutes), recheck the rhythm. If VT/VF persists, check to make sure the oxygen flow is off, clear everyone from the patient, and then give one shock with 4 J/kg (or equivalent biphasic energy). Resume CPR, and give epinephrine.
- If a shockable rhythm is not present:
  - Check a pulse if an organized rhythm is present on the monitor. If there is an organized rhythm on the monitor and a pulse is present, check the patient's blood pressure and other vital signs and begin postresuscitation care.
  - If there is an organized rhythm on the monitor but there is no pulse (pulseless electrical activity) or if the rhythm is asystole, resume CPR, consider possible causes of the arrest, and give medications and other emergency care as indicated.
- Possible reversible causes
  - Hypoxemia: give oxygen
  - Hypovolemia: replace volume
  - Hypothermia: use simple warming techniques
  - Hyperkalemia/hypokalemia and metabolic disorders: correct electrolyte and acid-base disturbances
  - Tamponade: pericardiocentesis
  - Tension pneumothorax: needle decompression
  - Toxins/poisons/drugs: antidote/specific therapy
  - Thromboembolism

Unacceptable Interventions: Absent/Pulseless Rhythms

- Failure to use personal protective equipment
- Failure to adequately assess the patient

CARDIAC ARREST ALGORITHM

First Impression: Sick or not sick?
Primary Survey
Unresponsive
Open airway, give 2 breaths
Give oxygen when available
If no pulse, begin CPR
Attach AED or monitor/defibrillator

S H O C K S

Defibrillation
*2 J/kg initially, then 4 J/kg or
equivalent biphasic energy
*AED: Per manufacturer

D R U G S

Vasopressors
Epinephrine IV/IO: 0.01 mg/kg
(1:10,000) every 3 to 5 min
Epinephrine ET: 0.1 mg/kg
(1:1000), max 10 mg

Antiarrhythmics
Amiodarone IV/IO 5 mg/kg or
Lidocaine IV/IO 1 mg/kg
Magnesium IV/IO 25 to 50 mg/kg,
max 2 g (consider for torsades)

M O N I T O R

Attempt/verify:
*Advanced airway placement
*Vascular access
Monitor and treat:
*Glucose
*Electrolytes
*Temperature
*CO_2

Electrical activity present?
Check pulse.
No pulse or asystole:
Resume CPR for about 2 min
During CPR, give vasopressor

Pulse present?
Assess vital signs,
begin postresuscitation care.

Algorithm assumes previous
step was unsucccessful

R E V E R S I B L E   C A U S E S

Hypoxemia - give oxygen
Hypovolemia - replace volume
Hypothermia - use simple
warming techniques
Hyper-/hypokalemia and
metabolic disorders - correct
electrolyte and acid-base
disturbances
Tamponade -
pericardiocentesis
Tension pneumothorax -
needle decompression
Toxins/poisons/drugs -
antidote/specific therapy
Thromboembolism

Assess ECG rhythm
Shockable?

NO   YES

Shock × 1
Resume CPR for about 2 min
Without interrupting CPR, start IV/IO
(if not already done)
During CPR, give vasopressor

NO

Assess ECG rhythm
Shockable?

YES

Shock × 1
Resume CPR for about 2 min
During CPR, consider antiarrhythmic
Consider reversible causes of arrest

R E A S S E S S

*Airway
*Oxygenation/ventilation
*Paddle/pad position/contact
*Effectiveness of CPR
*No O_2 flowing over patient
during shocks

- Administration of oxygen by a means other than positive-pressure ventilation
- Failure to reassess respiratory status after initiating positive-pressure ventilation
- Failure to correctly identify the ECG rhythm
- Failure to begin CPR
- Performing chest compressions or defibrillation before assessing pulses
- Unsafe operation of defibrillator (failure to clear self or others before shocking)
- Failure to recognize rhythm change
- Failure to establish vascular access
- Extended attempts to establish IV access when IO access could be established quickly
- Failure to use an accurate method for weight and medication dosage determination
- Medication errors
- Failure to confirm tracheal tube position using assessment and mechanical methods
- Failure to search for possible reversible causes of the arrest
- Ordering a dangerous or inappropriate intervention
- Performing any technique resulting in potential harm to the patient

Syncope

Description

Normal brain function and maintenance of a responsive state depend on a constant supply of oxygen and glucose. Because the brain is unable to store these nutrients, an interruption of cerebral blood flow for more than 5 to 10 seconds will result in unresponsiveness.

Syncope (fainting) is a brief loss of consciousness caused by transient cerebral hypoxia. In near-syncope (i.e., presyncope), signs and symptoms of imminent syncope occur, including dizziness with or without blackout (called a "gray-out"), anxiety, pallor, diaphoresis, thready pulse, low blood pressure, and may be accompanied by partial or complete loss of vision or hearing but no loss of consciousness.

The progression to syncope is marked by loss of consciousness, atony, and falling. The loss of consciousness typically occurs within a few seconds of the onset of symptoms and is associated with complete recovery shortly after the patient assumes a supine position. Syncope causes no residual neurologic problems.

Etiology

- Non–life-threatening causes
  - Increased vagal tone
  - Psychogenic reactions
  - Prolonged standing, fatigue, dehydration
- Potentially life-threatening causes
  - Dysrhythmias including SVT, bradycardia, prolonged QT syndrome
  - Cardiac abnormalities that decrease blood flow to the heart, lungs, brain, and body
  - Myocardial ischemia
  - Certain drug intoxications
  - Hypoglycemia, anemia, hypoxia, head trauma

Types of Syncope

- Circulatory causes
  - Vasovagal syncope
    - Also called vasodepressor, neurocardiogenic, or common syncope.
    - Warning signs and symptoms last a few seconds to a minute and consist of dizziness, lightheadedness, pallor, palpitations, nausea, and diaphoresis, followed by the loss of consciousness and muscle tone.
    - Unconsciousness does not last more than a minute and patient gradually awakens.
    - Usually occurs in association with anxiety or fright, pain, blood drawing or the sight of blood, fasting, hot and humid conditions, crowded places, prolonged and motionless standing, consuming a heavy meal or fasting, pain, or bearing down during urination or bowel movements.
  - Orthostatic hypotension
    - Normal vasoconstriction of the arterioles and veins in the upright position is absent or inadequate, resulting in hypotension without a reflex increase in HR.
    - Patient experiences only lightheadedness.
    - May be precipitated by prolonged bed rest, prolonged standing, and conditions that decrease the circulating blood volume (e.g., bleeding, dehydration).
    - Drugs that interfere with vasoconstriction (e.g., calcium channel blockers, antihypertensive drugs, vasodilators, phenothiazines) and diuretics may exacerbate orthostatic hypotension.
  - Inadequate venous return
    - May occur as a result of
      - Increased intrathoracic pressure (e.g., repetitive coughing, breath holding, tracheal obstruction)

- Decreased venous tone (may be caused by vasodilators)
- Decreased intravascular volume secondary to hemorrhage or dehydration
  - Cardiac syncope
    - May be caused by structural heart disease (e.g., aortic stenosis [AS], pulmonary stenosis [PS]) or may be secondary to dysrhythmias, including long QT syndrome
    - Consider a cardiac cause
      - Syncope occurs in a recumbent position.
      - Syncope is provoked by exercise.
      - Chest pain is associated with syncope.
      - Family history of fainting or sudden death.
  - Extremely fast or slow rates can result in insufficient CO, hypoperfusion, and increased cardiac workload.
    - SVT may cause syncope in children.
      - The HR in SVT is usually faster than 220 beats per minute in infants or 180 beats per minute in children.
      - WPW syndrome may be associated with SVT.
    - Prolonged QT syndrome
      - Characterized by sudden loss of consciousness during exercise or an emotional and stressful experience
      - Onset is typically in late childhood or adolescence, although onset in infancy may mimic sudden infant death syndrome (SIDS). During the period of syncope, various cardiac arrhythmias are evident, particularly VF. The child may recover within minutes or die during the event.[11]
    - Extreme bradycardia may occur in a child with complete heart block or a malfunctioning pacemaker. β-Blockers, calcium channel blockers, digoxin, and clonidine can also cause bradycardia.
- Metabolic causes
  - Hypoglycemia: preceded by confusion, altered mental status, weakness, nausea
- Respiratory causes
  - Hypoxia or hypocapnia (decreased carbon dioxide)
  - Cough syncope
    - Most common in asthmatic children.
    - Occurs shortly after the onset of sleep; coughing paroxysm abruptly awakens the child.
    - Child perspires, becomes agitated, and is frightened; loss of consciousness is associated with generalized muscle flaccidity, vertical upward gaze, and clonic muscle contractions lasting for several seconds.

- Urinary incontinence is frequent.
- Recovery begins within seconds, and consciousness is usually restored a few minutes later.
- Child has no recollection of the attack except for the events surrounding the paroxysm of coughing.

- Psychogenic causes
  - Often associated with experiencing or anticipating an unpleasant situation (e.g., feeling afraid, seeing blood, experiencing pain, witness to violence, or other disturbing experiences)
  - Initial temporary sympathetic response followed by a reflex vagal reaction

Epidemiology and Demographics

- Uncommon before age 10 to 12 years but is quite prevalent in adolescent girls
- Minor injuries are common (25%); serious injuries occur in 1% to 2%.
- If recurrent, may have a major effect on lifestyle and/or quality of life.
- Family history is positive for similar episodes in 90% of patients

History

- Frequently preceded by lightheadedness, nausea, gray-out, sweating, and pallor (presyncope)
- May occur while sitting, standing, walking, and occasionally during exercise

In addition to a SAMPLE or CIAMPEDS history, determine the following:
- What was the history of the event?
  - Patient's position and level of activity before the incident.
  - Were there any symptoms before the event (e.g., weakness, light-headedness, sweating, dizziness, visual disturbances, headache, chest pain, or palpitations)?
  - Were any observers present?
    - Caregivers should be questioned in an effort to identify a significant medical history and determine the sequence of events.
    - Question the caregiver about the following:
      - Duration of unresponsiveness
      - Occurrence of any involuntary movements
      - Duration of any confusion or disorientation after awakening
      - Possibility of a fall or other trauma
  - Is there any evidence of trauma?
  - What is the patient's past medical history? Medications?
  - Look for medical identification for conditions such as diabetes, seizures, or medications.

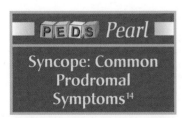

PEDS Pearl

Syncope: Common Prodromal Symptoms[14]

- Lightheadedness: 89%
- Visual disturbances: 71%
- Sensation of warmth: 39%
- Nausea: 35%
- Diaphoresis: 33%
- Altered hearing: 25%
- Sharp frontal headache: 15%
- Mild tachycardia: 13%

- Brief tonic-clonic activity observed in 6%
- Urinary incontinence in 2%
- Physical findings that suggest a life-threatening cause of syncope include the following:
  - Evidence of serious injury, particularly head trauma
  - Continuing altered mental status, particularly unresponsiveness
  - Sternal scar indicating cardiac surgery
  - Significant persistent abnormalities in vital signs
  - Prominent heart murmur
- Consider orthostatic vital signs if volume loss is suspected.
  - Do not perform if tachycardia or severe hypotension exists.
  - Perform orthostatic vital signs by moving the patient from a supine position to a sitting or standing position for 30 seconds.
  - A drop in systolic pressure of 20 mm Hg or a pulse increase of 20 per minute is considered significant.
  - A patient who becomes dizzy or develops near-syncope or syncope upon sitting or standing has a positive test.
  - No further attempts should be made to raise the patient.
- Assess skin condition.
  - Cool, moist, and pale skin results from the sympathetic nervous system's attempt to reestablish blood flow to the brain; should resolve when the patient is placed supine and blood pressure is restored.
  - Persistent cool, clammy skin suggests hypoperfusion caused by hypovolemia or a primary cardiac problem.
  - Hot or warm, dry skin may indicate a fever.
    - Can result in dehydration and hypovolemia
  - Assess for dry oral mucous membranes; assess skin turgor.

- Use personal protective equipment.
- If assessment reveals a potentially life-threatening cause of syncope
  - Secure the airway, provide high-concentration oxygen.
  - Initiate pulse oximetry and cardiac monitoring.
  - Establish vascular access if possible.
  - Check blood glucose levels and treat for hypoglycemia as indicated.
    - A child who is taking β-blockers is prone to hypoglycemia and may present with atypical signs.
- If the child appears stable and there are no findings to indicate a potentially life-threatening cause of syncope, allow the child to maintain a position of comfort, keep the child warm, and provide reassurance.

Physical Examination

Consider a cardiac cause of syncope if a loss of consciousness occurs in association with exercise or stress.

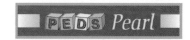

Syncope can usually be differentiated from a seizure because of its short duration, associated symptoms of nausea and diaphoresis, and complete orientation after the event.

Acceptable Interventions

The treatment of syncope is directed toward the underlying cause.

- An infant described as having been dusky or pallid during syncope, with apnea, hypotonia, and a lifeless look may have experienced an apparent life-threatening event (ALTE). These patients require physician evaluation.

Unacceptable Interventions

- Failure to use personal protective equipment
- Failure to recognize signs of respiratory distress and the need for interventions
- Failure to allow the child to assume a position of comfort
- Failure to administer supplemental oxygen
- Failure to measure oxygen saturation
- Failure to assist ventilation with a bag-valve-mask device and 100% oxygen if signs of respiratory failure or respiratory arrest are present
- Failure to reassess respiratory status after initiating assisted ventilations
- Failure to recognize signs of deterioration to respiratory failure or arrest and the need for more aggressive interventions
- Failure to monitor the cardiac rhythm if signs of respiratory failure or respiratory arrest are present

Chest Pain

Description

Chest pain in the pediatric patient, in the absence of associated symptoms, is not generally associated with a serious disorder.

Etiology

These three conditions account for 45% to 65% of chest pain in children.

- The following are the three most common causes of pediatric chest pain:
  - A pathologic condition of the chest wall (trauma or muscle strain)
  - Costochondritis (an inflammation of the cartilage that connects the inner end of each rib to the sternum)
  - Respiratory diseases, especially those associated with coughing.
- Chest pain in children younger than 12 years of age is usually the result of a cardiorespiratory cause such as coughing, asthma, pneumonia, or heart disease. Psychogenic causes are more likely in children more than 12 years of age.[7]

Epidemiology and Demographics

- Chest pain can occur in a child of any age, but rarely has a life-threatening cause.
- Chest pain is a relatively infrequent chief complaint in the young child, but increases in frequency as the child ages.

- No cause for chest pain can be found in 12% to 45% of patients, even after conducting a moderately extensive history, physical examination, and laboratory testing.

- Costochondritis
  - Characterized by tenderness over the costochondral junctions with palpation.
  - Pain is usually localized and increases with movement of the chest, deep inspiration, and/or exertion and is described as sharp, aching, or pressurelike.
- Esophageal reflux may present as substernal pain that is worse after eating or when supine.
- Chest trauma may result in a mild contusion or a rib fracture.
- Severe cough, asthma, or pneumonia may cause chest pain because of repeated stretching and strain at the costochondral junction and overuse of chest wall muscles.
- Acute myocardial infarction is rare in children. When it does occur, the child usually has an acute inflammatory condition of the coronary arteries, an anomalous origin of the left coronary artery, or a history of glue sniffing or cocaine use. Signs of myocardial infarction include respiratory distress, cardiac dysrhythmias, and cardiogenic shock.
- Cardiac dysrhythmias may cause palpitations or chest pain in some children. SVT, premature ventricular complexes (PVCs), or VT may cause episodes of brief, sharp chest pain.
- Marfan syndrome
  - Marfan syndrome is an inherited connective tissue disease that causes weakened blood vessel walls. Affected individuals are usually taller and thinner than their family members and have limbs that are disproportionately long compared with the trunk (Figure 6-31).
  - Cardiovascular involvement is the most serious problem associated with Marfan syndrome. The patient may experience chest pain or back pain due to dilation of the ascending aorta resulting in acute aortic dissection or rupture.
- The patient with pericarditis typically presents with sharp, stabbing pain that is exacerbated by inspiration, cough, or movement and improves when he or she sits up and leans forward. The child is usually febrile. Distant heart sounds and neck vein distention may be detected on physical examination.
- The child with myocarditis typically describes mild pain that has been present for several days. Physical examination may reveal muffled heart sounds, fever, or tachycardia.

History and Physical Examination

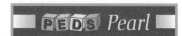

PEDS *Pearl*

Chest pain of possible cardiac origin must be considered when associated with known cardiac disease, exercise, syncope, palpitations, vertigo, or a change in skin color.

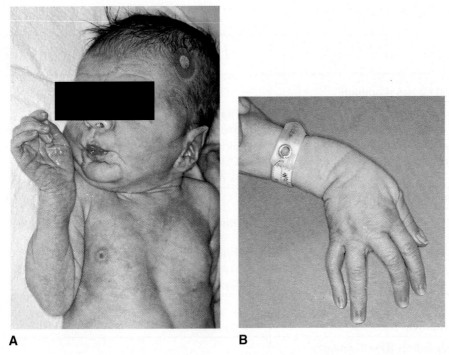

A   **B**

Figure 6-31   **Infant with Marfan syndrome. A,** Note the narrow elongated face, sunken chest (pectus excavatum), and long arms and fingers. **B,** A close-up view of the infant's hand.

Differential Diagnosis
Therapeutic Interventions

- Perform an initial assessment.
- If a cardiac cause for chest pain is suspected
  - Administer high-concentration oxygen.
  - Attach pulse oximeter and cardiac monitor.
  - Establish IV access if possible.
  - Consult a pediatric cardiologist.
- Reassess frequently.

TABLE 6-21 *Differential Diagnosis of Chest Pain in Pediatric Patients*

Musculoskeletal Causes (Common)

Trauma (accidental, abuse)	Fibrositis
Exercise, overuse injury (strain, bursitis)	Slipping rib
Costochondritis (Tietze syndrome)	Sickle cell anemia vaso-occlusive crisis
Herpes zoster (cutaneous)	Osteomyelitis (rare)
Pleurodynia	Primary or metastatic tumor (rare)

Pulmonary Causes (Common)

Pneumonia	Infarction (sickle cell anemia)
Pleurisy	Foreign body
Asthma	Embolism (rare)
Chronic cough	Pulmonary hypertension (rare)
Pneumothorax	Tumor (rare)

Idiopathic Causes (Common)

Anxiety, hyperventilation	Panic disorder

Gastrointestinal Causes (Less Common)

Esophagitis (gastroesophageal reflux)	Subdiaphragmatic abscess
Esophageal foreign body	Perihepatitis (Fitz-Hugh-Curtis syndrome)
Esophageal spasm	Peptic ulcer disease
Cholecystitis	

Cardiac Causes (Less Common)

Pericarditis	Marfan syndrome (dissecting aortic aneurysm)
Postpericardiotomy syndrome	Anomalous coronary artery
Endocarditis	Kawasaki disease
Mitral valve prolapse	Cocaine, sympathomimetic ingestion
Aortic or subaortic stenosis	Angina (familial hypercholesterolemia)
Arrhythmias	

Other Causes (Less Common)

Spinal cord or nerve root compression	Castleman disease (lymph node neoplasm)
Breast-related pathologic condition	

From History and physical examination. In: Behrman RE, Kliegman RM, Jenson HB, eds. *Nelson textbook of pediatrics*, 16th ed. Philadelphia: WB Saunders, 2000.

Congenital Heart Disease

Congenital cardiovascular defects are present in about one percent of live births and are the most frequent congenital malformations in newborns. Heart defects may obstruct blood flow in the heart or the vessels near it or cause an alteration in the normal pattern of blood flow through the heart. Although rare, defects may occur in which only one ventricle exists (single ventricle), both the pulmonary artery and aorta arise from the same ventricle (double outlet ventricle), or the right or left side of the heart is incompletely formed (hypoplastic right or left heart).

Acyanotic Heart Defects

Acyanotic heart defects are also called pink defects.

Acyanotic heart defects are congenital abnormalities in which oxygenated blood is shunted from the left (systemic) side of the heart to the right (pulmonary) side. This is called a left-to-right shunt.

Acyanotic defects may be classified according to their hemodynamic effects:

- Increased pulmonary blood flow
  - Atrial septal defect (ASD)
  - Ventricular septal defect (VSD)
  - Patent ductus arteriosus (PDA)
- Obstruction to blood flow from the ventricles
  - Coarctation of the aorta (COA)
  - Aortic stenosis (AS)
  - Pulmonary stenosis (PS)

Atrial Septal Defect

ASD is more common in females than males and accounts for 5% to 10% of all congenital heart defects.

- In ASD, an abnormal opening (i.e., hole/defect) exists in the wall (septum) separating the atrial chambers of the heart (Figure 6-32). This opening allows some of the oxygenated blood from the left atrium (higher pressure) to flow through the hole to the right atrium (lower pressure) instead of flowing through the left ventricle, out the aorta and to the body. The increased volume of blood flowing to the right atrium and ventricle causes enlargement of these chambers. If the defect is not repaired, pulmonary hypertension usually develops in adult life.
- Physical examination
  - Infants and children with ASD are usually asymptomatic, although height and weight are often below normal and endurance may be limited.
  - A characteristic murmur is present with ASD.
  - Patients are at risk for atrial dysrhythmias, probably due to atrial enlargement and stretching of conduction fibers.
- Small ASDs (less than 8 mm in size) often close spontaneously by 18

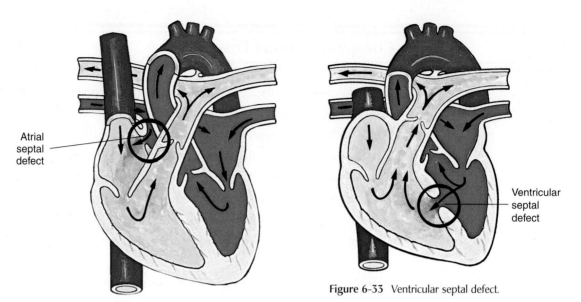

Figure 6-32 Atrial septal defect.

Figure 6-33 Ventricular septal defect.

months of age. Large defects frequently necessitate surgery, usually before school age.

Ventricular Septal Defect

- In VSD, an abnormal opening exists in the wall separating the right and left ventricles (Figure 6-33). This opening allows some of the oxygenated blood to flow from the left ventricle through the hole to the right ventricle and pulmonary artery, instead of being pumped into the aorta.

VSD is the most common (15% to 20%) congenital heart defect.

- Because less blood is pumped out of the left ventricle, SV is reduced, affecting CO. Because the right ventricle is under greater pressure and has to pump extra blood, it may enlarge. If the right ventricle is unable to accommodate the increased workload, the right atrium may also enlarge.
- Physical examination
  - If the opening is small, the patient is usually asymptomatic and growth and development are unaffected.
  - If the opening is of moderate to large size
    - Growth and development are often delayed. Height is usually normal but weight may be decreased.
    - Decreased exercise tolerance.
    - Repeated pulmonary infections.
    - Signs of CHF (e.g., tachypnea, grunting respirations, tachycardia, diminished pulses, fatigue with feeding, and diaphoresis) are common.
    - A characteristic murmur is present.
- Infants and children with a VSD are at risk for bacterial endocarditis and will need to take antibiotics before certain dental and surgical procedures.

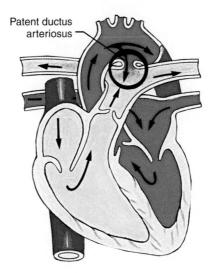

Figure 6-34   Patent ductus arteriosus.

- Many small defects close spontaneously during the first year of life. Moderate and large defects may require surgical closure.

Patent Ductus Arteriosus

The ductus arteriosus normally closes within a few hours of birth. Persistence of the ductus arteriosus beyond 10 days of life is considered abnormal.

- PDA occurs when the ductus arteriosus, a blood vessel present during fetal development that connects the pulmonary artery to the descending aorta, fails to close after birth (Figure 6-34). The hemodynamic consequences of PDA are determined by the diameter and length of the ductus and the level of peripheral vascular resistance.
- In PDA, oxygenated blood traveling through the aorta is shunted from the aorta, across the duct, to the pulmonary artery (instead of flowing from the aorta and on to the body) where it mixes with deoxygenated blood.
  - The workload of the left atrium and ventricle is increased because of the additional blood that is recirculated through the lungs to these heart chambers.
  - At the same time, less blood is delivered to the lungs to be oxygenated.

Symptoms depend on the size of the ductus and how much blood flow it carries.

- Physical examination
  - Small shunt
    - May be asymptomatic
  - Large shunt
    - Wide pulse pressure
    - Bounding peripheral pulses
    - A characteristic murmur is present.
    - Tachypnea, increased work of breathing, frequent respiratory infections, tires easily, and/or poor growth
- PDA is common in premature infants.
- An increased incidence of PDA exists with maternal rubella infection.
- PDA is more common in patients who were born at a high altitude.

- Closure of the ductus
  - In premature infants, an attempt is made to close the patent ductus by fluid restriction and prostaglandin inhibitors (e.g., indomethacin). Surgical tying (ligation) of the defect is usually performed if these steps do not close the ductus.
  - In term infants, surgical ligation of the patent ductus is recommended if CHF develops. If the infant is asymptomatic, surgery is postponed until 6 months to 3 years of age, unless the infant develops symptoms.
  - A small PDA may be closed using plugs or coils that are positioned by means of a catheter inserted in an artery in the groin during cardiac catheterization.

Coarctation of the Aorta

- Coarctation (narrowing, constriction) of the aorta (COA) is a common defect that affects males twice as often as females. COA may be associated with other cardiac defects, typically those involving the left side of the heart.

COA occurs in 8% to 10% of all cases of congenital heart defects.

- In COA, the aorta is pinched or constricted in the area of the ductus arteriosus, just beyond the aorta's branching vessels to the head and arms (Figure 6-35).
  - Because a segment of the aorta is narrowed, the left ventricle must work harder to force blood through the narrowed area to the lower part of the body. This results in increased blood pressure proximal to the defect (head and arms) and decreased blood flow distal to it (the body and legs).
  - In cases of severe narrowing, the left ventricle may not be strong enough to perform this extra work, resulting in CHF or poor perfusion.

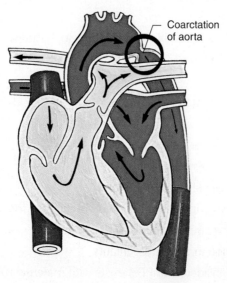

Figure 6-35 Coarctation of the aorta.

Most patients with COA are asymptomatic until later in childhood at which time the child presents with a heart murmur or systolic hypertension.

- Physical examination
  - Dyspnea, poor feeding, poor weight gain, and signs of shock may develop in the first 6 weeks of life.
  - High blood pressure and bounding pulses in the arms.
  - Lower blood pressure with weak or absent femoral pulses and cool lower extremities; differential cyanosis may be present (i.e., the lower half of the body is cyanotic).
  - Infants may show signs of CHF. Twenty percent to 30% of patients with COA develop CHF by 3 months of age.
  - Dizziness, frequent headaches, fainting, and epistaxis may be present in the older child due to hypertension.
- Patients are at risk for hypertension, ruptured aorta, aortic aneurysm, or stroke.
- Surgical repair is recommended within the first 2 years of life. There is a 15% to 30% risk of recurrence of COA in patients who undergo surgical repair as infants. Some of these cases can be treated by balloon angioplasty. The long-term results of this procedure are being studied.
- Before and after treatment, infants and children with COA are at risk for bacterial endocarditis and will need to take antibiotics before certain dental and surgical procedures.

Aortic Stenosis

AS occurs in 3% to 6% of all cases of congenital heart defects and is four times more common in males than in females.

- In AS, the aortic valve (located between the left ventricle and the aorta) is narrowed (Figure 6-36).
  - Narrowing may occur below the aortic valve, at the valve itself, or immediately above the valve. The most common form of AS is obstruction at the valve itself.
- A normal aortic valve consists of three cusps (valve leaflets) that spread apart when the left ventricle ejects blood into the aorta.
  - In AS, the valve may have only one cusp (unicuspid) or two cusps (bicuspid) that are thick and stiff.
  - The thick and stiffened valve does not open freely, causing the left ventricle to work harder to eject blood into the aorta. Over time, the muscle of the left ventricle thickens (hypertrophies) to compensate for the increased workload.
- Physical examination
  - Most children with mild to moderate AS have no symptoms. Some children may experience chest pain, dizziness, fainting, or unusual tiring with severe AS.
  - A characteristic murmur is present.
  - Blood pressure is usually normal, but a narrow pulse pressure may be present in cases of severe AS.

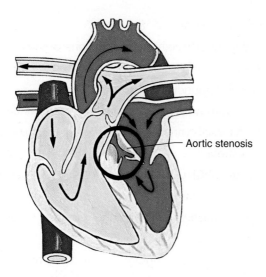

Figure 6-36 Aortic stenosis.

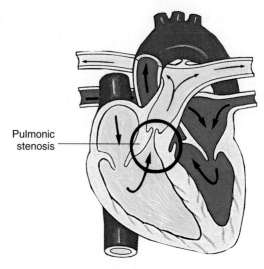

Figure 6-37 Pulmonic stenosis.

- Exercise restriction against sustained strenuous activity is recommended in children with moderate to severe AS. The need for surgical intervention is dependent on the severity of the stenosis.

Pulmonary Stenosis
- In PS, the pulmonic valve (located between the right ventricle and pulmonary artery) is narrowed (Figure 6-37).
  - Narrowing may occur below the pulmonic valve, at the valve itself, or immediately above the valve. The most common form of PS is obstruction at the valve itself.
- A normal pulmonic valve consists of three cusps that spread apart when the right ventricle ejects blood into the pulmonary artery.
  - In PS, the valve cusps are thickened and stiff, hindering blood flow from the right ventricle.
  - The right ventricle must overcome increased resistance to eject blood into the pulmonary artery and gradually hypertrophies because of its increased workload.
- Physical examination
  - Most children with mild PS have no symptoms. Children with moderate or severe PS may experience shortness of breath and chest pain or epigastric pain with exertion and diminished exercise tolerance.
  - A characteristic murmur is present.
  - Cyanosis and signs of CHF may be present in infants with severe PS.
  - Sudden death is possible in a child with severe stenosis during heavy physical activity.
- Mild PS rarely requires treatment. Moderate to severe PS usually requires treatment that may involve balloon dilation or open-heart surgery, depending on the type of valve abnormality present.

PS occurs in 8% to 12% of all cases of congenital heart defects.

• Before and after treatment, infants and children with PS are at risk for bacterial endocarditis and will need to take antibiotics before certain dental and surgical procedures.

Cyanotic Heart Defects

Cyanotic heart defects are also called blue defects.

Cyanotic heart defects are congenital abnormalities in which deoxygenated blood from the right (pulmonary) side of the heart mixes with oxygenated blood from the left (systemic) side and enters the systemic circulation, bypassing the pulmonary circulation. This is called a right-to-left shunt.

Cyanotic defects may be classified according to their hemodynamic effects:

• Decreased pulmonary blood flow
  ◦ TOF
  ◦ Tricuspid atresia
• Mixed blood flow
  ◦ Transposition of great vessels (TGV)
  ◦ Total anomalous pulmonary venous return or communication
  ◦ Truncus arteriosus
  ◦ Hypoplastic heart syndrome

TOF and TGV will be discussed here.

Tetralogy of Fallot

• TOF occurs in 10% of congenital heart defects and is the most common cyanotic heart defect seen in children beyond infancy.
• The four (tetra) elements of TOF are as follows:
  ◦ A large VSD (Figure 6-38)
    ▪ The defect allows blood to pass from the right ventricle to the left ventricle without going through the lungs.

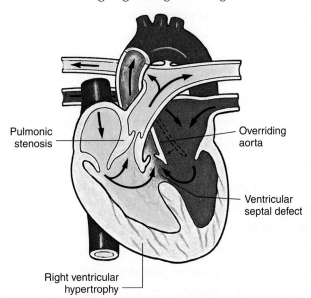

Figure 6-38 Tetralogy of Fallot.

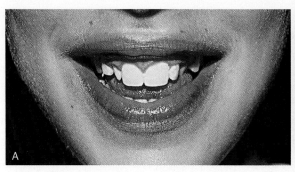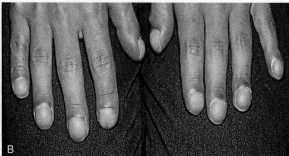

Figure 6-39 A, Severe cyanosis of the lips, tongue, and mucous membranes associated with marked clubbing and cyanosis of the nails (**B**).

- Narrowing (stenosis) at or just below the pulmonary valve (PS)
  - This narrowing partially obstructs the flow of blood from the right ventricle to the lungs.
- A right ventricle that is more muscular than normal (right ventricular hypertrophy)
  - Right ventricular hypertrophy occurs because the right ventricle is pumping at high pressure.
- The aorta lies directly over the VSD (overriding aorta)
- Physical examination
  - Most infants with TOF are pink at birth because they usually have a PDA that provides additional pulmonary blood flow. However, as the ductus closes in the first hours or days of life, cyanosis may develop or become more severe.
  - Clubbing occurs as PS becomes more significant, reducing blood flow to the lungs (Figure 6-39).
  - A characteristic murmur is present after the first few days of life.
- Therapeutic interventions
  - When there is a sudden decrease in arterial oxygen saturation, an infant or child may experience a "tetralogy spell." A hypoxic spell usually results from sudden, increased constriction of the outflow tract to the lungs, further restricting pulmonary blood flow.
  - During a hypoxic spell, the child becomes increasingly cyanotic and irritable in response to hypoxemia and breathes very deeply and rapidly (hyperpnea). If left untreated, a severe spell may result in syncope, seizures, stroke, or death.
  - In infants, a hypoxic spell often occurs in the morning after crying, feeding, or a bowel movement.
  - Acute management of a hypoxic spell should include the following:
    - Keep the infant or child as calm as possible.
      - An infant experiencing a hypoxic spell should be picked up and held in a knee-chest position (i.e., place the infant on the caregiver's shoulder with the knees tucked up underneath)

Tetralogy spells are also called "tet spells," "hypoxic spells," "hypercyanotic spells," or "blue spells."

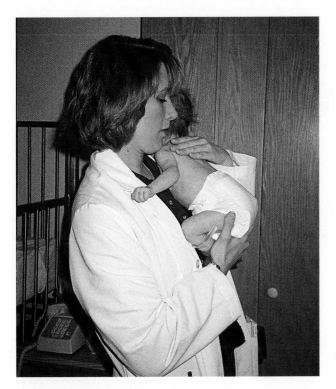

Figure 6-40 Infant held in knee-chest position.

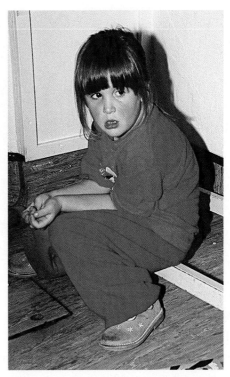

Figure 6-41 Squatting increases systemic vascular resistance and improves pulmonary blood flow in tetralogy of Fallot.

(Figure 6-40). This provides a calming effect and reduces systemic venous return.

- The older child experiencing a hypoxic spell will often squat to recover (Figure 6-41). Squatting compresses the superior vena cava and increases systemic vascular resistance, directing blood through the PS and into the lungs (rather than across the VSD).
  - Administer oxygen.
  - Give morphine 0.1 to 0.2 mg/kg IV, SC, or IM to suppress the respiratory center and resolve the hyperpnea.
  - Give a NS fluid bolus of 10 mL/kg to counteract morphine's vasodilating effects and ensure adequate preload.
  - Consider sodium bicarbonate 1 mEq/kg IV to reduce the respiratory center-stimulating effect of acidosis.[7]
  - Consider propranolol 0.1 to 0.2 mg/kg slow IV to slow the HR or phenylephrine 0.1 mg/kg IV followed by an infusion of 2 to 10 mcg/kg per minute to increase systemic vascular resistance.
  - General anesthesia may be necessary if the preceding measures do not terminate the hypoxic spell.
- Infants with TOF usually need surgery. A temporary shunt procedure may be used to allow more blood to reach the lungs until the defects can be completely corrected with surgery when he or she is older.

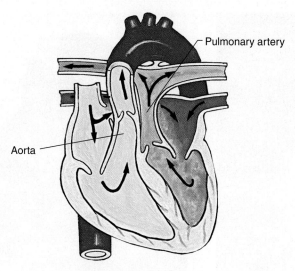

Figure 6–42 Transposition of the great vessels.

Transposition of the Great Vessels

- TGV is also called transposition of the great arteries (TGA). In this condition, the positions of the pulmonary artery and the aorta are reversed (Figure 6-42).
  - The aorta is connected to the right ventricle, so deoxygenated blood returning to the right atrium from the body is pumped out to the aorta and back to the body without first going to the lungs for oxygenation.
  - The pulmonary artery is connected to the left ventricle, so oxygenated blood returning from the lungs to the left atrium goes back to the lungs via the pulmonary artery without being sent to the body.
- An infant born with TGV can survive only if there is one or more associated defects that will permit oxygenated blood to reach the systemic circulation, such as an ASD, VSD, or PDA that allows mixing of oxygenated and deoxygenated blood.
- Physical examination
  - Cyanosis is usually present soon after birth.
    - At birth, a PDA may permit sufficient mixing of oxygenated and deoxygenated blood to prevent severe cyanosis. However, as the ductus closes in the first hours or days of life, cyanosis becomes increasingly severe.
  - Hypoglycemia and hypocalcemia may be present.
  - A murmur may be present depending on the type of associated cardiac defects, but many infants do not have a murmur.
  - Signs of CHF may be present.
- Without surgical intervention, death occurs in 90% of patients before 6 months of age.

TGV occurs in about 5% of all congenital heart defects and is three times more common in males than in females.

Other Cardiac Conditions

Congestive Heart Failure

CHF occurs when the heart is unable to generate enough CO to meet the body's metabolic needs.

Etiology

- Excessive workload
  - Volume overload
    - VSD
    - PDA
    - Single ventricle
  - Pressure overload
    - COA
    - Valvular stenosis
- Normal workload on damaged myocardium
  - Asphyxia
  - Myocarditis
  - CM
- Secondary heart failure
  - Sepsis (myocardial injury)
  - Renal failure (toxin, excessive volume, or both)
  - Severe hypertension
  - Sickle-cell anemia (volume overload)
- SVT
- Complete heart block associated with structural disease

History

- Poor feeding of recent onset due to fatigue and shortness of breath
- Tachypnea that worsens during feeding
- Diaphoresis on the forehead and/or back of the neck during sleep and feeding
- Poor weight gain
- Increased fatigue, long naps, easy fatigability
- Shortness of breath with activity
- Peripheral edema appearing first around the face and eyes, later in the hands and feet

Physical Examination

- Cyanosis that worsens with crying
- Tachypnea, often above 50 breaths per minute
- Tachycardia: resting HR above 150 beats per minute in infants or above 100 beats per minute in children
- Crackles (infrequent in infants and young children; presence suggests severe edema)

Drug Pearl
Furosemide (Lasix)

- Diuretics are used in the treatment of CHF to decrease extracellular fluid volume and increase excretion of sodium and water, thereby decreasing preload.
- Furosemide is a diuretic that acts on the ascending loop of Henle (loop diuretic) in the kidney, inhibiting the reabsorption of sodium and chloride and causing excretion of sodium, calcium, magnesium, chloride, water, and some potassium. Furosemide also has a vasodilatory effect that helps reduce vasoconstriction (afterload).
- Common side effects of diuretics are potassium depletion, low blood pressure, dehydration, and hyponatremia. Hypokalemia may increase the likelihood of digitalis toxicity.
- Monitor intake and output, daily weight, serum electrolytes, and hematocrit regularly.

- Wheezes (often confused with bronchospasm; poor response to bronchodilators)
- Increased work of breathing, retractions
- Diaphoresis
- Peripheral pulses may be diminished
  - Cool, mottled extremities with delayed capillary refill
  - Bounding pulses may be present in PDA
- Third heart sound
- Blood pressure may be elevated or low depending on the cause of CHF
- Hepatomegaly due to increased venous pressure; may or may not be present depending on the degree of failure; when present, does not always indicate CHF

Therapeutic Inventions

- Semi-Fowler position.
- Administer oxygen.
- Minimize stress and energy output.
- Monitor intake and output, electrolytes, hematocrit.
- Daily weight measurement.
- Administer a rapid-acting diuretic.
- Administer digoxin if directed by pediatric cardiologist.
- A rapid acting inotropic medication may be ordered if the infant is in severe distress and CO is compromised.

Endocarditis

Description

Endocarditis is an infection of the heart valves and the endocardium (the inner lining of the heart muscle) (Figure 6-43).

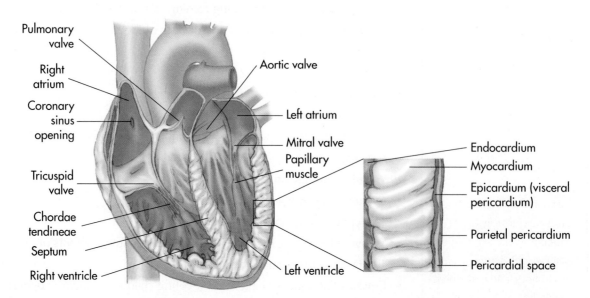

Figure 6-43 Cross-sectional view of the heart wall and tissue layers.

Drug Pearl
Digoxin (Lanoxin)

- Digoxin is a cardiac glycoside. Cardiac glycosides are a closely related group of medications that have common specific effects on the heart. *Digitalis* is a term that refers to the entire group of cardiac glycosides.
- Digoxin increases the force and velocity of myocardial contraction (a positive inotropic effect). It also slows conduction through the SA and AV node, slowing the heart rate.
- If the infant or child is in severe heart failure, the initial (i.e., loading or digitalizing) doses of digoxin are given parenterally and the heart rate is carefully monitored before, during, and after administration of the medication. Maintenance doses are given once daily or divided into two doses 12 hours apart. When digitalization occurs, the ECG will show slowing of the sinus rate and a prolonged PR interval.
- The toxic-to-therapeutic ratio is narrow. Before administering, ensure the child's apical pulse rate is more than 100 beats per minute and an older child's apical pulse rate is more than 70 beats per minute.
- Use of digoxin may result in toxicity in the infant or child with hypokalemia or hypomagnesemia because potassium or magnesium depletion sensitizes the myocardium to digoxin.
- Signs and symptoms of toxicity include visual disturbances, fatigue, weakness, nausea, loss of appetite, abdominal discomfort, psychological complaints, dizziness, abnormal dreams, headache, diarrhea, vomiting, and dysrhythmias.

Etiology

Endocarditis occurs when bacteria in the bloodstream lodge and begin to multiply on a heart valve or other damaged tissue in the heart. If untreated, the bacteria can damage the heart valve, causing it to malfunction.

Epidemiology and Demographics

- Most cases of endocarditis are caused by a bacterial infection.
- Predisposing factors
  - Artificial heart valve
  - Previous history of endocarditis
  - Heart valves damaged by rheumatic fever
  - Congenital heart or heart valve defects
  - Hypertrophic CM
  - Intravascular (i.e., arterial or venous) catheter

History

- History of underlying heart defect
- Central venous catheter
- History of recent toothache
- Recent dental or surgical procedure
- Fever
- Weakness, fatigue, poor feeding/appetite, weight loss

Physical Examination

- Fever, chills
- Enlarged spleen
- Petechiae on the skin, mucous membranes, or conjunctivae
- CHF (in 30% to 40% of patients)
- New or changed murmur
- Joint pain
- Clubbing
- Chest and abdominal pain
- Dyspnea
- Malaise
- Night sweats
- Weight loss
- Elevated temperature
- Tachycardia
- Heart failure
- Dysrhythmias

Therapeutic Inventions

- Supportive care
- Blood cultures
- IV antibiotics
- If a prosthetic valve is the site of infection, surgery may be necessary

Myocarditis is an inflammation of the middle and thickest layer of the heart, the myocardium. The myocardium contains the cardiac muscle fibers that cause contraction of the heart and contains the conduction system. Myocarditis may occur with or without involvement of the endocardium or pericardium.

The body responds to the extensive inflammation associated with myocarditis by infiltrating the area with white blood cells. Interstitial inflammation and myocardial injury result, leading to an increase in ventricular end-diastolic volume and enlargement of the heart. Contractility decreases and CO decreases. The sympathetic division of the ANS responds through vasoconstriction, increasing afterload and resulting in tachycardia. If a large portion of the heart is involved, CHF ensues, depriving body organs and tissues of oxygen and essential nutrients. If untreated, myocarditis may progress to cardiac failure and death.

Myocarditis

Etiology

- Viral infections are the most common cause, although myocarditis may be caused by any pathogen (e.g., bacteria, virus, fungus, protozoa, yeast, or parasite).
- Kawasaki disease
- Scleroderma

- Hypersensitivity or autoimmune disorders
- Medications, including antimicrobial medications
- Metabolic disorders

Epidemiology and Demographics

Viral myocarditis can occur as an epidemic that is usually seen in newborns in association with coxsackievirus B. Adenovirus and influenza A are transmitted mostly through the air.

History

- History of previous viral illness (usually 10 to 14 days earlier)
- Parents may mention a recent nonspecific flulike illness, gastrointestinal symptoms, poor feeding, or rapid breathing.
- In mild cases, the patient may have few or no symptoms. In severe cases, the infant or child may present with acute cardiac decompensation. Heart failure is the most common presentation.

Physical Examination

Tachycardia is often out of proportion to the degree of temperature elevation.

- Newborns or infants
  - Fever
  - Irritability or listlessness
  - Periodic episodes of pallor that precede tachypnea or respiratory distress
  - Diaphoresis
  - Poor feeding
  - Mild cyanosis
  - Cool, mottled skin due to decreased CO
  - Rapid, labored respirations; grunting
  - Crackles (uncommon)
  - Heart failure (tachycardia, gallop rhythm)
- Older child and adolescents
  - Low-grade fever
  - Lethargy
  - Pallor
  - Decreased appetite
  - Fatigue
  - Muscle aches/pain
  - Chest pain (usually of pleuritic type described as sharp, stabbing)
  - Dyspnea on exertion
  - Orthopnea and shortness of breath at rest
  - Palpitations (common)
  - Heart failure (tachycardia, gallop rhythm, muffled heart sounds [especially in the presence of pericarditis])

Therapeutic Inventions

- Interventions include evaluation and treatment of the underlying cause.

Drug Pearl
Angiotensin-Converting Enzyme Inhibitors

- In the body, the hormone angiotensin I is converted to angiotensin II (the active form of angiotensin) by the action of ACE. Angiotensin II causes vasoconstriction (more potent than norepinephrine) and increased aldosterone secretion from the kidneys. Aldosterone causes the kidneys to retain salt and water and to excrete potassium, leading to an increase in blood volume and blood pressure. ACE inhibitors prevent the conversion of angiotensin I to angiotensin II. As a result, the blood vessels dilate, reducing the pressure against which the heart must pump. This decreases myocardial workload and blood pressure. By increasing renal blood flow, ACE inhibitors help rid the body of excess sodium and fluid.
- Examples of ACE inhibitors include captopril (Capoten), enalapril (Vasotec), lisinopril (Prinivil, Zestril), and ramipril (Altace).
- Side effects include cough (common), elevated potassium levels, low blood pressure, dizziness, headache, drowsiness, weakness, abnormal taste (metallic or salty taste), rash, kidney failure, allergic reactions, a decrease in white blood cells, and angioedema.

Drug Pearl
Dobutamine (Dobutrex)

- Dobutamine is a direct-acting sympathomimetic/cardiac stimulant used for short-term management of patients with cardiac decompensation due to depressed contractility.
- Dobutamine stimulates α-, β_1-, and β_2-receptors. It has a potent inotropic effect (i.e., increased myocardial contractility, increased stroke volume, increased cardiac output), less chronotropic effect (heart rate), and minimal alpha effect (vasoconstriction).
- Dobutamine is administered by continuous IV infusion.

- In seriously ill infants and children, the following interventions may be necessary:
  - Mechanical ventilation
  - IV medications to improve myocardial contractility (e.g., dobutamine, dopamine)
  - IV diuretics
  - Antiarrhythmic therapy for ventricular dysrhythmias
  - IV medications to reduce afterload (e.g., sodium nitroprusside, amrinone, milrinone)
- Oral medications may be used in stable infants and children
  - Digoxin
  - Diuretics
  - Angiotensin-converting enzyme (ACE) inhibitors (to reduce afterload)
- Anticoagulation may be necessary in some children.
- Diagnostic studies
  - Cardiac monitoring
  - Chest radiograph
  - Ultrasound of the heart (echocardiogram); may show weak heart muscle, an enlarged heart, or fluid surrounding the heart.
  - Viral studies, CBC
  - Blood cultures for infection

○ Endomyocardial biopsy to obtain CO and intracardiac pressure measurements

Pericarditis

The **pericardium** is a double-walled sac that encloses the heart and helps to anchor the heart in place, preventing excessive movement of the heart in the chest when body position changes, and protect it from trauma and infection. **Pericarditis** is an inflammation of the pericardium that results in an increase in the volume of pericardial fluid that surrounds the heart.

The pressure within the pericardium increases as pericardial fluid accumulates. If the fluid accumulates slowly, the pericardium will expand gradually and can accommodate a large volume before signs and symptoms appear. If the fluid accumulates rapidly, the pressure within the pericardium increases significantly with a smaller volume of fluid. The accumulated fluid compresses the heart and impairs contraction and ventricular filling, resulting in decreased SV and CO.

Etiology

Pericarditis is usually the result of an infection that may be bacterial, viral (most common), or occasionally, fungal. Pericarditis may be caused by other disorders such as chest trauma, open-heart surgery, drugs and toxins (e.g., radiation and chemotherapy, penicillin, procainamide), kidney failure, autoimmune and other inflammatory disorders (e.g., rheumatoid arthritis, lupus), and tuberculosis (among other causes).

History

- History of recent upper respiratory infection common
- Poor feeding/loss of appetite
- Recent autoimmune disease, neoplastic disease (e.g., leukemia, Hodgkin disease, lymphoma), renal disease, chest trauma, or surgery

Physical Examination

The sound of a pericardial friction rub has been described as a train in the tunnel.

- Fever, tachycardia, tachypnea (most common signs of pericarditis)
- Chest pain (infrequent symptom in young children) or shoulder pain
- Pericardial friction rub (a grating/scratchy sound heard on the chest with a stethoscope)
- Pallor
- Possible JVD
- Muffled heart sounds
- Unable to lie flat; prefers to sit forward to alleviate pain
- Pulsus paradoxus

Therapeutic Inventions

- Supportive care
- Pericardiocentesis (analyze fluid to determine cause)
- Antiinflammatory medications (i.e., nonsteroidal antiinflammatory agents, steroids)

- Surgery for recurrent pericardial effusions
- Diagnostic studies
  - Cardiac monitoring
  - Chest radiograph
  - Blood studies include erythrocyte sedimentation rate
  - Echocardiogram
  - Possible cardiac catheterization

Cardiomyopathy (CM) is a disease of the heart muscle itself. The primary types of CM are dilated, hypertrophic, and restrictive—named by the type of muscle damage they cause.

Cardiomyopathy

In dilated CM, the heart muscle weakens, decreasing the heart's ability to pump sufficient blood to the rest of the body. The pressure of the blood within the left ventricle causes the heart to enlarge and stretch. In most cases, a specific cause is never identified (idiopathic).

In hypertrophic cardiomyopathy (HCM), the growth and arrangement of muscle fibers are abnormal. Individual heart muscle cells enlarge, leading to thickened heart walls. The greatest thickening tends to occur in the left ventricle, particularly in the septum. Thickened heart walls are usually stiff resulting in impaired ventricular filling that may lead to left atrial enlargement and pulmonary venous congestion. The patient may have a history of easy fatigability, dyspnea, palpitations, or chest pain. Most cases of HCM are inherited. In other cases, there is no clear cause.

Hypertrophy refers to thickening.

In restrictive CM, the walls of the ventricles stiffen because of abnormal substances that are deposited throughout the heart between heart muscle cells or because the inner surface of the heart is coated with a layer of scar tissue. The rigid ventricular walls impede ventricular filling and the heart eventually loses its ability to pump properly.

Restrictive CM usually results from a disease that originates elsewhere in the body such as amyloidosis, a condition in which amyloid (abnormal protein fibers) accumulates in the heart's muscle; sarcoidosis, a disease that causes the formation of small lumps in organs; or hemochromatosis (iron overload), a condition that is usually due to a genetic disease.

Physical Examination

The patient's presentation often depends on the type of CM the patient has. Signs of CHF are common, including tachypnea, tachycardia, diaphoresis, and pallor.

Therapeutic Interventions

Interventions depend on the type of CM the patient has and its cause.

- Dilated CM
  - Cardiac monitoring.
  - Low-salt diet, fluid restriction.

- Digoxin and diuretics may be used to increase contractility and eliminate excess fluid.
- β-Blockers to decrease myocardial workload.
- Antiarrhythmic therapy may be required for dysrhythmias.
- Anticoagulation may be necessary in some children.
- ACE inhibitors may be used to reduce afterload.
- Cardiac transplantation may be considered when medical therapy is unsuccessful.

- HCM
  - Cardiac monitoring.
  - β-Blockers.
  - Calcium channel blockers.
  - Digitalis, catecholamines, and nitrates are contraindicated.
  - Diuretics may worsen symptoms.

- Restrictive CM
  - Diuretics.
  - Anticoagulants.
  - Corticosteroids.
  - Permanent pacemaker insertion may be necessary for advanced heart block.
  - Cardiac transplantation.

- Diagnostic studies
  - Cardiac monitoring
  - Chest radiograph
  - Echocardiogram
  - Blood tests including CBC, electrolytes, thyroid studies, and bacterial, viral, and fungal cultures
  - Cardiac catheterization to evaluate myocardial function and hemodynamics
  - Endomyocardial biopsy

Kawasaki Disease

Kawasaki disease is an inflammation of the walls of small and medium-sized arteries throughout the body and is the leading cause of acquired heart disease in children. Bacteria, viruses, and environmental chemicals or pollutants have been considered as possible causes, but none has proven to be the cause of the disease.

Epidemiology and Demographics

- Usually occurs in children 6 months to 5 years of age; rare in patients younger than 3 months or older than 8 years.
- Occurs year round but is more common in the winter and spring.
- In North America, the highest incidence rates are in children of Asian ethnicity (especially those of Japanese or Korean background).

- Kawasaki disease is associated with coronary artery aneurysms in approximately 25% of cases, with an overall case fatality rate of 0.5% to 2.8%. These complications usually occur between the third and fourth weeks of illness during the convalescent stage. Vasculitis of the coronary arteries is seen in almost all the fatal cases that have been autopsied.[12]

History and Physical Examination

- Diagnostic criteria include a fever (usually exceeding 103° F) for 5 or more days and the presence of at least four of the following five principal features:
  - Skin rash.
  - Swollen, dry, cracked lips or a red tongue with small, raised bumps (papillae); a condition called "strawberry tongue" because the enlarged papillae resemble the seeds on the surface of a strawberry.
  - Red ("bloodshot") eyes (conjunctivitis).
  - Swollen lymph nodes in the neck.
  - Swelling and redness of the hands and feet; the skin of the hands and feet begins to peel off in large pieces or even a single piece (like a snake shedding its skin) 1 to 3 weeks after onset, especially around the tips of the fingers and toes.
- Extreme irritability
- Headache, vomiting, abdominal pain, diarrhea
- Tachycardia greater than expected from fever

Therapeutic Inventions

- Cardiac monitoring
- The usual treatment is IV immune globulin (IG) administered over 12 hours along with salicylate therapy. When given within the first 10 days of the illness, IVIG reduces the duration of fever and the incidence of coronary artery abnormalities.
- Aspirin is given in an antiinflammatory dose initially to control fever and symptoms of inflammation and then continued at an antiplatelet dose.
- IV methylprednisolone has been used in patients resistant to IVIG.
- Warfarin (Coumadin) may be indicated in those children with giant coronary artery aneurysms (larger than 8-mm diameter).
- Diagnostic studies
  - Cardiac monitoring
  - Chest radiograph
  - Echocardiogram
  - Blood tests including CBC, electrolytes, liver enzymes
  - Urinalysis

Case Study Resolution

This child is sick. Further assessment reveals a respiratory rate of 40 breaths per minute, HR of 136 beats per minute, and capillary refill of 4 seconds. His blood pressure is 62/44 mm Hg. The child's presentation suggests anaphylaxis. Move quickly. Ensure a patent airway. Be prepared to intubate if necessary. Administer high-concentration oxygen; ensure effective ventilation and oxygenation. Apply a pulse oximeter. Maintain oxygen saturation at above 95%. Attach a cardiac monitor. Check a glucose level. This child was given epinephrine 0.01 mL/kg of 1:1000 solution IM and diphenhydramine 1.0 mg/kg IM with prompt resolution of his symptoms.

Web Resources

- www.4hcm.org/home.php (Hypertrophic Cardiomyopathy Association)
- www.kdfoundation.org (Kawasaki Disease Foundation)

References

1. Barkin RM, Rosen P. *Emergency pediatrics: a guide to ambulatory care*, 5th ed. St. Louis: Mosby, 1999:39.

2. Hazinski MF. *Manual of pediatric critical care*. St. Louis: Mosby, 1999.

3. Carcillo JA, Fields AI, American College of Critical Care Medicine Task Force Committee Members. Clinical practice parameters for hemodynamic support of pediatric and neonatal patients in septic shock. *Crit Care Med* 2002;30:1365–1378.

4. Soileau-Burke M. Emergency management in Johns Hopkins. In: *The Harriet Lane handbook: a manual for pediatric house officers*, 16th ed., St. Louis: Mosby, 2002:8–9.

5. Behrman RE, Kliegman RM, Jenson HB, eds. *Disturbances of rate and rhythm of the heart in Nelson textbook of pediatrics*, 16th ed. Philadelphia: WB Saunders, 2000:1413–1423.

6. Park SC, Beerman LB. Cardiology. In: Zitelli BJ, Davis HW, eds. *Atlas of pediatric physical diagnosis*, 4th ed. St. Louis: Mosby, 2002:141–143.

7. Park MK. *Pediatric cardiology for practitioners*, 4th ed. St. Louis: Mosby, 2002:339.

8. Perron AD, Brady WJ, Erling BF. Commotio cordis: an underappreciated cause of sudden cardiac death in young patients: assessment and management in the ED. *Am J Emerg Med* 2001;19:406–409.

9. Maron BJ, Gohman TE, Kyle SB, et al. Clinical profile and spectrum of commotio cordis., *JAMA* 2002;287:1142–1146.

10. Link MS. Mechanically induced sudden death in chest wall impact (commotio cordis). *Prog Biophys Mol Biol* 2003;82:175–186.

11. Johnston MV. Conditions that mimic seizures. In: Behrman RE, Kliegman RM, Jenson HB eds. *Nelson's textbook of pediatrics*, 17th ed. Philadelphia: WB Saunders, 2004:2009–2012.

12. Fauci AS. The vasculitis syndromes. In: Braunwald E, Fauci AS, Isselbacher KJ, et al. *Harrison's principles of internal medicine*, 15th ed. New York: McGraw-Hill, 2003.

13. Vincent GM. Long QT syndrome. *Cardiol Clin* 2000;18:309–325.

14. Harris JP. Syncope, neurally mediated. In: Garfunkel LC, Kaczorowski J, Christy C, eds. *Mosby's pediatric clinical advisor: instant diagnosis and treatment*. St. Louis: Mosby, 2002:706–707.

Chapter Quiz

1. The most common type of shock in the pediatric patient is:
   A) Septic.
   B) Hypovolemic.
   C) Cardiogenic.
   D) Anaphylactic.

2. For the infant or child in early shock, the body attempts to compensate by:
   A) Increasing contractility.
   B) Decreasing capillary refill time.
   C) Increasing the heart rate.
   D) Decreasing the respiratory rate.

3. A 44-pound child presents with fever, irritability, mottled color, cool extremities, and a prolonged capillary refill time. The appropriate initial fluid bolus for administration to this child is:
   A) 100 mL of normal saline over 30 to 60 minutes.
   B) 200 mL of 5% dextrose in water in less than 20 minutes.
   C) 800 mL of normal saline or Ringer's lactate infused over 30 to 60 minutes.
   D) 400 mL of normal saline or Ringer's lactate in less than 20 minutes.

4. In the pediatric patient, cardiac arrest is most often due to:
   A) Myocardial trauma.
   B) Respiratory failure.
   C) Drug intoxication.
   D) Severe electrolyte or acid-base imbalance.

5. List the four essential questions to ask in the initial emergency management of a pediatric patient with a dysrhythmia.
   A) _____
   B) _____
   C) _____
   D) _____

6. Which of the following is the leading cause of acquired heart disease in children?
   A) Kawasaki disease
   B) Dilated cardiomyopathy
   C) Tetralogy of Fallot
   D) Marfan syndrome

7. True or False: Afterload is the force or resistance against which the heart must pump to eject blood.

8. What is meant by the term pulseless electrical activity (PEA)?
   A) PEA refers to a flat line on the cardiac monitor.
   B) PEA refers to a chaotic dysrhythmia that is likely to degenerate into cardiac arrest.
   C) PEA refers to an organized rhythm on the cardiac monitor, though a pulse is not present.
   D) PEA refers to a slow, wide-QRS ventricular rhythm.

9. Which of the following dysrhythmias is a normal phenomenon that occurs with respiration and changes in intrathoracic pressure?
   A) Supraventricular tachycardia.
   B) Sinus arrhythmia.
   C) Ventricular tachycardia.
   D) Complete AV block.

10. Identify the following rhythm. (Lead II)

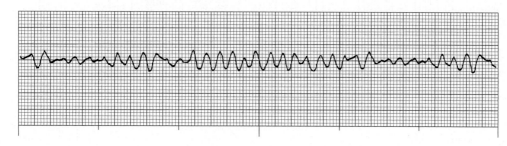

   Identification: _____

11. Identify the following rhythm. (Lead II)

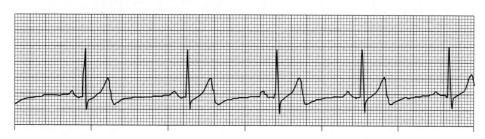

   Identification: _____

12. Identify the following rhythm. (Lead II)

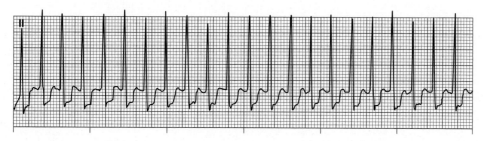

   Identification: _____

13. Identify the following rhythm. (Lead II)

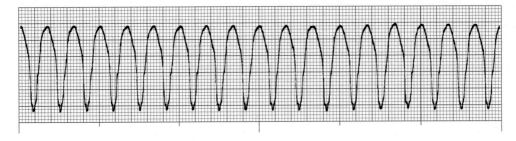

Identification: _____

14. Identify the following rhythm. (Lead II)

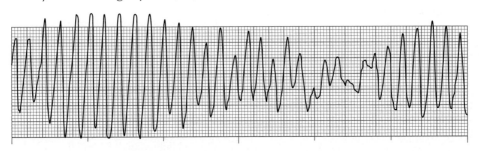

Identification: _____

15. Identify the following rhythm.

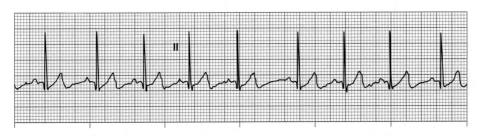

Identification: _____

16. Identify the following rhythm. (Lead II)

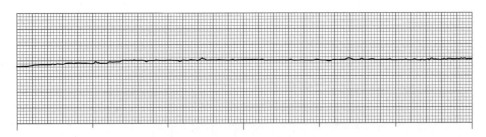

Identification: _____

17. Which of the following is the first medication administered in the management of a patient in cardiopulmonary arrest?
    A) Amiodarone
    B) Magnesium
    C) Lidocaine
    D) Epinephrine

18. The heart's primary pacemaker is the _____ , which is located in the _____ .
    A) SA node; right atrium
    B) SA node; left atrium
    C) AV node; right atrium
    D) AV node; left atrium

Questions 19 through 22 pertain to the following scenario.

You are called to see an 18-month-old child with difficulty breathing. Mom reports the child has had a cough and cold for the past two days and appears worse today. You note the child is cyanotic and appears limp in his mother's arms. His respiratory rate is rapid and shallow. Intercostal retractions are visible and wheezing is audible without a stethoscope.

19. From the information provided, complete the following documentation regarding the Pediatric Assessment Triangle.
    Appearance:
    Breathing:
    Circulation:

20. Your initial assessment reveals a patent airway. The child's respiratory rate is 60/min. Auscultation of the chest reveals wheezes bilaterally. A weak brachial pulse is present at a rate of 194 beats/min. The skin is cyanotic. Capillary refill is 2 to 3 seconds; temperature is 101.8°F; and the pulse oximeter reveals a SpO_2 of 80%. This child's presentation is most consistent with:
    A) Respiratory distress.
    B) Respiratory failure.
    C) Respiratory arrest.
    D) Cardiopulmonary arrest.

21. Is this child sick or not sick? Describe your approach to the initial management of this patient.

22. The child's condition worsens. Central cyanosis persists despite administration of 100% oxygen. The child's respiratory rate is now 8 to 14/min and shallow. The cardiac monitor reveals narrow QRS complexes at a rate of 32/min. You are unable to palpate a peripheral pulse, but a weak central pulse is present. An IV has been established. You should now:

   A) Begin chest compressions and give epinephrine.

   B) Give atropine.

   C) Continue to monitor the child closely for signs of deterioration.

   D) Give adenosine.

Chapter Quiz Answers

1. B. Hypovolemic shock is the most common type of shock in the pediatric patient.

2. C. For the infant or child in early shock, the body attempts to compensate by increasing the heart rate. Because of the immaturity of sympathetic innervation to the ventricles, infants and children have a relatively fixed stroke volume and are therefore dependent on an adequate heart rate to maintain adequate cardiac output.

3. D. Administer a bolus of 20 mL/kg of isotonic crystalloid solution (NS or LR) over 5 to 20 minutes. 44 pounds = 20 kilograms. For this child, the appropriate initial fluid bolus is 400 mL of normal saline or Ringer's lactate.

4. B. In children, cardiopulmonary arrest is usually the result of respiratory failure or shock that progresses to cardiopulmonary failure with profound hypoxemia and acidosis, and eventually cardiopulmonary arrest.

5. The initial emergency management of pediatric dysrhythmias requires a response to four important questions:

   A) Is a pulse (and other signs of circulation) present?

   B) Is the rate within normal limits for age, too fast, too slow, or absent?

   C) Is the QRS wide (ventricular in origin) or narrow (supraventricular in origin)?

   D) Is the patient sick (unstable) or not sick (stable)?

6. A. Kawasaki disease is an inflammation of the walls of small and medium-sized arteries throughout the body and is the leading cause of acquired heart disease in children.

7. True. Afterload is the force or resistance against which the heart must pump to eject blood.

8. C. In pulseless electrical activity (PEA), organized electrical activity is visible on the ECG, but central pulses are absent. The mnemonic "4 H's and 4 T's" can be used to memorize the possible causes of PEA. PEA has a poor prognosis unless the underlying cause can be rapidly identified and appropriately managed.

9. B. Sinus arrhythmia is a normal phenomenon that occurs with respiration and changes in intrathoracic pressure. The heart rate increases with inspiration (R-R intervals shorten) and decreases with expiration (R-R intervals lengthen). Sinus arrhythmia is commonly observed in infants and children.

10. Ventricular fibrillation (VF)

11. Sinus bradycardia

12. Supraventricular tachycardia (SVT)

13. Monomorphic ventricular tachycardia (VT)

14. Polymorphic ventricular tachycardia

15. Sinus arrhythmia

16. Asystole

17. D. Epinephrine (a vasopressor) is the first drug given in cardiac arrest. Amiodarone is the preferred antiarrhythmic in cardiac arrest due to pulseless VT or VF. Lidocaine may be used if amiodarone is not available. Magnesium may be used if the rhythm is Torsades de Pointes.

18. A. The heart's primary pacemaker is the SA node, which is located in the right atrium.

19. Pediatric Assessment Triangle (first impression) findings
    Appearance: Awake but appears limp
    Breathing: Respirations are rapid and shallow; audible wheezing is present; increased work of breathing evident
    Circulation: Skin is cyanotic; no evidence of bleeding

20. B. This child's presentation is most consistent with respiratory failure. The presence of tachypnea and tachycardia reflects compensatory mechanisms that are attempting to increase cardiac output. However, these mechanisms will fail (signifying the onset of cardiopulmonary failure) as oxygen demand increases and the child tires. Aggressive treatment is essential.

21. This child is sick. Move quickly. Open the airway and suction if necessary. Correct hypoxia by giving high-flow oxygen. Begin assisted ventilation if the patient does not improve. Provide further interventions based on assessment findings.

22. A. If there is no improvement after approximately 30 seconds of effective assisted ventilation and the child's heart rate is less than 60 beats/min with signs of poor perfusion, begin chest compressions, and give epinephrine. If the bradycardia persists, consider atropine and pacing. Adenosine is contraindicated in this situation because the patient is bradycardic. Adenosine is used to slow the heart rate in supraventricular tachycardia (SVT).

7 Cardiovascular Interventions

Case Study

On a warm summer day in mid June, a 3-year-old boy is found floating face down in the swimming pool of an apartment complex. The baby-sitter pulled the child from the pool. She states the child was last seen 10 to 15 minutes ago. She does not know how to perform cardiopulmonary resuscitation (CPR). Your first impression reveals a pale, motionless child with no obvious signs of breathing or circulation. Further assessment reveals the child is unresponsive, apneic, and pulseless. The child's chest is pale and his extremities are blue. CPR is started and a cardiac monitor is applied.

The monitor reveals asystole. What should you do next?

Objectives

1. Identify appropriate parameters for performing infant and child CPR.
2. Describe the differences in proper hand position when performing external chest compressions in infants and children.
3. State the proper ventilation and compression rates for infants and children when performing CPR.
4. Describe the indications for vascular access.
5. Discuss age-appropriate vascular access sites for infants and children.
6. List local and systemic complications of intravascular access.
7. State the indications for intraosseous (IO) infusion.
8. Identify the landmarks for IO infusion.
9. Describe the advantages and disadvantages of peripheral venous, central venous, and IO vascular access.
10. Define defibrillation and synchronized cardioversion.
11. Describe four factors affecting transthoracic resistance.
12. Describe proper placement of hand-held defibrillator paddles or self-adhesive monitoring/defibrillation pads.
13. Identify indications for defibrillation and synchronized cardioversion.

14. Describe the procedure for defibrillation and synchronized cardio-version.

15. Describe the differences in the delivery of energy relative to the cardiac cycle with synchronized cardioversion and defibrillation.

16. For each of the following dysrhythmias, identify the energy levels currently recommended and indicate if the shock should be delivered using synchronized cardioversion or defibrillation:

    A) Pulseless ventricular tachycardia (VT)/ventricular fibrillation (VF)

    B) Supraventricular tachycardia (SVT)

17. Discuss the indications and procedure for transcutaneous pacing (TCP).

18. List two examples of vagal maneuvers that may be used in the pediatric patient.

Basic Life Support

Basic Life Support skill components

According to the 2005 resuscitation guidelines, an infant is less than 1 year of age. A child is considered 1 to 12 to 14 years of age. Some hospitals may prefer to consider the age of a child from 1 to 16 to 18 years of age.

- Assess/alert/attend
- Assess responsiveness
- Position the victim
- Airway
- Breathing
- Circulation/chest compressions

Assess

- Assess the scene for safety. Is it safe to approach the victim? If the scene is not safe, alert emergency medical services (EMS) for help and make sure other bystanders are aware of existing danger.

- Assess the victim for life-threatening conditions and shout for help if necessary. For example, "I need help here!"

- Assess and make a quick determination regarding the nature of the emergency and the approximate age of the victim.

Alert and Attend

- If you are alone and the patient collapsed suddenly, phone for help, get an AED, and quickly return to the patient to begin CPR and use the AED.

- If you are alone and find the patient unresponsive, perform CPR for about 2 minutes (about 5 cycles). Briefly leave the patient to phone for help and get an AED. Then return to the patient to resume CPR and use the AED.

Assess Responsiveness

- Quickly assess the child's level of responsiveness by tapping the child and speaking loudly, "Are you OK?"

  ○ If head or neck trauma is suspected, to avoid spinal injury do not shake the child

- If the child is unresponsive but breathing, call EMS to facilitate transport of the child as rapidly as possible to an appropriate facility.
- The child with respiratory distress should be permitted to remain in the position he or she finds most comfortable to maintain patency of the partially obstructed airway.

Position the Victim

- Positioning or moving a victim may be necessary if
  - You find an unresponsive victim lying face down.
  - You must momentarily leave a breathing victim unattended.
  - The victim is breathing but unresponsive.
  - The victim is vomiting or has debris in his or her mouth.
  - The victim's life is in immediate danger in his or her current location.
- The following techniques are suggested for repositioning or moving a victim:
  - If you are alone and the victim is an unresponsive child:
    - Kneel at the victim's waist.
    - Attempt to roll the victim as a single unit. Grasp the victim's opposite shoulder and opposite hip and roll the victim toward you.
    - As soon as movement begins, remove your hand from the victim's shoulder and support his or her head and neck until the victim is flat on his or her back on a flat, hard surface, such as a sturdy table, the floor, or the ground.
  - If an assistant is available, one person should stabilize the head and neck while the other responder rolls the victim's body. Roll the victim's body as a single unit.
  - If the victim is an infant and trauma is not suspected, carry the infant with his or her head in your hand, torso supported by your forearm, and the infant's legs straddling your elbow.
- If the child is breathing and trauma to the head or neck is not suspected, place the child in the recovery position.
  - Kneel at the child's waist.
  - Position the child's arm that is closest to you up and away from the child's side.
  - Bend the child's leg that is opposite you upward.
  - Grasp the child's hip and shoulder and roll him or her toward you, resting the child's head on his or her extended arm. The child's bent leg should help keep him or her from rolling.
  - If the child is to be left in this position for an extended period, alternate the child's position to the opposite side every 30 minutes. Continue to monitor airway, breathing, and circulation.

A = Airway

The tongue is the most common cause of airway obstruction in the unresponsive pediatric victim. Because the tongue is attached to the lower jaw, displacing the jaw forward lifts the tongue away from the back of the throat, opening the airway.

- Kneel beside the victim.
- Place one hand on the child's forehead. Place the fingers of your other hand on the bony part of the child's chin. Tilt the child's head back and open the mouth (head tilt–chin lift maneuver).
- If you suspect a neck or spinal injury, lift the child's jaw without tilting the head (jaw thrust without head tilt maneuver).

B = Breathing

- Determine if the infant or child is breathing (assess for no more than 10 seconds).
  - LOOK for rise and fall of the chest and abdomen.
  - LISTEN for exhaled air.
  - FEEL for exhaled air.
- If the patient is breathing, maintain a patent airway.
- If the patient is not breathing or if breathing is inadequate:
  - Remove any obvious airway obstruction.
  - Begin rescue breathing while maintaining a patent airway with a chin lift or jaw thrust without head tilt.
  - Deliver two breaths (1 second per breath) with sufficient volume to cause gentle chest rise. Allow for exhalation between breaths.

C = Circulation

- Check for a pulse for up to 10 seconds.
- In infants, assess the brachial or femoral pulse.
  - To assess a brachial pulse, place your thumb on the outside of the infant's arm and your index and middle fingers on the inside of the infant's upper arm between the elbow and the shoulder (Figure 7-1).
  - Press gently and assess for a pulse for up to 10 seconds.
- Assess the carotid pulse in children older than 1 year.
  - Locate the child's thyroid cartilage (Adam's apple) with two to three fingers of one hand.
  - Using the side of the patient's neck closest to you, slide your fingers into the groove between the trachea and the sternocleidomastoid muscles and gently palpate the carotid artery (Figure 7-2). Assess for a pulse for up to 10 seconds.
- If a pulse is present but the infant or child is not breathing, give rescue breaths at a rate of one breath every 3 to 5 seconds (a rate of 12 to 20 breaths per minute) until breathing resumes.

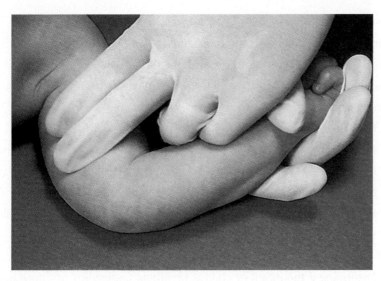

Figure 7-1   Locating the brachial pulse in an infant.

- ◦ If adequate breathing resumes and head or neck trauma is not suspected, place the child in the recovery position.
- Begin chest compressions if there is no pulse or if the heart rate is less than 60 beats per minute with signs of poor perfusion.

Chest Compressions: Infant

- Imagine a line between the nipples. Place the flat part of your middle and ring fingers about one finger's width below this imaginary line (Figure 7-3).
- Press down on the sternum and deliver five compressions at a rate of about 100 per minute. Apply firm pressure, depressing the sternum about 1/3 to 1/2 the depth of the chest (about to 1/2 to 1 inch). Do not apply pressure over the bottom tip of the sternum (xiphoid process) or over the upper abdomen.
- After 30 compressions, tilt the head, lift the chin, and deliver two breaths (or, if trauma is suspected, use the jaw thrust without head tilt maneuver).
- Continue compressions and breaths in a ratio of 30:2 until the infant shows obvious signs of life, advanced life support personnel arrive and take over, you are too exhausted to continue, or a physician instructs you to stop.

Chest Compressions: Child

- Find the lower half of the sternum (center of the chest between the nipples) and place the heel of one hand there (Figure 7-4). Using the heel of one hand, with the second hand on top (adult CPR technique) is also acceptable.

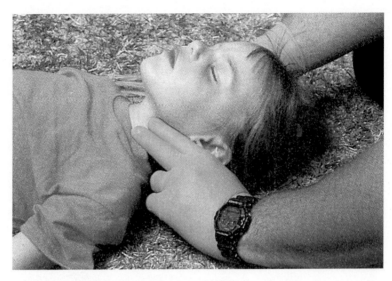

Figure 7-2   Locating the carotid pulse in a child.

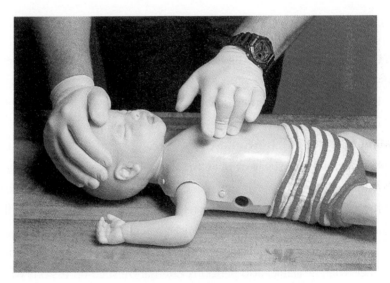

Figure 7-3   Locating finger position for infant chest compression.

- Position yourself directly over the child's chest. With your arms straight and your elbows locked, press down on the sternum and deliver compressions at a rate of about 100 per minute. Apply firm pressure, depressing the sternum about 1/3 to 1/2 the depth of the chest (about 1 to 1 1/2 inches). Do not apply pressure over the bottom tip of the sternum or over the upper abdomen.
- After 30 compressions, tilt the head, lift the chin, and deliver two breaths (or, if trauma is suspected, use the jaw thrust without head tilt maneuver).
- Continue compressions and breaths in a ratio of 30:2 until the victim shows obvious signs of life, advanced life support personnel arrive and

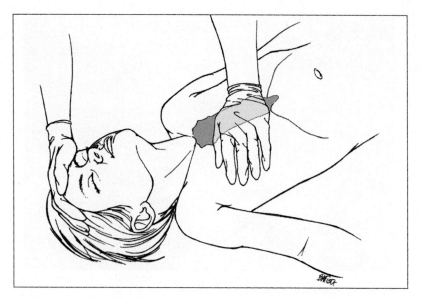

Figure 7-4   Locating hand position for child chest compression.

take over, you are too exhausted to continue, or a physician instructs you to stop.

- If an automated external defibrillator (AED) is available, attach the device and follow the machine's instructions/prompts.

Infant and Child CPR: Two Rescuers

EMS professionals usually work in teams of at least two and arrive simultaneously on the scene of an emergency. Typically, one rescuer establishes unresponsiveness, assesses and opens the airway, and proceeds with the indicated care. The other rescuer quickly prepares equipment such as suction, oxygen, and ventilation devices. The second rescuer (or third rescuer when available) also performs external chest compressions when indicated. Whenever two rescuers are present and are not responding EMS professionals, one rescuer should provide CPR while the second rescuer activates EMS.[1]

CPR Performed by Two (or More) Rescuers

- Establish unresponsiveness.
- Rescuer no. 1
    ◦ Open the airway (head tilt–chin lift or jaw thrust without head tilt maneuver).
    ◦ Look, listen, and feel for breathing.
    ◦ Give two breaths (1 second each) if breathing is absent or inadequate. Be sure the chest rises with each breath and allow for exhalation between breaths.
    ◦ Check for a pulse. Assess the brachial or femoral pulse in infants. Assess the carotid pulse in a child.

    ◦ If a pulse is present but the infant or child is not breathing, give rescue breaths at a rate of one breath every 3 to 5 seconds (a rate of approximately 12 to 20 breaths per minute) until breathing resumes.

- Rescuer no. 2
  - ◦ If no pulse is present or if the heart rate is less than 60 beats per minute with signs of poor perfusion, perform chest compressions.
    - For an infant, encircle the chest with both hands and compress the sternum between your opposing thumbs (or use the finger position previously described for single-rescuer infant CPR) at a rate of at least 100 per minute. Apply firm pressure, depressing the sternum about 1/3 to 1/2 the depth of the chest (about 1/2 to 1 inch). Your thumbs should be positioned about one finger's width below the nipple line (Figure 7-5).
    - For a child, use the same technique used for single-rescuer child CPR at a rate of about 100 per minute. Apply firm pressure, depressing the sternum about 1/3 to 1/2 the depth of the chest (about 1 to 1 1/2 inches).
    - Deliver 15 chest compressions, pausing for the breaths delivered by rescuer no. 1. Once an advanced airway is in place, it is not necessary to pause for a breath.
      - Do not apply pressure over the bottom tip of the sternum or over the upper abdomen.
- Rescuer no. 1 should provide oxygen by means of a pediatric bag-valve-mask device or CPR mask.
- Assess the pulse after about 2 minutes of CPR. If there is still no pulse, continue CPR with cycles of 15 compressions to 2 breaths

Once an advanced airway is in place, do not pause chest compressions for a breath. The rate of ventilations should then change to 8 to 10/minute.

PEDS Pearl

To ensure the effectiveness of compressions during CPR, periodically assess central pulses. If chest compressions are effective, you should be able to palpate a central pulse.

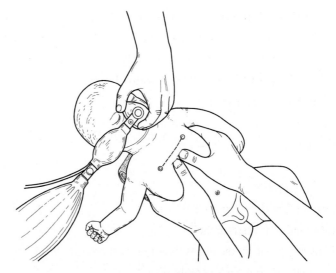

Figure 7-5   Two-rescuer infant cardiopulmonary resuscitation, two thumb–encircling hands technique.

TABLE 7-1 *Summary of Basic Life Support Interventions*

	Infant	Child	Adult
Age	Under 1 y	1 to 12 to 14 y	More than 12 to 14 y
Ventilation rate	1 breath every 3 to 5 seconds (12 to 20 breaths/min)	1 breath every 3 to 5 seconds (12 to 20 breaths/min)	1 breath every 5 to 6 seconds (10 to 12 breaths/min)
Assess pulse	Brachial or femoral	Carotid	Carotid
Compress with	Two fingers (one rescuer) or two thumbs encircling chest (two rescuers)	Heel of 1 hand; heels of two hands (adult technique) acceptable	Heels of two hands
Compression depth	$1/3$ to $1/2$ depth of chest ($1/2$ to 1 inch)	$1/3$ to $1/2$ depth of chest (1 to $1 1/2$ inches)	$1 1/2$ to 2 inches
Compression rate	About 100/min	About 100/min	About 100/min
Compression to ventilation ratio	1 rescuer = 30:2 2 rescuers = 15:2	1 rescuer = 30:2 2 rescuers = 15:2	1 or 2 rescuers = 30:2

(Table 7-1). Rescuer no. 1 should periodically check the brachial or femoral pulse.

Vascular Access

Various routes may be used for parenteral administration of fluid and/or medications including the intravenous (IV), IO, and cutdown. **IV cannulation** is the placement of a catheter into a vein to gain access to the body's venous circulation. IV access may be achieved by cannulating a peripheral or central vein.

When direct IV cannulation is unsuccessful or is taking too long, an IO infusion or venous cutdown are alternative methods of gaining access to the vascular system. An **IO infusion** is the infusion of fluids, medications, or blood directly into the bone marrow cavity.

A venous **cutdown** is a surgical procedure that is usually performed by a physician at the patient's bedside. The median cubital vein in the antecubital fossa or the long saphenous vein is most commonly used for this procedure.

Indications for Vascular Access

- Maintain hydration
- Restore fluid and electrolyte balance
- Provide fluids for resuscitation
- Administration of medications, volume expanders, blood and blood components, maintenance solutions
- Obtain venous blood specimens for laboratory analysis

General Principles

- In the management of cardiopulmonary arrest and decompensated shock, the preferred vascular access site is the largest, most readily accessible vein.
  - If no IV is in place at the onset of a cardiac arrest, attempt to establish vascular access using a site that will not interrupt resuscitation efforts.
  - If a central line is in place when an arrest occurs, it should be used for drug administration during the resuscitation effort.
- The preferred IV solutions in cardiac arrest are normal saline or lactated Ringer's solution. Large volumes of dextrose-containing solutions should not be infused because hyperglycemia may induce osmotic diuresis, produce or aggravate hyperkalemia, and worsen ischemic brain injury.

Peripheral Venous Access

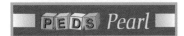

PEDS Pearl

Medications administered via a peripheral vein during CPR should be followed with a saline flush of 5 to 10 mL to facilitate delivery of the medication to the central circulation.

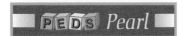

PEDS Pearl

Keep in mind that fluid flow rates are proportional to the length of the catheter and its diameter.
   When rapid volume expansion is needed, use the shortest and largest catheter possible.

Advantages

- Effective route for fluid and medication administration
- Does not require interruption of resuscitation efforts
- Easier to learn than central venous access techniques
- If IV attempt unsuccessful, site easily compressible to reduce bleeding
- Fewer complications than central venous access

Disadvantages

- In circulatory collapse, peripheral veins may be absent or difficult to access
- Small vessel diameter
- Greater distance from the central circulation
- Should be used only for administration of isotonic solutions; hypertonic or irritating solutions may cause pain and phlebitis

Needle Size

- Gauge: outside diameter of the venipuncture device
- Provides a "rough" indication of flow rate
- Thickness of the wall of the IV catheter varies from manufacturer to manufacturer, affecting actual flow rate.
- Although IV catheters are color-coded to aid in the visual recognition of the catheter's gauge, the color-coding system is not standard or universal in the medical device industry.[2]

Needle Types

Over-the-Needle Catheter

- Soft catheter commonly made of plastic or plastic-like material; rigid, plastic hub is color-coded (Figure 7-6)
- Hollow metal needle is preinserted into the catheter; the needle is used to perform the venipuncture. After venipuncture, the catheter is introduced and the needle removed, leaving the catheter in place through which fluid is administered.

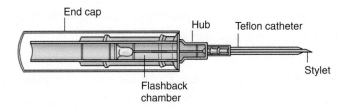

Figure 7-6   An over-the-needle catheter.

- Length of catheter limited by length of needle
- Puncture site in vein exactly size of catheter, which reduces possibility of bleeding around venipuncture site
- Available in 24- to 10-gauge sizes (24- to 22-gauge usually used for infants)
- Advantages
  - More comfortable for the patient than the hollow-needle because the catheter is pliable
  - Incidence of infiltration is lower because the blunt tip of the catheter reduces the chance of puncturing the vein
  - May be used to cannulate the veins on the back of the hands, feet, and antecubital fossa as well as the external jugular (EJ), femoral, and saphenous veins
- Disadvantages
  - Possibility of catheter-fragment embolism exists if proper insertion technique is not used

Through-the-Needle Catheter

- Primary use is for administration of medications and fluids into the central circulation
- Steel needle used to perform venipuncture; plastic catheter then slides through the needle and into the vein (Figure 7-7). After the venipuncture is performed, the needle is pulled out of the skin and left attached to the apparatus. A protective device (needle guard) is used to cover the needle to reduce the incidence of catheter shear or trauma to the patient.
- Advantages
  - Useful for accessing the central venous circulation when attempts to establish peripheral vascular access have proven futile
- Disadvantages
  - Risk of infection.
    - The diameter of the puncture wound from the needle is larger than the catheter providing a possible port of entry for organisms.
  - Risk of the sharp tip of the needle shearing off the end of the catheter and producing a catheter-fragment embolus.

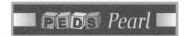

PEDS Pearl

When cannulating a large vein, the IV catheter is typically inserted with the bevel up. This position permits entry into the skin and vein in one step. Consider inserting the IV catheter with the bevel down if the vein to be cannulated is very small or fragile. This method allows a flashback of blood as the vein is entered and helps prevent puncturing the back wall of the vein.

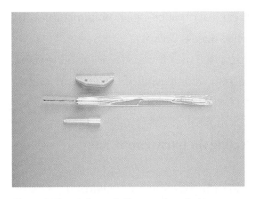

Figure 7-7   A through-the-needle catheter.

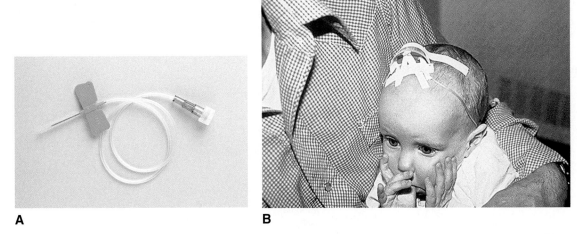

A   **B**

Figure 7-8   **A,** Hollow needle—butterfly type. **B,** Hollow needle secured in place.

- Never pull backward through the needle.
- If the catheter cannot be advanced through the needle, both the needle and catheter must be removed as a unit.

Hollow Needle

- "Butterfly" or "scalp vein" needle (also called a winged infusion set) common type of hollow needle—steel needle with flexible plastic wings (Figure 7-8).
- Available in 27- to 19-gauge sizes
- Advantages
  - May be easier to insert than other types of IV devices because there are no parts to manipulate.
  - Wings allow the needle to be taped securely in place.
- Disadvantages
  - Risk of infiltration higher than with other devices because steel needle tip may puncture vessel after placement.

Catheter-Introducing Sheath/Dilator

- A guidewire (Seldinger technique) is used to introduce a dilator and sheath into the central venous circulation after initial venipuncture with a small gauge needle or over-the-needle catheter.

- After the dilator and sheath are passed over the guidewire into the vein, the guidewire and dilator are removed, leaving the sheath in place. The sheath may then be attached to an administration set for fluid administration.

Factors to Consider when Selecting an Intravenous Site

- The purpose of the infusion
- The amount and type of IV fluid or medications to be infused
- The expected duration of IV therapy
- Accessibility, size, and condition of the vein
- The patient's age, development, mobility, hand dominance, and general health
- Presence of disease or prior surgery
- Your experience and skill at venipuncture

Venipuncture Sites

- Scalp veins (infants) (Figure 7-9)

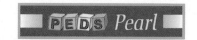

When a vein in an extremity is used for IV access, the tape used to secure the IV in place should never completely encircle the extremity.

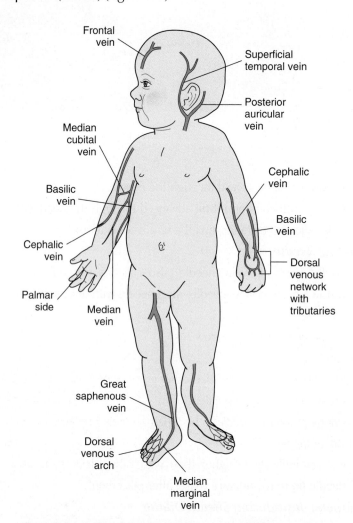

Figure 7-9   Preferred sites for venous access in infants.

- Very small veins found close to the surface and more easily seen than extremity veins
- Rarely useful during resuscitation efforts
- May be useful for fluid and medication administration after patient stabilization
- Upper extremity veins (Figure 7-10)
  - Forearm veins (may be difficult to locate in chubby babies)
    - Cephalic
    - Median basilica
    - Median antecubital
  - Dorsal hand veins

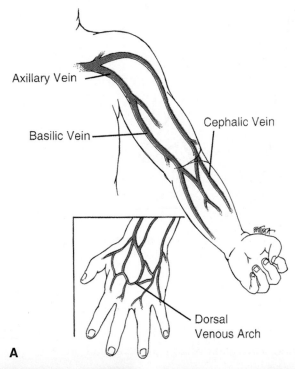

A

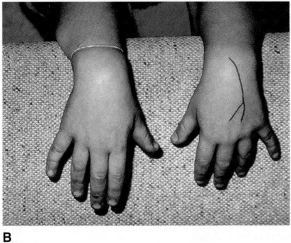

B

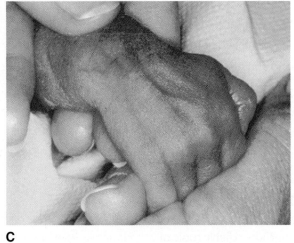

C

Figure 7-10 Veins of the forearm and hand.

- Tributaries of the cephalic and basilic veins
- Dorsal venous arch
- Lower extremity veins (Figure 7-11)
  - Saphenous
  - Median marginal
  - Dorsal venous arch

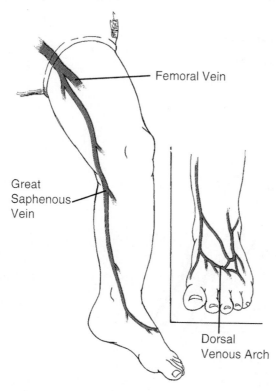

Femoral Vein

Great
Saphenous
Vein

Dorsal
Venous Arch

Figure 7-11   Lower extremity veins.

Indications

- Emergency access to venous circulation when peripheral sites are not readily accessible
- Need for long-term IV therapy
- Administration of large volumes of fluid
- Administration of blood products, hypertonic solutions, caustic medications, or parenteral feeding solutions
- Plasmapheresis, exchange transfusion, or dialysis
- Placement of transvenous pacemaker electrodes
- Central venous pressure monitoring or central venous blood sampling

Advantages

- Rapid volume expansion
- Delivery of medications closer to their sites of action
- More reliable route of venous access than peripheral venous cannulation
- Central venous pressure measurement

Central Venous Access

Disadvantages

- Special equipment (syringe, catheter, needle) required
- Excessive time may be required for placement
- Higher complication rate than with peripheral venipuncture
- Skill deterioration
- Inability to initiate procedure while other patient care activities in progress

Sites

External Jugular Vein

- The EJ vein lies superficially along the lateral portion of the neck (Figure 7-12). It extends from behind the angle of the jaw and passes downward across the sternocleidomastoid muscle until it enters the thorax at a point just above the middle third of the clavicle. It joins the subclavian vein just behind the clavicle.
- Advantages
  - Usually easy to cannulate because the vein is superficial and easy to visualize
  - Provides rapid access to the central circulation
- Disadvantages
  - May not be readily accessible during an arrest situation due to rescuers working to manage the airway
  - May be easily dislodged
  - May be positional with head movement
  - May be difficult to thread a guidewire or catheter into the central circulation because of the tortuous angle of entry into the subclavian vein
- Procedure
  - Use personal protective equipment.
  - Auscultate and document bilateral breath sounds to establish a baseline.
  - Restrain the child in a supine, head-down position of 30 degrees.

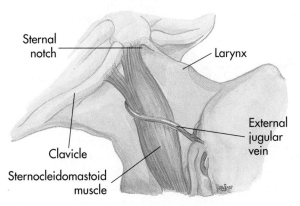

Figure 7-12 Anatomy of the external jugular vein.

- ◦ If no head or neck trauma is suspected, turn the child's head to the left (the right side is preferred for venipuncture), away from the venipuncture site. Cleanse the site. If time permits, use local anesthesia with 1% lidocaine.

- ◦ For peripheral cannulation, insert a short over-the-needle catheter into the vein. For central venous cannulation, insert a through-the-needle catheter or catheter-over-guidewire.

- ◦ Apply pressure to the EJ vein just above the clavicle (Figure 7-13). This temporarily occludes the vessel and causes it to distend, making cannulation easier.

- ◦ Apply slight traction to the vein to stabilize it. Advance the needle at a small angle from the skin plane (about 10 degrees) until a "pop" is felt as the needle enters the lumen of the vein. Advance the needle or catheter slightly after feeling the pop to ensure placement within the vessel lumen. Attach a prepared IV infusion set.

- ◦ Reassess breath sounds. If central venous cannulation was attempted, obtain a chest radiograph to verify the tip of the catheter is correctly positioned at or above the junction of the superior vena cava and right atrium and rule out pneumothorax.

Internal Jugular Vein

- The internal jugular (IJ) vein runs from the base of the skull downward along the carotid artery and then through the triangle formed by the clavicle and the two heads of the sternocleidomastoid muscle before it meets the subclavian vein behind the clavicle.

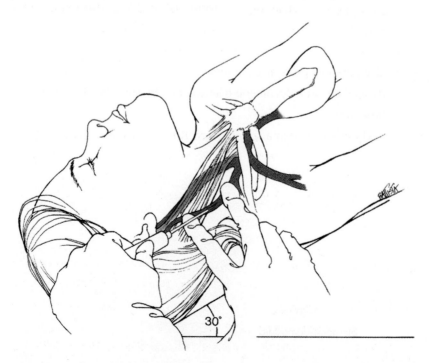

Figure 7-13 Cannulating the external jugular vein.

- Cannulation of the right side of the neck is preferred because:
  - The dome of the right lung and pleura are lower than on the left side.
  - There is more or less a straight course to the right atrium.
  - The thoracic duct is not in the way (empties on the LEFT side).
- Advantages
  - Less risk of pneumothorax with this technique versus subclavian
  - Hematomas in the neck are visible and more easily compressible
  - Easier access during CPR than subclavian
  - Usually remains patent even when peripheral veins are collapsed
- Disadvantages
  - Adjacent structures easily damaged
  - More training required than peripheral venipuncture
  - May interrupt resuscitation efforts
  - Higher complication rate than with peripheral venipuncture
  - Limits patient neck movement
- Procedure: Central (Middle) Approach
  - Use personal protective equipment.
  - Auscultate and document bilateral breath sounds to establish a baseline.
  - Restrain the child in a supine, head-down position of 30 degrees. If no head or neck trauma is suspected, turn the child's head to the left (the right side is preferred for venipuncture), away from the venipuncture site.
  - Attach a 3-mL syringe to a large-gauge catheter, lining up the bevel of the needle with the numbers on the syringe.
  - Identify landmarks by observation and palpation (clavicle and the triangle formed by the two lower heads of the sternocleidomastoid muscle) (Figure 7-14). Cleanse the site. If time permits, use local anesthesia with 1% lidocaine.
  - Insert the needle at a 30- to 45-degree angle, bevel up, into the center of the triangle formed by the two heads of sternomastoid muscle and the clavicle. With the needle directed toward the feet, slowly advance the needle aiming toward the ipsilateral nipple, while applying gentle negative pressure to the syringe (Figure 7-15).
  - When a free flow of blood appears in the syringe, remove the syringe and occlude the needle hub with a gloved finger to prevent air embolism. (Newer catheter packaging makes this step unnecessary because the guidewire is advanced through the syringe or from a Y port.)
  - Advance a guidewire through the needle. Remove the needle and advance the appropriate central venous catheter over the guidewire

---

PEDS Pearl

Inadvertent puncture of the carotid artery can occur when attempting cannulation of the jugular vein. If a hematoma occurs on one side of the neck, it is hazardous to attempt venipuncture on the opposite side because of the possibility of bilateral hematomas severely compromising the airway.

If bright red blood forcibly fills the syringe, it is probable that the carotid artery has punctured. Remove the needle and apply firm pressure for at least 10 minutes.

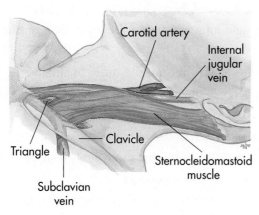

Figure 7-14 Anatomy of the internal jugular vein.

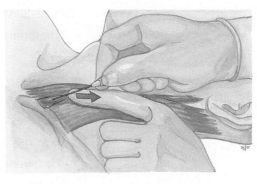

Figure 7-15 Cannulation of the internal jugular vein – central approach.

to the junction of the superior vena cava and right atrium during exhalation. Remove the guidewire and connect the catheter to a prepared IV infusion set.

- Secure the catheter in place. Reassess breath sounds. Obtain a chest radiograph to ensure the catheter tip is correctly positioned and rule out pneumothorax.

Femoral Vein

- The femoral vein lies directly medial to the femoral artery (Figure 7-16). If a line is drawn between the anterior superior iliac spine and the symphysis pubis, the femoral artery runs directly across the midpoint. Medial to that point is the femoral vein.
- If the femoral artery pulse is palpable, the artery can be located with a finger and the femoral vein will lie immediately medial to the pulsation.
- Advantages
  - Distant from major sites of activity during resuscitation efforts
  - Vein does not collapse like peripheral veins
  - Once cannulated, easy access to the central circulation
  - In case of bleeding, the neck of the femur and pelvis provide hard surfaces against which direct pressure may be applied.
- Disadvantages
  - If a pulse is absent, the vein may be hard to locate.
  - Injury to the femoral artery, femoral nerve, and hip capsule may occur; however, injury is unlikely if proper technique is used.
- Procedure
  - Use personal protective equipment.
  - Restrain the patient's lower extremities with slight external rotation.
  - Attach a 3-mL syringe to a large-gauge catheter, lining up the bevel of the needle with the numbers on the syringe.
  - Identify the femoral vein medial to the femoral artery. Cleanse the site thoroughly. If time permits, use local anesthesia with 1% lidocaine.

An acronym used to recall relevant anatomy is NAVEL (Nerve, Artery, Vein, Empty space, Ligament).

The right femoral vein may be easier to cannulate than the left because of a straighter path to the inferior vena cava.

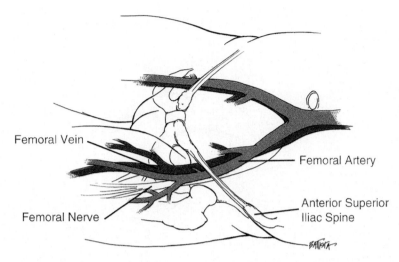

Figure 7-16　Anatomy of the femoral vein.

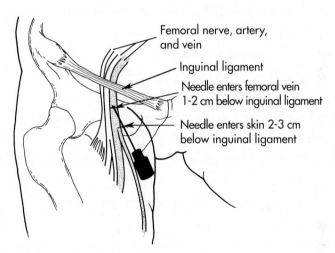

Figure 7-17　Cannulation of the femoral vein.

A finger should remain on the artery to assist in landmark identification and avoid insertion of the catheter into the artery.

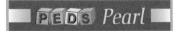

PEDS *Pearl*

During CPR, pulsations may be palpable in the femoral area that may originate from either the femoral vein or femoral artery. If CPR is in progress and femoral vein cannulation is attempted, insert the needle directly over the pulsations.

○ Insert the needle 2 to 3 cm below the inguinal ligament and just medial to the femoral artery (Figure 7–17). Slowly advance the needle parallel to the femoral artery while gently withdrawing the plunger of the syringe. When a free flow of blood appears in the syringe, remove the syringe and occlude the needle hub with a gloved finger to prevent air embolism.

○ Advance a guidewire through the needle. Remove the needle and advance the appropriate central venous catheter over the guidewire. Remove the guidewire and connect the catheter to a prepared IV infusion set.

○ Secure the catheter in place. Obtain a radiograph to ensure the catheter tip is correctly positioned.

Subclavian Vein

• The subclavian vein is a continuation of the axillary vein at the outer border of the first rib. It joins the IJ vein behind the medial end of the

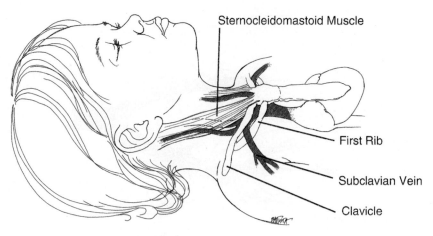

Sternocleidomastoid Muscle

First Rib

Subclavian Vein

Clavicle

Figure 7-18 Anatomy of the subclavian vein.

clavicle to form the brachiocephalic (innominate) vein (Figure 7-18). The subclavian vein is immobilized by small attachments to the first rib and clavicle. It lies anterior to the subclavian artery and is separated from it by the anterior scalene muscle.

- Advantages
  - Usually remains patent even when peripheral veins are collapsed
  - More subsequent patient neck movement with prolonged cannulation
- Disadvantages
  - Significant risk of pneumothorax, hemothorax, subclavian artery puncture
  - More training required than peripheral venipuncture
  - May interrupt resuscitation efforts
  - Higher complication rate than with peripheral venipuncture
- Procedure: Infraclavicular Approach
  - Use personal protective equipment.
  - Auscultate and document bilateral breath sounds to establish a baseline.
  - Restrain the child in a supine, head-down position of 30 degrees. If no head or neck trauma is suspected, turn the child's head to the left (the right side is preferred for venipuncture), away from the venipuncture site.
  - Attach a 3-mL syringe to a large-gauge catheter, lining up the bevel of the needle with the numbers on the syringe.
  - Identify landmarks—the suprasternal notch and the junction of the middle and medial thirds of the clavicle. Cleanse the site. If time permits, use local anesthesia with 1% lidocaine.
  - Firmly press a fingertip into suprasternal notch to establish a point of reference.
  - Introduce the needle, bevel up, just under the clavicle at the junction of the middle and medial thirds of the clavicle.

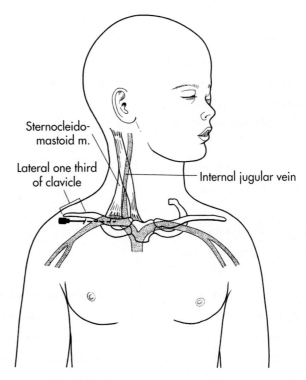

Figure 7-19 Cannulation of the subclavian vein–infraclavicular approach.

- ◦ Holding the syringe and needle parallel to frontal plane, slowly advance the needle while applying gentle negative pressure to the syringe, aiming the needle at the suprasternal notch (Figure 7-19).
- ◦ When a free flow of blood appears in the syringe, remove the syringe and occlude the needle hub with a gloved finger to prevent air embolism. (Newer catheter packaging makes this step unnecessary because the guidewire is advanced through the syringe or from a Y port.)
- ◦ Advance a guidewire through the needle. Remove the needle and advance the appropriate central venous catheter over the guidewire to the junction of the superior vena cava and right atrium during exhalation. Remove the guidewire and connect the catheter to a prepared IV infusion set.
- ◦ Secure the catheter in place. Reassess breath sounds. Obtain a chest radiograph to ensure the catheter tip is correctly positioned and rule out pneumothorax.

Atrial or ventricular dysrhythmias may be observed on the cardiac monitor if the guidewire or catheter enters the right atrium. If a dysrhythmia is observed, withdraw the guidewire or catheter a few centimeters and reassess.

Complications of Vascular Access

Local Complications

- Pain and irritation
- Cellulitis
- Phlebitis
- Thrombosis

- Bleeding
- Hematoma formation
- Inadvertent arterial puncture
- Nerve, tendon, ligament, and/or limb damage
- Infiltration and extravasation

Systemic Complications

- Sepsis
- Fluid overload/electrolyte imbalance
- Hypersensitivity reactions
- Air embolism
- Catheter-fragment embolism
- Pulmonary thromboembolism

Intraosseous infusion (IOI) is the process of infusing medications, fluids, and blood products into the bone marrow cavity. Because the marrow cavity is continuous with the venous circulation, fluids and medications administered by the IO route are subsequently delivered to the venous circulation.

In the presence of cardiac arrest or decompensated shock, an IOI should be established in any patient when IV access cannot be rapidly achieved. IOI is a temporary means of vascular access. The duration of the infusion should be limited to a few hours. Venous access is often easier to obtain after initial fluid and medication resuscitation via the IO route.

Indications

- Cardiopulmonary arrest or decompensated shock where vascular access is essential and venous access is not readily achieved
- Multisystem trauma with associated shock and/or severe hypovolemia
- Unresponsive patient in need of immediate medications or fluid resuscitation (e.g., burns, sepsis, near-drowning, anaphylaxis, status epilepticus)
- Presence of burns or a traumatic injury preventing access to the venous system at other sites

Advantages

- Skill is easily mastered, even if done infrequently; healthcare professionals experienced in the technique can often establish IO access in 60 seconds or less.
- Preferred access sites are distant from major sites of activity during resuscitation efforts.
- Low incidence of complications.
- Medications and fluids administered IV can be administered IO.
- Absorption of medications administered via the IO route is more rapid than medications administered via the subcutaneous or rectal routes.

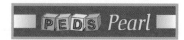

PEDS Pearl

Infusion pumps should be used for all IV infusions in infants and children to avoid inadvertent circulatory overload unless large volumes of fluid are deliberately administered as part of the resuscitation effort.

Minidrip infusion sets should be used and closely monitored if infusion pumps are not available.

Intraosseous Infusion

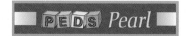

PEDS Pearl

Comparisons of IO and IV infusion of medications have shown that the drugs reach the central circulation by both routes in similar concentrations and at the same time.[18]

- Blood sampling for laboratory studies is possible.
- Venous access is often easier to obtain after initial fluid resuscitation via the intraosseous route.

Disadvantages

- Short-term intervention until venous access can be obtained
- Causes extreme pain in the responsive patient

Contraindications

- Femoral fracture on the ipsilateral side
- Osteopetrosis (high fracture potential)
- Osteogenesis imperfecta (high fracture potential)
- Fracture at or above the insertion site
- Severe burn overlying the insertion site (unless this is the *only* available site)
- Infection at insertion site (unless this is the *only* available site)
- Use of the same bone in which an unsuccessful IO attempt was made

Procedure

The preferred site for IOI is the anteromedial surface of the proximal tibia. This site is preferred because of the broad flat surface of the bone, the thin layer of skin that covers it, the ease of palpation of this bony landmark, and use of the proximal tibia does not interfere with airway management and CPR.

- Use personal protective equipment.
- Place the infant or child in a supine position. Place a towel roll or small sandbag in the popliteal fossa to provide support, optimize positioning, and minimize the risk of fractures (Figure 7-20).
- Identify the landmarks for needle insertion. Palpate the tibial tuberosity. The site for IO insertion lies 1 to 3 cm (1 finger's width) below this tuberosity on the medial flat surface of the anterior tibia.
- Cleanse the intended insertion site. If the child is responsive and time permits, use local anesthesia with 1% lidocaine.
- Stabilize the patient's leg. With the needle angled away from the joint, insert the needle using firm pressure.
  ◦ Angling away from the joint reduces the likelihood of damage to the epiphyseal growth plate.
  ◦ Firm pressure pushes the needle through the skin and subcutaneous tissue.
- Advance the needle using a twisting motion at an angle of 60 to 90 degrees away from the epiphyseal plate (i.e., toward the toes).
  ◦ A twisting or boring motion is necessary to advance the needle through the periosteum of the bone.
- Advance the needle until a sudden decrease in resistance or a "pop" is felt as the needle enters the marrow cavity.

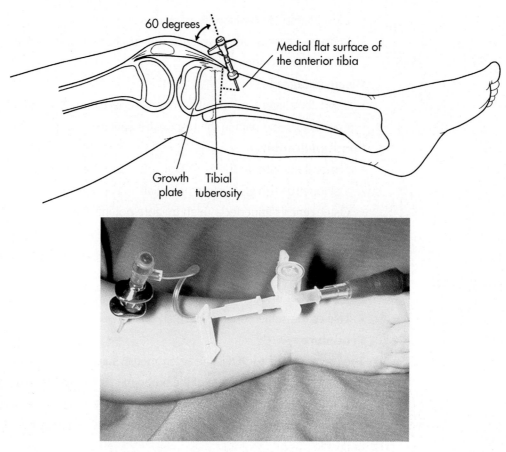

Figure 7-20 Anterior tibial approach for intraosseous infusion.

- Unscrew the cap, remove the stylet from the needle, attach a 10-mL, saline-filled syringe to the needle, and attempt to aspirate bone marrow into the syringe.
  - If aspiration is successful, slowly inject 10 to 20 mL of saline to clear the needle of marrow, bone fragments, and/or tissue. Observe for any swelling at the site.
  - If aspiration is unsuccessful, consider other indicators of correct needle position:
    - The needle stands firmly without support.
    - A sudden loss of resistance occurred on entering the marrow cavity (this is less obvious in infants than in older children because infants have soft bones).
    - Fluid flows freely through the needle without signs of significant swelling of the subcutaneous tissue.
  - If signs of infiltration are present, remove the IO needle and attempt the procedure at another site.
  - If no signs of infiltration are present, attach standard IV tubing. A syringe, pressure infuser, or IV infusion pump may be needed to infuse fluids.

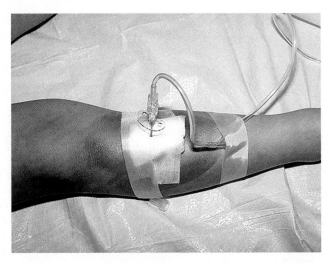

Figure 7-21 Secure the intraosseous needle and tubing in place with a sterile dressing and tape. Observe the site every 5 to 10 minutes for the duration of the infusion. Monitor for signs of infiltration and assess distal pulses.

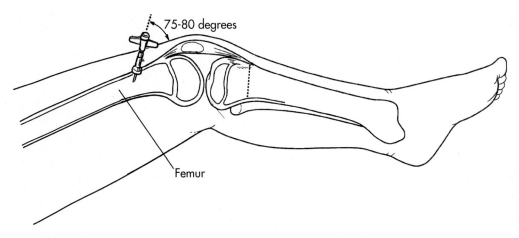

75-80 degrees

Femur

Figure 7-22 Distal femur approach. Insert the intraosseous needle 2 to 3 cm proximal to the external condyle in the midline and direct it superiorly at a 75- to 80-degree angle.

- Secure the needle and tubing in place with a sterile dressing and tape (Figure 7-21). Observe the site every 5 to 10 minutes for the duration of the infusion. Monitor for signs of infiltration and assess distal pulses.
- Attempt to establish venous access as soon as possible and discontinue the IOI. After the IO needle is removed, hold manual pressure for at least 5 minutes and then apply a sterile dressing to the site.

Alternate Intraosseous Infusion Sites

- Distal femur, 2 to 3 cm above the lateral condyle in the midline (Figure 7-22)
- Medial surface of the distal tibia 1 to 2 cm above the medial malleolus (may be a more effective site in older children) (Figure 7-23)
- Anterior superior iliac spine (may be a more effective site in older children) (Figure 7-24)

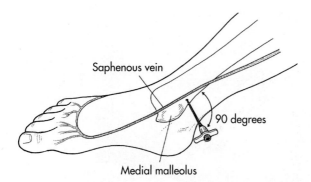

Figure 7-23   Distal tibia approach. Insert the intraosseous needle at a 90-degree angle, just proximal to the medial malleolus and posterior to the saphenous vein.

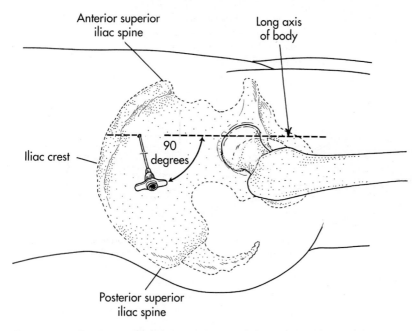

Figure 7-24   Anterior superior iliac spine approach. Insert the intraosseous needle at a 90-degree angle to the long axis of the body.

Possible Problems Encountered with Intraosseous Infusion

- Incomplete penetration of the bony cortex (Figure 7-25A)
- Penetration of the posterior cortex (Figure 7-25B,C)
- Fluid or medications escaping around the needle through the puncture site (Figure 7-25D)
- Fluid leaking through a nearby previous cortical puncture site (Figure 7-25E)
- Fracture of the tibia
- Local abscess or cellulitis
- Lower extremity compartment syndrome
- Osteomyelitis
- Loss of vascular access site may occur due to needle obstruction by marrow, bone fragments, or tissue

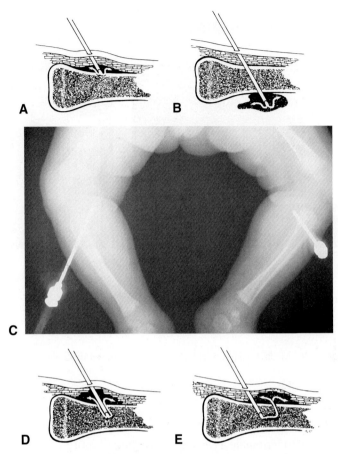

Figure 7-25 **Possible problems encountered with intraosseous (IO) infusion. A,** Incomplete penetration of the bony cortex. **B,** Penetration of the posterior cortex. **C,** Radiograph of bilaterally misplaced IO needles with penetration through the posterior tibial cortices. **D,** Fluid or medications escaping around the needle through the puncture site. **E,** Fluid leaking through a nearby previous cortical puncture site.

Electrical Therapy

Defibrillation

Definition and Purpose

Defibrillation is the therapeutic delivery of an unsynchronized electrical current (the delivery of energy has no relationship to the cardiac cycle) through the myocardium over a very brief period to terminate a cardiac dysrhythmia.

Defibrillation does not "jump start" the heart. The shock attempts to deliver a uniform electrical current of sufficient intensity to simultaneously depolarize ventricular cells, including fibrillating cells, causing momentary asystole. This provides an opportunity for the heart's natural pacemakers to resume normal activity. The pacemaker with the highest degree of automaticity should then assume responsibility for pacing the heart.

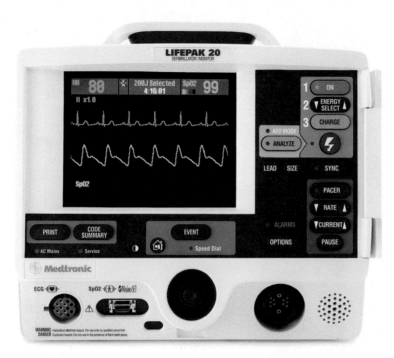

Figure 7-26   Medtronic PhysioControl LIFEPAK 20 monitor/defibrillator.

A **defibrillator** is a device used to administer an electrical shock at a preset voltage to terminate a cardiac dysrhythmia (Figure 7-26). A defibrillator consists of a **capacitor** that stores energy, an adjustable high-voltage power supply that allows the operator to select an energy level, a charge switch/button that allows the capacitor to charge, discharge switches/buttons that allow the capacitor to discharge, and hand-held paddles (Figure 7-27A) or self-adhesive monitoring/defibrillator pads (Figure 7-27B) that deliver the energy from the defibrillator to the patient.

Self-adhesive pads record and monitor the cardiac rhythm and are used to deliver the shock. These pads are used during "hands-free" or "hands-off" defibrillation and consist of a flexible metal "paddle," a layer of conductive gel, and an adhesive ring that holds them in place on the patient's chest. Hands-free defibrillation enhances operator safety by physically separating the operator from the patient. Instead of leaning over the patient with hand-held paddles, the operator delivers a shock to the patient by means of discharge buttons located on a remote cable, an adapter, or on the defibrillator itself.

Defibrillators deliver energy or current in "waveforms" that flow between two electrode patches (or paddles). Waveforms are classified by whether the current flow delivered is in one direction, two directions, or multiple directions. Monophasic waveforms use energy delivered in one (mono) direction through the patient's heart. With biphasic waveforms, energy is delivered in two (bi) phases—the current moves in one direction for a

If available, use combination pads instead of hand-held paddles for electrical therapy. Combination pads are disposable and have multiple functions. They are applied to a patient's bare chest for ECG monitoring and then used for defibrillation and synchronized cardioversion (and in some cases, pacing) if necessary. Not all combination pads are alike. Some pads can used for defibrillation, synchronized cardioversion, ECG monitoring, and pacing. Others can be used for defibrillation, synchronized cardioversion, and ECG monitoring, but not for pacing. Be sure you are familiar with the capabilities of the pads you are using.

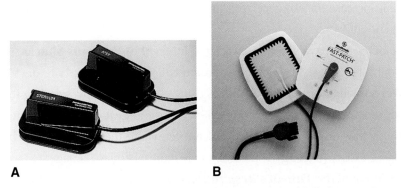

A   **B**

Figure 7-27 **A**, Hand-held paddles. **B**, Self-adhesive monitoring/defibrillation pads.

specified period, stops, and then passes through the heart a second time in the opposite direction. When delivered at appropriate energy levels, biphasic success rates can equal those of conventional devices.[3,4]

Transthoracic Resistance (Impedance)

Energy (joules) = Current (amperes) × Voltage (volts) × Time (seconds)

The strength of the electrical shock delivered is expressed in joules (J). **Impedance** refers to the resistance to the flow of current. **Transthoracic impedance** (resistance) refers to the natural resistance of the chest wall to the flow of current.

Factors Known to Affect Transthoracic Resistance

Paddle Size

To a point, transthoracic resistance decreases with increased paddle size. The largest size paddle that allows good skin contact but maintains separation between the two paddles is preferred. Infant paddles should be used for patients up to 1 year of age or 10 kg. However, larger paddles may be used as long as contact between the paddles is avoided. Adult paddles should be used for patients older than 1 year or weighing more than 10 kg.[5]

Use of Conductive Media (Electrode Interface)

Do not use alcohol-soaked pads for defibrillation—they may ignite!

Never use ultrasound gel for defibrillation.

Use of a conductive medium aids the passage of current at the interface between the defibrillator paddles/electrodes and the body surface. Types of conductive material available include gels, pastes, and prepackaged defibrillator pads. Failure to use conductive material results in very high transthoracic impedance, a lack of penetration of current, and burns to the skin surface. Use of improper pastes, creams, gels, or pads can cause burns or sparks and pose a risk of fire in an oxygen-enriched environment.[6] Use of excessive gel may result in spreading of the material across the chest wall during resuscitation, leading to arcing of the current between paddles and an insufficient delivery of current to the heart. Damp skin and air pockets beneath hand-held paddles or self-adhesive defibrillation pads increase transthoracic resistance and may cause an uneven delivery of current.[7]

Selected Energy, Number, and Time Interval of Previous Shocks

Defibrillation is the definitive treatment for pulseless VT or VF. When treating cardiac dysrhythmias using electrical therapy, selecting the appropriate energy (joules) is important. If the energy and current selected is too low, the shock delivered will not terminate the dysrhythmia. The use of excessive energy and current may induce cardiac damage.[8]

Phase of the Patient's Respiration

Inspiration increases transthoracic resistance and resistance is lowered during exhalation. Because air is a poor conductor of electricity, the greater the volume of air in the lungs when a shock is delivered, the greater the resistance to the flow of current.[9,10] Resistance may be lowest when a shock is delivered during the expiratory phase of respiration because the distance between the paddles and the heart is decreased.

Paddle Position

Location of defibrillation paddles (electrodes) affects the magnitude of the shock necessary to defibrillate the heart. Hand-held paddles or self-adhesive defibrillator pads may be placed in one of the following positions for transthoracic defibrillation:

* Sternum-apex (anterolateral) position. Place the sternum paddle to the right of the upper sternum below the clavicle. Place the other (apex) paddle to the left of the patient's left nipple with the center of the paddle in the left anterior axillary line (Figure 7-28). This paddle position is most commonly used during resuscitation because the anterior chest is usually readily accessible.

* Anteroposterior position. Place one paddle (or self-adhesive monitoring/defibrillation pad) immediately to the left of the sternum and the other on the back behind the heart (Figure 7-29).

Paddle Pressure

When using hand-held paddles for defibrillation, firm paddle-to-chest contact pressure lowers transthoracic resistance by improving contact between the skin surface and the paddles and decreasing the amount of air in the lungs. No pressure is applied when using self-adhesive monitoring/defibrillation pads. Despite the absence of pressure, these pads appear to be as effective as hand-held paddles.[11]

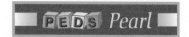
PEDS Pearl

If one of the shocks delivered successfully terminates pulseless VT/VF but the dysrhythmia recurs, begin defibrillation at the last energy level used that resulted in successful defibrillation.

Defibrillation: Indications

* Pulseless VT
* Ventricular fibrillation

Operating the Defibrillator

Before using a defibrillator, become familiar with standard defibrillator components. Locate the following:

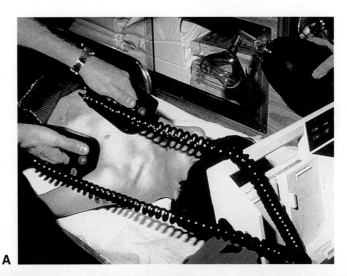

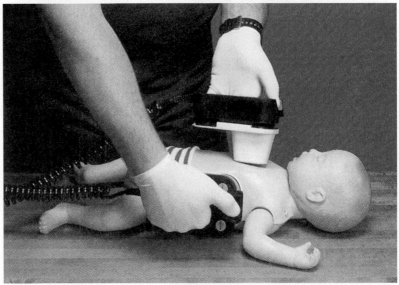

Figure 7-28 **A**, Sternum-apex (anterolateral) paddle position for a child using large (adult) paddles. **B**, Sternum-apex paddle position using infant paddles.

- On/off switch
- Energy selector
- Charge button (on paddles and/or on machine)
- Discharge buttons
- Lead-select switch
- Synchronization button
- Electrocardiogram (ECG) size (gain) control

Defibrillation Procedure

- Turn the power on to the monitor/defibrillator.
- If hand-held paddles are used, apply conductive gel to the paddles or place disposable pre-gelled defibrillator pads to the patient's bare

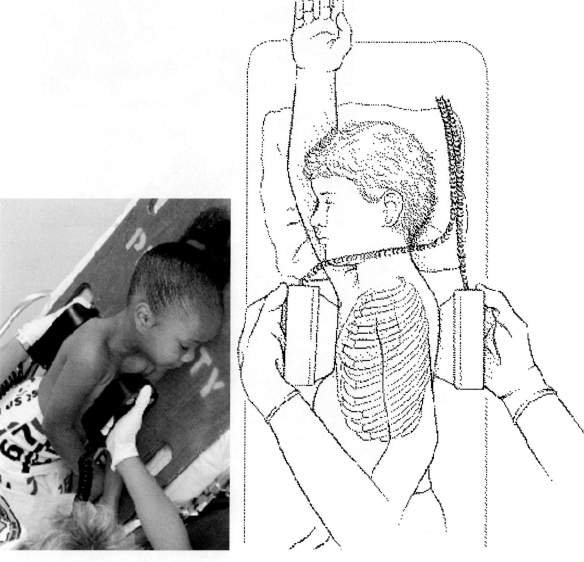

Figure 7-29 Anteroposterior paddle position.

PEDS *Pearl*

When a "flat line" is observed on an ECG:	If the rhythm appears to be asystole, confirm the rhythm in second lead
• Ensure the power to the monitor is on	because it is possible (although rare)
• Check the lead/cable connections	that coarse VF may be present in
• Ensure the correct lead is selected	some leads.
• Turn up the gain (ECG size) on the monitor	

In cardiac arrest due to pulseless VT/VF, defibrillation and CPR are more important than starting an IV, inserting an advanced airway, and giving drugs.

If the defibrillator's lowest dose exceeds the calculated dose, use the lowest dose available. When the calculated dose is between two available energy levels, choose the higher level.

If defibrillation terminates pulseless VT/VF and then recurs, begin defibrillation at the last energy setting that resulted in an ECG rhythm change.

torso. Place the defibrillator paddles on the patient's torso and apply firm pressure. If self-adhesive monitoring/defibrillation pads are used, place them in proper position on the patient's bare torso.

- Verify the presence of VT or VF on the monitor.
- While the defibrillator is readied, instruct the IV/medication team member to prepare the initial drugs that will be used and start an IV after the first shock is delivered.
- Select 2 J/kg on the defibrillator (or equivalent biphasic energy), charge the defibrillator, and recheck the ECG rhythm.
- If the rhythm is unchanged, call "Clear!" and look (360 degrees). Make sure everyone is clear of the patient, bed, and any equipment connected to the patient. As the airway team member clears the patient, he or she should be reminded to turn off the oxygen flow (oxygen flow over the patient's torso during electrical therapy increases the risk of spark/fire). If the area is clear, press the SHOCK buttons to discharge energy to the patient. After the shock has been delivered, release the buttons.
- Instruct the resuscitation team to immediately resume CPR, beginning with chest compressions. Instruct the IV/medications team member to start an IV and give a vasopressor (epinephrine). *CPR should not be interrupted to start an IV or give medications.* Give epinephrine every 3 to 5 minutes as long as the patient does not have a pulse. After 5 cycles of CPR (about 2 minutes), recheck the rhythm.
- If a shockable rhythm is present:
  - Select 4 J/kg on the defibrillator (or equivalent biphasic energy), charge the defibrillator and then call "Clear!" Check to be certain everyone is clear and the oxygen flow is off. Deliver a shock and then immediately resume CPR, starting with chest compressions. Consider giving an antiarrhythmic. Give amiodarone (or lidocaine if amiodarone is not available). Consider magnesium sulfate if the rhythm is torsades. Consider placement of an advanced airway and possible causes of the arrest. After 5 cycles of CPR (about 2 minutes), recheck the rhythm.
  - If VT/VF persists, check to make sure the oxygen flow is off, clear everyone from the patient, and then given one shock with 4 J/kg (or equivalent biphasic energy). Resume CPR, and give epinephrine.
- If a shockable rhythm is not present:
  - Check a pulse if an organized rhythm is present on the monitor. If there is an organized rhythm on the monitor and a pulse is present, check the patient's blood pressure and other vital signs and begin postresuscitation care.

◦ If there is an organized rhythm on the monitor but there is no pulse (pulseless electrical activity) or if the rhythm is asystole, resume CPR, consider possible causes of the arrest, and give medications and other emergency care as indicated.

If the patient's rhythm changes, run a rhythm strip for placement in the patient's medical record.

An **automated external defibrillator** (AED) is an external defibrillator with a computerized cardiac rhythm analysis system. The patient's cardiac rhythm is analyzed by a microprocessor in the defibrillator that uses an algorithm to distinguish rhythms that should be shocked from those that do not require defibrillation. Some AEDs require the operator to press an "analyze" control to initiate rhythm analysis whereas others automatically begin analyzing the patient's cardiac rhythm when the electrode pads are attached to the patient's chest.

Depending on the type of AED used, the AED will defibrillate or advise the operator (by means of visual and/or audible signals) to deliver a shock if a shockable rhythm is present. The shock is delivered by means of two self-adhesive monitoring/defibrillation pads applied to the patient's chest. Safety "filters" check for false signals (e.g., radio transmissions, poor electrode contact, 60-cycle interference, and loose electrodes).

Standard AEDs should be used for patients who are apneic, pulseless, and at least 8 years old (approximately 25 kg body weight or more) (Figure 7-30A). Several AED manufacturers have designed pediatric pad/cable systems for use with AEDs designed for use in adults to reduce the energy delivered to patients younger than 8 years (Figure 7-30B). Any

Automated External Defibrillation

If an AED with a special pediatric pad/cable system is not available, use a standard AED.

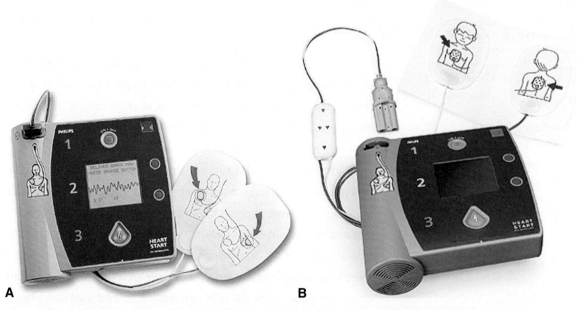

A   **B**

Figure 7-30 A, A standard automated external defibrillator (AED) should be used for patients who are apneic, pulseless, and 8 years of age or older (approximately 25 kg body weight or more). **B,** This defibrillation pad and cable system reduces the energy delivered by a standard AED to that appropriate for a child.

AED that is to be used on a patient under the age of 8 years must be approved by the Food and Drug Administration (FDA) for that age group. The FDA has given several AED manufacturers clearance to advertise, distribute, and sell this new system to physicians (or physicians' agents).

Children represent less than 10% of all resuscitation attempted outside the hospital by professional rescuers. Out-of-hospital survival from cardiac arrest in children ranges from 4% to 9%. However, the death of a child is an enormous emotional and social loss. Because of their life expectancy, the number of years of a child's life lost may rival that for all adult arrests. Two studies reported VF as the initial rhythm in 19% to 24% of out-of-hospital pediatric cardiac arrests if sudden infant death syndrome (SIDS) deaths were excluded.[12,13] In studies that included SIDS victims, however, the frequency dropped to 6% to 10%.[14,15] The rationale for exclusion of SIDS patients is that SIDS is not amenable to treatment; thus, patients with SIDS should not be included in studies that may influence potential treatment strategies for cardiac arrest.[16] Many children who survive cardiac arrest have significant neurologic problems, but when VF is promptly treated, survival rivals that of adults.[12,15]

Medical science now supports early defibrillation for children with a pediatric-ready AED. However, there is currently insufficient evidence to support a recommendation for or against the use of AEDs in children less than 1 year of age.[16] Always follow the AED manufacturer's guidelines for the application, use, and maintenance of the AED.[17]

AED Operation

- Use personal protective equipment.
- Assess responsiveness.
- Open the airway and check for breathing. If the patient is not breathing, deliver two slow breaths.
- Assess for the presence of a pulse. If the patient is pulseless, begin chest compressions and attach the AED.
- Turn the power on to the AED. Depending on the brand of AED, this is accomplished by either pressing the "on" button or lifting up the monitor screen or lid.
  - Open the package containing the self-adhesive monitoring/defibrillation pads. Connect the pads to the AED cables (if not preconnected), and then apply the pads to the patient's torso in the locations specified by the AED manufacturer. Momentarily stop CPR to allow placement of the pads.
  - Some models require connection of the AED cable to the AED before use.
- Analyze the ECG rhythm.
  - AEDs take multiple "looks" at the patient's rhythm—each lasting a

few seconds. If several "looks" confirm the presence of a shockable rhythm, the AED will signal that a shock is indicated.

○ Artifact due to motion or 60-cycle interference may simulate VF and interfere with accurate rhythm analysis. While the AED is analyzing the patient's cardiac rhythm, all movement (including chest compressions, artificial ventilations, and the movement associated with patient transport) must cease.

• Clear the area surrounding the patient. Be sure to look around you.

○ Ensure everyone is clear of the patient, bed, and any equipment connected to the patient.

○ Ensure oxygen is not flowing over the patient's torso (increases risk of spark/fire).

• If the area is clear, press the shock control to deliver the shock. After delivering the shock, immediately resume CPR, beginning with chest compressions.

AED: Advantages

• Voice prompts the user
• Easy to learn; memorizing treatment protocol is easier than recalling the steps of CPR
• Less training required to operate and maintain skills than conventional defibrillators
• Promotes rescuer safety by permitting remote, "hands-free" defibrillation

AEDs: Special Considerations

• If the patient is lying in water or on a wet surface, remove the patient from contact with the water and quickly dry the patient's torso before attaching the AED.
• If the patient is lying on a metal surface, remove the patient from contact with the metal surface before attaching the AED.

Description and Purpose

Synchronized cardioversion is the delivery of a shock to the heart to terminate a rapid dysrhythmia that is timed to avoid the vulnerable period during the cardiac cycle. On the ECG, this period occurs during the peak of the T wave to approximately the end of the T wave. When the "sync" control is pressed, the machine searches for the highest (R wave deflection) or deepest (QS deflection) part of the QRS complex. When a QRS complex is detected, the monitor places a "flag" or "sync marker" on that complex that may appear as an oval, square, line, or highlighted triangle on the ECG display, depending on the monitor used. When the shock controls are pressed while the defibrillator is charged in "sync" mode, the machine will discharge energy only if both discharge buttons are pushed

Depending on the manufacturer and battery condition, the time required for charging of the AEDs capacitors is approximately 10 to 30 seconds.

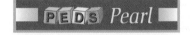

Both monophasic and biphasic AEDs are currently available. Depending on the manufacturer, biphasic waveform AEDs may deliver nonescalating shocks.

Synchronized Cardioversion

When discussing synchronized cardioversion, the QRS complex is often simply referred to as the "R wave."

and the monitor tells the defibrillator that a QRS complex has been detected.

Indications

Synchronized cardioversion may be used to treat the "sick" (unstable) patient in SVT, atrial flutter with a rapid ventricular response, or VT with a pulse. Signs of hemodynamic compromise include poor perfusion, hypotension, or heart failure. This procedure may also be performed electively in a child with stable SVT or VT at the direction of a pediatric cardiologist.

Procedure

- If the patient is awake and time permits, administer sedation unless contraindicated.

Place ECG electrodes away from defibrillator paddle sites.

- Turn the monitor/defibrillator on.
- Attach ECG electrodes to monitor the patient's ECG.
  - Some devices allow monitoring and synchronized cardioversion via disposable self-adhesive monitoring/defibrillation pads. In this case, additional ECG electrodes are not necessary.
  - If self-adhesive monitoring/defibrillation pads are to be used, place them in proper position on the patient's bare torso.

Hand-held paddles should not be used to monitor the ECG during this procedure because artifact caused by paddle movement on the chest may be mistakenly identified by the monitor as an R wave.

- Select a lead with an optimum QRS complex amplitude (positive or negative) and no artifact, or if monitoring through disposable defibrillation electrodes, select the "paddles" lead. Run an ECG strip to document the patient's rhythm.
- Press the "sync" control on the defibrillator. Verify the machine is "marking" or "flagging" each QRS complex. If sync markers do not appear, or appear elsewhere on the ECG display, adjust the gain (ECG size) until the markers occur within each QRS complex. If adjusting the gain does not result in sync markers within each QRS complex, select another lead or reposition the ECG electrodes.
- If hand-held paddles are used, apply conductive gel to the paddles or place disposable pre-gelled defibrillator pads to the patient's bare torso. Place the defibrillator paddles on the patient's torso and apply firm pressure.
- Ensure the machine is in "sync" mode, select 0.5 to 1 J/kg on the defibrillator (or equivalent biphasic energy), charge the defibrillator, and recheck the ECG rhythm. If the rhythm is unchanged, call "clear!" and look (360 degrees).
  - Ensure everyone is clear of the patient, bed, and any equipment connected to the patient.
  - Ensure oxygen is not flowing over the patient's torso.
- If the area is clear, press and hold both discharge buttons simultaneously until the shock is delivered. There may be a slight delay while the machine detects the next QRS complex. Release the shock controls after the shock has been delivered.

- Reassess the ECG rhythm. If the tachycardia persists, ensure the machine is in sync mode before delivering another shock. The energy dose may be increased to 2 J/kg for the second and subsequent attempts if necessary.
- If VF occurs during the course of synchronization, check the patient's pulse and rhythm (verify all electrodes and cable connections are secure), turn off the sync control, and defibrillate.

Defibrillation and Synchronized Cardioversion: Special Considerations

- Keep monitoring electrodes and wires away from the area where defibrillator pads or self-adhesive monitoring/defibrillation pads will be placed. Contact may cause electrical arcing and patient skin burns during defibrillation.
- Remove transdermal patches, bandages, necklaces, or other materials from the sites used for paddle placement—do not attempt to defibrillate through them.
- Wipe the area clean where defibrillator pads or self-adhesive monitoring/defibrillation pads will be placed—do not use alcohol or alcohol-based cleansers.
- Correct hypoxemia, acidosis, hypoglycemia, or hypothermia if the patient does not respond to cardioversion.

Defibrillation and Synchronized Cardioversion: Possible Complications

- Skin burns due to lack of conductive medium, gel "bridging" (i.e., the gel forms a "bridge" on the skin), risk of fire from combination of electrical and oxygen sources
- Myocardial damage/dysfunction
- Dysrhythmias including asystole, atrioventricular (AV) block, bradycardia, or VF following cardioversion
- Injury to the operator and/or team members if improper technique used

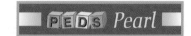

PEDS Pearl

Some defibrillators revert to the defibrillation mode after the delivery of a synchronized shock to allow immediate defibrillation in case synchronized cardioversion produces VF. Other defibrillators remain in the synchronized mode after a synchronized shock. If VF occurs when using this type of defibrillator, ensure the sync button is off before attempting to defibrillate.

Transcutaneous Pacing

Transcutaneous pacing (TCP) is the use of electrical stimulation through pacing pads positioned on a patient's torso to stimulate contraction of the heart. Most transcutaneous pacemakers provide an output current of 0 to 200 milliamperes (mA) and have a heart rate selection that ranges from 30 to 180 beats per minute.

TCP requires the use of two pacing electrodes that are attached to the patient's chest. Small or medium pediatric electrodes should be used for a child weighing less than 15 kg. Adult electrodes should be used for a child weighing more than 15 kg.

Indications

TCP may be used for the patient with profound symptomatic bradycardia refractory to basic and advanced life support therapy.

Procedure

Do not place the pads over open cuts, sores, or metal objects.

Pacer pad positioning varies by manufacturer. Follow the manufacturer's recommendations for proper pacer pad placement.

Sedation or analgesia may be needed to minimize the discomfort associated with this procedure.

Mechanical capture occurs when pacing produces a measurable hemodynamic response (e.g., palpable pulse, measurable blood pressure).

- Position the pacing pads so that current passes from the negative pacing pad through the heart to the positive pad.
  - ○ Place the negative (anterior) pad on the anterior chest over the heart. Place the positive (posterior) pad on the patient's back, behind the heart (Figure 7-31).
  - ○ If the posterior pad cannot be placed on the patient's back, the anterior-lateral position may be used. Place the negative pacing pad on the left side of the patient's chest over the fourth intercostal space in the midaxillary line and the positive pad on the anterior chest under the right clavicle (Figure 7-32).
- Connect the patient to an ECG monitor and obtain a rhythm strip. Connect the pacing cable to the pacemaker and to the adhesive electrodes on the patient.
- Turn the power on to the pacemaker and set the pacing rate to the desired number of paced pulses per minute (ppm). Set the initial pacing rate at 100. After the rate has been regulated, start the pacemaker (Figure 7-33).
  - ○ Increase the stimulating current (output or milliamperes [mA]) until pacer spikes are visible before each QRS complex.
  - ○ Observe the cardiac monitor for electrical capture (usually evidenced by a wide QRS and broad T wave). Evaluate mechanical capture by assessing the patient's femoral pulse.
  - ○ Once capture is achieved, continue pacing at an output level slightly higher (approximately 2 mA) than the threshold of initial electrical capture.
- Assess the patient's blood pressure, SpO_2, and level of responsiveness. Monitor the patient closely, including assessment of the skin for irritation where the pacing pads have been applied. Document and record the ECG rhythm.

Complications

- Skin burns.
- Interference with sensing due to patient agitation or muscle contractions.
- Pain from electrical stimulation of the skin and muscles.
- Tissue damage, including third-degree burns, has been reported in pediatric patients with improper or prolonged TCP.

Contraindications

- Major chest trauma that precludes placement of the pacing pads

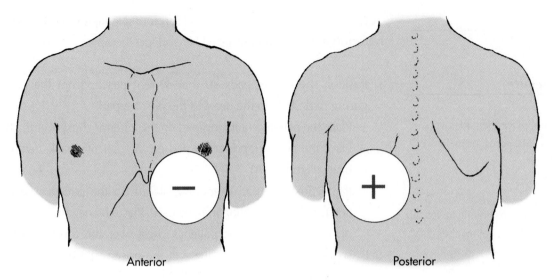

Anterior   Posterior

Figure 7-31   Anteroposterior positioning of transcutaneous electrodes.

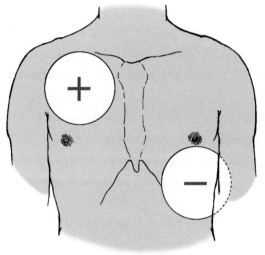

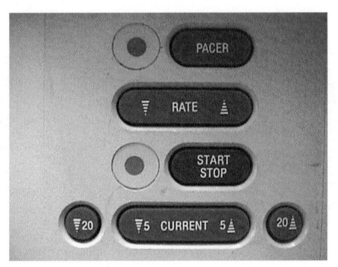

Figure 7-32   Anterolateral positioning of transcutaneous electrodes.

Figure 7-33   Transcutaneous pacemaker controls.

PEDS Pearl

Documentation should include the date and time pacing was initiated (including baseline and pacing rhythm strips), the current required to obtain capture, the pacing rate selected, the patient's responses to electrical and mechanical capture, medications administered during the procedure, and the date and time pacing was terminated.

TABLE 7-2 *Electrical Therapy—Summary*

Intervention	Dysrhythmia	Recommended Energy Levels
Defibrillation	Pulseless VT/VF	2 J/kg to 4 J/kg (or equivalent biphasic energy)
Synchronized cardioversion	SVT Atrial flutter with a rapid ventricular response VT with a pulse	0.5 to 1 J/kg (or equivalent biphasic energy)
Transcutaneous pacing	Severe bradycardia (e.g., complete AV block)	Set initial rate at 100 pulses/min Increase the output (mA) until pacer spikes are visible before each QRS complex. Verify capture. The final mA setting should be slightly above where capture is obtained to help prevent the loss of capture.

AV, atrioventricular; SVT, supraventricular tachycardia; VF, ventricular fibrillation; VT, ventricular tachycardia.

Vagal Maneuvers

Vagal maneuvers are methods used to stimulate baroreceptors located in the internal carotid arteries and the aortic arch. Stimulation of these receptors results in reflex stimulation of the vagus nerve and release of acetylcholine. Acetylcholine slows conduction through the AV node, resulting in slowing of the heart rate.

Indications

Vagal maneuvers may be tried in the stable but symptomatic child in SVT or during preparation for cardioversion or drug therapy for this dysrhythmia. Success rates with vagal maneuvers vary and depend on the patient's age, level of cooperation, and the presence of underlying conditions.

Techniques

Vagal maneuvers that may be used in the pediatric patient include the following:

- Application of a cold stimulus to the face (e.g., a washcloth soaked in iced water, cold pack, or crushed ice mixed with water in a plastic bag or glove) for up to 10 seconds. This technique is often effective in infants and young children. When using this method, do not obstruct the patient's mouth or nose or apply pressure to the eyes.
- Valsalva maneuver. Instruct the child to blow through a straw or take a deep breath and bear down as if having a bowel movement for 10 seconds. This strains the abdominal muscles and increases intrathoracic

pressure. In the younger child, abdominal palpation may be used to create the same effect. Abdominal palpation causes the child to bear down in an attempt to resist the pressure.

- Gagging. Use a tongue depressor or culturette swab to briefly touch the posterior oropharynx.

When using vagal maneuvers, keep the following points in mind: **Special Considerations**

- Ensure oxygen, suction, a defibrillator, and crash cart are available before attempting the procedure.
- Obtain a 12-lead ECG before and after the vagal maneuver.
- Continuous monitoring of the patient's ECG is essential. Note the onset and end of the vagal maneuver on the ECG rhythm strip.
- In general, a vagal maneuver should not be continued for more than 10 seconds.
- Application of external ocular pressure may be dangerous and should not be used because of the risk of retinal detachment.
- Carotid massage is less effective in children than in adults and is not recommended.

Hemodynamically unstable tachycardia when immediate synchronized cardioversion is imperative.   **Contraindications**

- Syncope   **Complications**
- Bradydysrhythmias (e.g., sinus arrest, AV block, asystole)
- Ventricular dysrhythmias

Case Study Resolution

Continue CPR. Confirm the rhythm in a second lead. Attempt tracheal intubation. Confirm the position of the tracheal tube position with primary (assessment) and secondary (mechanical) techniques. Establish vascular access and give epinephrine. Provide further interventions on the basis of the child's response to therapy.

References

1. *CPR Pro for the Professional Rescuer.* Holiday, FL: National Instructor's Resource Center, 2003: 18.

2. Terry J, Baranowski L, Lonsway RA, et al. *Intravenous therapy: clinical principles and practice.* Philadelphia: WB Saunders, 1995.

3. Schneider T, Martens PR, Paschen H, et al. Multicenter, randomized, controlled trial of 150-J biphasic shocks compared with 200- to 360-J monophasic shocks in the resuscitation of out-of-hospital cardiac arrest victims. *Circulation* 2000;102:1780–1787.

4. Gliner BE, Jorgenson DB, Poole JE, et al. Treatment of out-of-hospital cardiac arrest with a low-energy impedance-compensating biphasic waveform automatic external defibrillator: the LIFE Investigators. *Biomed Instrum Technol* 1998;32:631–644.

5. Atkins DL, Kerber RE. Pediatric defibrillation: current flow is improved by using "adult" electrode paddles. *Pediatrics* 1994;94:90–93.

6. Hummell RS, Ornato JP, Wienberg SM, et al. Spark-generating properties of electrode gels used during defibrillation: a potential fire hazard. *JAMA* 1988;260:3021–3024.

7. Crockett PJ, Droppert BM, Higgins SE, et al. *Defibrillation: what you should know.* Redmond, WA: PhysioControl Corporation, 1996.

8. Kerber RE. Transthoracic cardioversion of atrial fibrillation and flutter: standard techniques and new advances. *Am J Cardiol* 1996;78:22–26.

9. Ewy GA, Hellman DA, McClung S, et al. Influence of ventilation phase on transthoracic impedance and defibrillation effectiveness. *Crit Care Med* 1980;8:164–166.

10. Sirna SJ, Ferguson DW, Charbonnier F, et al. Factors affecting transthoracic impedance during electrical cardioversion. *Am J Cardiol* 1988;62:1048–1052.

11. Stults KR, Brown DD, Cooley F, et al. Self-adhesive monitor/defibrillation pads improve prehospital defibrillation success. *Ann Emerg Med* 1987;16:872–877.

12. Mogayzel C, Quan L, Graves JR, et al. Out-of-hospital ventricular fibrillation in children and adolescents: causes and outcomes. *Ann Emerg Med* 1995;25:484–491.

13. Hickey RW, Cohen DM, Strausbaugh S, et al. Pediatric patients requiring CPR in the prehospital setting. *Ann Emerg Med* 1995;25:495–501.

14. Eisenberg M, Bergner L, Hallstrom A. Epidemiology of cardiac arrest and resuscitation in children. *Ann Emerg Med* 1983;12:672–674.

15. Sirbaugh PE, Pepe PE, Shook JE, et al. A prospective, population-based study of the demographics, epidemiology, management, and outcome of out-of-hospital pediatric cardiopulmonary arrest. *Ann Emerg Med* 1999;33:174–184.

16. Samson RA, Berg RA, Bingham R, Pediatric Advanced Life Support Task Force, International Liaison Committee on Resuscitation for the American Heart Association; European Resuscitation Council. Use of automated external defibrillators for children: an update—an advisory statement from the Pediatric Advanced Life Support Task Force, International Liaison Committee on Resuscitation. *Pediatrics* 2003;112[Pt 1]:163–168.

17. *The Use of AEDs for Children. CPR Pro for the Professional Rescuer.* Holiday, FL: National Instructor's Resource Center, 2003: 20.

18. Stanley R. Intraosseous infusion. In: Roberts JR, Hedges JR, eds. *Clinical procedures in emergency medicine,* 4th ed. New York: Elsevier, 2004:475–484.

Chapter Quiz

Questions 1 – 12 refer to the following scenario.

A 6-year-old boy is complaining of stomach pain. The child's father says his son has had frequent vomiting and diarrhea for the past 72 hours. He is seeking medical care because his son vomited immediately on awakening this morning and then had diarrhea. Dad put his son in the shower to wash him and his son "collapsed" for about 10 to 15 seconds. You observe the child sitting in a chair with his hand over his stomach. He appears uncomfortable and restless, but is aware of your presence. The child has listened intently to the conversation between you and his father. His face and lips appear pale. Some mottling of the extremities is present. His breathing is unlabored at a rate that appears normal for his age.

1. Which of the following statements is true of your interactions with a child of this age?
   A) Speak to the child in a respectful, friendly manner, as if speaking to an adult.
   B) When speaking with the caregiver, include the child.
   C) Avoid frightening or misleading terms such as shot, deaden, germs, etc.
   D) Establish a contract with the child—tell him that if he does not cooperate with you, you are certain he will have to have surgery.

2. From the information provided, complete the following documentation regarding the Pediatric Assessment Triangle.
   Appearance:
   Breathing:
   Circulation:

Your initial assessment reveals a patent airway. The child's respiratory rate is 20/min. Auscultation of the chest reveals clear breath sounds bilaterally. A radial pulse is easily palpated at a rate of 157 beats/min. The skin is pale and dry. The child's capillary refill is 3 seconds, temperature is 99.4°F, and his blood pressure is 82/56.

3. The normal heart rate range for a 6-year-old child at rest is _____ beats/min.
    A) 60 to 100
    B) 70 to 120
    C) 80 to 140
    D) 90 to 150

4. You have applied the cardiac monitor and observe the ECG shown below.

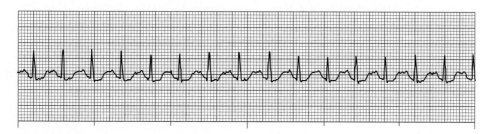

    This rhythm is:
    A) Atrial flutter.
    B) Supraventricular tachycardia.
    C) Sinus tachycardia.
    D) Ventricular tachycardia.

5. Assessment of the child's skin turgor reveals an elapsed time of 4½ seconds for the skin to return to normal. You estimate the child's degree of dehydration to be:
    A) < 5% of the child's body weight.
    B) 5 to 8% of the child's body weight.
    C) 9 to 10% of the child's body weight.
    D) > 10% of the child's body weight.

6. The lower limit of a normal systolic blood pressure for a child of this age is:
    A) About 60 mm Hg.
    B) About 70 mm Hg.
    C) About 80 mm Hg.
    D) About 90 mm Hg.

7. This child's history and presentation is consistent with:
    A) Compensated hypovolemic shock.
    B) Irreversible cardiogenic shock.
    C) Decompensated anaphylactic shock.
    D) Preterminal distributive shock.

8. Select the **incorrect** statement:
   A) Hypotension is an early sign of shock in a child.
   B) The diastolic blood pressure is usually two-thirds of the systolic pressure.
   C) A child may be in shock despite a normal blood pressure.
   D) Blood pressure is one of the least sensitive indicators of adequate circulation in children.

9. The presence of compensated shock can be identified by:
   A) Assessment of heart rate, ECG rhythm, and skin temperature.
   B) Assessment of the presence and strength of peripheral pulses, mental status, and pupil response to light.
   C) Assessment of heart rate, presence and strength of peripheral pulses, and the adequacy of end-organ perfusion.
   D) Assessment of end-organ perfusion, ECG rhythm, and pupil response to light.

10. Which of the following methods of vascular access should be attempted first in this child?
    A) Establish an intraosseous infusion.
    B) Establish an internal jugular intravenous (IV) line.
    C) Establish an IV using the saphenous vein.
    D) Establish an IV in the antecubital fossa.

11. True or False: As you prepare to establish vascular access, the child becomes uncooperative. A reasonable approach in this situation would be to ask the child's father to assist in restraining his son in order to accomplish the procedure as quickly as possible.

12. Vascular access has been successfully established. You should begin volume resuscitation with a fluid bolus of:
    A) 10 mL/kg.
    B) 20 mL/kg.
    C) 30 mL/kg.
    D) 50 mL/kg.

Questions 13 – 19 refer to the following scenario.

A 2-year-old near-drowning victim is apneic and pulseless. CPR is in progress.

13. The cardiac monitor reveals the rhythm below.

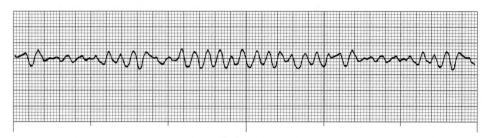

This rhythm is:

A) Ventricular tachycardia.

B) Atrial fibrillation.

C) Ventricular fibrillation.

D) Asystole.

14. CPR is in progress. Your next intervention should be to:

A) Establish vascular access, insert a tracheal tube, and then perform synchronized cardioversion followed by immediate defibrillation.

B) Insert a tracheal tube, establish vascular access, and then prepare to defibrillate.

C) Perform synchronized cardioversion followed by immediate defibrillation.

D) Prepare to defibrillate.

15. The initial energy dose used for defibrillation should be:

A) 0.5 joule/kg.

B) 1.0 joule/kg.

C) 2.0 joules/kg.

D) 4.0 joules/kg.

16. After delivery of the shock, you should:

A) Attempt a vagal maneuver.

B) Establish vascular access.

C) Attempt transcutaneous pacing.

D) Resume CPR immediately, starting with chest compressions.

17. An endotracheal tube has been inserted. To confirm proper positioning of the tube, you should first listen:

A) Over the epigastrium.

B) Over the posterior chest.

C) Over the left lateral chest in the axilla.

D) Over the right lateral chest in the axilla.

18. Attempts to establish vascular access have been unsuccessful. Proper positioning of the tracheal tube has been confirmed. You should now administer _____ via the tracheal tube.
    A) 1 mg/kg of lidocaine
    B) 0.02 mg/kg of atropine
    C) 0.1 mg/kg of epinephrine (1:1000 solution)
    D) 1.0 mg/kg of epinephrine (1:10,000 solution)

19. A 6-year-old is found unresponsive, not breathing, and pulseless. A standard AED can be used if an AED with a pediatric pad/cable system is not available.
    A) True
    B) False

Chapter Quiz Answers

1. B. When the patient is a school-age child (6 to 12 years of age), include the child when speaking with the caregiver. If the patient is an adolescent, speak to him in a respectful, friendly manner, as if speaking to an adult. Although it is reasonable to make a contract with a child of this age ("I promise to tell you everything I am going to do if you will help me by cooperating"), it is inappropriate and unprofessional to threaten him.

2. Pediatric Assessment Triangle (first impression) findings:
   Appearance: Awake and restless; aware of surroundings; listening intently
   Breathing: Respirations appear normal for age; normal respiratory effort
   Circulation: Pale face and lips. Some mottling of the extremities is present.

3. B. The normal heart rate for a 6 to 12 year old at rest is 70 to 120 beats/min.

4. C. The rhythm shown is sinus tachycardia at 157 beats/min.

5. D. When evaluating skin turgor to estimate dehydration, if it takes < 2 seconds for the skin to return to normal, suspect the approximate degree of dehydration to be $< 5\%$ of the child's body weight; 2–3 seconds $= 5$ to 8% of the child's body weight; 3–4 seconds $= 9$ to 10% of the child's body weight; and > 4 seconds $= > 10\%$ of the child's body weight.

6. C. The lower limit of a normal systolic blood pressure for a child between 1 and 10 years of age can be estimated using the formula $70 + (2 \times \text{age in years})$. This child's minimum systolic blood pressure should be about 82 mm Hg.

7. A. This child's history and presentation is consistent with compensated hypovolemic shock.

8. A. Hypotension is a late sign of shock in a child. Tachycardia and signs of poor perfusion such as pale, cool, mottled skin occur earlier and are more reliable indicators than hypotension.

9. C. The presence of compensated shock can be identified by evaluation of heart rate, the presence and volume (strength) of peripheral pulses, and the adequacy of end-organ perfusion. (Brain—assess mental status; skin—assess capillary refill and skin temperature; and kidneys—assess urine output.)

10. D. In this situation, you should first attempt to establish a peripheral IV line in the antecubital fossa. If the child was in decompensated shock or cardiac arrest, intraosseous access could be attempted if IV access was not rapidly achieved.

11. False. Because a child expects his or her caregiver to protect them, do not ask a caregiver to restrain a child or participate in any way other than to comfort the child.

12. B. Administer a bolus of 20 mL/kg of isotonic crystalloid solution (NS or LR) over 5 to 20 minutes. Assess response (i.e., mental status, capillary refill, heart rate, respiratory effort, blood pressure).

13. C. The rhythm shown is ventricular fibrillation.

14. D. Defibrillation is the definitive treatment for pulseless VT/VF. Defibrillation takes priority over establishing vascular access and placement of a tracheal tube. Synchronized cardioversion is used to shock hemodynamically compromising tachycardias with a pulse.

15. C. The initial energy dose used to defibrillate pulseless VT/VF is 2 J/kg.

16. D. After delivery of a shock, immediately resume CPR, starting with chest compressions. A vagal maneuver may be tried in the stable but symptomatic child in supraventricular tachycardia or during preparation for cardioversion or drug therapy for SVT. Transcutaneous pacing may be used for the patient with profound symptomatic bradycardia refractory to basic and advanced life support therapy.

17. A. To confirm proper positioning of the tube, listen first over the epigastrium. The presence of bubbling or gurgling sounds during auscultation of the epigastrium suggests the tube is incorrectly positioned in the esophagus. To correct this problem, deflate the tracheal tube cuff (if a cuffed tube was used), remove the tube, and preoxygenate before reattempting intubation. In infants, breath sounds may be heard over the stomach but should not be louder than midaxillary sounds.

18. C. If vascular access is unavailable, epinephrine may be administered via the tracheal tube. The tracheal dose is 0.1 mg/kg (1:1000 solution) or 0.1 mL/kg (10 times the IV/IO dose).

19. A. If an AED with a pediatric pad/cable system is not available, a standard AED may be used.

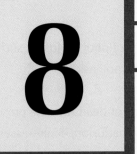

8 Fluids and Medications

Case Study

An 11-year-old boy presents with shoulder pain. The child's wrestling coach states the boy was taken down hard by his opponent in a wrestling match and complained of a sudden, severe pain in his right shoulder. Your first impression reveals the boy is awake and alert. He is holding his right extremity close to his chest. There is no evidence of respiratory distress. His skin is pink. Deformity of the right shoulder is visible.

How will you assess the intensity of this child's pain?

Objectives

1. Define the following terms: *chronotrope, dromotrope, inotrope, pain, sedation, analgesia, amnesia,* and *anesthesia.*
2. Identify the primary neurotransmitter for the sympathetic and parasympathetic divisions of the autonomic nervous system (ANS).
3. Describe the location and effects of stimulation of α-, β-, and dopaminergic receptors.
4. Describe advantages and disadvantages associated with pediatric medication administration routes.
5. Describe two tools that may be used to assess pain in the pediatric patient.
6. Explain the importance of pain management.
7. Describe techniques for nonpharmacologic management of pain in infants and children.
8. Discuss common pharmacologic agents used in pain management and sedation.
9. Describe the levels of sedation/analgesia.
10. Explain the preprocedural, procedural, and postprocedural care of patients who receive sedation/analgesia.
11. Identify factors that may increase the risk of complications during sedation/analgesia.
12. Explain the importance of postsedation monitoring.

Pharmacology Review

Review of the Autonomic Nervous System

The ANS consists of sympathetic and parasympathetic divisions. The sympathetic division mobilizes the body, allowing the body to function under stress ("fight or flight" response). The parasympathetic division is responsible for the conservation and restoration of body resources ("feed and breed" or "resting and digesting" response) (Table 8-1).

Baroreceptors

Baroreceptors (pressoreceptors) are specialized nerve tissues (sensors) located in the internal carotid arteries and the aortic arch. These sensory receptors detect changes in blood pressure and cause a reflex response in either the sympathetic or the parasympathetic division of the ANS (Figure 8-1).

Chemoreceptors

Chemoreceptors in the internal carotid arteries and aortic arch detect changes in the concentration of hydrogen ions (pH), oxygen, and carbon dioxide in the blood. The response to these changes by the ANS can be sympathetic or parasympathetic. Decreased pH or oxygen levels in the blood or increases in carbon dioxide levels cause a sympathetic response, resulting in increased heart rate, contractility, and vasoconstriction.[1] Increased pH or decreased carbon dioxide levels in the blood cause a decrease in vasoconstrictor effects, leading to a general vasodilatory effect.

Parasympathetic Stimulation

Acetylcholine, a **neurotransmitter**, is released when parasympathetic

TABLE 8-1 *Overview of the Divisions of the Autonomic Nervous System*

	Sympathetic Division	Parasympathetic Division
	"Fight or flight" response Mobilizes the body Allows the body to function under stress	"Feed and breed" or "resting and digesting" response Conservation of body resources Restoration of body resources
Neurotransmitter	Norepinephrine	Acetylcholine
Synonymous terms	Adrenergic, sympathomimetic, catecholamine, anticholinergic, parasympatholytic, cholinergic blocker	Cholinergic, parasympathomimetic, sympathetic blocker, cholinomimetic, sympatholytic, adrenergic blocker
Opposite terms	Sympatholytic, antiadrenergic, sympathetic blocker, adrenergic blocker	Parasympatholytic, anticholinergic, cholinergic blocker, vagolytic

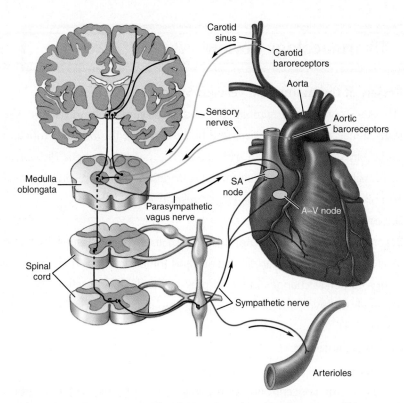

Figure 8-1   **Baroreceptor reflex.** Baroreceptors keep blood pressure within normal limits. The reflex consists of baroreceptors (aortic arch and carotid sinuses); nerves that carry sensory information to the brain; the medulla in the brain, which evaluates the information; and the nerves of the autonomic nervous system (sympathetic and parasympathetic), which carry the decision from the medulla to the heart and blood vessels.

(cholinergic) nerve fibers are stimulated. Acetylcholine binds to parasympathetic receptors. The two main types of cholinergic receptors are nicotinic and muscarinic receptors. Nicotinic receptors are located in skeletal muscle. Muscarinic receptors are located in smooth muscle.

Parasympathetic stimulation slows the rate of discharge of the sinoatrial (SA) node, slows conduction through the atrioventricular (AV) node, decreases the strength of atrial contraction, and can cause a small decrease in the force of ventricular contraction. (There is little effect on the strength of ventricular contraction because of minimal parasympathetic innervation of these chambers.) The net effect of parasympathetic stimulation is slowing of the heart rate.

Sympathetic Stimulation

Activation of the sympathetic division of the ANS results in the following:

- Increased blood flow to skeletal muscle.
- Release of glucose from the liver to ensure an adequate supply of oxygen and nutrients during a time of mental or physical stress.
- Narrowing of **splanchnic** (internal organ) blood vessels diverts blood into vascular beds in muscles.

Parasympathetic stimulation often involves a response by only one organ.

The effects of sympathetic stimulation are often widespread, affecting many organs.

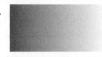

TABLE 8-2 *Organ Responses to Sympathetic and Parasympathetic Stimulation*

	Sympathetic	Parasympathetic
Eyes	Pupillary dilation	Accommodation for near vision
Saliva	Decreased secretions; viscous	Increased secretions; watery
Bronchial smooth muscle	Dilation	Constriction, increased secretion
Heart	Increased rate and force of contraction (β-receptors)	Decreased rate Minimal effect on force of contraction
Liver	Glucose release (β-receptors)	No effect
Gastrointestinal tract	Decreased peristalsis (β-receptors) Sphincter constriction (α-receptors) Decreased blood flow	Increased peristalsis Sphincter relaxation Increased secretion
Bladder	Relaxation (β-receptors) Sphincter constriction (α-receptors)	Contraction Relaxation
Sweat glands	Increased	No effect
Smooth muscle of blood vessels		
Abdominal	Constriction (α-receptors)	No effect
Coronary	Constriction (α-receptors) Dilation (β-receptors)	Dilation
Skeletal muscle	Dilation (β-receptors)	No effect
Skin	Constriction (α-receptors)	No effect

- In the lungs, smooth muscles of the bronchi dilate, allowing an increase in the uptake of alveolar oxygen and tidal volume.
- In the heart, sympathetic (accelerator) nerve fibers supply the SA node, AV node, atrial muscle, and ventricular myocardium.

Table 8-2 shows organ responses to sympathetic and parasympathetic stimulation.

Stimulation of sympathetic nerve fibers results in the release of norepinephrine. Norepinephrine binds to receptor sites located in the plasma membrane of cells. Sympathetic (adrenergic) receptor sites are divided into α-, β-, and dopaminergic receptors (Table 8-3).

Dopaminergic receptor sites are located in the coronary arteries, renal, mesenteric, and visceral blood vessels. Stimulation of dopaminergic receptor sites results in dilation.

Different body tissues have different proportions of α- and β-receptors. In general, α-receptors are more sensitive to norepinephrine and β-receptors are more sensitive to epinephrine. Stimulation of α-receptor sites results in constriction of blood vessels in the skin, cerebral, and splanchnic circulation.

Remember: β_1-receptors affect the heart (you have one heart); β_2-receptors affect the lungs (you have two lungs).

β-receptor sites are divided into β_1- and β_2. β_1-receptors are found in the heart. Stimulation of β_1-receptors results in an increased heart rate, contractility, and, ultimately, irritability of cardiac cells. β_2-receptor sites

TABLE 8-3 *Sympathetic (Adrenergic) Receptors*

	α_1	α_1	β_1	β_2	Dopaminergic
Location	Vascular smooth muscle	Skeletal blood vessels	Myocardium	Predominantly in bronchiolar and arterial smooth muscle	Coronary arteries, renal, mesenteric, and visceral blood vessels
Effects of Stimulation	Vasoconstriction ↑ peripheral vascular resistance	Inhibits norepinephrine release	↑ heart rate ↑ myocardial contractility ↑ oxygen consumption	Relaxation of bronchial smooth muscle; arteriolar dilation	Dilation

---

Important Terms to Remember

A chronotrope is a substance that affects heart rate.
- Positive chronotrope = ↑ heart rate
- Negative chronotrope = ↓ heart rate

An inotrope is a substance that affects myocardial contractility.
- Positive inotrope = ↑ force of contraction
- Negative inotrope = ↓ force of contraction

A dromotrope is a substance that affects AV conduction velocity.
- Positive dromotrope = ↑ AV conduction velocity
- Negative dromotrope = ↓ AV conduction velocity

---

are found in the lungs and skeletal muscle blood vessels. Stimulation of these receptor sites results in dilation of the smooth muscle of the bronchi and blood vessel dilation. Smooth muscle is located in the walls of many hollow organs including organs of the digestive, urinary, and reproductive tracts. Smooth muscle is also found in blood vessels, the bronchi, the hair follicles, and the iris and ciliary muscles of the eye.

Volume Expansion

TABLE 8-4 *Volume Expansion—Summary*

	Crystalloid Solutions
Description	Isotonic solutions that provide transient expansion of the intravascular volume
Examples	Normal saline—contains sodium chloride in water Ringer's lactate—contains sodium chloride, potassium chloride, calcium chloride, and sodium lactate in water
Advantages	Inexpensive, readily available, free from allergic reactions
Disadvantages	Effectively expand the interstitial space and correct sodium deficits but do not effectively expand the intravascular volume because approximately three fourths of the infused crystalloid solution will leave the vascular space in about 1 h.
	Colloid Solutions
Description	Contain molecules (typically proteins) that are too large to pass out of the capillary membranes. As a result, they remain in the vascular compartment and draw fluid from the interstitial and intracellular compartments into the vascular compartment to expand the intravascular volume.
Examples	5% albumin, fresh-frozen plasma; synthetic colloids include hetastarch and Dextran
Advantages	More efficient than crystalloid solutions in rapidly expanding the intravascular compartment; remain in the intravascular space for h.
Disadvantages	Expensive, short shelf-life, potential for adverse reactions; can produce dramatic fluid shifts
	Blood
Indications	Correction of a deficiency or functional defect of a blood component that has caused a clinically significant problem; severe acute hemorrhage
Notes	Red blood cells are the most frequently transfused blood component. They are given to increase the oxygen-carrying capacity of the blood and to maintain satisfactory tissue oxygenation. If blood is administered, it should be warmed before transfusion; otherwise, rapid administration may result in significant hypothermia.

Medication Administration

Although the terms *drug* and *medication* are often used interchangeably, a **drug** is any chemical compound that produces an effect on a living organism. **Medication** refers to drugs used in the practice of medicine as a remedy.

A drug is administered to create a desired effect (therapeutic effect) at a target organ or tissue. All drugs undergo the following processes from the time it is administered until it produces an effect:

- Entry into the body and then the bloodstream (absorption)
- Movement through the bloodstream to the target organ (distribution)
- Production of a drug effect
- Chemical breakdown (metabolism)
- Removal from the body (elimination)

Administering medications to the pediatric patient is challenging because of changes that occur from birth through adolescence in body size, physiology, and general health. These changes affect the way in which the drug is absorbed, distributed, metabolized, and eliminated, where and how much of the drug is deposited in the body, and the therapeutic effects and side effects of the drug.

In the pediatric patient, medications may be administered via the oral, transmucosal, intranasal, rectal, pulmonary, subcutaneous, intramuscular, intravenous (IV), intraosseous, or tracheal route. The route by which a drug is administered affects the rapidity with which the drug's onset of action occurs and may affect the therapeutic response that results.

TABLE 8-5 *Oral Medication Administration*

Advantages	Readily available route of administration Patient acceptance; painless Convenient, noninvasive Does not generally require special equipment for administration No risk of fluid overload, infection, or embolism as with IV medications
Disadvantages	Requires functioning GI tract and sufficient GI tract for absorption to occur Slow or erratic absorption following ingestion Limited value in an emergent situation Requires a responsive, cooperative patient with an intact gag reflex May cause gagging or aspiration if administered too rapidly
Examples	Activated charcoal, antibiotics, steroids
Notes	Do not administer oral medications in solid form (i.e., pills, capsules, tablets) to young children because of the danger of aspiration. A tuberculin syringe (needle removed) is ideal for administering liquid medications of 1 mL or less. A medicine cup can be used for older infants who are able to drink from a cup. Place an infant in a semireclining position or a child in a sitting or semireclining position. Position the infant or child securely. Place the syringe (or plastic dropper) along the side of the child's tongue, toward the back of the mouth. Administer the medication slowly and in small amounts, allowing the child sufficient time to swallow (Figure 8-2). If available, follow the medication with water, juice, or a frozen juice bar.

GI, gastrointestinal; IV, intravenous.

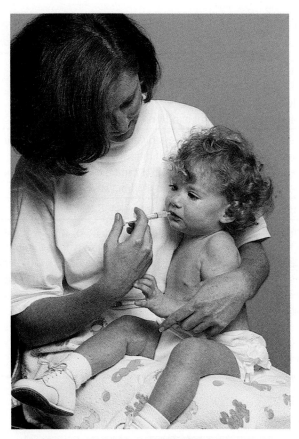

Figure 8-2   This child is partially restrained to ensure easy and comfortable administration of an oral medication using a tuberculin syringe.

TABLE 8-6 *Oral Transmucosal (Sublingual, Buccal) Medication Administration*

Advantages	Readily available route of administration Ease of administration Painless Rapid onset of action
Disadvantages	Requires a responsive, cooperative patient with an intact gag reflex Unsuitable for very young patients who may not understand your instructions Limited number of medications that can be administered via this route Variable absorption
Examples	Sedatives
Notes	Mucosal surfaces typically have a rich blood supply, allowing rapid drug transport to the systemic circulation

TABLE 8-7 *Intranasal Medication Administration*

Advantages	Easy to administer Rapid, reliable onset of action Relatively painless Obviates need for painful injections
Disadvantages	Some medications (e.g., midazolam) are associated with a burning sensation and lacrimation when administered intranasally Limited number of medications that can be administered via this route May cause gagging or aspiration if administered too rapidly
Examples	Fentanyl, midazolam, lorazepam, steroids
Notes	Intranasal medications are administered via spray, drops, or aerosol into the nasal cavity. The child should be placed in a supine position with the head tilted back so that the opening to the nares is almost horizontal (Figure 8-3). The child should remain in this position for approximately 1 min after the medication has been instilled to ensure the medication reaches the nasal mucosa. The medication is being given too quickly if the child sputters, coughs, or swallows during administration. Do not administer medications via this route if the child has respiratory distress, copious nasal secretions, or nasal bleeding because of the increased risk of airway obstruction and aspiration.

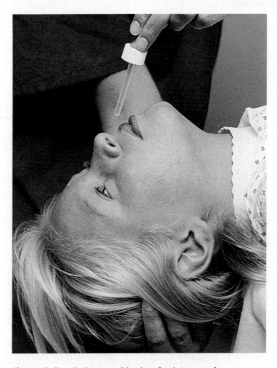

Figure 8-3   Patient positioning for intranasal medication administration.

TABLE 8-8 *Rectal Medication Administration*

Advantages	Route is always available More easily accessible route during active seizures than intravenous route Rapid absorption Relatively painless
Disadvantages	Limited number of medications that can be administered via this route If the rectum is not empty when the medication is inserted, drug absorption may be delayed, diminished, or prevented Most children dislike this route of administration
Examples	Anticonvulsants, antipyretics, antiemetics, analgesics, sedatives
Notes	Rectal medication administration should be avoided in patients with rectal trauma and immunosuppressed patients in whom even minimal trauma could lead to formation of an abscess. To administer, draw up the appropriate drug dose into a lubricated 1-mL disposable tuberculin syringe. Insert the syringe (without the needle) into the rectum to the end of the syringe and inject the medication (Figure 8-4). Remove the syringe.

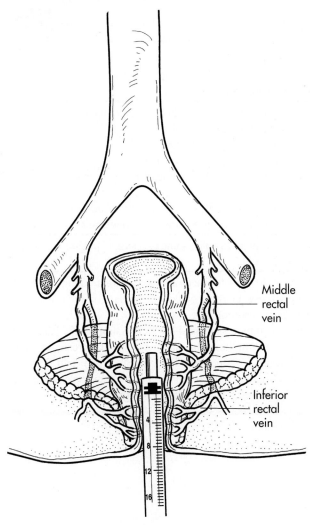

Middle
rectal
vein

Inferior
rectal
vein

Figure 8-4   Venous drainage of the middle and inferior rectum
and syringe insertion.

TABLE 8-9 *Pulmonary (Inhaled) Medication Administration*

Advantages	Painless Ease of administration Rapid onset of action
Disadvantages	Limited use with respiratory failure Medications used are limited to those with actions on or absorption through the respiratory tract
Examples	Oxygen, bronchodilators, nitrous oxide, steroids, antibiotics, antivirals
Notes	Administration may be difficult if the child is uncooperative; however, crying may improve medication delivery because of the child's deeper and more rapid respiratory rate. Medication delivery is affected by airway size and the degree of obstruction within the airways due to mucous plugs, bronchoconstriction, and inflammation.

TABLE 8-10 *Subcutaneous Medication Administration*

Advantages	Readily available route Allows delivery of a variety of medications Less painful than IM injection
Disadvantages	Painful; creates fear and anxiety in children and may cause a child to deny pain to avoid further injections of analgesics Inconvenient, time consuming Requires technical expertise to perform Volume of medication that can be delivered is limited to 0.5 to 1.0 mL (maximum of 1.0 mL in all age groups) Slower onset and lower peak effects than IV administration Can cause local tissue injury and nerve damage if improper technique used
Examples	Heparin, morphine, insulin, some vaccines, epinephrine, allergy desensitization, hormone replacement
Notes	Inappropriate route for medications that are irritating and are not water-soluble. Absorption may be rapid or slow depending on the water solubility of the drug and blood flow to the injection site. The most common sites used for SC injection are the lateral aspect of the upper arms, the abdomen from the costal margins to the iliac crests, and the anterior thighs (Figure 8-5). Use a 25-gauge 1/2-inch needle for infant or thin child; 25-gauge 5/8-inch needle for larger child. Insert the needle at a 90-degree angle, using a quick, dartlike motion. Some clinicians insert the needle at a 45-degree angle if the child has little SC tissue.

IM, intramuscular; IV, intravenous; SC, subcutaneous.

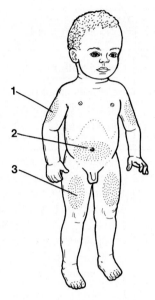

Figure 8-5   The most common
sites used for
subcutaneous
injection are the
lateral aspect of
the upper arms, the
abdomen from
the costal margins
to the iliac crests,
and the anterior
thighs.

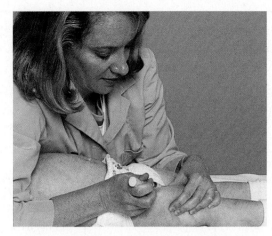

Figure 8-6   When administering an intramuscular (IM)
injection, grasp the muscle between your
thumb and index finger to isolate and
stabilize the muscle and ensure IM delivery
of the medication.

TABLE 8-11 *Intramuscular Medication Administration*

Advantages	Readily available route Allows delivery of a variety of medications
Disadvantages	Painful; creates fear and anxiety in children and may cause a child to deny pain to avoid further injections of analgesics Erratic absorption may cause discontinuous levels of analgesia Requires technical expertise to perform Volume of medication that can be delivered is limited by the site chosen and child's size More painful than SC injection Medication is given more slowly than SC injection Can cause local tissue injury and nerve damage if improper technique used Chronic injections may damage tissue (fibrosis, abscesses)
Examples	Antibiotics, some vaccines, sedatives, analgesics
Notes	Absorption may be rapid or slow depending on the water solubility of the drug and blood flow to the injection site. When administering an IM injection, grasp the muscle between your thumb and index finger to isolate and stabilize the muscle and ensure IM delivery of the medication (Figure 8-6). If the child is obese, spread the skin with your thumb and index finger to displace SC tissue and then grasp the muscle on each side.

IM, intramuscular; SC, subcutaneous.

TABLE 8-12 *Intramuscular Injection Sites in Children*

Site	Age	Needle	Considerations
Vastus lateralis (Figure 8-7)	Preferred site for infants and children younger than 3 y, but may be used in all ages	Use 22- to 25-gauge, 5/8- to 1-inch needle inserted at a 90-degree angle to site	No nearby major nerves or vessels Large, easily accessible muscle Can inject up to 0.5 mL of fluid in infant, 2.0 mL in child
Ventrogluteal (Figure 8-8)	Consider for children older than 3 y	Use 22- to 25-gauge, 1/2- to 1-inch needle inserted almost perpendicular to site but angled slightly (10 to 15 degrees) toward iliac crest	No nearby major nerves or vessels Prominent bony landmarks Thin layer of SC tissue Can inject up to 0.5 mL of fluid in infant, 2.0 mL in child Less painful than vastus lateralis Healthcare professional is often unfamiliar with site
Dorsogluteal (Figure 8-9)	Contraindicated in children younger than 3 y and in nonambulatory patients	Use 20- to 25-gauge 1/2- to 1½-inch needle inserted perpendicular to surface on which the child is lying when prone	Risk of damage to sciatic nerve Depth of overlying SC tissue varies between patients Advantage: child does not see needle and syringe Well-developed muscle in older child can tolerate fluid volume of up to 2 mL
Deltoid (Figure 8-10)	Toddler, preschooler, older child, adolescent	Use 22- to 25-gauge 1/2- to 1-inch needle inserted at a 90-degree angle to site	Small muscle mass can tolerate only small fluid volume (0.5 to 1 mL) Faster absorption than gluteal sites Easily accessible Less pain than vastus lateralis Possible damage to radial and axillary nerves

SC, subcutaneous.

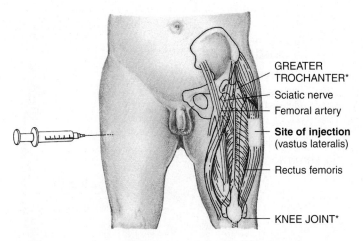

GREATER
TROCHANTER*

Sciatic nerve

Femoral artery

Site of injection
(vastus lateralis)

Rectus femoris

KNEE JOINT*

Figure 8-7   Vastus lateralis intramuscular injection site.

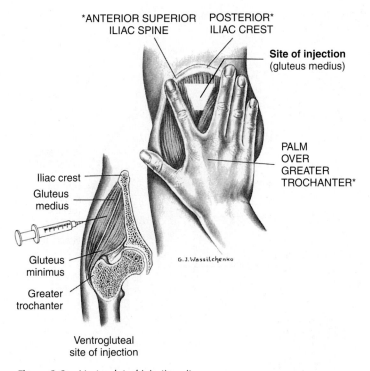

*ANTERIOR SUPERIOR
ILIAC SPINE

POSTERIOR*
ILIAC CREST

Site of injection
(gluteus medius)

PALM
OVER
GREATER
TROCHANTER*

Iliac crest

Gluteus
medius

Gluteus
minimus

Greater
trochanter

G. J. Wassilchenko

Ventrogluteal
site of injection

Figure 8-8   Ventrogluteal injection site.

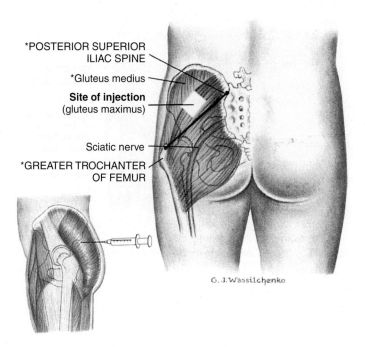

Figure 8-9   Dorsogluteal injection site.

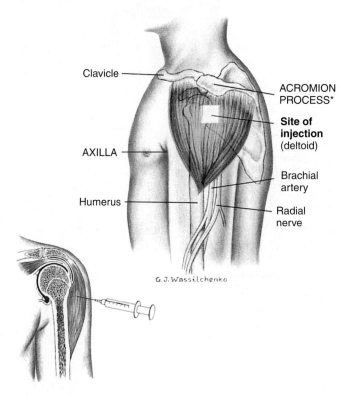

Figure 8-10   Deltoid injection site.

TABLE 8-13 *Intravenous Medication Administration*

Advantages	Rapid onset of action for medications administered via this route Route is easily accessible Control over the level of the drug in the blood Particularly useful for resuscitation medications and fluids
Disadvantages	Painful Limits patient mobility Time consuming Requires technical expertise to perform
Examples	Antiarrhythmics, sedatives, analgesics, antibiotics
Notes	No barriers to absorption since the drug is administered directly into the circulatory system Do not attempt IV access in a child experiencing respiratory distress unless the procedure is necessary for immediately lifesaving interventions.

IV, intravenous.

TABLE 8-14 *Intraosseous Medication Administration*

Advantages	Rapid onset Control over the level of the drug in the blood Effective route when venous access is difficult or time consuming Useful for resuscitation medications and fluids
Disadvantages	Painful Limits patient mobility Requires technical expertise to perform
Examples	Antiarrhythmics
Notes	No barriers to absorption

TABLE 8-15 *Tracheal Medication Administration*

Advantages	Permits delivery of lipid-soluble medications into the pulmonary alveoli and systemic circulation via lung capillaries
Disadvantages	Limited number of medications that can be administered via this route Medication absorption may be negatively affected by the presence of blood, emesis, or secretions in the trachea or tracheal tube No fluid resuscitation possible via this medication route
Examples	Remember "NAVEL": Naloxone, Atropine, Vasopressin, Epinephrine, Lidocaine
Notes	Use the tracheal route for medication administration during resuscitation efforts if a tracheal tube is in place but IV or IO access is not available. Tracheal medications should be diluted with approximately 5 mL of sterile normal saline When administering medications by means of a tracheal tube, temporarily stop chest compressions and instill the medication down the tracheal tube. Follow the medication with five positive-pressure ventilations to ensure adequate distribution of the drug, and then resume CPR. Some medications may cause false end-tidal carbon dioxide detector readings when administered via the tracheal route[1]

Considerations in Pediatric Medication Administration

- When possible, use a length-based resuscitation tape to determine the correct dosage for medication administration or fluid resuscitation in children.
- Check each medication at least three times before administering it.
  - Check the medication when removing it from its storage container (i.e., drug box, code cart).
  - Check the medication again when preparing it for administration.
  - Check it once more at the patient's side before administering it.
- Question any medication dosage that is outside the normal range.
- Using age-appropriate language, explain to the child (and caregiver) why a medication is necessary.
- Children should always be praised for cooperating in taking their medications.
- If the child is uncooperative, restrain the child as necessary.

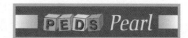

PEDS Pearl

Medication errors are common and preventable. Make it a habit to have a co-worker double-check your medication and dosage before administering it to an infant or child. This is particularly important for controlled substances (e.g., narcotics, sedatives), antiarrhythmics, heparin, insulin, and medications used during resuscitation.

Pain Management and Sedation

Barriers to Pain Assessment and Management

Pain is a subjective experience that is underestimated and inadequately treated by many healthcare professionals despite the availability of effective medications and other therapies. Factors contributing to the inadequate treatment of pain include the following[2]:

- The attitudes, beliefs, and behaviors of healthcare professionals. Some do not view pain relief as important or do not want to "waste time" assessing pain.
- Inappropriate or exaggerated concerns and inadequate or inaccurate clinical knowledge (Table 8-16). Concerns often relate to aspects of pharmacologic treatment such as regulatory scrutiny, analgesic side effects, and iatrogenic addiction.
- Failure of some healthcare organizations to adopt a standard pain assessment tool or provide their personnel with sufficient time and/or chart space for documenting pain-related information. Others have failed to provide clinicians with practical tools and training to improve pain management, such as clinical practice guidelines, algorithms, or protocols.
- A lack of accountability for pain management practices.
- Patient characteristics (e.g., age, language, cognitive abilities, coexisting physical or psychological illness, and cultural traditions) that may impair the patient's ability to communicate his or her needs to a healthcare professional.

TABLE 8-16 *Fallacies and Facts about Children and Pain*

Fallacy	Fact
Infants do not feel pain.	Infants demonstrate behavioral (especially facial) and physiologic (including hormonal) indicators of pain. Fetuses have the neural mechanisms to transmit noxious stimuli by 20 wk of gestation.
Children tolerate pain better than adults do.	A child's tolerance for pain increases with age. Younger children tend to rate procedure-related pain higher than older children do.
Children cannot tell you where they hurt.	By 4 y of age, children can accurately point to the body area or mark the painful site on a drawing. Children as young as 3 y can use pain scales, such as FACES.
Children always tell the truth about pain.	Children may not admit having pain to avoid an injection. Because of constant pain, they may not realize how much they are hurting. Children may believe that others know how they are feeling and not ask for analgesia.
Children become accustomed to pain or painful procedures.	Children often demonstrate *increased* behavioral signs of discomfort with repeated painful procedures.
Behavioral manifestations reflect pain intensity.	A child's developmental level, coping abilities, and temperament (e.g., activity level and intensity of reaction to pain) influence pain behavior. Children with more active, resisting behaviors may rate pain lower than children with passive, accepting behaviors.
Narcotics are more dangerous for children than they are for adults.	Narcotics (opioids) are no more dangerous for children than they are for adults. Addiction to opioids used to treat pain is extremely rare in children. Reports of respiratory depression in children are also uncommon. By 3 to 6 mo of age healthy infants can metabolize opioids like other children.

Adapted from Hockenberry MJ, Wilson D, Winkelstein ML, et al. *Wong's nursing care of infants and children*, 7th ed. St. Louis: Mosby, 2003:1049.

The safe and effective relief of pain should be a priority in the management of a patient of any age.

Pain Terminology

The following list of terms and definitions related to pain are from the International Association for the Study of Pain.[3]

- Pain: An unpleasant sensory and emotional experience associated with actual or potential tissue damage or described in terms of such damage. The inability to communicate verbally does not negate the possibility that an individual is experiencing pain and is in need of appropriate pain-relieving treatment.
- Pain threshold: The least experience of pain that a subject can recognize.
- Pain tolerance level: The greatest level of pain that a subject is prepared to tolerate.
- Analgesia: Absence of pain in response to stimulation that would normally be painful.

PEDS Pearl

Because no individual can feel another's pain, "Pain is whatever the experiencing person says it is, existing whenever s/he says it does."[10] The *patient*, not the healthcare professional, is the authority regarding his or her pain.

Pain Assessment in Infants and Children

The American Pain Society created the phrase "Pain: the fifth vital sign" to increase awareness of the importance of pain assessment.[5] The rationale for this initiative is that healthcare professionals should assess (and treat) pain with the same diligence and seriousness as evaluation of a patient's pulse, respiratory rate, temperature, and blood pressure.

Pain should be assessed in *all* patients; however, the methods for assessing pain in the pediatric patient will vary according to the age of the child. Adequate pain management requires ongoing assessment of the presence and severity of pain and the child's response to treatment. If pain is unrelieved, determine whether the cause is related to a new cause of pain, the progression of disease, procedure-related pain, or treatment-related pain.

- Obtain a pain history from the child and his or her caregivers.
  - The answers a patient provides in response to questions about his or her pain is called a "self-report."
    - The patient's self-report is considered the most reliable method for assessing pain (in patients who can communicate verbally) because it is the *child's* verbal statement and description of pain.
    - Self-reporting is appropriate for most children 3 years and older.
  - Ascertain information related to the following:
    - Characteristics of the pain (e.g., duration, location, intensity, quality, exacerbating/alleviating factors)
    - Type of previous painful experiences
    - Present and past pain management strategies and their outcomes
      - Analgesic use
      - Nonpharmacologic comfort measures
    - Past and present medical problems that may influence the pain and/or its management
    - Medication allergies and side effects
    - Relevant family history
    - Current and past psychosocial issues or factors that may influence the pain and its management
  - Children may have difficulty verbally reporting their pain due to the following:
    - Immaturity (infants and children younger than 3 years)
    - Nonverbal or critically ill child
    - Cognitive impairment, severely emotionally disturbed, or sensory or motor impairment
    - Language of the child differs from that of the healthcare provider
- Use an age-appropriate pain rating scale.
  - Many assessment tools are available. The same scale should be used consistently by all providers caring for the child.

The most common reason for the undertreatment of pain in U.S. hospitals is the failure of clinicians to assess pain and pain relief.[4]

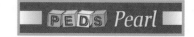

PEDS Pearl

Methods for assessing pain in the pediatric patient vary according to the age of the child. One approach to pain assessment is QUESTT[11]:

Question the child
Use pain-rating scales
Evaluate behavior and physiologic changes
Secure parents' involvement
Take cause of pain into account
Take action

Use physiologic or behavioral measures to assess pain if self-report is not available.

Some pain scales are difficult to use because of the length of time required for their use and their scoring complexity.

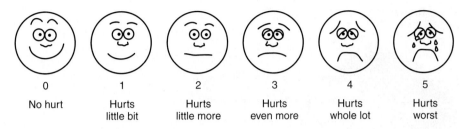

0	1	2	3	4	5
No hurt	Hurts little bit	Hurts little more	Hurts even more	Hurts whole lot	Hurts worst

Figure 8-11   Wong, DL, Hockenberry-Eaton, M, Wilson, D, Winkelstein, ML, Schwartz, P.: Wong's Essentials of Pediatric Nursing, ed. 6, St. Louis, 2001, p. 1301. Copyrighted by Mosby, Inc. Reprinted by permission.

- Assessment tools include but are not limited to the following:
  - The Children's Hospital of Eastern Ontario Pain Scale (CHEOPS) was one of the earliest tools developed to assess pain behaviors in young children. CHEOPS incorporates six categories of behavior that are scored individually (range of 0 to 2 or 1 to 3) and then totaled for a pain score ranging from 4 to 13.
  - Wong-Baker FACES Pain Rating Scale. This scale combines three scales in one: facial expressions, numbers, and words. The scale consists of six cartoon faces ranging from a smiling face depicting "no hurt" to a tearful, sad face illustrating "worst hurt" (Figure 8-11). The FACES scale is best used for children 3 years or older.
  - The Oucher Scale consists of a vertical numeric scale (10 to 100) for children who can count to 100 and a vertical photographic scale of a child with expressions of no hurt to worst hurt.
  - The Color Scale. Using markers or crayons, the child is asked to select a color that is like their "worst or most hurt," a color that is like "a little less hurt," a color for even less hurt, and finally, a color for "no hurt." A numeric value is then placed on each color.

Remember that a child often regresses when stressed.

- Observe the behavior and physiologic responses of the infant or child for cues regarding the intensity of pain (Figure 8-12).
  - Behavioral observations should be used for pain assessment of pre-verbal and nonverbal children and as an adjunct to the self-report of an older verbal child.
  - Specific behaviors associated with pain in young children include crying, facial grimaces, body posture, rigidity, changes in sleep, and level of consolability. Physiologic parameters evaluated in pain assessment include heart rate, respiratory rate, oxygen saturation, restlessness, and diaphoresis.
  - Events other than pain (e.g., fear, anxiety, loneliness, and overstimulation) can cause alterations in many of these behavioral and physiologic signs and may be misinterpreted. For example, healthcare professionals may misinterpret sleeping, watching television, and

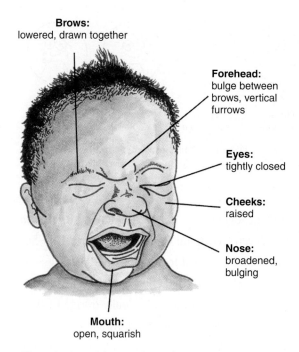

Brows:
lowered, drawn together

Forehead:
bulge between
brows, vertical
furrows

Eyes:
tightly closed

Cheeks:
raised

Nose:
broadened,
bulging

Mouth:
open, squarish

Figure 8-12   Facial expression is the most consistent
behavioral indicator of pain in infants.

using humor as indicators of an absence of pain when in fact the
child is using these behaviors to cope with and control pain.

° Because heart rate, respiratory rate, blood pressure, and diaphoresis
alter with a variety of stress-arousal events, they should not be used
as measures of pain in the absence of other pain assessment
methods or clinical indicators.[6]

° FLACC is a behavioral scale that can be used for scoring pain in
children age 3 months to 7 years, cognitively impaired patients, and
patients unable to use other scales. FLACC targets five categories for
pain evaluation: *F*ace, *L*egs, *A*ctivity, *C*rying, and *C*onsolability. Each
area is scored from 0 to 2. The subtotal from each category is added
to create a total score between 0 and 10 (10 = severe pain, 0 = no
pain) (Table 8-17).

° Reassess behavior and vital signs after administration of an analgesic. Decreased irritability, cessation of crying, and decreased pulse,
respirations, and blood pressure are important parameters to assess
when evaluating the effectiveness of pain management.

• Secure the caregiver's involvement.

° Encourage the child's caregiver to take an active role in the assessment and management of the child's pain. The caregiver is often
adept at noticing subtle changes in their child that could indicate
pain, particularly in the preverbal or nonverbal child.

° Studies have shown that although caregivers may be able to identify
the presence of pain, they often underestimate the pain severity of

Physiologic and behavioral
measures must be used with
caution because discrepancies
often exist between these
measures and the child's
self-report of pain.

TABLE 8-17 FLACC Pain Assessment Tool[2]

Category	0	1	2
Face	No particular expression or smile	Occasional grimace or frown, withdrawn, disinterested	Frequent to constant quivering chin, clenched jaw
Legs	Normal position or relaxed	Uneasy, restless, tense	Kicking, or legs drawn up
Activity	Lying quietly, normal position, moves easily	Squirming, shifting back and forth, tense	Arched, rigid or jerking
Cry	No cry (awake or asleep)	Moans or whimpers; occasional complaint	Crying steadily, screams or sobs, frequent complaints
Consolability	Content, relaxed	Reassured by occasional touching, hugging or being talked to, distractible	Difficult to console or comfort

From Merkel SI, Voepel-Lewis T, Shayevitz JR, et al. The FLACC: A behavioral scale for scoring postoperative pain in young children *Pediatr Nurse* 1997;23:293–297.

others. Underestimation of pain may contribute to inadequate pain control.

- Take the cause of the pain or emotional distress into account.
  - Identify sources of anxiety or discomfort. Anxiety can increase the severity and intensity of pain and cause physical tension, which can generate pain.
  - Possible causes include the following:
    - Pathology (e.g., sickle cell disease, sore throat)
    - Absence of the child's caregiver or a familiar toy or blanket
    - An overstimulating environment
- Take action and evaluate results.
  - Select appropriate therapeutic interventions on the basis of the initial pain assessment. The treatment goal should be complete relief of pain.
  - Therapeutic interventions may include child-parent teaching, analgesics, and nonpharmacologic techniques (e.g., coping strategies, guided visual imagery, distraction).

Sedation

Terminology

- Anxiolysis: relief of apprehension and uneasiness without alteration of awareness
- Amnesia: lack of memory about events occurring during a particular period
- Analgesia: absence of pain in response to stimulation that would normally be painful
- Anesthesia: a state of unconsciousness

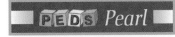

Analgesics used to manage severe pain usually cause sedation, but most sedatives do not provide analgesia.

- Sedation: depression of an individual's awareness of the environment and reduction of his or her responsiveness to external stimulation

Sedation: Indications

- Sedation may be used for the following[7]:
  - Help control anxiety or fear
  - Combat effects of toxic ingestions or withdrawal syndromes
  - Promote sleep
  - Decrease physical activity, metabolism, or oxygen consumption
  - Provide amnesia during procedures and neuromuscular paralysis
  - Facilitate management of mechanical ventilation
- If a procedure is not painful, a sedative is typically used. If pain is expected, analgesics are used, usually in conjunction with a sedative. When selecting medications, consider the duration of action of the sedatives/analgesics and the duration of procedure.

Levels of Sedation/Analgesia

Sedation is a dose-dependent continuum from minimal sedation to general anesthesia (Table 8-18). Individual patient responses to a given dosage of a drug vary and the potential for serious adverse effects exists regardless of the medications selected or the route of administration. Because of this variation in patient response, the American Society of Anesthesiologists prefers the term *sedation-analgesia*[8] and the American College of Emergency Physicians (ACEP) uses the term *procedural sedation* instead of *conscious sedation*.

With each level of sedation/analgesia, the risk of the patient slipping into the next deeper level of sedation exists. The practitioner responsible for the procedure must have the skills and equipment necessary to safely manage patients who are sedated.

Nonpharmacologic Methods of Pain Management

Nonpharmacologic techniques used to reduce pain and anxiety depend on the child's age, pain intensity, and abilities. Examples of nonpharmacologic techniques are listed in Table 8-19.

Pharmacologic Methods of Pain Management and Sedation

Sedation and analgesia may be provided by a variety of pharmacologic agents that differ in pharmacologic classification and effects. A partial list of commonly used medications is shown in Table 8-20.

Procedural Guidelines for Sedation and Analgesia

The following steps should be completed before a procedure necessitating sedation/analgesia is begun.

Preprocedure Assessment

The preprocedure assessment focuses on evaluation of the respiratory and cardiovascular systems and is performed to determine how the patient's condition might alter his or her response to sedation/analgesia. The

TABLE 8-18 *Levels of Sedation/Analgesia*

Level of Sedation/Analgesia	Description	Comments
Minimal sedation/analgesia	Anxiety reduction; cognitive function and coordination may be impaired Protective reflexes present Able to maintain patent airway independently and continuously Able to respond appropriately to verbal command (e.g., "Open your eyes") Ventilatory and cardiovascular functions intact	Equivalent to anxiolysis Examples of minimal sedation/analgesia include peripheral nerve blocks, local or topical anesthesia or a single, oral sedative or analgesic medication administered in doses appropriate for the unsupervised treatment of insomnia, anxiety, or pain
Moderate sedation/analgesia	Minimally depressed level of consciousness Protective reflexes present; able to maintain patent airway independently and continuously Spontaneous ventilation is adequate Able to respond purposefully to verbal command (e.g., "Open your eyes"), either alone or accompanied by light tactile stimulation; reflex withdrawal from a painful stimulus is NOT considered a purposeful response Cardiovascular function is usually maintained	Moderate sedation/analgesia is equivalent to the term "conscious sedation" Risk of potential loss of protective reflexes exists
Deep sedation/analgesia	Drug-induced state of depressed consciousness Cannot be easily aroused but responds purposefully following repeated or painful stimulation; reflex withdrawal from a painful stimulus is NOT considered a purposeful response Ability to maintain ventilatory function independently may be impaired Spontaneous ventilation may be inadequate Cardiovascular function is usually maintained	May be accompanied by loss of protective reflexes and ventilatory drive Assistance may be required to maintain a patent airway Positive pressure ventilation may be required
General anesthesia	Drug-induced state of unconsciousness Unable to maintain patent airway independently Not arousable, even by painful stimulation Ability to maintain ventilatory function independently is often impaired Cardiovascular function may be impaired	Assistance often required to maintain a patent airway Positive pressure ventilation may be required

clinician performing the procedure must obtain a history and physical examination that includes the following:

- Patient age, weight, and mental status
- AMPLE history
  - *A*llergies to food, medications, or latex
  - *M*edications (e.g., anticonvulsant medications [barbiturates, benzodiazepines], cardiac medications [digoxin, β-blockers, calcium channel blockers])

Allergies and medications may affect the choice of medications used during the procedure.

TABLE 8-19 Nonpharmacologic Methods of Pain Management

Age	Nonpharmacologic Technique
Infant (1 to 12 mo)	Allow caregiver to remain with the child Promote relaxation with rocking, holding, light massage Allow the infant to suck on a pacifier Distract the infant with finger puppets, a rattle, plastic keys, music box, singing Cover injuries or deformities
Toddler (1 to 3 y)	Allow caregiver to remain with the child Promote relaxation with rocking, holding, light massage Distract the child with singing, listening to music, making funny faces, playing with a favorite toy, finger puppets, telling a story, using pop-up books or books with sound effects Cover injuries or deformities
Preschooler (4 to 5 y)	Allow caregiver to remain with the child Promote relaxation with rocking, holding, light massage Deep breathing exercises Cover injuries or deformities Distract the child with singing, listening to music, making funny faces, playing with a favorite toy, finger puppets, telling a story, using pop-up books or books with sound effects
School-aged (6 to 12 y)	Allow caregiver to remain with the child Have the child visualize himself in a "safe" or beautiful place Deep breathing exercises Cover injuries or deformities Progressive muscle relaxation Distract the child with humor, telling stories, watching cartoons, playing games, or listening to familiar music on a tape or CD
Adolescent (13 to 18 y)	Allow caregiver to remain with the child, if child and caregiver desire Have the child visualize himself in a tranquil place Deep breathing exercises, rhythmic breathing Progressive muscle relaxation Distract the child with humor, watching a favorite movie, playing games, or listening to familiar music on a tape or CD Cover injuries or deformities

- *P*ast medical history
  - Airway abnormalities (e.g., snoring, sleep apnea)
  - History of adverse reaction to sedation/analgesia, as well as regional and general anesthesia
  - History of tobacco, alcohol, or substance use or abuse
  - Pregnancy status
  - *L*ast oral intake (Table 8-21)
  - *E*vents leading to the need for the procedure
- A focused physical examination
  - Obtain vital signs including pulse, blood pressure, respiratory rate, and oxygen saturation.

A focused physical examination is performed to determine the patient's physiologic status and identify factors that may increase the risk of complications during the procedure.

TABLE 8-20 *Pharmacologic Agents Used in Pain Management and Sedation*

Drug Classification	Indications and Uses	Remarks
Adjuvant Analgesics or Coanalgesics		
Antiepileptic drugs (carbamazepine, phenytoin)	Neuropathic pain (especially shooting, stabbing pain) from peripheral nerve syndromes	Side effects limit use
Tricyclic antidepressants (amitriptyline, nortriptyline, imipramine)	Used in the treatment of a variety of pain types including migraines, cancer pain, and fibromyalgia	Well-established analgesic efficacy; anticholinergic side effects; sedation common; use with caution in children with increased risk for cardiac dysfunction
Local anesthetics (EMLA [eutectic mixture of lidocaine and prilocaine], TAC [tetracaine, adrenaline, cocaine] solution)	EMLA: Indicated for procedures in which intact skin is punctured (e.g., venipuncture, circumcision, lumbar puncture, bone marrow aspiration) TAC: Provides topical local anesthesia for dermal lacerations	EMLA: Do not use in areas with limited circulation because of vasoconstrictive properties TAC: Contraindicated in areas supplied by end arteries, on mucous membranes, and on areas adjacent to mucous membranes
Nonopioid Analgesics		
Nonopioids (NSAIDs, including aspirin and other salicylic acid derivatives)	Relief of acute and chronic mild to moderate pain of nonvisceral origin	Can be administered alone or in combination with opiates; when used alone, do not produce tolerance, physical dependence, or addiction
Opioid Analgesics		
Opioids/narcotics (morphine, fentanyl, meperidine, codeine, hydrocodone, oxycodone)	Used to treat moderate to severe pain unresponsive to nonopioids alone; often combined with nonopioids to lower opioid dose required	Common side effects include respiratory depression (particularly when combined with a benzodiazepine) and hypotension
Sedatives/Hypnotics		
Barbiturates (pentobarbital, thiopental, methohexital)	Can cause CNS depression ranging from mild sedation to deep coma; no analgesic properties	May cause significant respiratory depression
Benzodiazepines (diazepam, lorazepam, midazolam)	Provide sedation and amnesia but possess no analgesic properties	May cause respiratory and/or cardiovascular depression; reversible with flumazenil
Chloral hydrate	Sedative-hypnotic; no analgesic properties	Use with caution in neonates; irregular absorption may lead to prolonged effect
Propofol (Diprivan)	Short-acting sedative-hypnotic that rapidly produces a state of general anesthesia	Continuous infusion required to maintain sedation
Other Agents		
Diphenhydramine (Benadryl)	Antihistamine that can produce sedation ranging from mild drowsiness to deep sleep	May cause paradoxic excitement
Ketamine (Ketalar)	Provides sedation, amnesia, and analgesia	Derivative of phencyclidine; use with anticholinergic agent (e.g., atropine) to decrease secretions

CNS, central nervous system; NSAID, nonsteroidal antiinflammatory drug.

TABLE 8-21 *American Society of Anesthesiologists Fasting Recommendations Before Elective Procedures**

Ingested Material	Minimum Fasting Period
Clear liquids Examples of clear liquids: water, fruit juices without pulp, carbonated beverages, clear tea, black coffee	2 h
Breast milk	4 h
Infant formula	6 h
Nonhuman milk Because nonhuman milk is similar to solids in gastric emptying time, the amount ingested must be considered when determining an appropriate fasting period.	6 h
Light meal A light meal typically consists of toast and clear liquids. Meals that include fried or fatty foods or meat may prolong gastric emptying time. Both the amount and type of foods ingested must be considered when determining an appropriate fasting period.	6 h

* These recommendations apply to healthy patients who are undergoing elective procedures. Following these recommendations does not guarantee complete gastric emptying has occurred.

- ◦ Auscultate the heart and lungs.
- ◦ Perform a general assessment of the patient's airway. Identify characteristics that suggest the possibility of a difficult tracheal intubation and/or increased risk of airway obstruction during the procedure.
  - Significant obesity, especially when the neck and facial structures are involved
  - Large tongue
  - Short neck
  - Small lower jaw (micrognathia)
  - Conditions that limit the range of motion of the neck or jaw
  - Excessive airway secretions
  - Decreased airway protective reflexes
- ◦ Identify risk factors.
  - Upper respiratory infection (increased risk of upper airway obstruction due to secretions, laryngospasm)
  - Altered mental status (increased risk of tongue displacement into posterior pharynx)
  - Respiratory problems (e.g., asthma with active wheezing) (increased risk of apnea, hypoxemia, respiratory depression)
  - Cardiac disease with poor cardiac output (increased risk of hypotension, poor perfusion)
  - Seizure disorders (increased risk of depressed mental status with resultant airway and ventilation problems)

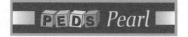
PEDS Pearl

Extended observation of the newly born and infants younger than 6 months old is necessary because they metabolize medications differently than older children and appear to be more prone to the respiratory depression associated with sedatives and analgesics (particularly narcotics).

PEDS Pearl

In urgent, emergent, or other situations where gastric emptying is impaired, the potential for pulmonary aspiration of gastric contents must be considered in determining the following:
- The target level of sedation
- Whether the procedure should be delayed or
- Whether the trachea should be protected by intubation.[8]

Necessary age-appropriate and size-appropriate emergency equipment should be immediately available whenever medications capable of causing cardiorespiratory depression are administered.

Oxygen is usually administered to patients receiving sedation/analgesia to reduce the incidence of hypoxia associated with some sedatives.

- Newly born or young infant (increased risk of respiratory depression, apnea)
- Preprocedure laboratory testing should be guided by the patient's underlying medical condition and the likelihood that the results will affect the management of sedation/analgesia.
- Obtained informed consent.

Equipment and Personnel

Before administering a sedative or analgesic, ensure that age-appropriate and size-appropriate equipment is **immediately** available.

- Equipment
  - Visor or protective eyewear, disposable mask, and gloves
  - Length-based resuscitation tape or emergency medication sheet listing appropriate dosages for resuscitation
  - Airway equipment including oxygen and an oxygen source with regulator/flowmeter, oropharyngeal and nasopharyngeal airways, suction catheters (soft and Yankauer types), suction tubing, and a vacuum source; bag-valve-mask with oxygen attachments and face masks of appropriate sizes; intubation equipment including laryngoscope, blades, tubes, and stylets; pediatric laryngeal mask airways
  - IV equipment including gloves, tourniquet, alcohol wipes, gauze pads, IV catheters, tubing, and fluids; needles, syringes, and tape; intraosseous needles
  - Resuscitation medications (e.g., atropine, epinephrine) and reversal agents (e.g., naloxone, flumazenil)
  - Pulse oximeter, electrocardiogram (ECG) monitor/defibrillator
  - Noninvasive blood pressure monitor
- Personnel
  - The individual performing the procedure must have an understanding of the pharmacologic agents administered, the ability to monitor the patient's response to the medications given, and the skills necessary to intervene in managing all potential complications.
    - Sedative or anxiolytic medications should not be administered at home as part of a preprocedural sedation plan or administered by anyone who is not medically skilled or supervised by skilled medical personnel.
  - In addition to the individual performing the procedure, it is imperative to designate a qualified individual whose sole responsibility is to monitor the child during the procedure.
    - This individual must be capable of providing pediatric basic life support and skilled in airway management and cardiopulmonary resuscitation; training in pediatric advanced life support is strongly encouraged.[9]

- This individual
  - Is responsible for monitoring the child's airway patency, work of breathing, vital signs including oxygen saturation levels, mental status, circulatory status, and ECG
  - Must be able to recognize signs of airway compromise and be able to open the child's airway, administer oxygen, and begin positive-pressure ventilation if required
  - Should have an understanding of the pharmacologic agents administered including the role and actions of antagonists and possible adverse effects of these agents
  - If available, another qualified individual should be designated to assist with the procedure.

Patient Monitoring and Documentation

Patient monitoring should begin before medications are administered and continue until the patient returns to his or her presedation level and recovery is complete (discharge criteria are met).

The following must be monitored and documented:

- Vital signs (pulse, blood pressure, respiratory rate, oxygen saturation)
  - Document preprocedure (baseline) vital signs.
  - Monitor and document every 5 to 10 minutes during minimal and moderate sedation/analgesia.
  - Monitor and document at least every 5 minutes during deep sedation/analgesia.
  - Continue until the patient returns to his or her presedation level.
- Medication names, dosages, route, time, and effects of administration
- Sedation level and level of consciousness
- Airway patency, work of breathing, respiratory pattern
- Any adverse effects including apnea, hypoxia, tachycardia or bradycardia, hypotension, and emesis
- Any necessary interventions and resolutions

Postsedation Monitoring and Discharge

Monitoring the patient in the immediate postprocedure period is imperative because the patient is at risk of complications from the medications used. Some patients may become more deeply sedated after the stimulus of the procedure is discontinued. Others may experience prolonged sedative effects because of the medications used. Children who received medications with a long half-life may require extended observation.

The patient can be discharged to a less intensely monitored level of care:

- When the patient has returned to his or her preprocedure/presedation state with regard to airway, breathing, circulation, and mental status:

TABLE 8-22 *Medications Used for Sedation/Analgesia*

Barbiturates	Sedation	Amnesia	Analgesia
	☺ ☺ ☺	–	–
Methohexital (Brevital)	Administered rectally Faster onset of action and recovery time than thiopental, and twice as potent May precipitate seizures Use with extreme caution in patients in status asthmaticus Onset 5 to 15 min; duration 30 to 90 min		
Pentobarbital (Nembutal)	Can increase pain perception; not useful as a sedative during painful procedures Onset IV 1 to 5 min, duration 15 to 60 min; onset IM 5 to 15 min, duration 2 to 4 h; onset PO 15 to 60 min, duration 2 to 4 h		
Thiopental (pentothal)	Administered rectally Onset 5 to15 min; duration 60 to 90 min		

Benzodiazepines	Sedation	Amnesia	Analgesia
	☺ ☺ ☺	☺ ☺ ☺	–
Diazepam (Valium)	Sedative effects reversible with flumazenil Fat soluble Respiratory depressant effects are potentiated when administered in conjunction with opioids Slow administration decreases incidence of respiratory side effects and venous irritation Onset IV 2 to 3 min, duration 30 to 90 min; half-life about 30 h Onset per rectum 5 to 15 min, duration 2 to 4 h		
Lorazepam (Ativan)	Sedative effects reversible with flumazenil Respiratory depressant effects are potentiated when administered in conjunction with opioids IV administration can cause venous irritation Onset IV 3 to 5 min, duration 2 to 6 h Onset IM 10 to 20 min, duration 2 to 6 h Onset PO 60 min, duration 2 to 6 h		

Midazolam (Versed)	Sedative effects reversible with flumazenil
	Water soluble
	Two to four times more potent than diazepam and provides deeper sedation and more
	    amnesia than diazepam
	Respiratory depressant effects are potentiated when administered in conjunction with
	    opioids; respiratory depression is related to dosage given and rate of administration–
	    the faster the drug is given, the more likely apnea will result
	Compatible with many IV solutions and other medications; IV administration does not
	    result in venous irritation
	Onset IV 1 to 2 min, duration 30 to 60 min; onset IM 5 to 15 min, duration 30 to 60 min;
	    onset per rectum 5 to 10 min, duration 30 to 60 min; onset PO 10 min, duration 1 to 2 h		

Opioids (Narcotics)	Sedation	Amnesia	Analgesia
	☺ ☺	–	☺ ☺ ☺
Fentanyl (Sublimaze)	Respiratory depression reversible with naloxone Synthetic opioid used for pain or anxiety associated with short procedures 50 to 100 times more powerful than morphine–recheck dosage carefully before administering Causes minimal or no release of histamine Infants younger than 3 mo may be more sensitive to respiratory depressant effects		

TABLE 8-22 *cont'd*

Opioids (Narcotics)	Sedation	Amnesia	Analgesia
	☺ ☺	–	☺ ☺ ☺

Respiratory depressant effects are potentiated when administered in conjunction with benzodiazepines
Chest wall rigidity may occur with large doses given rapidly
Onset IV 2 min; duration IV 20 to 60 min; half-life about 20 min

Morphine

Respiratory depression reversible with naloxone
Used as a standard of comparison for all opioids
Can stimulate histamine release
Respiratory depressant effects are potentiated when administered in conjunction with benzodiazepines
Hypovolemia makes the occurrence of hemodynamic side effects more common
Onset IV 5 to 10 min; duration IV 2 to 4 h

Other Agents

Chloral hydrate	Sedation	Amnesia	Analgesia
	☺ ☺	–	–

Sedative/hypnotic used for pediatric sedation for more than 100 y
Used primarily for sedation for painless diagnostic procedures (e.g., MRI scan)
Has CNS, respiratory, and cardiovascular depressant effects
Increased risk of respiratory depression when administered concurrently with opioids or benzodiazepines
Paradoxic agitation may occur; more likely in children with underlying developmental delays or neurologic disorders
Onset PO or per rectum 15 to 30 min, duration 2 to 3 h

Ketamine (Ketalar)	Sedation	Amnesia	Analgesia
	☺ ☺ ☺	☺	☺ ☺ ☺

Used for sedation during painful procedures
Derivative of phencyclidine
Child may appear awake with eyes open despite deep sedation
May cause hypertension, hypotension, emergence reactions, tachycardia, laryngospasm, respiratory depression, and stimulation of salivary secretions.
Onset IV 1 to 2 min, duration 15 to 60 min; onset IM 3 to 10 min, duration 15 to 60 min

Ketorolac (Toradol)	Sedation	Amnesia	Analgesia
	–	–	☺ ☺ ☺

NSAID used for moderate to severe pain
IV route of administration in children is not yet recommended by the manufacturer, although it is well supported in the literature and in clinical practice
Onset IV 10 to 15 min; duration IV 3 to 6 h

Propofol (Diprivan)	Sedation	Amnesia	Analgesia
	☺ ☺ ☺	☺	–

Used for sedation during procedures not associated with pain
Potent vasodilator, cardiac depressant, and respiratory depressant
Short duration of action necessitates administration by continuous IV infusion
Insoluble in water
Onset IV 1 to 2 min, duration 3 to 5 min

☺ = minimal; ☺ ☺ = moderate; ☺ ☺ ☺ = heavy
CNS, central nervous system; IM, intramuscular; IV, intravenous; MRI, magnetic resonance imaging; NSAID, nonsteroidal anti-inflammatory drug; PO, by mouth.

TABLE 8-23 *Pharmacologic Antagonists (Reversal Agents)*

Agent	Remarks
Naloxone (opioid antagonist)	Effective for all opioids (narcotics) Effects of narcotics are usually longer than naloxone: thus, respiratory depression may return when naloxone has worn off. Monitor the patient closely and observe continuously for resedation for at least 2 h after the last dose of naloxone.
Flumazenil (benzodiazepine antagonist)	Effective for all benzodiazepines Observe continuously for resedation for at least 2 h after the last dose of flumazenil. Administer as a series of small injections (not as a single bolus injection) to control the reversal of sedation to the approximate endpoint desired and minimize the possibility of adverse effects. Safety and efficacy in reversal of moderate sedation/analgesia in pediatric patients younger than 1 y have not been established.

- ○ The patient is conscious and responds appropriately.
- ○ Vital signs are stable and within acceptable limits for that patient.
- ○ The patient's respiratory status is not compromised.
- When the patient's pain and discomfort have been addressed.
- If there are no new signs, symptoms, or problems.
- If there is minimal nausea.
- When hydration status is adequate.
- When sufficient time (up to 2 hours) has elapsed following the last administration of reversal agents (naloxone, flumazenil) to ensure that the child does not become resedated after reversal effects have worn off.

Common Medications used in Pediatric Emergency Care

Medication	Indication(s)	Dosage	Precautions	Special Considerations
Adenosine (Adenocard)	SVT	IV/IO: Initial dose 0.1 mg/kg (up to 6 mg) as rapidly as possible IV push followed by a NS flush Second dose 0.2 mg/kg rapid IV push Maximum single dose is 12 mg.	Dysrhythmias at time of rhythm conversion Use with caution in patients with asthma; severe bronchospasm has been reported in several asthmatic patients following adenosine administration Discontinue in any patient who develops severe respiratory difficulty Do not use in second-degree or third-degree heart block or sick sinus syndrome	Constant ECG monitoring is essential. Onset of action 10 to 40 sec; duration 1 to 2 min Higher doses may be needed when a patient is taking methylxanthine preparations.
Albuterol (Proventil, Ventolin)	Bronchospasm, status asthmaticus	Nebulized albuterol (0.5% solution) 0.15 mg/kg/dose up to 5 mg diluted in 2 to 3 mL of NS Severe airflow obstruction may benefit from continuous albuterol nebulization (0.6 to 1 mg/kg/h) The patient in severe distress may require albuterol nebulizations every 20 min for up to 1 h. Repeated dosing produces incremental bronchodilation.	Watch for tachycardia, nausea, vomiting, tremor	The onset of action of inhaled bronchodilators is within 5 min. Their duration of action in severe asthma is unknown and may vary with the severity of the disease. Evaluate the patient's response to the initial inhaled albuterol treatments. Assess clinical signs of respiratory distress including pulse and respiratory rate, oxygen saturation, and PEFR. Any deterioration may require prompt intervention.
Amiodarone (Cordarone)	Pulseless VT/VF Perfusing tachycardias—particularly ectopic atrial tachycardia, junctional ectopic tachycardia, and VT	IV/IO pulseless VT/VF: 5 mg/kg IV/IO perfusing tachycardias: IV/IO 5 mg/kg loading dose over 20 to 60 min. Repeat as needed to max dose of 15 mg/kg/d.	Like all antiarrhythmic agents, amiodarone may cause a worsening of existing arrhythmias or precipitate a new arrhythmia. Common side effects include hypotension (most common), bradycardia, and AV block. Slow infusion rate or discontinue if seen. Forms a precipitate when mixed with sodium bicarbonate or heparin	Maximum dose 15 mg/kg/d Cordarone IV contains the preservative benzyl alcohol. Benzyl alcohol has been associated with "gasping syndrome" characterized by metabolic acidosis, CNS depression, respiratory distress, and death in neonates. Concerns about benzyl alcohol exposure and the lack of safety and efficacy data in children have prompted the manufacturer to state that the use of amiodarone IV in pediatric patients is not recommended.

Medication	Indication(s)	Dosage	Precautions	Special Considerations
Atropine sulfate	Symptomatic bradycardia Anticholinesterase poisoning To reduce secretions during RSI or block reflex bradycardia induced by succinylcholine and laryngoscopy during RSI	Symptomatic bradycardia IV/IO: 0.02 mg/kg. Minimum single dose 0.1 mg. Maximum single dose 0.5 mg for child, 1.0 mg for adolescent. Maximum total dose 1.0 mg in a child and 2.0 mg in an adolescent. ET dose 0.03 mg/kg; follow with 5 mL normal saline flush and 5 ventilations Anticholinesterase poisoning IV: 0.05 mg/kg Repeat as needed for clinical effect. RSI 0.02 mg/kg IV or 0.02 to 0.04 mg/kg IM just before or simultaneously with succinylcholine	Do not administer in less than minimum recommended dose – may cause paradoxic bradycardia (particularly in infants) with lower doses Monitor for tachycardia	Anticholinesterase poisonings may require large doses of atropine. Symptomatic bradycardia should first be treated with oxygenation and ventilation. Epinephrine is the drug of choice if bradycardia is due to hypoxia and oxygenation and ventilation do not correct the bradycardia. Give atropine before epinephrine if the bradycardia is due to increased vagal tone or if AV block is present.
Calcium	Ionized hypocalcemia Hyperkalemia Hypermagnesemia Calcium channel blocker toxicity	Calcium chloride 10% IV/IO: 20 mg/kg (0.2 mL/kg) slowly	Bradycardia with rapid IV injection. Stop administration if symptomatic bradycardia occurs. Precipitates with sodium bicarbonate. Do not administer IM or SubQ – can cause severe tissue necrosis, sloughing or abscess formation. Administration may be accompanied by peripheral vasodilation, with a moderate fall in blood pressure.	Ensure patency of IV line before administering. Monitor IV site closely. Patient may experience pain, burning at the IV site, severe venous thrombosis, and severe tissue necrosis if solution extravasates. Patient may complain of "heat waves," tingling, and/or a metallic taste if administered too rapidly. Incompatible with all medications. Flush line before and after administration.
Charcoal, activated	Acute ingestion of selected toxic substances	PO or via nasogastric tube: Children up to 1 year of age: 1 g/kg; Children 1 to 12 years: 25 to 50 g; Adolescents and adults: 25 to 100 g	Fatal hypernatremic dehydration has been reported after repeated doses of charcoal with sorbitol (a cathartic). Use products that do not contain sorbitol if repeated doses are necessary.	Iron, lithium, alcohols, ethylene glycol, alkalis, fluoride, mineral acids, and potassium do not bind to activated charcoal.

Medication	Indication(s)	Dosage	Precautions	Special Considerations
Chloral hydrate	Sedation	PO or rectally: 25 to 100 mg/kg; maximum 2 g	Avoid in liver or kidney failure. Use with caution in patients with large tonsils/adenoids or other abnormalities of the upper airway. Toxicity worsens when used concurrently with benzodiazepines, ethanol, or barbiturates; overdose can be fatal	Possesses CNS, respiratory, and cardiovascular depressant effects. Gastric irritant. Primary reason for failure of successful sedation is inadequate initial dose
Dexamethasone (Decadron)	Moderate to severe croup	IV/IM/PO: 0.6 mg/kg as a single dose (maximum dose 8 mg).	Use of corticosteroids is controversial. Some data show early treatment with dexamethasone may shorten the course and prevent the progression of croup to complete obstruction.	Further dosing and route of administration determined by clinical course.
Diazepam (Valium)	Status epilepticus Extreme anxiety or agitation	IV: 0.1 mg/kg every 2 min; maximum dose 0.3 mg/kg (maximum 10 mg/dose); administer at a rate no faster than 2 mg/min. Rectal: 0.5 mg/kg up to 20 mg. Onset after rectal administration is 5 to 10 min.	Do NOT give IM. Do not dilute with solutions or mix with other drugs in syringe, tubing, or IV container – incompatible. May cause local irritation when given rectally.	Does not provide analgesia Monitor oxygen saturation. Monitor IV site frequently for phlebitis, which may occur rapidly.
Digoxin (Lanoxin)	Heart failure due to poor left-sided ventricular contractility	IV digitalizing dose: Premature infant 15–25 mcg/kg Full-term infant 20–30 mcg/kg 1–24 months 30–50 mcg/kg 2–5 years 25–35 mcg/kg 5–10 years 15–30 mcg/kg Over 10 years 8–12 mcg/kg	Common adverse effects of chronic digoxin toxicity are visual disturbances and fatigue followed by weakness, nausea, loss of appetite, abdominal discomfort, psychological complaints, dizziness, abnormal dreams, headache, diarrhea, and vomiting. Visual disturbances include distorted yellow, red, and green color perception; blurred vision, and halos around solid objects.	Toxic-to-therapeutic ratio is narrow May result in toxicity in patients with hypokalemia or hypomagnesemia, because potassium or magnesium depletion sensitizes the myocardium to digoxin
Diphenhydramine (Benadryl)	Anaphylaxis Dystonic reactions	IM/IV: 1 mg/kg deep IM or slow IV push over 1 to 4 min; maximum dosage 50 mg	Should not be used in newborn or premature infants May cause hypotension. Do not give SC due to irritating effects.	May cause paradoxic CNS excitation, palpitations, and seizures in young children

Medication	Indication(s)	Dosage	Precautions	Special Considerations
Dobutamine (Dobutrex) infusion	Impaired cardiac contractility Cardiogenic shock	IV/IO: 2 to 20 mcg/kg/min; titrate to desired effect. For the child in shock, consider a starting dosage of 5 to 10 mcg/kg/min. To prepare a dobutamine infusion: 6 times body weight in kilograms = the number of milligrams of dobutamine to be added to an IV solution for a total volume of 100 mL (6 × kg = mg). Then: 1 mL/h = 1 mcg/kg/min 2 mL/h = 2 mcg/kg/min	Tachycardia may occur with high doses. Other side effects include nausea, vomiting, hypertension, and hypotension. Extravasation may cause tissue ischemia and necrosis. Should only be infused via an infusion pump.	Correct hypovolemia before treatment with dobutamine. Patient response varies widely – continuously monitor ECG and blood pressure.
Dopamine (Intropin, Dopastat) infusion	Persistent hypotension or shock after volume resuscitation and stable cardiac rhythm Inadequate cardiac output Cardiogenic shock, septic shock	IV/IO: 2 to 20 mcg/kg/min; titrate to desired effect. For the child in shock, consider a starting dosage of 10 mcg/kg/min. To prepare a dopamine infusion: 6 times body weight in kilograms = the number of milligrams of dopamine to be added to an IV solution for a total volume of 100 mL (6 × kg = mg). Then: 1 mL/h = 1 mcg/kg/min 2 mL/h = 2 mcg/kg/min	Gradually taper drug before discontinuing the infusion. Tachycardia, palpitations, dysrhythmias (due to increased myocardial oxygen demand) Extravasation may cause necrosis and sloughing. Should only be infused via an infusion pump.	Monitor blood pressure, ECG, and drip rate closely. Dose-related effects: **Low dose** (0.5 to 5 mcg/kg/min), mesenteric, renal, and coronary vessel vasodilation. **Moderate dose** (5 to 10 mcg/kg/min), increases myocardial contractility and stroke volume, increasing cardiac output. **High dose** (10 to 20 mcg/kg/min), systemic vasoconstriction
Epinephrine for bradycardia	Symptomatic bradycardia unresponsive to oxygenation and ventilation	IV/IO: 0.01 mg/kg (0.1 mL/kg) of 1:10,000 solution ET: 0.1 mg/kg (0.1 mL/kg) of 1:1000 solution Max IV/IO dose = 1.0 mg; max ET dose 10 mg	Should not be administered in the same IV line as alkaline solutions – inactivates epinephrine Follow ET dose with 5 mL normal saline flush and 5 ventilations.	ET absorption is unpredictable.

Medication	Indication(s)	Dosage	Precautions	Special Considerations
Epinephrine for bronchospasm	Asthma/reactive airway disease Anaphylaxis	SVN: 0.5 mL/kg of 1:1000 (1 mg/mL) in 3 mL NS (maximum dose is 2.5 mL for 4 y or younger, 5 mL for older than 4 y) **Racemic** epinephrine 2.25% inhalation solution 0 to 20 kg: 0.25 mL in 2 mL with NS via nebulizer 20 to 40 kg: 0.50 mL in 2 mL with NS via nebulizer Above 40 kg: 0.75 mL in 2 mL with NS via nebulizer SC/IM: 0.01 mL/kg (0.01 mL/kg) of 1:1000 solution, maximum single dose 0.5 mL in anaphylaxis, 0.35 mL in asthma. May be administered every 15 min up to three doses if necessary while attempting IV access.	Side effects include transient, moderate anxiety, apprehensiveness, restlessness, tremor, weakness, dizziness, sweating palpitations, pallor, nausea and vomiting, headache	After inhalation, the patient's sputum may be pink in color due to a chemical reaction between mucous secretions and the epinephrine solution. Large doses of epinephrine may be required in the treatment of some anaphylactic reactions (e.g, latex allergy). A continuous epinephrine infusion may be necessary.
Epinephrine for cardiac arrest	Pulseless VT VF Asystole Pulseless electrical activity	IV/IO: 0.01 mg/kg (0.1 mL/kg) of 1:10,000 solution. May repeat every 3 to 5 min. ET: 0.1 mg/kg (0.1 mL/kg) of 1:1000 solution Max IV/IO dose = 1.0 mg; max ET dose 10 mg	Should not be administered in the same IV line as alkaline solutions – inactivates epinephrine. Follow ET dose with 5 mL normal saline flush and 5 ventilations.	
Epinephrine infusion	Continued shock after volume resuscitation	IV/IO: Start at 0.1 mcg/kg/min. Titrate according to patient response up to 1 mcg/kg/min. To prepare infusion: 0.6 mg × body weight (kg) = no. of mg of epinephrine to be added to a solution for a total volume of 100 mL (0.6 × kg = mg). Then: 1 mL/h = 0.1 mcg/kg/min 2 mL/h = 0.2 mcg/kg/min	Increases myocardial oxygen demand Check IV site frequently for evidence of tissue sloughing Extravasation may cause necrosis and sloughing. Should only be infused via an infusion pump	Low-dose infusions (less than 0.3 mcg/kg/min) primarily produce effects. Infusions larger than β-adrenergic 0.3 mcg/kg/min produce a mix of β-adrenergic and α-adrenergic effects.

Medication	Indication(s)	Dosage	Precautions	Special Considerations
Etomidate (Amidate)	Sedative used in RSI	0.2 to 0.6 mg/kg (child > 10 yrs)	Use with caution in asthmatics. Myoclonus (jerky, muscular contractions) may be seen after administration. Monitor oxygen saturation.	Possesses no analgesic or amnestic properties May cause minor pain during administration Produces little alteration in hemodynamics, cerebral blood flow, respiratory function, or coronary oxygenation Rapid onset with a very short duration of action
Fentanyl (Sublimaze)	Pain Sedative used in RSI	Pain IV: 0.5 to 2 mcg/kg. Administer slowly over several minutes. Repeat dose as necessary for clinical effect. Sedation in RSI: IV: 2 to 3 mcg/kg slowly over several minutes; give 1 to 3 min before intubation	Respiratory depression is common and dose dependent; reversible with naloxone Chest wall rigidity with large doses given rapidly Do not use with MAO inhibitors Increased incidence of apnea when combined with other sedative agents, particularly benzodiazepines	Fentanyl is an opiate. 50 to 100 times more powerful than morphine but causes minimal or no release of histamine No significant cardiovascular effects at usual therapeutic doses Provide respiratory support as necessary
Flumazenil (Romazicon)	Benzodiazepine intoxication	IV: Initial dose: 0.01 mg/kg (max. dose: 0.2 mg), then 0.005–0.01 mg/kg (max. dose: 0.2 mg) given Q 1 min to a max. total cumulative dose of 1 mg. Doses may be repeated in 20 min up to a maximum of 3 mg in 1 hr.	Seizure activity after flumazenil administration has occurred in patients physically dependent on benzodiazepines and those receiving benzodiazepines for control of seizures. May precipitate acute withdrawal in dependent patients. Safety and efficacy in reversal of moderate sedation/analgesia in pediatric patients below the age of 1 y has not been established.	Observe continuously for resedation for at least 2 h after the last dose of flumazenil. Administer as a series of small injections (not as a single bolus injection) to control the reversal of sedation to the approximate endpoint desired and minimize the possibility of adverse effects.

Medication	Indication(s)	Dosage	Precautions	Special Considerations
Furosemide (Lasix)	Congestive heart failure Fluid overload	IV/IO/IM: 1 mg/kg; if given IV/IO, give slowly	Potassium depletion, low blood pressure, dehydration, hyponatremia Because furosemide is a sulfonamide derivative, it may induce allergic reactions in patients with sensitivity to sulfonamides (sulfa drugs).	Monitor intake and output, daily weight, and serum electrolytes regularly. Ototoxicity and transient deafness can occur with rapid administration.
Glucose	Hypoglycemia	IV/IO: Newly born: 200 mg/kg (2 mL/kg of a $D_{10}W$ solution) slow IV push Newborn: 0.5 to 1 g/kg (5 to 10 mL/kg) of $D_{10}W$ over 20 min For patient one mo to two y: 0.5 to 1 g/kg (2 to 4 mL/kg) of $D_{25}W$ For children older than 2 y: 0.5 to 1 g/kg (1 to 2 mL/kg) of $D_{50}W$	Administer through a large vein. Determine glucose levels before and during administration. Extravasation can cause severe local tissue damage.	If large volumes of dextrose are administered, include electrolytes to prevent hyponatremia and hypokalemia. Diluting a 50% dextrose solution 1:1 with sterile water or NS = $D_{25}W$. Diluting 50% dextrose solution 1:4 with sterile water or NS = $D_{10}W$.
Glycopyrrolate (Robinul)	Adjunctive medication that may be used during RSI	IV: 0.005 to 0.01 mg/kg; maximum 0.2 mg	Occurrence of CNS related side effects is lower than with atropine Safety and efficacy in children has not been established	Anticholinergic effects similar to atropine Do not combine in the same syringe with methohexital, chloramphenicol, pentobarbital, dimenhydrinate, thiopental, secobarbital, sodium bicarbonate, or diazepam. A gas will evolve or precipitate may form.
Ipratroprium bromide (Atrovent)	May be beneficial for moderate to severe exacerbations of asthma	Nebulized treatments: Infants and children: 250 mcg/dose TID–QID >12 yr and adults: 250–500 mcg/dose TID–QID Onset 30 to 60 min to maximum effect	Side effects include nervousness, dizziness, drowsiness, headache, upset stomach, constipation, cough, dry mouth or throat irritation, skin rash, and blurred vision.	Anticholinergic. Anticholinergics produce preferential dilation of the larger central airways, in contrast to β-agonists, which affect the peripheral airways.

Medication	Indication(s)	Dosage	Precautions	Special Considerations
Ketamine (Ketalar)	Sedation/analgesia Adjunct to RSI	Sedation/analgesia IM: 1 to 2 mg/kg IV: 0.5 to 1 mg/kg Adjunct to RSI IV: 1 to 2 mg/kg Rate of IV infusion should not exceed 0.5 mg/kg/min and should not be administered in less than 60 sec.	May increase blood pressure, heart rate, and oral secretions Contraindicated in eye injuries, increased intracranial pressure Emergence reactions (hallucinations, nightmares) common in children older than 11 y Higher doses and rapid IV administration can result in apnea	A PCP derivative that is rapid acting in producing a "dissociative" anesthesia Provides amnesia, analgesia, and sedation Often used for RSI in children with respiratory failure due to asthma because this drug causes bronchodilation Monitor oxygen saturation. Be prepared to provide respiratory support.
Ketorolac (Toradol)	Moderate to severe pain	Children 2–16 years of age should receive only a single dose of Toradol injection, as follows: IM dosing: One dose of 1 mg/kg up to a maximum of 30 mg. IV: One dose of 0.5 mg/kg up to a maximum of 15 mg.	Anaphylactoid reactions may occur in patients without a known previous exposure or hypersensitivity to aspirin, ketorolac, or other NSAIDs, or in individuals with a history of angioedema, asthma, and nasal polyps.	NSAID Possesses no amnesic or sedative properties
Lidocaine	VT, VF Adjunctive agent in RSI	Ventricular dysrhythmias IV/IO: 1 mg/kg Adjunctive agent in RSI IV/IO/ET: 1 to 2 mg/kg Maximum IV bolus dose is 3 mg/kg.	Signs and symptoms of lidocaine toxicity are primarily CNS related (e.g., drowsiness, disorientation, muscle twitching, seizures) Give IV dose over 1–2 min if the patient has a pulse	Diminishes the cough and gag reflexes, and may diminish the rise in ICP associated with intubation. If indicated, administer 2 to 5 min before RSI procedure.
Lidocaine infusion	VT, VF	IV/IO: 20 to 50 mcg/kg/min To prepare a lidocaine infusion: 60 × body weight in kg = no. of mg of lidocaine to be added to a solution with a total volume of 100 mL (60 × kg = mg). Then: 1 mL/h = 10 mcg/kg/min. 2 mL/h = 20 mcg/kg/min, etc.	Metabolized (90%) in the liver; decrease infusion rate in congestive heart failure or liver impairment (infusion rate should not exceed 20 mcg/kg/min)	If there is a delay of more than 15 min between the initial dose of lidocaine and the start of the infusion, consider giving a second bolus of 0.5 to 1 mg/kg to reestablish a therapeutic level.

Medication	Indication(s)	Dosage	Precautions	Special Considerations
Lorazepam (Ativan)	Status epilepticus Adjunct for intubation	IV/IM: 0.05 to 0.1 mg/kg Repeat doses every 10 to 15 min for clinical effect. Maximum single dose 4 mg. Onset of action IV is about 15 to 30 min, IM is 30 to 60 min	Increased incidence of apnea when combined with other sedative agents	Does not provide analgesia. Monitor oxygen saturation. Be prepared to provide respiratory support.
Magnesium sulfate	TdP Severe asthma Documented hypo–magnesemia	TdP: IV/IO: 25 to 50 mg/kg slow bolus over 10 to 20 min. Maximum dose 2 g. Severe asthma: 75 mg/kg (maximum dose 2g) IV over 20 min every 6 h	Rapid administration may result in hypotension, bradycardia, and decreased cardiac contractility Contraindicated in renal failure, heart block, or myasthenia gravis	While treating TdP, search for possible reversible causes of the dysrhythmia, such as an electrolyte disturbance. Monitor magnesium levels.
Methohexital (Brevital)	Sedation	Rectally: 20 to 30 mg/kg	May worsen or precipitate seizures Adverse reactions include respiratory depression, apnea, dyspnea, hypotension (from direct myocardial depression and vasodilation), dysrhythmias, cardiac arrest, and respiratory arrest	Short-acting barbiturate Children are more likely than adults to react with paradoxic excitement to methohexital
Methyl-prednisolone (Solu-Medrol)	Reactive airway disease Anaphylaxis Croup	Reactive airway disease/ anaphylaxis IV: 1 to 2 mg/kg every 6 h Croup IV: 1 to 2 mg/kg then 0.5 mg/kg every 6 to 8 h	Rapid administration of large doses may result in hypotension and cardiovascular collapse	Contraindicated in premature infants because the Act-O-Vial system and the accompanying diluent contain benzyl alcohol. Benzyl alcohol is reportedly associated with a fatal "gasping syndrome" in premature infants.
Midazolam (Versed)	Sedative used in RSI Sedation/anxiolysis	6 mo to 5 yrs: 0.05–0.1 mg/kg; total dose up to 0.6 mg/kg 6–12 yrs: 0.025–0.05 mg/kg; total dose up to 0.4 mg/kg 12–16 yrs: 0.3–0.35 mg/kg; total dose up to 0.6 mg/kg	May cause decreased blood pressure, heart rate, respiratory depression Monitor oxygen saturation.	Midazolam is a benzodiazepine reversible with flumazenil. Possesses antianxiety, amnesic, anticonvulsant and sedating properties but possesses no analgesic properties.

Medication	Indication(s)	Dosage	Precautions	Special Considerations
Morphine sulfate	Pain "Tet spell"	IV (slowly) or IM: 0.05 to 0.1 mg/kg. Repeat dose as necessary until desired effect is achieved.	Watch closely for bradycardia, CNS depression, nausea/vomiting, respiratory depression, hypotension. Histamine release can cause bronchospasm, hypotension, and facial itching. Hypovolemia makes the occurrence of hemodynamic side effects more common.	Monitor the patient's vital signs and oxygen saturation. Be prepared to provide respiratory support. Ensure naloxone and airway equipment is readily available before administration. Respiratory depressant effects are potentiated when administered in conjunction with benzodiazepines.
Naloxone (Narcan)	Coma of unknown etiology to rule out (or reverse) opioid-induced coma Opiate-induced respiratory depression	Acute opiate intoxication IV/IO/IM/ET: If 5 y or younger or 20 kg or less: 0.1 mg/kg. If older than 5 y or more than 20 kg: 2 mg minimum dose. Repeat as needed to maintain opiate reversal. ET: Dilute dose with 5 mL of NS and follow with 5 positive-pressure ventilations. Respiratory depression during pain management IV/IO/IM/ET: 0.01 mg/kg titrated to effect	May induce acute withdrawal in opioid dependency resulting in nausea, vomiting, sweating, tachycardia, increased blood pressure, tremor, seizures, or cardiac arrest. IM absorption may be erratic in the hypoperfused patient.	Effects of narcotics are usually longer than naloxone; thus, respiratory depression may return when naloxone has worn off. Monitor the patient closely and observe for at least 2 h after the last dose of naloxone.
Nitrous oxide	Moderate to severe pain	Self-administered and self-regulated by the patient who must hold the mask to the face to create an airtight seal until the pain is significantly relieved or the patient drops the mask. The child must be old enough to follow the instructions for use and large enough so that the mask creates an airtight seal. Give oxygen during intervals that nitrous oxide is not being used.	Contraindications: Unresponsive patient Inability to comply with instructions Head injury with altered mental status Abdominal pain, unless intestinal bowel obstruction has been completely ruled out Possible drug overdose Respiratory compromise or distress (pulmonary edema, pneumothorax) Otitis, air embolism, decompression sickness (expands air pockets and can exacerbate these problems) Administration by a healthcare provider or anyone other than the patient	Produces CNS depression and decreases sensitivity to all types of pain. Effects dissipate within 2 to 5 min after cessation of administration. Produces sedation and some amnesia.

Medication	Indication(s)	Dosage	Precautions	Special Considerations
Nitroprusside (Nipride) infusion	Immediate reduction of blood pressure in a hypertensive emergency or hypertensive urgency	IV: 0.5 to 8 mcg/kg/min Begin infusion at 0.1 mcg/kg/min and titrate slowly upward to desired clinical response (up to 8 mcg/kg/min). To prepare infusion: 6 mg × body weight in kg = no. of milligrams of nitroprusside to be added to D_5W with a total volume of 100 mL (6 × kg = mg). Then: 1 mL/h = 1 mcg/kg/min	Cover the bottle, burette, or syringe pump (but not the IV tubing) with protective foil to avoid breakdown by light. Can cause precipitous decreases in blood pressure: monitor continuously. Cyanide toxicity can result from large doses and/or prolonged infusions.	Do not mix with NS. Onset of action is 1 to 2 min. Effects stop quickly upon discontinuation of infusion. Administer via an infusion pump.
Norepinephrine (Levophed) infusion	Inadequate cardiac output Septic shock, neurogenic shock, anaphylaxis, drug overdose with significant α-adrenergic blocking effects (e.g, tricyclic antidepressants)	IV/IO: 0.1 to 2 mcg/kg/min Begin infusion at 0.1 mcg/kg/min and titrate slowly upward to desired clinical response (up to 2 mcg/kg/min).	Extravasation into surrounding tissue may cause necrosis and sloughing.	Correct volume depletion with appropriate fluid and electrolyte replacement therapy before administration of norepinephrine. Should be administered via an infusion pump into a central vein or a large peripheral vein to reduce the risk of necrosis of the overlying skin from prolonged vasoconstriction.
Oxygen	All arrest situations Hypoxemia and/or respiratory distress Carbon monoxide poisoning Shock	In the spontaneously breathing patient: nasal cannula, simple face mask, blow-by or other device as tolerated In cardiac or respiratory arrest, positive-pressure ventilation with 100% oxygen	With prolonged administration of high-concentration oxygen, concern regarding toxic effects on the lungs and, in premature infants, on the eyes	Supplemental oxygen should be considered during EVERY pediatric emergency. Do NOT withhold oxygen if signs of hypoxemia are present.

Medication	Indication(s)	Dosage	Precautions	Special Considerations
Pancuronium (Pavulon)	Nondepolarizing agent used during RSI	IV: 0.06 to 0.1 mg/kg; 0.02 mg/kg in neonates Conditions satisfactory for intubation are usually present within 2 to 3 min of administration.	Tachycardia Contraindicated in renal failure, tricyclic antidepressant use Does not alter the level of responsiveness; provide analgesia or amnesia Monitor oxygen saturation.	Long-acting neuromuscular blocker that requires ventilatory assistance for at least 1 hour. For neonates, it is recommended that a test dose of 0.02 mg/kg be given first to measure responsiveness. Can be used when succinylcholine is contraindicated.
Pentobarbital (Nembutal)	Sedation	IV: 1 to 3 mg/kg; may repeat up to 6 mg/kg; administer at a rate no faster than 50 mg/min IM: 2 to 5 mg/kg PO: 2 to 3 mg/kg Maximum dose: 150 mg	Avoid in hypotensive or hypovolemic patients Respiratory depression is dose-related	Barbiturate with an intermediate duration of action; no analgesic effects When given IV, may rapidly induce general anesthesia No advantage over phenobarbital for seizure control
Procainamide (Pronestyl)	VT with a pulse	IV/IO: 15 mg/kg over 30 to 60 min Maintenance infusion: 20 to 80 mcg/kg/min (0.02 to 0.08 mg/kg/min); maximum 2 g/24 h	Contraindicated in complete AV block in the absence of an artificial pacemaker, patients sensitive to procaine or other ester-type local anesthetics, patients with a prolonged QRS duration or QT interval because of the potential for heart block; preexisting QT prolongation/TdP; digitalis toxicity (procainamide may further depress conduction) If the QRS widens to > 50% of its original width or hypotension occurs, stop the infusion.	During administration, carefully monitor the patient's ECG and blood pressure. Observe ECG closely for increasing PR and QT intervals, widening of the QRS complex, heart block, and/or onset of TdP
Propofol (Diprivan)	Sedation Sedative/hypnotic used in RSI	Sedation dosage: IV: 0.5 to 1 mg/kg; may repeat in 0.5 mg/kg boluses; may give as a titrated continuous infusion of 25 to 100 mcg/kg/min RSI dosage: IV: 2.5–3.5 mg/kg (3 to 6 years of age)	Has been associated with laryngospasm and bronchospasm Hypotension may occur, particularly in hypovolemic patients The FDA recommends propofol not be used to sedate critically ill or injured children. Contraindicated in patients with soybean or egg allergies	Lowers intracranial pressure but also decreases intracranial blood flow Potent vasodilator, cardiac depressant, and respiratory depressant A white, milky, alcohol emulsion that consists of 1% propofol, 10% soybean oil, 2.25% glycerol, and 1.25% egg lecithin; contaminates easily. Use quickly after opening.

Medication	Indication(s)	Dosage	Precautions	Special Considerations
Prostaglandin E₁ infusion	Possible ductal-dependent cardiac malformation in a neonate	IV/IO: 0.05 to 0.1 mcg/kg/min in D₅W	Apnea, hyperthermia, hypotension, hypoglycemia, and seizures may occur.	Monitor oxygen saturation. Be prepared to provide respiratory support.
Rocuronium (Zemuron)	Nondepolarizing agent used during RSI	IV: 0.6 to 1.2 mg/kg Satisfactory conditions for intubation usually occur 45 to 60 sec after administration.	The use of rocuronium bromide injection in pediatric patients younger than 3 mo and older than 14 y has not been studied. Ventilatory support is necessary. Monitor oxygen saturation.	Minimal effect on heart rate or blood pressure Precipitates when in contact with other medications so flush IV line before and after use Does not alter level of responsiveness or provide analgesia or amnesia
Sodium bicarbonate	Severe metabolic acidosis Tricyclic antidepressant overdose Hyperkalemia	IV/IO: 1 mEq/kg (1 mL/kg of 8.4% solution) per dose slowly—administer only after ensuring ventilation is adequate.	Extravasation may lead to tissue inflammation and necrosis Do not mix with parenteral drugs because of the possibility of drug inactivation or precipitation.	Administer slowly. The solution is hyperosmotic. The 0.5-mEq/mL concentration (4.2% solution) should be used for newborns.
Succinylcholine (Anectine)	Depolarizing agent used during RSI	IV: 2 mg/kg infants/small children; 1 mg/kg older children/adolescent IM: Double the IV dose Satisfactory conditions for tracheal intubation generally occur 30 to 45 sec after IV administration and 3 to 5 min after IM administration.	Muscle fasciculations Hypertension, life-threatening hyperkalemia Increased intracranial, intraocular, intragastric pressure Contraindications for use include known or suspected hyperkalemia, penetrating eye injuries, burns or crush injuries several hours old, history of malignant hyperthermia, rhabdomyolysis.	Monitor oxygen saturation Atropine administration should be standard for all children younger than 1 year, children who are bradycardic, children younger than 5 y who are to receive succinylcholine, and adolescents who receive a second dose of succinylcholine.
Thiopental (Pentothal)	Sedative used in RSI Sedation	Dosage in RSI: IV: 2 to 4 mg/kg Dosage for sedation: 25 mg/kg rectally; maximum 1 g/dose	May cause respiratory depression, histamine release, hypotension; monitor oxygen saturation. Decreases ICP and cerebral blood flow May increase oral secretions, cause bronchospasm and laryngospasm; contraindicated in status asthmaticus	Thiopental is a short-acting barbiturate that possesses no analgesic properties. Rapid onset; short duration Cerebroprotective effect During RSI, avoid or use reduced dose (1 to 2 mg/kg) in patients with known or suspected shock or hypovolemia.

Medication	Indication(s)	Dosage	Precautions	Special Considerations
Vecuronium (Norcuron)	Nondepolarizing agent used during RSI	IV/IM: 0.08–0.10 mg/kg	Safety and effectiveness in pediatric patients less than 7 wk of age have not been established	Possesses no analgesic properties Minimal effect on blood pressure or heart rate
Verapamil (Isoptin, Calan)	SVT	IV/IO: 0.1 mg/kg/dose (maximum: 5 mg/dose); may repeat in 30 min	Contraindicated in patients younger than 1 y or with ventricular dysfunction, sick sinus syndrome, second-degree or third-degree heart block, atrial fibrillation or flutter Monitor blood pressure and heart rate closely	Administer slowly and in small doses; continuous ECG monitoring is essential Extreme bradycardia and hypotension may occur if used in infants younger than 1 y; avoid use

AV, atrioventricular; ECG, echocardiogram; ET, endotracheal; FDA, Food and Drug Administration; ICP, intracranial pressure; IM, intramuscular; IO, intraosseous; IV, intravenous; MAO, monoamine oxidase; NS, normal saline; NSAID, nonsteroidal antiinflammatory drug; PCP, phencyclidine; PEFR, peak expiratory flow rate; RSI, rapid sequence intubation; SC, subcutaneous; SVN, Small Volume Nebulizer; SVT, supraventricular tachycardia; TdP, torsades de pointes; VF, ventricular fibrillation; VT, ventricular tachycardia.

Case Study Resolution

Pain should be assessed in *all* patients; however, the methods for assessing pain in the pediatric patient will vary according to the age of the child. In this situation, ask the child to rate his degree of discomfort using a tool such as the Wong–Baker FACES Pain Rating Scale. Observe the child's behavior and physiologic responses (e.g., heart rate, respiratory rate, blood pressure) as adjuncts to his verbal statement and description of pain.

Web Resources

www.painfoundation.org (American Pain Foundation)

www.ampainsoc.org (American Pain Society)

www.cityofhope.org/prc (City of Hope Pain Resource Center)

www.iasp-pain.org (International Association for the Study of Pain)

www.npecweb.org (National Pain Education Council)

References

1. Thibodeau GA, Patton KT. *Anatomy and physiology,* 2nd ed. St. Louis: Mosby–Year Book, 1993.

2. Berry PH, Chapman CR, Covington EC, et al. Current Understanding of Assessment, Management, and Treatments. Reston, VA: National Pharmaceutical Council and the Joint Commission on Accreditation of Healthcare Organizations; December, 2001. Available at: www.jcaho.org. Accessed October, 2004.

3. Merskey H, Bogduk N, eds. *Classification of chronic pain,* 2nd ed. Seattle, WA: IASP Press, 1994:209–214.

4. Max MB, Payne R, Edwards WT. *Principles of analgesic use in the treatment of acute pain and cancer pain,* 4th ed. Glenview, IL: American Pain Society, 1999.

5. Campbell J. Pain: the fifth vital sign. Presidential address to the American Pain Society; November 11, 1995; Los Angeles, CA.

6. McGrath PA, de Veber LL, Hearn MT. Multidimensional pain assessment in children. In: Fields HL, Dubner R, Cervero F, eds. *Proceedings of the Fourth World Congress on Pain,* New York: Raven Press, 1985:387–393.

7. Sherif M, Mokhtar MS, Carlson RW. Sedation monitoring. In: Kruse JA, Fink MP, Carlson RW, eds. *Saunders manual of critical care.* Philadelphia: Elsevier, 2003:800–802.

8. Task Force on Sedation and Analgesia by Non-Anesthesiologists. Practice guidelines for sedation and analgesia by non-anesthesiologists: a report by the American Society of Anesthesiologists task force on sedation and analgesia by non-anesthesiologists. *Anesthesiology* 2002;96:1004–1017.

9. American Academy of Pediatrics Committee on Drugs. Guidelines for monitoring and management of pediatric patients during and after sedation for diagnostic and therapeutic procedures (addendum). *Pediatrics* 2002;110:836–838.
10. McCaffery M, Pasero CL. When the physician prescribes a placebo. *Am J Nurs* 1998;98:52–53.
11. Wong DL, Hess CS. *Wong and Whaley's clinical manual of pediatric nursing*, 5th ed. St. Louis: Mosby, 2000.

Chapter Quiz

1. When administering medications by means of a tracheal tube you should:
   A) Continue chest compressions throughout administration of the medication.
   B) Insert a needle through the wall of the tracheal tube to administer the medication.
   C) Temporarily stop chest compressions, instill the medication down the tracheal tube, ventilate 5 times with a bag-valve device, then resume CPR.
   D) Temporarily stop chest compressions, instill the medication down the tracheal tube, ventilate the patient for a minimum of 5 minutes with a bag-valve device to ensure the drug is dispersed through the alveoli, and then resume CPR.

2. Anxiolysis is:
   A) Relief of apprehension and uneasiness without alteration of awareness.
   B) Lack of memory about events occurring during a particular period.
   C) Absence of pain in response to stimulation that would normally be painful.
   D) A state of unconsciousness.

3. The drug of choice for a stable but symptomatic child in supraventricular tachycardia is:
   A) Atropine.
   B) Amiodarone.
   C) Adenosine.
   D) Procainamide.

4. Which of the following medications can be administered by the endotracheal route?
   A) Epinephrine, atropine, naloxone, amiodarone.
   B) Naloxone, atropine, vasopressin, epinephrine, and lidocaine.
   C) Atropine, dopamine, naloxone, and sodium bicarbonate.
   D) Diazepam, adenosine, sodium bicarbonate, and verapamil.

5. Medications used to maintain cardiac output include:
   A) Midazolam, epinephrine, and naloxone.
   B) Lorazepam, midazolam, and naloxone.
   C) Diazepam, dopamine, and dobutamine.
   D) Dopamine, epinephrine, and dobutamine.

6. The term "conscious sedation" is equivalent to:
   A) Minimal sedation/analgesia.
   B) Moderate sedation/analgesia.
   C) Deep sedation/analgesia.
   D) General anesthesia.

7. Bronchodilation and vasodilation are effects that occur with stimulation of:
   A) β-1 receptors.
   B) β-2 receptors.
   C) α-1 receptors.
   D) Dopaminergic receptors.

8. Select the **incorrect** statement regarding benzodiazepines.
   A) The respiratory depression associated with benzodiazepines may be reversed with naloxone.
   B) Benzodiazepines have potent amnestic effects.
   C) Diazepam, lorazepam, and midazolam are examples of benzodiazepines.
   D) Benzodiazepines decrease patient anxiety.

9. Activation of the parasympathetic division of the autonomic nervous system:
   A) Prepares the body for emergencies (i.e., the "fight-or-flight" response).
   B) Results in an increase in blood pressure.
   C) Results in a decrease in heart rate.
   D) Results in bronchodilation and peripheral vasoconstriction.

10. Which of the following medications should be administered first to an infant or child with severe symptomatic bradycardia that persists despite effective oxygenation and ventilation?
    A) Epinephrine
    B) Atropine
    C) Dopamine
    D) Amiodarone

11. Which of the following is **NOT** a common site used for subcutaneous injections in the pediatric patient?
    A) The lateral aspect of the upper arms.
    B) The abdomen from the costal margins to the iliac crests.
    C) The anterior thighs.
    D) The buttocks.

12. Medications used for moderate sedation/analgesia most often include:
    A) Paralytics, barbiturates, and benzodiazepines.
    B) Benzodiazepines, opioids, and barbiturates.
    C) Paralytics, barbiturates, and opioids.
    D) Paralytics, opioids, and benzodiazepines.

13. Indications for the use of amiodarone include:
    A) Asystole.
    B) Severe bradycardia.
    C) Ventricular fibrillation.
    D) Sinus tachycardia.

14. The minimum recommended single dose of atropine in the pediatric patient is:
    A) 0.03 mg/kg.
    B) 0.04 mg/kg.
    C) 0.1 mg.
    D) 1.0 mg.

15. What is the recommended dose of naloxone for infants and children from birth to 5 years of age (or up to 20 kg of body weight)?
    A) 0.1 mg
    B) 0.1 mg/kg
    C) 2.0 mg
    D) 3.0 mg/kg

Chapter Quiz Answers

1. C. When administering medications by means of a tracheal tube, temporarily stop chest compressions, instill the medication down the tube, ventilate 5 times with a bag-valve device, then resume CPR.

2. A. Anxiolysis is relief of apprehension and uneasiness without alteration of awareness. Amnesia is a lack of memory about events occurring during a particular period. Analgesia is the absence of pain in response to stimulation that would normally be painful. Anesthesia is a state of unconsciousness.

3. C. In stable patients with SVT, adenosine is the drug of choice because of its rapid onset of action and minimal effects on cardiac contractility.

4. B. Medications that can be administered by the tracheal route can be remembered by using the acronym NAVEL: Naloxone, Atropine, Vasopressin, Epinephrine, and Lidocaine.

5. D. Dopamine, epinephrine, and dobutamine are medications used to maintain cardiac output. Midazolam (Versed), lorazepam (Ativan), and diazepam (Valium) are benzodiazepines used for sedation. Naloxone (Narcan) is an opioid (narcotic) antagonist.

6. B. Sedation is a dose-dependent continuum from minimal sedation to general anesthesia. Individual patient responses to a given dosage of a drug vary. Because of this variation in patient response, the American Society of Anesthesiologists (ASA) prefers the term "sedation-analgesia" and the American

College of Emergency Physicians (ACEP) uses the term "procedural sedation" instead of "conscious sedation."

7. B. Bronchodilation and vasodilation are effects of β-2 adrenergic receptor stimulation.

8. A. The respiratory depression associated with benzodiazepines may be reversed with flumazenil. Benzodiazepines such as diazepam, lorazepam, and midazolam are sedative-hypnotic agents with potent amnestic effects that decrease patient anxiety.

9. C. Activation of the parasympathetic division of the autonomic nervous system (ANS) prepares the body for the ingestion and digestion of food, resulting in a decrease in heart rate and the strength of myocardial contractions, a decrease in blood pressure, and an increase in blood flow to the stomach and intestines. Activation of the sympathetic division of the ANS prepares the body for emergencies (i.e., the "fight-or-flight" response).

10. A. After oxygen, epinephrine is the first medication that should be administered to an infant or child with severe symptomatic bradycardia that persists despite effective oxygenation and ventilation.

11. D. In the pediatric patient, the most common sites used for a subcutaneous injection are the lateral aspect of the upper arms, the abdomen from the costal margins to the iliac crests, and the anterior thighs.

12. B. Medications used for moderate sedation/analgesia most often include benzodiazepines, opioids, and barbiturates. Paralytics are not routinely used for moderate sedation/analgesia.

13. C. Amiodarone may be used in the treatment of pulseless VT/VF and perfusing tachycardias – particularly ectopic atrial tachycardia, junctional ectopic tachycardia, and ventricular tachycardia.

14. C. The minimum recommended single dose of atropine in the pediatric patient is 0.1 mg.

15. B. For total reversal of narcotic effects, the recommended dose of naloxone for infants and children from birth to 5 years of age (or up to 20 kg of body weight) is 0.1 mg/kg. Smaller doses may be used if complete reversal is not required.

Trauma and Burns

9

Case Study

A 12-year-old girl has fallen from a third-story window in an apartment complex. At the scene, the child was found lying on her side on a sidewalk. Neighbors placed pillows under her head and instructed her not to move. Witnesses said she landed on her feet and then fell over, striking the concrete sidewalk.

Emergency Medical Technician-Basics (EMT-Bs) immobilized the child on a long backboard. She has arrived at your facility by ambulance. The child is awake. She knows her name and where she is, but does not remember the fall or events immediately preceding it. She says nothing hurts. There is an abrasion over the child's left eye, blood oozing from her left ear, and an open fracture of her left tibia/fibula.

What would you do next?

Objectives

1. Identify common mechanisms and types of injury in infants and children.
2. Explain the difference between primary and secondary brain injury.
3. Compare and contrast an epidural hematoma and subdural hematoma.
4. Explain the initial management of the patient with a head injury.
5. Explain mechanisms of injury that indicate spinal stabilization may be required.
6. Differentiate the clinical presentation of neurogenic shock from hypovolemic shock.
7. Explain the pathophysiology and initial management of a flail chest, open pneumothorax, tension pneumothorax, pulmonary contusion, and traumatic asphyxia.
8. State the immediately life-threatening and potentially life-threatening thoracic injuries.
9. Predict abdominal injuries based on blunt and penetrating mechanisms of injury.

10. Discuss mechanisms of burn injuries.
11. Identify and describe the depth classifications of burn injuries.
12. Describe how to determine the body surface area (BSA) percentage of a burn injury by using the "rule of nines" and the "rule of palms."
13. Describe the initial management of a thermal burn injury.

Mechanism of Injury/Anatomic and Physiologic Considerations

- Acute injury occurs when there is a transfer of energy from an external source to the human body that exceeds the ability of one or more body tissues to absorb that energy without loss of cellular or structural integrity.[1]
- The extent of injury is determined by the type of energy applied, how quickly it is applied, and to what part of the body it is applied.
- Recognizing the anatomic differences and injury patterns in children and the child's response to injury can assist healthcare professionals in the delivery of appropriate emergency care.
- Common childhood injuries by age group are shown in Table 9-1.
- The most common factor in acute traumatic injuries is kinetic energy (the energy of motion), and the dissipation of that energy. A child's small size and shape permits distribution of intense force over a smaller area.
- "Children are small, with less fat and elastic connective tissue, and have multiple organs in close proximity to a very pliable skeleton. Because of the smaller body mass, the transmitted injury from whatever mechanism is distributed over a smaller body that is ill-equipped to withstand this intense force, resulting in transmission of injury throughout the body and multisystem injuries in almost 50% of children with serious trauma."[2]

With the exception of burns, poisonings, and foreign bodies, trauma may be divided into two broad categories—blunt and penetrating. Because the

Blunt trauma is the most common mechanism of serious injury in the pediatric patient.

Kinematics is the process of predicting injury patterns.

TABLE 9-1 Common Childhood Injuries by Age Group

Age Group	Common Childhood Injuries
Infant	Child abuse, burns, falls, drowning
Toddler	Burns, drowning, falls, poisonings
School-age	Pedestrian injuries, bicycle-related injuries (the most serious usually involve motor vehicles), motor vehicle occupant injuries, burns, drowning
Adolescent	Motor vehicle occupant trauma, drowning, burns, intentional trauma, work-related injuries

Firearm Facts	
• In the United States, firearms are the fifth-ranking cause of death from nonintentional injury among children younger than 18 years.	• Homicide is the most common cause of death among nonwhite teenagers. Almost 80% of homicides among males involve firearms, 75% of which are handguns.
• Eighty-five percent of firearm-related deaths occur in the home.	
• Firearms are the most common means of suicide in males of all ages.	

extent and seriousness of a child's injuries may not be readily apparent on initial evaluation, knowledge of specific mechanisms of trauma is important to predict resultant injury.

Penetrating Trauma

• **Penetrating trauma** is any mechanism of injury that causes a cut or piercing of the skin. A penetrating injury typically results from a gunshot, stab wound, or blast injury, but may also result from a child's toy or foreign body. Penetrating trauma usually affects organs and tissues in the direct path of the wounding object (Figure 9-1).

• The severity of a knife wound depends on the length of the blade, angle of penetration, the area of the body pierced with the knife, and the motion applied to the blade (Figure 9-2). The severity of a firearm injury is related to the size or caliber of the bullet, alteration in the trajectory of the bullet within the body, the bullet's velocity, and the distance of the victim from the weapon.

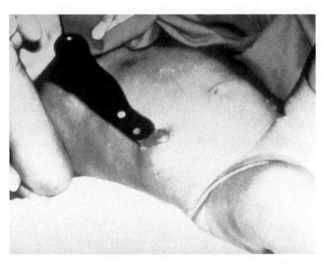

Figure 9-1   Penetrating trauma usually affects organs and tissues in the direct path of the wounding object.

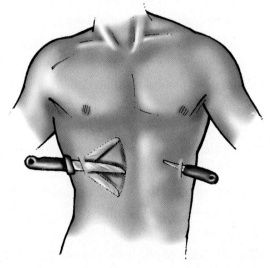

Figure 9-2   The severity of a knife wound depends on the length of the blade, angle of penetration, the area of the body pierced with the knife, and the motion applied to the blade.

- Penetrating trauma is less common in young children but is becoming an increasing problem in adolescents, particularly in urban areas.

- **Blunt trauma** is any mechanism of injury that occurs without actual penetration of the body and typically results from motor vehicle crashes (MVCs), falls, sports injuries, or assaults with a blunt object. Blunt trauma produces injury first to the body surface and then to the body's contents, resulting in compression and/or stretching of the tissue beneath the skin. The amount of injury depends on the length of time of compression, the force of compression, and the area compressed.
- Examples of compression injuries include the following:
  - Contusions and lacerations of solid organs, resulting in severe bleeding
  - Rupture of hollow (air filled) organs with subsequent spillage of the organ's contents into the abdominal cavity
- Secondary injury may occur following blunt trauma and can be more severe than the initial injury. For example, failure to successfully manage the airway of a head-injured patient can result in anoxic brain damage.

Motor Vehicle Crashes

MVCs include those involving automobiles, motorcycles, all-terrain vehicles, and tractors. An MVC may be classified by the type of impact. These include head-on (frontal), lateral, rear end, rotational, and rollover. In a MVC, three separate impacts occur as kinetic energy is transferred:

- The vehicle strikes an object.
- The occupant collides with the interior of the vehicle. This includes a seat belt, airbag, or the dashboard.
- Internal organs collide with other organs, muscle, bone, or other supporting structures inside the body. The lungs, brain, liver, and spleen are particularly vulnerable to this trauma.
- A fourth impact may occur if loose objects in the vehicle become projectiles.

The injuries that result depend on the following:

- The type of collision
- The position of the occupant inside the vehicle
- The use or nonuse of active or passive restraint systems

Child safety seats are available in several shapes and sizes to adapt to the different stages of physical development, including infant carriers, toddler seats, and booster seats. Safety seats use a combination of lap belts, shoulder belts, full-body harnesses, and harness and shield apparatus to protect the child during vehicle crashes. When used properly, the restraints

Blunt Trauma

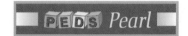

Hollow organs include the stomach, intestines, gallbladder, and urinary bladder. Solid organs include the kidneys, pancreas, liver, and spleen.

The use of lap belts alone (without a shoulder restraint) has been associated with a marked rise in seat belt–related injuries, especially fractures of the lumbar spine and hollow-viscus injuries of the abdomen.

- An unrestrained child involved in a front-end crash at 30 miles per hour hits the dashboard with the same force as that in a three-story fall.
- The potential for death of occupants ejected from a vehicle is 25 times greater than for occupants who remain with the vehicle. For occupants remaining within a vehicle, the potential for death is greatest in side impacts, followed by impact with the steering wheel and dashboard.[1]

In the United States, left-sided injuries are more common because automobiles are driven on the right side of the road.

The injury pattern experienced by a child involved in a pedestrian injury is referred to as Waddell's triad because the child experiences (a) extremity trauma, (b) thoracic and abdominal trauma, and (c) head trauma.

transfer the force of the impact from the patient's body to the restraint belts and restraint system.

An improperly worn restraint may not protect against injury in the event of a crash and may even cause injury. For example, if an infant is properly restrained in a car seat but the car seat is not properly secured to the vehicle, the infant may be ejected from the vehicle or strike various parts of the vehicle during a crash.

Predictable injuries that may occur even with proper use of a child safety seat include blunt abdominal trauma, change-of-speed injuries from deceleration forces, and neck and spinal injury.

Motor Vehicle/Pedestrian Crashes

Among children 5 to 9 years of age, pedestrian injuries are the most common cause of death from trauma. Children younger than 5 years are at risk of being run over in the driveway. Most pedestrian injuries occur during the day, peaking in the after-school period. Approximately 30% of pedestrian injuries occur while the child is in a marked crosswalk. Pedestrian injuries are the most important cause of traumatic coma in children and are a frequent cause of serious lower extremity fractures, particularly in the school-aged child.[3]

Adults will typically turn away if they are about to be struck by an oncoming vehicle, resulting in lateral or posterior injuries. In contrast, a child will usually face an oncoming vehicle, resulting in anterior injuries. Factors affecting the severity of injury include the following:

- The speed of the vehicle.
- The point of initial impact.
- Additional points of impact.
- The height and weight of the child.
- The surface on which the child lands.

Pedestrian versus MVCs have three separate phases, each with its own injury pattern.

- Initial impact (Figure 9-3)
  - Because a child is usually shorter, the initial impact of the automobile occurs higher on the body than in adults.
  - The bumper typically strikes the child's pelvis or legs (above the knees) and the fender strikes the abdomen.
  - Predictable injuries from the initial impact include injuries to the chest, abdomen, pelvis, or femur.
- Second impact (Figure 9-4)
  - The second impact occurs as the front of the vehicle's hood continues forward and strikes the child's thorax. The child is thrown backward, forcing the head and neck to flex forward.
  - Depending on the position of the child in relation to the vehicle, the

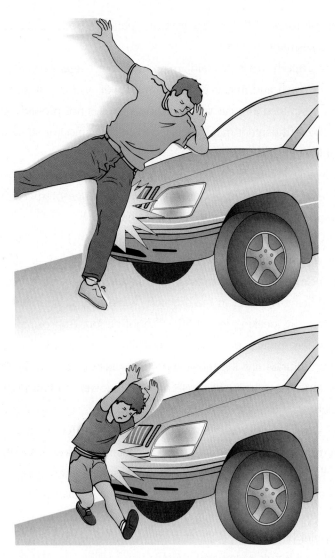

Figure 9-3   The initial impact on a child occurs when the vehicle strikes the child's upper leg or pelvis.

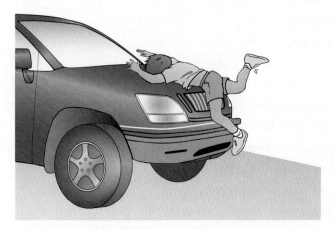

Figure 9-4   The second impact occurs when the child's head and face strike the top of the vehicle's hood.

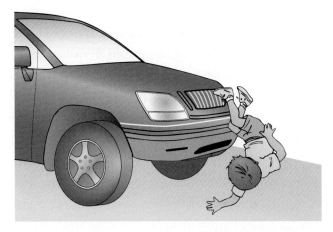

Figure 9-5   The third impact occurs as the child is thrown to ground. The child may fall under vehicle and be trapped and dragged for some distance, fall to side of vehicle and the child's lower limbs run over by a front wheel, or fall backward and end up completely under the vehicle.

child's head and face may strike the front or top of the vehicle's hood. An impression from the child's head may be left on the hood or windshield. Primary and contrecoup injuries to the head are common in this situation.

- Predictable injuries from the second impact include facial, abdominopelvic, and thoracic trauma and head and neck injury.
- Third impact (Figure 9-5)
  - The third impact occurs as the child is thrown to the ground.
  - Because of the child's smaller size and weight, the child may
    - Fall under the vehicle and be trapped and dragged for some distance
    - Fall to the side of the vehicle and the child's lower limbs run over by a front wheel
    - Fall backward and end up completely under the vehicle. In this situation, almost any injury can occur (e.g., run over by a wheel, being dragged).

Falls

- Falls are the single most common cause of injury in children. Consider the following factors in a fall:
- The height from which the child fell
- The mass of the child
- The surface the child landed on
- The part of the child's body that struck first
- The incidence of death resulting from accidental falls is low, but morbidity is high with more than 60% of children sustaining a fracture. In general, the greater the height from which the child falls, the more

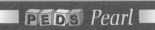

The velocity of a motor vehicle need only be 40 miles per hour for the force of impact to knock a child out of his or her shoes.[1]

Baby walkers do not help an infant develop walking skills. Thirty five percent of infants using walkers have accidents requiring emergency care.

The radius, ulna, and femur are most frequently fractured.

severe the injury. However, the type of surface onto which the child falls (concrete and trash are the most common) and the degree to which the fall is broken on the way down affect the type and severity of injuries.

- The average age of patients injured in falls from heights is approximately 5 years. Infants fall from low objects such as changing tables, high chairs, countertops, and beds. Preschool children usually fall from windows. Older boys fall from dangerous play areas, such as rooftops and fire escapes.[4]

- Children younger than 3 years are much less likely to have serious injuries than older children who fall the same distance. It is thought that younger children may better dissipate the energy transferred by the fall because they have more fat and cartilage and less muscle mass than older children.[5]

- Fatalities occur primarily when a child falls from a height of more than two stories or 22 feet (e.g., a fall from a roof, window, or balcony) or when the head of a child hits a hard surface (e.g., concrete).

- Because witnessed falls of two stories or less usually do not result in serious injury, consider the possibility of child abuse in a child with serious injuries from a fall that was reportedly from a low height, particularly if the fall was unwitnessed.[4] Some children jump to avoid beatings or fires, and some are pushed by siblings or parents.[6]

Falls from greater heights tend to occur in warm weather, probably because windows are more likely to be open.

Bicycle Injuries

- In the United States, children from age 5 to 14 are seen in emergency departments more often for injuries associated with bicycles than with any other sport. Most severe and fatal bicycle injuries involve head trauma. Other injuries associated with bicycle crashes include facial and extremity trauma and abdominal injuries (from striking the handle bars).

- The use of helmets can reduce the risk of head injury. A helmet absorbs some of the energy and dissipates the blow over a larger area for a slightly longer time. The skull provides another layer of protection and absorbs additional energy.[7]

- Studies indicate that helmets are very effective, reducing the risk of head injury by 85% and serious brain injury by 88%.[3] Helmets also protect against injuries to the mid and upper face.

- All young children should wear a bicycle helmet, whether they are riding a bicycle, a tricycle, or are a passenger on a parent's bicycle. Bicycle helmets for children ages 1 to 5 cover a larger portion of the head than helmets for older individuals.

A child younger than 1 year should never be carried on a bicycle.

- Any helmet involved in a crash or otherwise damaged should be discarded and replaced. Otherwise, all helmets should be replaced at least every 5 years or sooner if recommended by the manufacturer.

Assessment of the Pediatric Trauma Patient

Detailed information regarding patient assessment has been discussed in a previous chapter. Specific points to consider during assessment of the pediatric trauma patient are presented here.

Scene Safety

On arrival, assess the scene for safety, mechanism of injury, and other victims. Ensure the scene is safe before proceeding with your assessment of the patient.

The Pediatric Assessment Triangle (PAT)

From a distance, evaluate the child's appearance, work of breathing, circulation, and the presence of obvious injuries to determine the severity of the child's injury and assist you in determining the urgency for care. If the child's condition is urgent, proceed immediately with rapid assessment of airway, breathing, and circulation. Treat problems as you find them.

Primary Survey

Airway and Cervical Spine Protection

- Assume spinal injury if the child is unresponsive or has an altered mental status, has experienced blunt trauma above the nipple line, has a significant mechanism of injury, complains of neck or back pain, numbness or tingling, loss of movement or weakness, or has multiple injuries of any cause.
- If cervical spine injury is suspected (by examination, history, or mechanism of injury), manually stabilize the head and neck in a neutral in-line position or maintain spinal stabilization if already completed.
  - If the patient's spine has not already been stabilized, do not take the time to apply a cervical collar until the primary survey is finished. Maintain manual in-line cervical spine stabilization throughout the assessment and management of the patient until cervical spine injury has been ruled out or until the patient has been properly secured to a backboard.
  - Do NOT apply traction to the neck. In a child with possible cervical spine trauma, the application of traction can exacerbate an existing injury or convert a stable cervical fracture to an unstable fracture. If an attempt to move the head and neck into a neutral in-line position results in any of the following, STOP any movement and stabilize the head in that position:
    - Compromise of the airway or ventilation
    - Neck muscle spasm
    - Increased pain

- Onset or increase of a neurologic deficit such as numbness, tingling, or loss of motor ability
- The prominent occiput of infants and young children often causes passive flexion of the neck when the child is placed in a supine position on a flat surface (Figure 9-6). Flexion of the neck may compromise air exchange or aggravate an existing spinal cord injury (SCI).
- To maintain the cervical spine in a neutral position, it is often necessary to place padding under the child's torso. The padding should be firm, evenly shaped, and extend from the shoulders to the pelvis (Figure 9-7). Use of irregularly shaped or insufficient padding or placing padding only under the shoulders can result in movement and misalignment of the spine.

For an infant or small child, the padding should be of appropriate thickness so that the child's shoulders are in horizontal alignment with the ear canal.

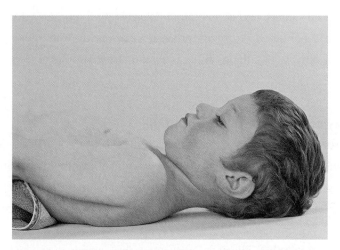

Figure 9-6   The prominent occiput of an infant or young child often causes passive flexion of the neck when the child is placed in a supine position on a flat surface.

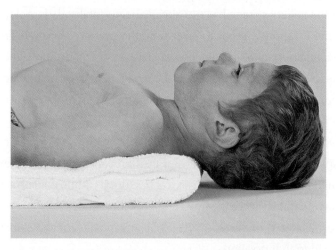

Figure 9-7   To maintain the cervical spine in a neutral position, it is often necessary to place padding under the torso of an infant or young child. The padding should be of appropriate thickness so that the child's shoulders are in horizontal alignment with the ear canal.

If blood, vomitus, or other secretions are visible, suction the oropharynx with a rigid (tonsil tip) suction catheter before manually opening the airway.

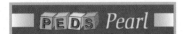

After intubation, remember to confirm placement of the tracheal tube with both primary (assessment) methods and at least one secondary (mechanical) method (e.g., end-tidal carbon dioxide, chest radiograph).

Intubation can be performed with simultaneous in-line stabilization of the cervical spine.

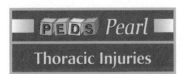

Thoracic Injuries

Immediately life-threatening injuries that must be identified and managed in the primary survey include the following:
- **Airway obstruction**
- **Open pneumothorax**
- **Tension pneumothorax**
- **Massive hemothorax**
- **Flail chest**
- **Cardiac tamponade**

Gastric distention is a cause of ventilatory compromise that is frequently overlooked.

- If the child is unresponsive and trauma is suspected, use the jaw thrust without head tilt maneuver to open the airway. If the airway is open, move on to evaluation of the patient's breathing. If the airway is not open, assess for sounds of airway compromise (snoring, gurgling, or stridor). Look in the mouth for blood, broken teeth, gastric contents, and foreign objects (e.g., loose teeth, gum). Suction as needed.
- Insert an oropharyngeal airway as needed to maintain an open airway.
  - Use of a nasopharyngeal airway (NPA) is not recommended if trauma to the mid face is present or in cases of a known or suspected basilar skull fracture. If a basilar or cribriform plate fracture is present, the NPA may enter the cranial vault during insertion.
- Perform tracheal intubation if airway patency cannot be maintained by other means.
  - Rapid sequence intubation (RSI) should be considered for those patients in whom intubation may otherwise be difficult due to combativeness, seizures, clenched teeth, or posturing.
  - RSI provides a controlled method of achieving airway access while limiting the risk of complications, such as aspiration of stomach contents.
- Indications for tracheal intubation in the injured child include the following[8]:
  - Inability to ventilate the child by bag-valve-mask methods
  - The need for prolonged control of the airway
  - Prevention of aspiration in a comatose child
  - The need for controlled hyperventilation in patients with serious head injuries
  - Flail chest with pulmonary contusion
  - Shock unresponsive to fluid volume replacement
- Although rarely necessary in the pediatric patient, cricothyroidotomy may be necessary if less invasive airway methods have been unsuccessful. Needle cricothyroidotomy is preferred over surgical cricothyroidotomy in a child younger than 10 years.

Breathing and Ventilation

Expose the child's chest and abdomen. Look for surface trauma, penetrating wounds, paradoxic motion, and retractions. If the patient is breathing, determine if breathing is adequate or inadequate.

Look at the rate and depth of respiration.

- Assess the chest and abdomen for respiratory movement.
- Evaluate the depth (tidal volume) and symmetry of movement with each breath.
- Determine if the patient's respiratory rate is within normal limits for the child's age.

Listen for the presence and quality of bilateral breath sounds and briefly listen to heart sounds.

- To minimize the possibility of sound transmission from one side of the chest to the other, listen along the midaxillary line (under each armpit) and in the midclavicular line under each clavicle. Alternate from side to side and compare your findings.
- Briefly listen to heart sounds to establish a baseline from which to compare (e.g., development of muffled heart sounds).

Feel for air movement from the nose or mouth against your chin, face, or palm. Palpate the chest for tenderness, instability, and crepitation. Assess for the presence of respiratory distress/failure. Note signs of increased work of breathing (respiratory effort).

If breathing is adequate, provide supplemental oxygen and move on to assessment of circulation. If breathing is inadequate:

- Ensure the airway is clear of blood, vomitus, and foreign material.
- Provide supplemental oxygen and, if necessary, positive-pressure ventilation.
- Ensure the patient's chest wall rises with each ventilation. Continue the primary survey.

If breathing is absent:

- Insert an airway adjunct (if not previously done and not contraindicated) and deliver two slow breaths with a pocket mask or bag-valve-mask with supplemental oxygen.
- Ensure the patient's chest wall rises with each ventilation. Continue the primary survey.

If an open pneumothorax is present (i.e., sucking chest wound), cover the wound with a sterile occlusive dressing taped on three sides (Figure 9-8).

All injured children should receive supplemental oxygen. Attempt to keep the SpO_2 at greater than 95%.

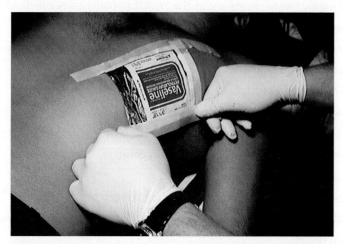

Figure 9-8   If an open pneumothorax is present (i.e., sucking chest wound), cover the wound with a sterile occlusive dressing taped on three sides.

If signs of a tension pneumothorax are present, needle decompression is indicated.

Circulation and Bleeding Control

Heart rate, capillary refill (in children younger than 6 years), and mental status are signs that are particularly helpful in detecting shock.

Internal bleeding should be suspected if the child shows signs of shock but there is no evidence of external volume loss.

- Rapidly assess the child for signs of shock.
  - Look for visible external hemorrhage.
    - Control major bleeding, if present. Apply direct pressure over the bleeding site with sterile dressings. Elevate the extremity (unless contraindicated). Apply pressure over arterial pressure points if necessary.
  - Consider possible areas of major internal hemorrhage.
    - Significant internal hemorrhage may occur in the chest, abdomen, pelvis, retroperitoneum, and femoral areas. Pain or swelling in any of these areas may signal possible internal hemorrhage.
  - Compare the strength and quality of central and peripheral pulses.
    - If a pulse is absent, begin chest compressions immediately and consider possible causes of the arrest (e.g., hypovolemia, tension pneumothorax, cardiac tamponade). Begin appropriate interventions.
    - If a pulse is present, determine if the patient's heart rate is within normal limits for the child's age. Note the quality of the pulse (thready, bounding, weak, or irregular).
  - Evaluate skin color, temperature, moisture, and capillary refill.

If signs of shock are present, establish vascular access. If decompensated shock is present, establish access in two sites using large-bore catheters. In the field, the presence of shock in an infant or child indicates rapid stabilization and transport are needed immediately. Obtain intravenous (IV)/intraosseous (IO) access quickly or on the way to an appropriate receiving facility. Transport must not be delayed for multiple vascular access attempts at the scene. Begin fluid resuscitation with 20 mL/kg of an isotonic crystalloid solution (e.g., normal saline [NS] or lactated Ringer's [LR]).

Disability (Mental Status)

To rapidly assess the patient's level of responsiveness, use the AVPU scale. This version of the Glasgow Coma Scale (GCS) modified for pediatric use (see Chapter 3) provides a more thorough assessment of the patient's neurologic status and can be used to document the patient's progress over time.

Avoid vague terms such as *lethargic or obtunded* when describing a patient's level of responsiveness. Use descriptive phrases that describe the child's awareness of his or her environment and the appropriateness of his or her response. For example, "cries vigorously and fights attempts at venipuncture."

PEDS Pearl

In an injured patient, tachycardia may be a compensatory response to hypovolemia, but may also be a response to fear, pain, anxiety, or stress. Prolonged capillary refill and cool extremities may indicate poor perfusion, but may also occur as a result of fright or cold weather. Be sure to correlate your patient's vital signs with your assessment findings when considering your treatment plan.

Expose/Environment

Undress the patient. Preserve body heat and maintain appropriate temperature. Respect the child's modesty. Keep the child covered if possible and replace clothing promptly after examining each body area.

Cervical Spine Stabilization

- After completing the primary survey, apply a rigid cervical collar if a device of appropriate size is available. Maintain the neck in a neutral position before and during application of the collar. A rigid cervical collar should be applied *only if it fits properly*. Estimate the distance between the angle of the jaw and the top of the shoulder and use a collar of that width. The collar should be measured in width from the top of the shoulder to the chin when the head is in a neutral position.

- A collar that is too tight may cause airway compromise or compress the veins of the neck, causing circulatory compromise. A collar that is too loose may accidentally cover the anterior chin, mouth, and nose, resulting in an airway obstruction. A collar that is too short will permit significant flexion, ineffectively limiting motion. A collar that is too large may cause hyperextension or full motion if the chin is inside of it, or push the jaw posteriorly, occluding the airway.

- If a properly fitting device is not available, use towels, washcloths, or blanket rolls (depending on the child's size) and adhesive tape across the forehead to immobilize the head as best as possible. Avoid the use of IV bags or sand bags; their weight may push the cervical spine out of alignment.

Spinal stabilization: possible contraindications[9]:

- Combative child
  - Efforts to forcefully immobilize a combative child with a possible head or spinal injury may result in further manipulation of the spine and exacerbate the injury.
  - If the risks of agitation and increased spinal movement from full spinal stabilization are greater than the benefits, defer the stabilization procedure and consider other stabilization options. For example, enlist the assistance of the child's parent or caregiver to hold the child in a position the child can tolerate that has a neutral effect on the spine and minimizes movement.
- Penetrating foreign body to the neck with hemorrhage
- Massive cervical swelling
- Presence of a tracheal stoma that is integral to the management of the patient's airway
- Requirement for any maneuver to ensure adequate oxygenation and ventilation

Before applying the cervical collar, assess the neck veins and palpate the position of the trachea to determine if it is in a midline position.

If full spinal stabilization is indicated but not performed, be sure to clearly document the circumstances in the patient's medical record.

Manual stabilization is better in these situations.

PEDS Pearl

Spinal Stabilization: Indications

- Mechanisms of injury involving blunt or penetrating trauma directly to the spine or forces applied to the spine involving flexion, extension, or rotation of the head and neck (e.g., sports injuries, falls from heights)
- If the mechanism of injury may have resulted in rapid, forceful head movement
- Consider in any child with an altered mental status and no history available, found in setting of possible trauma, or near drowning with history or probability of diving
- Neurologic deficit in the arms or legs
- Significant helmet damage
- Local tenderness or deformity in the cervical, thoracic, or lumbar region

PEDS Pearl

When used alone, a rigid cervical collar does not immobilize. A rigid collar is for the following:

- Temporarily splint the head and neck in a neutral position
- Limit movement of the cervical spine
- Support the weight of the head while the patient is in a sitting position
- Help maintain alignment of the cervical spine when the patient is in a supine position

- Remind the patient and healthcare professionals that the integrity of the patient's cervical spine is questionable because of the mechanism of injury

For effective stabilization, a rigid collar must be used with manual stabilization or mechanical stabilization provided by a suitable spine stabilization device.

Transfer/Transport Decision

At the end of the primary survey, you should have sufficient information to make important decisions about your patient's care.

- In the field, it is important to remember that definitive care for a trauma patient requires physician evaluation of the patient at an appropriate facility. With this in mind, limit scene time to 10 minutes or less if the patient's condition is critical. The patient should be rapidly packaged after initiating essential field interventions and transported to the closest appropriate facility.

- In an urgent care or hospital setting, the physician evaluating the patient should determine if the patient requires transfer to another facility for definitive care. If this decision is made, additional patient care and evaluation can be performed while preparations are made for the patient's transfer. Communication between the referring physician and receiving physician is essential.

Suggestions for Radiographic Evaluation of the Cervical Spine[18]	
Preverbal or Precooperative Child at Risk of Cervical Spine Injury **High Risk** • Fall in which the body weight lands on the head • Head-on MVC with child in a forward-facing seat • Abnormal posture of the head and neck • Anomaly of the face, head, or neck • Any suspicion of nonaccidental trauma • Evidence of intracranial injury or significant facial trauma • High-speed, rear-end impact with an infant in a rear-facing seat • Risky mechanism with distracting pain • Neck tenderness • Neurologic deficit • Fall while in an infant walker	**Low Risk** • Head-on MVC with child in a rear-facing seat • Short fall in which impact is evenly distributed between trunk and head • Unwitnessed short fall with no scalp hematoma or soft-tissue injury • Lateral impact MVC with the child in appropriate restraint and no evidence of intracranial injury or concussion Verbal and Cooperative Child at Risk for Cervical Spine Injury • Neck tenderness • Neurologic abnormality • Distracting pain with adequate mechanism • Altered mental status • High-energy impact involving a child younger than 8 years

Pediatric Trauma Score

The Pediatric Trauma Score (PTS) is a scoring tool used to evaluate the severity of injury in the pediatric patient and assist in pediatric triage decisions. The PTS consists of six parameters that are evaluated during the initial assessment of an injured child. Each parameter is assessed and given a numeric score based on three variables: +2 (no injury or non–life-threatening), +1 (minor injury or potentially life-threatening), or −1 (life-threatening). The scores are then added together. Children with a PTS of less than 8 should be treated in a designated trauma center.

TABLE 9-2 Pediatric Trauma Score

Clinical Category	Score		
	+2	+1	−1
Size	Child/adolescent above 20 kg (44 lb)	Toddler 10 to kg (22 to 44 lb)	Infant Less than 10 kg (22 lb)
Airway	Patent; no assistance required	Maintainable by patient but observation needed to adequate airway (e.g., positioning, suctioning)	Unmaintainable; airway devices needed to maintain airway (e.g., oral airway, tracheal tube, cricothyroidotomy)
Mental status (AVPU)	Awake; no loss of consciousness	Obtunded; responds to verbal or painful stimulus; any loss of consciousness	Coma, unresponsive, decerebrate
Systolic blood pressure (or central pulse)	Above 90 mm Hg Good peripheral pulses	50 to 90 mm Hg Weak carotid/femoral pulse palpable	Below 50 mm Hg Very weak or no pulses
Skeletal (fractures)	None seen or suspected	Single closed fracture anywhere or suspected	Open or multiple fractures
Open wounds	No visible injury	Minor contusion, abrasion, laceration smaller than 7 cm not through fascia, burns less than 10% and not involving hands, face, feet, or genitalia	Major/penetrating; tissue loss, any gunshot wound or stab through fascia; burns more than 10% or involving hands, face, feet, or genitalia

Scoring: 9–12, minor trauma; 6–8, potentially life-threatening; 0–5, life threatening; below 0, usually fatal.
Adapted from Tepas JJ III, Mollitt DL, Talbert JL. The pediatric trauma score as a predictor of injury severity in the injured child. *J Pediatr Surg* 1987;22:14–18.

Secondary Survey

Remember to use age-appropriate language when asking questions of the patient.

The history is often obtained simultaneously during the physical examination and while interventions are performed.

Focused History

In addition to the SAMPLE or CIAMPEDS history, consider the following questions when obtaining a focused history for a pediatric trauma patient. This list will require modification based on the patient's age, mechanism of injury, and patient's chief complaint.

Mechanism of Injury

- How did the injury occur? When?
- Circumstances of the incident: Does the explanation for how the trauma occurred fit the injury and the child's abilities?

Fall Injury

- Height of the fall?
- What type of surface did the child land on?

Motor Vehicle Crash

- Site of impact (e.g., lateral, frontal)? Estimated speed? What was struck (e.g., moving or stationary object)? Amount of damage to the vehicle?

- Where was the child located in the vehicle? Was the child restrained? Was the child's safety seat properly secured?
- Was the vehicle equipped with an air bag? If so, did the air bag deploy (open)?
- Ejected from the vehicle? Prolonged extrication required? Scene fatalities?

Pedestrian Injury

- If the child was struck by a car and thrown while walking, roller-skating, or bicycling, was a helmet worn? If so, is it still in place or was it knocked off the head on impact? Is there damage to the helmet?
- How fast was the car traveling?
- Where was the child struck?
- How far was the child thrown?
- What type of surface did the child land on?

Bicycle Injury

- If struck by a motor vehicle, was the vehicle moving or stationary? If moving, estimated speed?
- Was the child wearing a helmet? If so, is it still in place or was it knocked off the head on impact? Is there damage to the helmet?

Burns

- Location of the burn?
- What caused the burn (e.g., fire, scalding, electrical shock, chemicals)?
- How long ago did the injury occur?
- What treatment has been given?

Penetrating Trauma

- Location of the wound(s)?
- Type/caliber/velocity of the weapon
- Distance from which the child was shot (close range or long range) or stabbed?
- Presence of powder burns surrounding the wounds?
- Number of shots or stab wounds?
- Estimated blood loss at the scene?

Chronology

- Initial GCS?
- Behavior immediately after the incident (e.g., crying, stunned, seizure, unconscious)?
- LOC immediately or shortly after the incident? Duration?
- Any breathing problems following the injury?

Physical Examination

A detailed physical examination is presented here; however, a focused physical examination may be more appropriate, based on your patient's presentation and chief complaint.

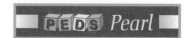

PEDS *Pearl*

In the prehospital setting, perform the secondary survey en route to an appropriate facility if you have a priority (critical) patient. If the patient is stable, the secondary survey can be performed on the scene; however, factors such as time of day, traffic and weather conditions, and distance from an appropriate receiving facility may affect your decision to do so.

- Obtain vital signs, attach a pulse oximeter, electrocardiogram (ECG) monitor, and blood pressure monitor. Evaluate the information obtained and determine if it is within normal range for the patient's age.
- Inspect and palpate each of the major body areas for DCAP-BLS-TIC (**D**eformities, **C**ontusions, **A**brasions, **P**enetrations/punctures, **B**urns, **L**acerations, **S**welling/edema, **T**enderness, **I**nstability, **C**repitus)

Head and Face

A scalp laceration can result in significant blood loss in an infant or child. If present, control bleeding as quickly as possible.

- Inspect the scalp and skull for DCAP-BLS. Palpate for DCAP-BLS-TIC, depressions, protrusions.
  - In a child younger than 14 months, gently palpate the anterior and posterior fontanelles. Feel for any bulging beyond the level of the skull. A bulging fontanelle in a quiet infant may indicate increased intracranial pressure (ICP)
  - Assess for other signs of a head injury. If brain tissue is visible, cover it with a saline-moistened sterile dressing.
- Inspect the ears for DCAP-BLS, postauricular ecchymosis (Battle's sign), blood, or clear fluid in the ears. Palpate for tenderness or pain.
- Inspect the face for DCAP-BLS, singed facial hair, symmetry of facial expression. Palpate the orbital rims, zygoma, maxilla, and mandible for DCAP-BLS-TIC, neurovascular impairment, muscle spasm, false motion, or motor impairment.

In a trauma patient, unequal or fixed and dilated pupils suggest severe brain injury.

- Inspect the eyes for DCAP-BLS, foreign body, blood in the anterior chamber of the eye (hyphema), presence of eyeglasses or contact lenses, periorbital ecchymosis (raccoon eyes), color of sclera and conjunctiva, periorbital edema, pupils (size, shape, equality, reactivity to light), eye movement (dysconjugate gaze, ocular muscle function).
- Inspect the nose for DCAP-BLS, blood or fluid from the nose, singed nasal hairs, nares for flaring. Palpate the nasal bones.

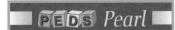

To quickly assess the cranial nerves in a child who can follow commands, ask the child to close his or her eyes, open his or her eyes wide, follow a finger with his or her eyes, open his or her mouth, and stick out his or her tongue.

- Inspect the mouth for DCAP-BLS, blood, absent or broken teeth, gastric contents, foreign objects (e.g., loose teeth, gum, small toys); injured or swollen tongue, color of the mucous membranes of the mouth, note presence and character of fluids, vomitus; note sputum color, amount, and consistency (Figure 9-9). Listen for hoarseness, inability to talk. Note unusual odors (e.g., alcohol, acetone, almonds).

Neck

- Inspect the neck for DCAP-BLS, neck veins (flat or distended), use of accessory muscles, presence of a hematoma, presence of a stoma, and presence of a medical identification device.
- Palpate for DCAP-BLS-TIC, subcutaneous emphysema, and tracheal position. Subcutaneous emphysema feels like "Rice Krispies" or bubble wrap.

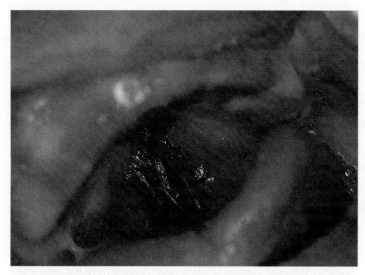

Figure 9-9　This infant's soft palate was shredded by repeated stabs with a sharp object. He presented with a report of spitting up blood and no history of trauma.

Chest

- Inspect the chest. Assess work of breathing, symmetry of movement, use of accessory muscles, and presence of retractions. Note abnormal breathing patterns, DCAP-BLS, and presence of vascular access devices.
- Auscultate the chest. Assess the equality of breath sounds and presence of adventitious breath sounds (e.g., crackles, wheezes). Evaluate heart sounds for rate, rhythm, murmurs, bruits, gallops, friction rub, and muffled heart tones.
- Palpate for DCAP-BLS-TIC, chest wall tenderness, symmetry of chest wall expansion, and subcutaneous emphysema.

Abdomen, Pelvis, and Genitalia

- Inspect the abdomen for DCAP-BLS, distention, scars from healed surgical incisions or penetrating wounds, feeding tubes, use of abdominal muscles during respiration, signs of injury, discoloration, tire marks, and signs of seat belt injury.
- Auscultate the presence or absence of bowel sounds in all quadrants
- Palpate all four quadrants for DCAP-BLS, guarding or distention, rigidity, masses
- In the hospital setting, examine the perineum for lacerations, hematomas, or active bleeding and examine the rectum for integrity of the wall, muscle tone, prostatic injury, and occult gastrointestinal (GI) bleeding.
- Assess the integrity of the pelvis.
  - First, gently palpate for point tenderness.
  - Next, place your hands on each iliac crest and press gently inward. If pain, crepitation, or instability is elicited, suspect a fracture of the

PEDS *Pearl*

Assessment of an infant or young child's abdomen can be difficult. The abdomen of a young child is naturally protuberant and may appear somewhat distended. An infant will naturally tense his or her abdominal muscles when palpated, simulating guarding. A toddler may scream throughout the examination. It may be necessary to evaluate the abdomen more than once for a more accurate assessment.

Intraabdominal bleeding is a common cause of reversible shock.

pelvic ring. No further assessment is necessary if this assessment reveals positive findings.

  ◦ If this assessment is negative, simultaneously push down on both iliac crests. Then place one hand on the pubic bone (over the symphysis pubis) and apply gentle pressure.

Extremities

Assess and document pulses, motor function, and sensory function before and after splinting.

Examine each extremity for five P's: pain, pallor, paralysis, paresthesia, and pulses. Compare an injured extremity to an uninjured extremity and document your findings.

- Inspect each extremity for DCAP-BLS and abnormal extremity position.
- Palpate for DCAP-BLS-TIC.
  ◦ Assess skin temperature, moisture, and capillary refill in each extremity.
  ◦ Assess the strength and quality of pulses, motor function, and sensory function (PMS) in each extremity.
  ◦ If the child is alert, assess sensation by lightly touching the extremity and asking, "Do you feel me brushing your skin? Where?"
  ◦ Assess motor function in an upper extremity in an alert patient by instructing the child to "Squeeze my fingers in your hand." To assess motor function in a lower extremity, instruct the child to "Push down on my fingers with your toes."
  ◦ When assessing a child's sensory function, carefully consider the method you will use. A pinch in a child may result in more distress, distrust, and/or a lack of cooperation. Consider a less distressing method such as, "Can you feel my hand touching your toes?"

PEDS Pearl

Because they can be a source of significant blood loss, long bone fractures can contribute to the development of hypovolemic shock.

Posterior Body

Ensure manual in-line stabilization of the head and spine during examination of the posterior body.

- Inspect the posterior body for DCAP-BLS, purpura, petechiae, rashes, and edema.
- Auscultate the posterior thorax.
- Palpate the posterior trunk for DCAP-BLS.

Ongoing Assessment

Perform an ongoing assessment (also called monitoring and reassessment) to reevaluate the patient's condition, assess the effectiveness of emergency care interventions provided, identify any missed injuries or conditions, observe subtle changes or trends in the patient's condition, and alter emergency care interventions as needed.

An ongoing assessment should be

- Performed on EVERY patient

- Performed after assuring completion of critical interventions
- Performed after the detailed physical examination, if one is performed. (In some situations, the patient's condition may preclude performance of the detailed physical examination.)
- Repeated and documented every 5 minutes for an unstable patient
- Repeated and documented every 15 minutes for a stable patient

Head Trauma

The head of the pediatric patient is vulnerable to injury because of the following:

- The skull of an infant and child is thin and pliable and is more likely to transfer force to the brain beneath it instead of fracturing and absorbing some of the force along the fracture line.
- The disproportionately large size and weight of the head (Figure 9-10) adds to the momentum of acceleration-deceleration forces and accounts for the fact that infants and children tend to "lead with their head" when falling or when thrown (whether bodily or ejected from a motor vehicle).
- Underdeveloped cervical ligaments, relatively weak neck muscles, and anteriorly wedged cervical vertebrae make an infant susceptible to extreme hyperflexion and hyperextension of the neck and greater head motion when subjected to acceleration-deceleration forces.[10]

Brain Perfusion

- The brain is sensitive to decreases in glucose, oxygen, and perfusion.
- Brain perfusion must be maintained to optimize a child's chances of a good recovery after a head injury.

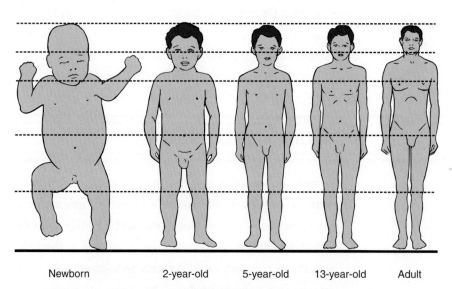

Newborn   2-year-old   5-year-old   13-year-old   Adult

Figure 9-10 Changes in the proportions of body parts from birth to maturity. Note the dramatic differences in head size.

CPP = MAP − ICP

Edema, hypotension, and bleeding can interfere with CPP.

Maintenance of an adequate blood volume and blood pressure is critical for brain perfusion. If the blood pressure is reduced, so is CPP.

- Cerebral perfusion pressure (CPP) is determined by the difference between mean arterial blood pressure (MAP) and ICP.
- A mechanism called autoregulation regulates the body's blood pressure to maintain CPP. It is generally believed that attempts to maintain the CPP above 70 mm Hg improves outcome; however, there are no systematic scientific studies to validate this.[11]
- The brain can compensate for changes in ICP by manipulating one of three major components of the skull (a decrease in any one of these will lower ICP):
  - Brain tissue (occupies 78% of the skull)
  - Blood volume (occupies 12%)
  - Cerebrospinal fluid (CSF) (occupies 10%)

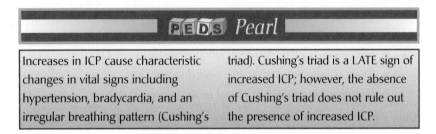

PEDS Pearl

Increases in ICP cause characteristic changes in vital signs including hypertension, bradycardia, and an irregular breathing pattern (Cushing's triad). Cushing's triad is a LATE sign of increased ICP; however, the absence of Cushing's triad does not rule out the presence of increased ICP.

General Categories of Injury

- Coup injuries: injury directly below point of impact
- Contrecoup injuries: injury at another site, usually opposite the impact
- Diffuse axonal injury (DAI): shearing, tearing, stretching force of nerve fibers with axonal damage
- Focal injury: an identifiable site of injury limited to a particular area or region of the brain

Causes of Brain Injury

Primary (direct) injury

- Refers to the direct damage incurred during the actual injury/impact to the head.
- Damage resulting in dysfunction occurs to the scalp and skull, neurons, axons, and blood vessels.
- Examples of primary injuries include skull fractures, concussions, contusions, lacerations, axon-shearing injuries, and neuronal and vascular damage.

If left untreated, secondary injuries can exacerbate the primary injury.

Secondary or tertiary (indirect) injury

- Secondary injury: the result of metabolic events precipitated by the trauma that produce damage to the brain minutes, hours, or days after the initial event.
- Examples of secondary injuries include cerebral ischemia and brain edema, which may result from systemic hypotension, hypercapnia, and hypoxemia.

- Vasospasm, seizures, meningitis, and hydrocephalus may also produce secondary injury.
- Tertiary injury: caused by apnea, hypotension, pulmonary resistance, and change in ECG.

Head injury

- Definition: a traumatic insult to the head that may result in injury to soft tissue, bony structures, and/or brain injury
- Categories: blunt (closed) trauma and open (penetrating trauma)
  - Blunt head trauma (common)
    - Dura remains intact during the injury and brain tissue is not exposed to the environment (Figure 9-11)
    - May result in fractures, focal brain injuries, and/or diffuse axonal injuries
  - Penetrating head trauma (less common)
    - Dura and cranial contents penetrated (Figure 9-12)
    - Brain tissue exposed to the environment
    - Results in fractures and focal brain injury

Brain injury

- Defined by the National Head Injury Foundation as "a traumatic insult to the brain capable of producing physical, intellectual, emotional, social, and vocational changes"
- Categories: focal injury, subarachnoid hemorrhage, or DAI

GCS

- GCS score is a reliable indicator of the severity of injury and deterioration or improvement. The initial GCS score often influences treatment/transport/transfer decisions.
  - GCS score of 3 to 7 = severe injury
  - GCS score of 8 to 12 = moderate injury
  - GCS score of 13 to 15 = mild injury

Concussion (Mild Diffuse Axonal Injury)

- A brain insult with transient impairment of consciousness followed by rapid recovery to baseline neurologic activity
- Most common result of blunt trauma to the head
- Infrequently associated with structural brain injury and rarely lead to significant long-term sequelae
- Concussion grades
  - Grade 1 definition: transient confusion, no loss of consciousness (LOC), and duration of mental status abnormalities less than 15 minutes.
  - Grade 2 definition: transient confusion, no LOC, and duration of mental status abnormalities of more than 15 minutes.
  - Grade 3 definition: concussion involving LOC.

Categories of Head and Brain Injury

Diffuse Axonal Injury

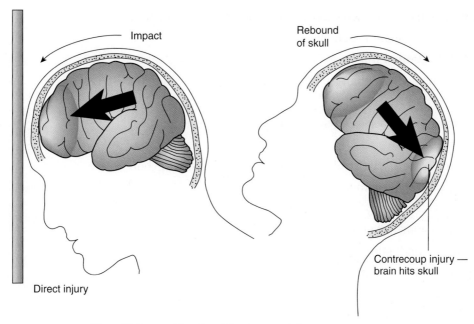

Closed Injury — Direct and Contrecoup Injury

Figure 9-11   A closed head injury occurs when the dura remains intact during the injury and brain tissue is not exposed to the environment, but the brain tissue is injured. Blood vessels may rupture because of the force exerted against the skull.

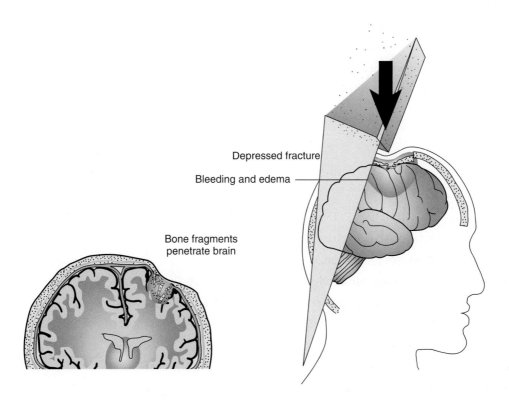

Open Injury

Figure 9-12   In an open head injury, the dura is penetrated, exposing the cranial contents to the environment.

- Assessment: confusion, disorientation, amnesia of the event; anorexia, vomiting, or pallor common soon after the insult

Moderate Diffuse Axonal Injury

- Shearing, stretching, or tearing results in minute petechial bruising of brain tissue.
- Brainstem and reticular activating system may be involved leading to unresponsiveness.
- Commonly associated with basilar skull fracture, most survive but neurologic impairment common.
- Assessment
  - May result in immediate unresponsiveness or persistent confusion, disorientation, and amnesia of the event extending to amnesia of moment-to-moment events.
  - May have focal deficit.
  - Residual cognitive (inability to concentrate), psychologic (frequent periods of anxiety, uncharacteristic mood swings), and sensori-motor deficits (sense of smell altered) may persist.

Severe Diffuse Axonal Injury

- Formerly called brainstem injury
- Involves severe mechanical disruption of many axons in both cerebral hemispheres and extending to the brainstem
- Assessment: unresponsiveness for prolonged period, posturing common, other signs of increased ICP occur depending on various degrees of damage

Skull Fractures

Types

- Linear
  - Line crack in the skull (Figures 9-13 and 9-14).
  - Most common type of skull fracture; make up approximately 60% to 90% of skull fractures in children.
  - Most linear fractures have an overlying hematoma or soft-tissue swelling, although the swelling may not be detectable if the child is evaluated within a short period of the trauma or if the swelling is underlying the patient's hair.
  - Larger hematomas or hematomas in the temporal or parietal regions are more likely to indicate fracture.
  - Rarely require therapy and are often associated with good outcomes; uncomplicated linear skull fractures heal spontaneously within 6 months without surgical treatment.
  - Linear fractures that may be associated with a less favorable outcome include those that overlie a vascular channel, a fracture

Focal Injuries

Significance is in the amount of force involved.

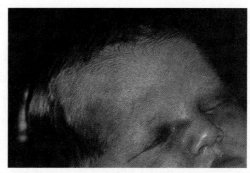

Figure 9-13   Bilateral black eyes are seen in this 12-day-old. His father reported that he had fallen on the stairs while holding the baby in a football hold and that, in the fall, the baby hit the steps face first with the father landing on top of him. The absence of an associated forehead hematoma or frontal fracture and the presence of an occipital fracture consistent with impact against a hard surface (not the father's chest) belied this story. Nevertheless, abuse was not suspected and the baby was sent home. He returned 3 months later in extremis with massive intracranial injury and died. On this occasion, the father said he had found the infant choking and gasping for breath and that he picked him up and shook him to revive him.

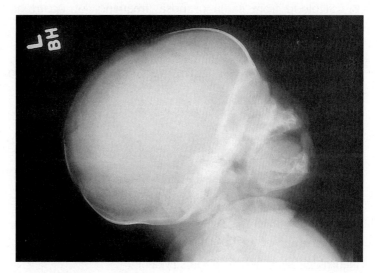

Figure 9-14   This linear skull fracture was found in the infant in Figure 9-13.

that extends through a suture line, or a fracture that extends over the area of the middle meningeal artery.

- Depressed
  - Pieces of bone are pushed inward pressing on, and sometimes causing tearing of, brain tissue.
  - Most commonly seen in the parietal area; a fracture in this area causes concern because the underlying brain may have been

bruised or lacerated and there is a higher likelihood of intracranial hemorrhage.

- In some cases, the fracture is open (a compound fracture) or comminuted, and requires neurosurgical débridement and inspection.
  - A neurosurgeon may consider surgical elevation of the bony edges if the depression is greater than either the thickness of the skull or 5 mm.
- Neurologic signs and symptoms evident.
- Cover the depressed area with a sterile dressing moistened with sterile saline.
- Monitor closely for signs of increased ICP.
- Basilar
  - Extension of linear fracture to floor of skull; may not be seen on radiograph or computed tomography (CT) scan.
  - Frequently involve the temporal bone with resultant bleeding into the middle ear, but may occur anywhere along the base of the skull
  - Fracture may cause a dural tear, which can lead to CSF leak and exposure to microorganisms of the upper airway (with potential for meningitis)
  - Signs and symptoms depend on amount of damage
  - Clinical signs and symptoms
    - CSF/blood from ear(s) or nose (frequency of occurrence is approximately 15% to 30%)
    - Bilateral black eyes: raccoon's eyes
    - Bruising behind ear(s): Battle's sign; usually presents 12 to 24 hours after the injury
    - Hemotympanum
    - Hearing loss occurs in up to half of patients and may be permanent in a small number of patients
    - May have seizures due to irritation of blood on brain tissue
  - Most heal spontaneously within 7 to 10 days
- Open skull fractures
  - Severe force involved, brain tissue may be exposed
  - Neurologic signs and symptoms evident

Assessment

- Linear fractures may be missed.
  - Depressed and open skull fractures usually found on palpation of head
  - Use balls of fingers to palpate
- Airway patency and breathing adequacy are a priority; vomiting and inadequate respirations are common.
- Assess for signs and symptoms of increased ICP.

Children are particularly prone to basilar skull fractures.

Leakage of CSF from the ear (otorrhea) or nose (rhinorrhea) is evidence that a basilar fracture communicates with the subarachnoid space and indicates the presence of a pathway for infection from the exterior to the subarachnoid space.

- ◦ Infant
  - ▪ Full fontanelle, altered mental status, paradoxic irritability, persistent vomiting, and inability to fully open the eyes (referred to as the "setting sun" sign).
- Child
  - ▪ Headache, stiff neck, photophobia, altered mental status, persistent vomiting, cranial nerve involvement, Cushing's triad, and decorticate or decerebrate posturing.
  - ▪ In decorticate posturing, the legs are extended and the arms are flexed (Figure 9-15). In decerebrate posturing, all extremities are extended and rotated inward. Progression from decorticate to decerebrate posturing is an ominous sign.
- Current data do not indicate that prophylactic antibiotic therapy significantly reduces the incidence of meningitis in a child with a basilar skull fracture.

Cerebral Contusion

- A focal brain injury in which brain tissue is bruised and damaged in a local area; may occur at both the area of direct impact (coup) and/or on the side opposite (contrecoup) the impact.
- Assessment
  - ◦ Airway patency and breathing adequacy a priority
  - ◦ Alteration in level of responsiveness
  - ◦ Confusion or unusual behavior common
  - ◦ May complain of progressive headache and/or photophobia
  - ◦ May be unable to lay down memory; repetitive phrases common
  - ◦ Assess for signs and symptoms of increased ICP

Intracranial Hemorrhage

Epidural Hematoma

- An epidural hematoma is a rapidly accumulating hematoma between the dura and the cranium (Figure 9-16).

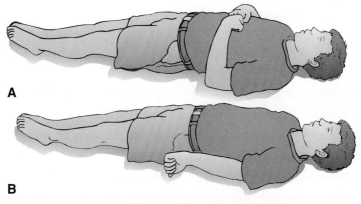

A

B

Figure 9-15 **Decorticate and decerebrate posturing. A,** In decorticate posturing, the legs are extended and the arms are flexed. **B,** In decerebrate posturing, all extremities are extended and rotated inward.

TYPES OF HEMATOMAS AND THE MENINGES

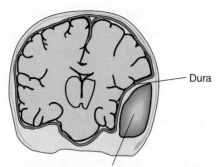

A. EXTRADURAL OR EPIDURAL HEMATOMA
Blood fills space between
dura and bone

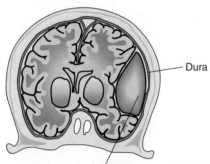

B. SUBDURAL HEMATOMA
Blood fills space between dura
and arachnoid

C. INTRACEREBRAL HEMATOMA

Figure 9-16 **Types of cerebral hematomas and the meninges. A,** Epidural
hematoma. **B,** Subdural hematoma. **C,** Intracerebral hematoma.

- Eighty-five percent are associated with an overlying skull fracture; the most serious lacerate the middle meningeal artery.
  - In adults, an epidural hematoma is usually from an arterial tear, usually of the middle meningeal artery.
  - Occasionally, a pediatric epidural hematoma may be the result of *venous* bleeding, which predisposes the infant or child to a subtle and more subacute presentation over days.[12]
- Most patients experience an LOC followed by a lucid, awake interval

often associated with a severe headache. If untreated, this abruptly evolves to deterioration and death within 15 to 60 minutes.

- Not all patients experience a lucid interval. The patient may initially remain conscious or regain consciousness after trauma to the head and then experience an increasing headache and a progressive decline in level of consciousness. This occurs as the hematoma accumulates between the skull and the dura and ICP increases.

The hallmark sign is a dilated and fixed pupil on the same side as the impact.

- Other signs and symptoms include headache, vomiting, and altered mental status, early dilation of the ipsilateral pupil, and contralateral hemiparesis.
- Early diagnosis and treatment results in a good prognosis; delayed treatment results in a poor prognosis and possible death. Emergent surgical evacuation is usually necessary.

Subdural Hematoma

- Usually results from tearing of the bridging veins between the cerebral cortex and dura; blood fills the space between the dura and the arachnoid.
- A subdural hematoma may be acute or chronic.

Subdural hematomas most commonly occur in patients younger than 2 years of age, with 93% of cases involving children younger than 1 year.[13]

  - Most frequent, identifiable focal brain injury in sports and the most common cause of death in sports-related head injuries because it is also associated with cerebral contusion and edema.[13]
  - Chronic subdural hematomas are most often seen in patients who have been subjected to shaken baby syndrome.
- A newborn or infant often presents with focal seizures, decreased level of consciousness, bulging fontanelle, weak cry, pallor, and vomiting. Retinal hemorrhages, which may occur as a result of the primary injury, are common.
- In children older than 2 to 3 years, signs and symptoms often include pupillary changes, hemiparesis, restlessness, focal neurologic signs, and altered mental status.

Subarachnoid Hematoma

- Usually confined to the CSF space along the surface of the brain
- Results in bloody CSF and meningeal irritation

Intracerebral Hematoma

- Occurs within the brain substance; many small, deep intracerebral hemorrhages are associated with other brain injuries (especially DAI).
- Neurologic deficits depend on the associated injuries and the region involved, the size of the hemorrhage, and whether bleeding continues.

Assessment

- May be impossible to tell which type of hematoma is present.
  - History is important. What were they doing? What happened? What is wrong now? What doesn't seem right?
  - More important to recognize the presence of brain injury.

- Signs/symptoms of increasing ICP
  - Headache that becomes increasingly severe
  - Vomiting
  - Lethargy
  - Confusion
  - Changes in consciousness
  - Comatose
  - Pupil changes
  - Pulse slows or becomes irregular
  - Respirations become irregular
  - Posturing
  - Seizures
- Signs/symptoms of neurologic deficit: early signs and symptoms of alterations in level of consciousness
- Signs of brain irritation: change in personality, irritability, lethargy, confusion, repeating words or phrases, changes in consciousness, paralysis of one side of the body, seizures
- GCS

- Suspect cervical spine injury; cervical spine precautions.
- Maintain airway and adequate ventilation.
  - Hypoxia must be prevented to prevent secondary injury to brain tissue.
  - Tracheal intubation is often necessary for the severely head-injured child. Consider RSI and the use of lidocaine before the procedure to reduce ICP.
  - Ensure the availability of suction. Spontaneous emesis in the first 30 to 60 minutes following head injury is common in children. Consider placement of an orogastric tube.
- Elevate the head of the backboard 30 degrees.
- Establish vascular access.
  - Start IV of isotonic fluid (NS or LR) and titrate to blood pressure.
  - Prevent hypotension to preserve CPP.
  - If hypotension present, look for internal bleeding.
  - Stop external bleeding.
- Pharmacologic treatment
  - Possible use of diuretics (e.g., mannitol and/or furosemide). Because mannitol can cross the blood-brain barrier in areas of cerebral injury, some neurosurgeons do not recommend it for initial management of the head-injured patient.
  - Paralytics/sedation.
  - Avoid glucose unless hypoglycemia confirmed.

General Management of Head/Brain Injuries

Repeated assessment is crucial to detect signs of increasing ICP.

- Nonpharmacologic treatment
  - Position: Elevate the head of the backboard 30 degrees.
  - Decrease central nervous system (CNS) stimulation: Quiet, calm atmosphere; avoid bright lights due to photophobia.
- Perform serial neurologic checks including vital signs, arousability, size and reactivity of the pupils to light, and extent and symmetry of motor responses. Assessment should be performed as follows:
  - Every 15 to 30 minutes until the child is alert
  - Then every 1 to 2 hours for 12 hours
  - Then every 2 to 4 hours thereafter
  - Use the GCS for serial comparisons
    - A GCS score that falls two points suggests significant deterioration, urgent patient reassessment is required.
- Treat seizures if present.
- Consider CT scan. Do not send for CT without adequate stabilization. Minimum requirements include heart rate and pulse oximetry monitoring.
- Psychological support for patient and family.
- If the child is not admitted to the hospital, provide after-care instructions to the parent. Instruct the parent to notify the child's physician if any of the following signs or symptoms appear:
  - The headache becomes severe.
  - Vomiting occurs three or more times.
  - The child's vision becomes blurred or double.
  - The child becomes difficult to awaken or confused.
  - Walking or talking becomes difficult.
  - The child's neurologic condition worsens in any other way.

PEDS Pearl

If a penetrating object is present, do not remove it. The only indications for nonsurgical removal of an impaled object are the following:
- It is not possible to ventilate the child without removing the foreign body (e.g., the object is impaled in the patient's cheek)

- The presence of the object would interfere with chest compressions
- The presence of the object interferes with patient transport.

Manually secure the object, expose the wound area, control bleeding if present, and use a bulky dressing to help stabilize the object in place.

Spinal Trauma

- Children can have spinal nerve injury without damage to the vertebrae, a condition called Spinal Cord Injury without Radiographic Abnormality (SCIWORA). SCIWORA is thought to be attributable to the increased mobility of a child's spine due to the relatively large size of the child's head, weakness of the soft tissues of the neck, incomplete development of the bony spine, and frequency with which ligamentous injuries occur without cervical spine injury.

Hypotension can contribute to secondary injury after acute SCI by further reducing spinal cord blood flow and perfusion.

- Although spinal cord and spinal column injuries are uncommon in the pediatric patient, children younger than 8 years tend to sustain injury to the upper (C1 and C2) cervical spine region. Adults and older children tend to have cervical spine injuries in the lower cervical spine area (between C5 and C6 and between C6 and C7). As a child approaches 8 to 10 years of age, the spinal anatomy and injury pattern more closely approximate those of adult injuries.

Nearly 80% of injuries in children younger than 2 years affect the upper cervical spine region.

Causes of Spinal Trauma

- Direct trauma
- Excessive movement: acceleration, deceleration, deformation
- Directions of force
  - Flexion or hyperflexion (Figure 9-17)
    - Excessive forward motion of the head
    - May cause wedge fracture of anterior vertebrae, stretching or rupturing of interspinous ligaments, compression injury to spinal cord, disruption of disk with forward dislocation of vertebrae, fracture of pedicle and disruption of interspinous ligament

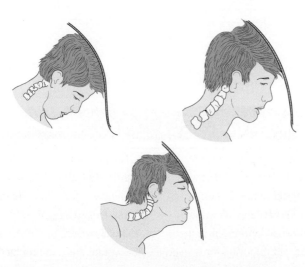

Figure 9-17 The spine can be compressed directly along its own axis or angled into either hyperextension or hyperflexion.

PEDS *Pearl*

Since the high cervical region is the most likely area of spinal injury in a pediatric patient, it is particularly dangerous to have a child's neck in a flexed position. Proper stabilization requires either a special board with a recess for the back of the head, allowing the head to rest in line with the body, or placement of padding under the shoulders to elevate the neck in line with the head.

- Extension or hyperextension
  - Excessive backward movement of the head
  - May cause disruption of the intervertebral disks, compression of the spinal cord, compression of the interspinous ligament, fracture
- Rotational
  - Usually from acceleration forces
  - May cause flexion-rotation dislocation, fracture or dislocation of vertebrae, rupture of supporting ligaments
- Lateral bending
  - Often caused by direct blow to the side of the body
  - May cause lateral compression of the vertebral body, lateral displacement of the vertebra, stretching of ligaments
- Vertical compression
  - Force applied along spinal axis, usually from top of cranium to vertebral body from sudden deceleration (e.g., diving accident)
  - May cause compression fracture without SCI, crushed vertebral body with SCI
- Distraction
  - Force applied to spinal axis to distract or pull apart (e.g., hanging injury)
  - May cause stretching of spinal cord, stretching of supporting ligaments
- It is possible to have a spinal **column** injury (i.e., bony injury) with or without SCI. It is also possible to have SCI with or without spinal **column** injury.

Types of Spinal Cord Injuries

Half of all children with SCI die immediately or within the first hour of injury, and another 20% of survivors succumb to complications within 3 months.[14]

- Primary injury
  - Occurs at time of impact/injury
  - Causes
    - Cord compression
    - Direct cord injury
      - Sharp or unstable bony structures
    - Interruption in the cord's blood supply
- Secondary injury
  - Occurs after initial injury
  - Causes
    - Swelling
    - Ischemia
    - Movement of bony fragments
  - Cord concussion: results from temporary disruption of cord-mediated functions
- Cord contusion

- ○ Bruising of the cord's tissues
- ○ Temporary loss of cord-mediated function
- Cord compression
  - ○ Pressure on the cord
  - ○ Causes tissue ischemia
  - ○ Must be decompressed to avoid permanent loss/damage to cord
- Laceration
  - ○ Tearing of the cord tissue
  - ○ May be reversed if only slight damage
  - ○ May result in permanent loss if spinal tracts are disrupted
- Hemorrhage
  - ○ Bleeding into the cord's tissue due to injured blood vessels
  - ○ Injury related to amount of hemorrhage
  - ○ Damage or obstruction to spinal blood supply results in local ischemia
- Cord transection
  - ○ Complete
    - All tracts of the spinal cord completely disrupted
    - Cord-mediated functions below transection are permanently lost
    - Accurately determined after at least 24 hours after injury
    - Results in the following:
      - Quadriplegia
        - ○ Injury at the cervical level
        - ○ Loss of all function below injury site
      - Paraplegia
        - ○ Injury at the thoracic or lumbar level
        - ○ Loss of lower trunk only
  - ○ Incomplete
    - Some tracts of the spinal cord remain intact
    - Some cord-mediated functions intact
    - Potential for recovery; function may only be temporarily lost
    - Types
      - Anterior cord syndrome (Figure 9-18)
        - ○ Caused by bony fragments or pressure on spinal arteries
        - ○ Symptoms include loss of motor function and pain, temperature, and light touch sensations
        - ○ Some light touch, motion, position, and vibration sensations are spared
      - Central cord syndrome (Figure 9-19)
        - ○ Usually occurs with a hyperextension of the cervical region
        - ○ Symptoms include weakness or paresthesia in upper extremities but normal strength in lower extremities
        - ○ May have varying degrees of bladder dysfunction

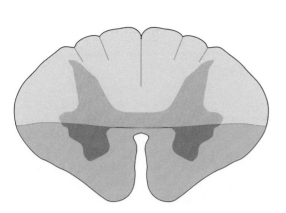

Figure 9-18 Anterior cord syndrome.

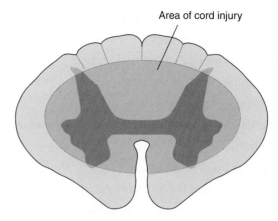

Area of cord injury

Figure 9-19 Central cord syndrome.

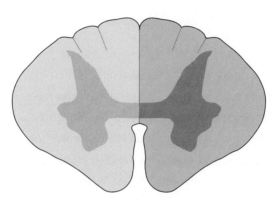

Figure 9-20 Brown-Séquard syndrome.

- Brown-Séquard syndrome (Figure 9-20)
  ○ Caused by penetrating injury and involves hemitransection of the cord involving only one side of the cord
  ○ Symptoms include complete cord damage and loss of function (e.g., motor pain, temperature, motion, position) on the affected side with loss of pain and temperature sensation on the side opposite the injury
- Neurogenic shock
  ○ Occurs secondary to SCI
  ○ Injury disrupts the body's sympathetic compensatory mechanism.
    ▪ Loss of sympathetic tone to the vessels
      • Arteries and arterioles dilate, enlarging the size of the vascular container and producing a relative hypovolemia
      • Skin will be warm and dry due to cutaneous vasodilation
    ▪ Relative hypotension
    ▪ Relative bradycardia
  ○ Shock presentation is usually the result of hidden volume loss (e.g., chest injuries, abdominal injuries).
  ○ Treatment focus primarily on volume replacement.

Differentiate neurogenic shock (↓ blood pressure, ↓ heart rate) from hypovolemic shock (↓ blood pressure, ↑ heart rate).

Signs and symptoms of possible spinal trauma include the following:

- Pain to the neck or back
- Pain on movement of the neck or back
- Pain on palpation of the posterior neck or midline of the back
- Deformity of the spinal column
- Guarding or splinting of the muscles of the neck or back
- Priapism
- Signs and symptoms of neurogenic shock (peripheral vasodilation, bradycardia, and hypotension)
- Paralysis, paresis, numbness, or tingling in the arms or legs at any time after the incident
- Diaphragmatic breathing

- Consider methylprednisolone.
  - Controversy currently exists concerning the effectiveness of steroids in SCI. Several studies have looked at the effectiveness of pharmacologic interventions after spine injury. The current recommendation based on these studies is to administer high-dose steroids for 24 hours if they are started within 3 hours of SCI and to administer for 48 hours if they started 3 to 8 hours after injury. Methylprednisolone is commonly used for this purpose. An initial IV dose of 30 mg/kg is given over 15 minutes and followed in 45 minutes by an infusion at a rate of 5.4 mg/kg per hour.
  - The effectiveness of this protocol remains controversial. Of special significance is that no children were involved in the National Acute Spinal Cord Injury Study studies. In a recent publication of the Congress of Neurologic Surgeons and American Association of Neurologic Surgeons, it was stated that, "methylprednisolone for either 24 or 48 hours is recommended as an option in the treatment of patients with acute spinal cord injuries that should be undertaken only with the knowledge that the evidence suggesting harmful side effects is more consistent than any suggestion of clinical benefit." No additional specific recommendations were made regarding pediatric patients.[15]
- Principles of spinal stabilization
  - Primary goal is to prevent further injury.
  - Treat the spine as a long bone with a joint at either end.
    - Stabilize the joint above (head) and the joint below (pelvis) the injury.
    - Always use "complete" spine stabilization; impossible to isolate and splint specific injury site.
  - Stabilization of the spine begins in the primary survey and continues

Signs and Symptoms of Spinal Trauma

General Management of Spinal Injuries

until the spine is completely immobilized on a long backboard or evidence of spinal injury has been definitively ruled out.

◦ The head and neck should be placed in a neutral in-line position unless contraindicated.

◦ Backboards

- To stabilize a pediatric patient on a backboard:
  - Manually stabilize the child's head and neck.
  - Apply a properly sized rigid cervical collar (Figure 9-21A). If a properly sized device is not available, use towels, washcloths, or other material to stabilize the head as best as possible.
  - Log roll the child onto a rigid board (Figure 9-21B).
    - ◦ To maintain the cervical spine in a neutral position, it is often necessary to place padding under the child's torso.
    - ◦ The padding should be firm, evenly shaped, and extend from the shoulders to the pelvis. For an infant or young child, the padding should be of appropriate thickness so that the child's shoulders are in horizontal alignment with the ear canal.
  - Secure the child to the board with straps around the chest, pelvis, and legs to restrict patient movement from side to side and to prevent the child from sliding up and down on the

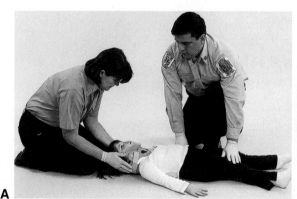

A

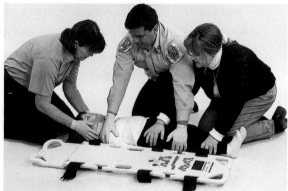

B

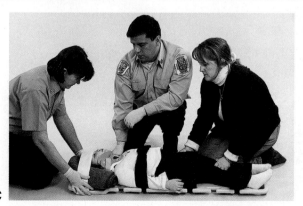

C

Figure 9-21 **Immobilizing a pediatric patient on a backboard. A,** Apply a properly sized rigid cervical collar. **B,** Log roll the child onto a rigid board. **C,** Secure the child to board with straps around the chest, pelvis, and legs. Secure the head to the board last.

backboard. Secure the torso to the board first and the head to the board last (Figure 9-21C).

- ○ Manual stabilization can be discontinued after the head has been secured to the board.
- ○ Additional padding may be necessary along the torso and between the legs.

- Secure the board to the stretcher and reassess the patient.

○ Child safety seats

- If a child is critically injured or the child's condition has the potential to worsen, a safety seat should NOT be used for stabilization. Instead, the child should be removed from the seat onto a rigid board.

- Place the seat on its back onto a long backboard.
- Unstrap the child and slide him or her onto the long backboard using a padded board splint to keep the child's spine in a neutral, in-line position (Figure 9-22A).
- Slide the child along the backboard and remove the safety seat (Figure 9-22B).
- Stabilize the child to the backboard.

> Do NOT pull on the child's head or neck. Slide the child out of the seat as a unit.

- If the child's condition is stable, a child safety seat can be used for stabilization only after a brief inspection to ensure the seat has not sustained any major structural damage and only if the safety seat can be secured appropriately in the ambulance.

- Manually stabilize the child's head and neck (Figure 9-23A).
- If the seat includes a protection plate over the child's chest, remove it to enable easy visualization and assessment of the child's chest.
  - ○ If a chest plate is not present, use the chest straps to secure the child in place whenever possible.
  - ○ Additional padding and/or cravats between the straps and the child or tightening of the straps may be needed.

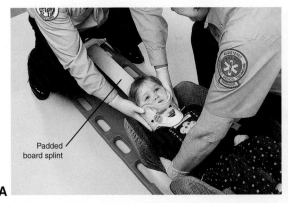
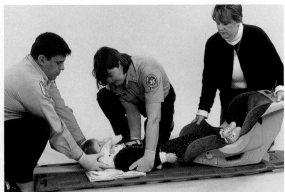

Padded board splint

A

B

Figure 9-22 **A,** Place the seat on its back onto a long backboard. Unstrap the child and slide him or her onto the long backboard using a padded board splint to keep the child's spine in a neutral, in-line position. **B,** Slide the child along the board and remove the safety seat. Immobilize the child to the backboard.

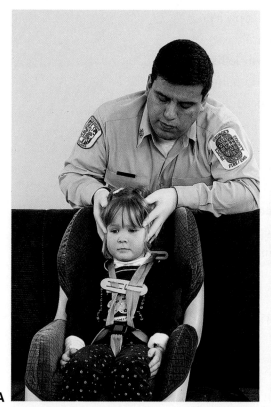

A

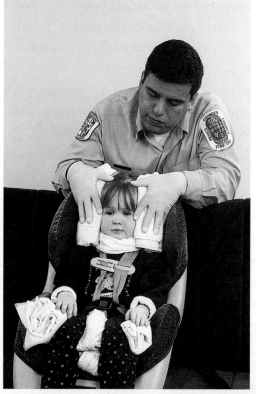

B

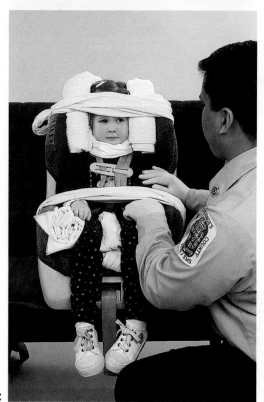

C

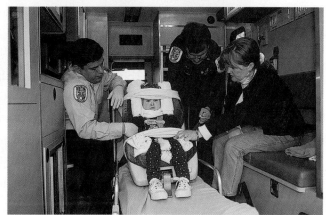

D

Figure 9-23 A, Manually stabilize the child's head and neck. Use the safety seat's chest straps to secure the child in place whenever possible. **B,** If a properly fitting rigid cervical collar is not available, use towels, washcloths, or small blankets (depending on the child's size) and adhesive tape across the forehead to immobilize the head. **C,** Use a cravat or similar material around the head to prevent forward movement. Use small blankets, towels, or similar materials to pad all open areas around the child's body so the child does not move. **D,** Secure the safety seat in place for transport.

- If a properly fitting rigid cervical collar is available, apply it and use towel rolls to limit movement. If a rigid cervical collar of appropriate size is not available, use towels, washcloths, or small blankets (depending on the child's size) and adhesive tape across the forehead to immobilize the head (Figure 9-23B). Use a cravat or similar material around the head to prevent forward movement (Figure 9-23C).
- Use small blankets, towels, or similar materials to pad all open areas around the child's body so the child does not move.
- Once adequately stabilized, the patient and seat should be transferred to the ambulance and carefully secured to the stretcher or captain's seat so that it is not mobile during transport (Figure 9-23D).

- Helmeted patients
  - Special assessment needs for patients wearing helmets
    - Airway and breathing
    - Fit of helmet and movement within the helmet
    - Ability to gain access to airway and breathing
  - Indications for leaving the helmet in place
    - Good fit with little or no head movement within helmet
    - No impending airway or breathing problems
    - Removal may cause further injury
    - Proper spinal stabilization could be performed with helmet in place
    - No interference with ability to assess and reassess airway
  - Indications for helmet removal
    - Inability to assess or reassess airway and breathing
    - Restriction of adequate management of the airway or breathing
    - Improperly fitted helmet with excessive head movement within helmet
    - Proper spinal stabilization cannot be performed with helmet in place (Figure 9-24)
    - Cardiac arrest

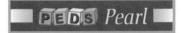

PEDS *Pearl*

A young child's vertebral column may withstand traction and torsion without evidence of deformity while the spinal cord tears. In longitudinal traction, the cadaveric infant spine is able to withstand up to 2 inches of stretch without disruption, whereas the spinal cord ruptures after only 1/4 inch of stretching.[14]

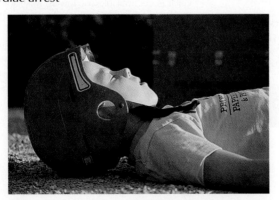

Figure 9-24 Neck flexion caused by a helmet on a child.

Thoracic Trauma

The most common thoracic injuries seen in children are pulmonary contusion/laceration (53%), pneumothorax/hemothorax (38%), rib/sternal fractures (36%), cardiac (5%), diaphragm (2%), and major blood vessel (1%).[16]

In children, thoracic trauma is associated with a high mortality rate. The greater elasticity and resilience of the chest wall in children makes rib and sternum fractures less common than in adults; however, force is more easily transmitted to the underlying lung tissues, resulting in pulmonary contusion, pneumothorax, or hemothorax.

Pathophysiology

- Impairments in cardiac output
  - Blood loss
  - Increased intrapleural pressures
  - Blood in pericardial sac
  - Myocardial valve damage
  - Vascular disruption
- Impairments in ventilatory efficiency
  - Bellows action of the chest compromised
  - Pain restricting chest excursion
  - Air entering pleural space
  - Chest wall fails to move in unison
  - Bleeding in pleural space
  - Ineffective diaphragmatic contraction
- Impairments in gas exchange
  - Atelectasis
  - Contused lung tissue
  - Disruption of respiratory tract

Chest Wall Injuries

Rib Fractures

- Children are less likely to sustain rib fractures than adults are because a child's chest wall is more flexible than that of an adult. The presence of a rib fracture suggests significant force caused the injury.
- Most frequently caused by blunt trauma and may be associated with injury to the underlying lung (pulmonary contusion) or the heart (myocardial contusion). The seriousness of the injury increases with age, the number of fractures, and the location of the fractures.
  - Left lower rib injury associated with splenic rupture.
  - Right lower rib injury associated with hepatic injury.
  - Multiple rib fractures may result in inadequate ventilation and pneumonia.

- Signs and symptoms
  - Localized pain at the fracture site that worsens with deep breathing, coughing, or moving. Pain often causes the patient to "splint" the injury by holding his or her arm close to the chest.
  - Pain on inspiration.
  - Shallow breathing (to decrease the pain associated with breathing).
  - Tenderness on palpation.
  - Deformity of chest wall.
  - Crepitus (grating sound produced by bone fragments rubbing together).
  - Swelling and/or bruising at the fracture site.
  - Possible subcutaneous emphysema (a crackling sensation felt under the fingers during palpation). The presence of subcutaneous emphysema suggests laceration of a lung and the leakage of air into the pleural space.
- Management
  - Airway and ventilation
    - Oxygen therapy
    - Positive-pressure ventilation
    - Encourage coughing and deep breathing
  - Pharmacologic: analgesics
  - Nonpharmacologic
    - Splint, but avoid circumferential splinting
    - Do not apply tape or straps to the ribs or chest wall
      - Limits chest wall motion
      - Reduces effectiveness of ventilation

Flail Chest

- Flail chest is a life-threatening injury.
- Most commonly occurs because of a vehicle crash but may also occur because of falls from a height, assault, and birth trauma.
  - Because a child's ribs are flexible, flail chest is uncommon in children.
- Pathophysiology
  - Three or more ribs fractured in two or more places producing a free floating segment of chest wall
    - The section of the chest wall between the fractured ribs becomes free-floating because it is no longer in continuity with the thorax. This free-floating section of the chest wall is called the "flail segment."
    - The injured portion of the chest wall (flail segment) does not move with the rest of the rib cage when the patient attempts to breathe (paradoxic movement). When the patient inhales, the flail

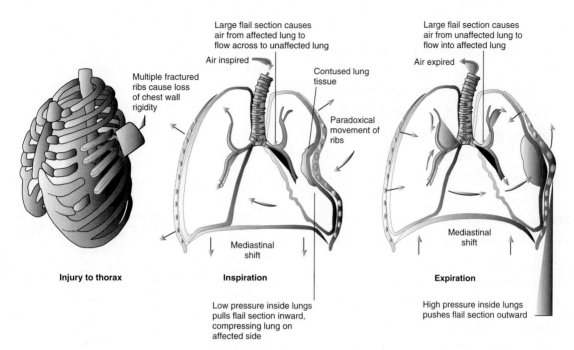

Multiple fractured ribs cause loss of chest wall rigidity

Large flail section causes air from affected lung to flow across to unaffected lung

Air inspired

Contused lung tissue

Paradoxical movement of ribs

Mediastinal shift

Injury to thorax

Inspiration

Low pressure inside lungs pulls flail section inward, compressing lung on affected side

Large flail section causes air from unaffected lung to flow into affected lung

Air expired

Mediastinal shift

Expiration

High pressure inside lungs pushes flail section outward

Figure 9-25 Flail chest.

segment is drawn inward instead of moving outward. When the patient exhales, the flail segment moves outward instead of moving inward (Figure 9-25).

- ○ Respiratory failure may occur due to the following
  - ▪ Bruising of the underlying lung and associated hemorrhage of the alveoli, reducing the amount of lung tissue available for gas exchange
  - ▪ Instability of the chest wall and pain associated with breathing, leading to decreased ventilation and hypoxia
  - ▪ Interference with the normal "bellows" action of the chest, resulting in inadequate gas exchange
  - ▪ Associated chest injuries
- ○ Paradoxic movement of the chest (may be minimal because of muscle spasm)
- ○ Pain: reduces thoracic expansion, decreases ventilation
- ○ Pulmonary contusion
  - ▪ Decreased lung compliance
  - ▪ Intraalveolar-capillary hemorrhage
  - ▪ Alveolar hemorrhage
- ○ Decreased ventilation
- ○ Impaired venous return with ventilation-perfusion mismatch
- ○ Hypercapnia, hypoxia
- • Signs and symptoms: chest wall contusion, respiratory distress, paradoxic chest wall movement, pleuritic chest pain, crepitus, pain and splinting of affected side, tachypnea, tachycardia

- Management
  - Oxygen (high concentration); positive-pressure ventilation may be needed
  - Evaluate the need for tracheal intubation
  - Positive end-expiratory pressure (PEEP)
  - Pharmacologic: analgesics
  - Nonpharmacologic: positioning; tracheal intubation, and positive-pressure ventilation

Pulmonary Contusion

A pulmonary contusion is one of the most frequently observed chest injuries in children.

- Potentially life-threatening injury
- Frequently missed due to presence of other associated injuries
- Pathophysiology
  - Alveoli fill with blood and fluid because of bruising of the lung tissue
  - Area of the lung available for gas exchange is decreased
  - Severity of signs and symptoms depends on the amount of lung tissue injured
- Signs and symptoms
  - Evidence of blunt chest trauma, apprehension, anxiety, tachypnea, tachycardia, cough, hemoptysis, dyspnea, wheezes, crackles, decreased breath sounds, subcutaneous emphysema may or may not be present
  - Arterial blood gas changes precede clinical symptoms; reflect increased $PaCO_2$ level and decreased PaO_2 level.
- Management
  - If no cervical spine injury, elevate head of bed
  - Mild contusion: observation and supportive care
  - More severe contusion: tracheal intubation and mechanical ventilation with PEEP
  - Maintain normal blood volume

Simple Pneumothorax

- Pathophysiology
  - Air enters the chest cavity causing a loss of negative pressure and a partial or total collapse of the lung
  - Air may enter the chest cavity through a hole in the chest wall (sucking chest wound) or a hole in the lung tissue, bronchus, or the trachea
  - As air enters and fills the pleural space, lung tissue is compressed, reducing the amount of lung tissue available for gas exchange
  - Signs and symptoms will depend on the size of the pneumothorax

Injury to the Lung

The child may initially be asymptomatic but develop symptoms a few hours later.

A simple pneumothorax may occur as a result of blunt or penetrating chest trauma (i.e., rib fractures or central line placement).

- Small tears may self-seal, resolving by themselves; patient may not experience dyspnea or other signs of respiratory distress
- Larger tears may progress, resulting in signs and symptoms of respiratory distress
  - If the child is sitting or standing, air will accumulate in the apices, check there first for diminished breath sounds; if the child is supine, air will accumulate in the anterior chest
  - Trachea may tug towards the affected side
  - Ventilation/perfusion mismatch
- Signs and symptoms: tachypnea, tachycardia, respiratory distress, absent or decreased breath sounds on affected side, decreased chest wall movement, dyspnea, slight pleuritic chest pain
- Management
  - Small pneumothorax (less than 15%) may not require treatment other than observation.
  - Positive-pressure ventilation if necessary.
  - Monitor for development of tension pneumothorax.

Open Pneumothorax

- Pathophysiology
  - Open defect in the chest wall (Figure 9-26).
    - Allows communication between pleural space and atmosphere
    - Prevents development of negative intrapleural pressure
    - Produces collapse of ipsilateral lung
    - Inability to ventilate affected lung
    - Ventilation/perfusion mismatch
  - Severity of an open pneumothorax depends on the size of the wound.

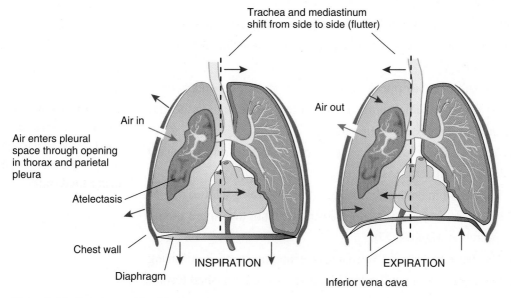

Figure 9-26 Open pneumothorax.

- If the diameter of the chest wound is more than two thirds of the diameter of the patient's trachea, air will enter the chest wound rather than through the trachea with each breath.
- A sucking or gurgling sound is heard as air moves in and out of the pleural space through the open chest wound.
- If the flap of chest wall closes during expiration, air will become trapped inside the pleural space. As air collects in the pleural space, pressure will build with each inspiration, eventually resulting in a tension pneumothorax.
  ○ Direct lung injury may be present.
  ○ Vena cava kinked from swaying of mediastinum; decreased preload.
- Signs and symptoms: defect in the chest wall, penetrating injury to the chest that does not seal itself, sucking sound on inhalation, tachycardia, tachypnea, respiratory distress, subcutaneous emphysema, decreased breath sounds on affected side
- Management
  ○ Positive-pressure ventilation if necessary
  ○ Monitor for development of tension pneumothorax
  ○ Nonpharmacologic
    - Promptly close the chest wall defect with an occlusive (airtight) dressing (e.g., plastic wrap, petroleum gauze, or a defibrillation pad are examples of dressings that may be used).
      - Tape the dressing on three sides (flutter-valve effect: The dressing is sucked over the wound as the patient inhales, preventing air from entering; the open end of the dressing allows air to escape as the patient exhales)
    - Tube thoracostomy: in-hospital management

Tension Pneumothorax

- Life-threatening chest injury that can occur because of blunt or penetrating trauma or as a complication of treatment of an open pneumothorax
- Pathophysiology
  ○ May result from an opening through the chest wall and parietal pleura (open pneumothorax) or from a tear in the lung tissue and visceral pleura (closed pneumothorax)
  ○ Air enters the pleura during inspiration and progressively accumulates under pressure.
    - The flap of injured lung acts as a one-way valve, allowing air to enter the pleural space during inspiration, but trapping it during expiration (Figure 9-27).
    - The injured lung collapses completely and pressure rises, forcing the trachea, heart, and major blood vessels to be pushed toward the opposite side.

Tension pneumothorax is common in children.

Shifting of the trachea to the side opposite the injury is called **tracheal deviation**. Shifting of the heart and major blood vessels to the side opposite the injury is called **mediastinal shift**.

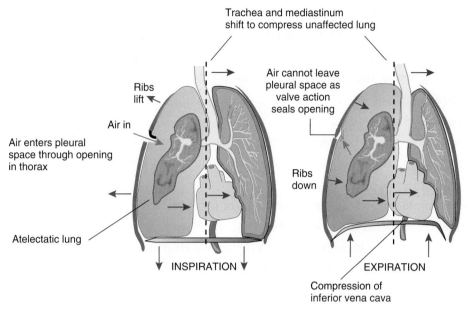

Trachea and mediastinum shift to compress unaffected lung

Ribs lift

Air in

Air enters pleural space through opening in thorax

Atelectatic lung

Air cannot leave pleural space as valve action seals opening

Ribs down

INSPIRATION

EXPIRATION

Compression of inferior vena cava

Figure 9-27   Tension pneumothorax.

A tracheal shift is difficult to detect in young children. JVD may not be prominent if hypovolemia is present.

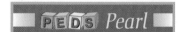 *Pearl*

Diagnosis of tension pneumothorax in children is complicated by false transmission of breath sounds. Uncertainty as to the side of the tension pneumothorax should not prohibit initiation of empirical treatment if the patient is deteriorating. Decompression of the other side should be performed if immediate improvement is not seen with the initial needle or tube thoracostomy.[17]

- Shifting of the major blood vessels causes them to kink, resulting in a backup of blood into the venous system.
- The backup of blood into the venous system results in jugular venous distention (JVD), decreased blood return to the heart, and signs of shock.
- Signs and symptoms: cool, clammy skin; increased pulse rate, cyanosis (a late sign), JVD, hypotension, severe respiratory distress; agitation, restlessness, anxiety; bulging of intercostal muscles on the affected side, decreased or absent breath sounds on the affected side, tracheal deviation toward the unaffected side (late sign), and possible subcutaneous emphysema in the face, neck, or chest wall.
- Management
  - Positive-pressure ventilation if necessary
  - Relieve tension pneumothorax to improve cardiac output
  - Nonpharmacologic
    - If the patient has an open chest wound with signs of a tension pneumothorax:
      - Remove the dressing over the wound for a few seconds.
      - If the wound in the chest wall has not sealed under the dressing, air will rush out of the wound.
      - Reseal the wound with the occlusive dressing once the pressure has been released.
      - This procedure may need to be repeated periodically if pressure again builds up in the chest.
      - If this procedure does not relieve the signs of a tension pneumothorax, needle decompression should be performed.

- Needle decompression
- Tube thoracostomy: in-hospital management

Hemothorax

- Life-threatening injury that frequently requires urgent chest tube and/or surgery
- Pathophysiology
  - Occurs because of blunt or penetrating trauma when large amounts of blood accumulate in the pleural space and compress the lung (Figure 9-28).
  - Massive hemothorax indicates great vessel or cardiac injury.
    - Massive hemothorax is rare in children.
    - Usually associated with high-speed MVC, fall from a great height, or a high-powered or close-range gunshot wound.
    - Produces both respiratory failure and circulatory collapse.
  - Respiratory insufficiency dependent on amount of blood.
  - Hypotension and inadequate perfusion may result from blood loss.
- Signs and symptoms: tachypnea, tachycardia, dyspnea, respiratory distress, hypotension, narrowed pulse pressure, flat neck veins, pleuritic chest pain; pale, cool, moist skin; decreased breath sounds and dullness to percussion on affected side with or without obvious respiratory distress
- Management
  - Positive-pressure ventilation if necessary
  - Tracheal intubation if necessary
  - Treat hypovolemia and shock with IV fluids, blood administration as indicated

A hemothorax requires a minimum of 10 mL/kg of blood to be visualized on chest radiograph.[17]

Signs of shock are often the initial indicators of a large hemothorax.

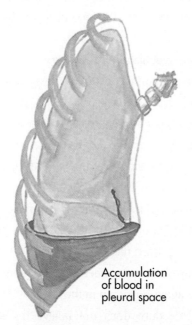

Accumulation
of blood in
pleural space

Figure 9-28 Hemothorax.

        ○ Tube thoracostomy: in-hospital management (ensure IV fluid resuscitation is initiated before procedure)

Traumatic Asphyxia

- Pathophysiology
  - Sudden compression force to the chest or upper abdomen, with the lungs full of air and glottis closed, causes a sudden increase in intrapleural and intraabdominal pressure.
  - This raises the pressure in the superior vena cava, causing the blood in the veins of the thorax and neck to be forced into the chest, lungs, neck, head, and brain.
  - Increased venous pressure causes rupture of capillaries, which results in violet color of skin in the head and neck area, bilateral subconjunctival hemorrhages, and facial edema.
- Signs and symptoms: cyanosis of the face and upper neck, JVD, swelling or hemorrhage of the conjunctiva, skin below area remains pink, tachypnea, disorientation, hemoptysis, epistaxis, signs of respiratory insufficiency
- Management
  - Manage associated injuries (e.g., pulmonary contusion)
  - Supportive care

Pericardial Tamponade

- Pathophysiology
  - Rapid accumulation of fluid in the pericardial sac over a period of minutes to hours leads to increases in intrapericardial pressure
  - Compresses heart and decreases cardiac output due to restricted diastolic expansion and filling (Figure 9-29)
  - Hampers venous return

Beck's triad is not often evident in the pediatric patient. If profound hypovolemia is present, JVD will be absent. If bradycardia occurs, the patient is about to arrest.

- Signs and symptoms: tachycardia, respiratory distress, pulsus paradoxus, cyanosis of head, neck, upper extremities, Beck's triad (narrowing pulse pressure, neck vein distention, muffled heart tones), dysrhythmias (e.g., bradycardia, pulseless electrical activity, asystole)
- Management
  - Airway and ventilation
  - IV fluid challenge (may transiently increase cardiac output by increasing the filling pressure of the heart)
  - Nonpharmacologic management (in hospital)
    - Echocardiographically guided pericardiocentesis
    - Percutaneous balloon pericardiotomy
    - Emergency department thoracotomy
    - Operative intervention

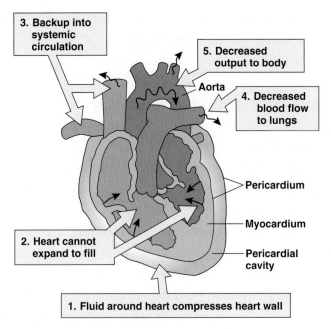

Figure 9-29   Pericardial tamponade.

Abdominal and Pelvic Trauma

Abdominal trauma is the third leading cause of traumatic death, after head and thoracic injuries and is the most common cause of unrecognized fatal injury in children. The abdominal organs of an infant or child are susceptible to injury for several reasons.

- The abdominal wall is thin, so the organs are closer to the surface of the abdomen.
- Children have proportionally larger solid organs, less subcutaneous fat, and less protective abdominal musculature than adults do.
- The liver and spleen of a small child are lower in the abdomen and less protected by the rib cage.
  1. Blunt mechanisms (85% of cases)
     A) Blunt abdominal trauma in an infant or child is primarily caused by motor vehicle collisions, motorcycle collisions, falls, sports-related injuries, pedestrian crashes, and child abuse.
        1) Blunt trauma related to motor vehicle collisions causes more than 50% of the abdominal injuries in children and is the most lethal.
        2) The effects of bicycle injuries may not be seen on initial presentation, with the mean elapsed time to onset of symptoms being nearly 24 hours.[12]
  2. Penetrating mechanisms (15% of cases)

Mechanism of Injury

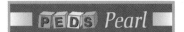

In children younger than 13 years old, penetrating injuries are likely to be caused by accidental impalement on objects such as scissors, picket fences, or by accidental discharge of a weapon. In patients older than 13 years, 75% of penetrating trauma injuries are knife or handgun wounds inflicted by an assailant.[20]

A) Energy imparted to the body

B) Low velocity: knife, ice pick, and scissors

C) Medium velocity: gunshot wounds, shotgun wounds

D) High velocity: high-power hunting rifles, military weapons

Pathophysiology of Abdominal Injuries

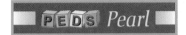

Serious injuries in children from blunt abdominal trauma (with frequency of injury) include splenic contusion/laceration (30%), liver contusion/laceration (28%), renal injury (28%), GI tract/duodenal hematoma (14%), GU tract injury (4%), pancreatic injury (3%), and disruption of major blood vessels (3%).[16]

Solid Organ Injuries

The spleen plays a major role in fighting infection.

All patients with suspected splenic injury should be evaluated by a surgeon.

1. Hemorrhage

A) No external signs

B) Rapid blood loss

C) Hypovolemic shock

D) Blood is not chemical irritant to peritoneum (therefore, no peritonitis)

2. Spillage of contents

A) Enzymes

B) Acids

C) Bacteria

D) Chemical irritation to peritoneum (peritonitis)

E) Localized pain sensation via somatic nerve fibers

F) Muscular spasm secondary to peritonitis (rigid abdomen)

- Splenic injuries
  - Most frequently injured abdominal organ during blunt trauma (e.g., MVCs, sudden-deceleration injuries, and contact sports–related injuries)
    - The spleen is completely protected by the rib cage in adolescents and adults but in infants and small children, the rib cage does not extend down far enough to provide adequate protection.
    - The rib cage of the infant and small child is also very pliable and does not provide the same degree of protection as the rib cage of an adult.
  - Commonly associated with other intraabdominal injuries
  - May present with left upper quadrant abdominal pain radiating to the left shoulder (Kehr's sign; result of diaphragm irritation)
  - Patient presentation may range from stable to persistent hypotension to cardiovascular collapse. Stable patients may undergo CT for radiologic evaluation or bedside ultrasound.
  - Bleeding from a minor splenic injury often stops spontaneously without requiring operative intervention; however, spontaneous splenic rupture 3 to 5 days after the injury has been described.
  - Patients with splenic injury should be admitted to the hospital, with frequent repeated assessments.
- Liver injuries
  - The liver is vulnerable to injury because of its large size and fragility.

- Second most commonly injured solid organ in the pediatric patient with blunt abdominal trauma but the most common cause of lethal hemorrhage.
- Mortality 10% to 20% in severe liver injury.
- Injuries may be the result of blunt or penetrating trauma; a firm blow to the right upper quadrant or right-sided rib fractures may cause liver injury.
- Absence of localized bruises or abrasions does not rule out the possibility of serious laceration or rupture.

- Kidney injuries
  - Children are more susceptible to renal injuries because
    - The kidneys are large in proportion to the abdomen.
    - The lower ribs do not shield the kidneys from injury.
    - Underdevelopment of abdominal wall muscles and a lack of extensive perirenal fat provide less protection for the kidneys.
    - Their kidneys are mobile; may be contused or lacerated by ribs or spinal transverse process.
  - Kidney injury is usually caused by blunt trauma (e.g., deceleration forces) and is rarely caused by penetrating trauma.
  - Often present with hematuria, back pain.
  - Most injuries are minor and can be managed without surgical intervention.

- Pancreas
  - Contusion most common type of injury to the pancreas.
    - Common mechanisms include falling from a bicycle with injury caused by the handlebars, pedestrian traffic collisions, MVCs, and child abuse.
  - Lacerations cause hemorrhage and release of enzymatic contents toxic to surrounding tissues.
  - Penetrating trauma requires surgical evaluation

- Morbidity/mortality secondary to blood loss and content spillage
- May result from blunt or penetrating injuries
  - Common mechanisms include lap-belt injuries (Figure 9-30), bicycle handlebar injuries, and child abuse
- Small and large intestines
  - Most often injured as a result of penetrating injuries
  - Can occur with deceleration injuries
- Stomach
  - Most often injured as a result of blunt trauma
  - Full stomach before incident increases risk of injury
- Duodenum

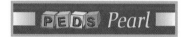

PEDS Pearl

Early placement of an orogastric or nasogastric tube (if not contraindicated) to decompress the stomach is very important in a child. The anxious and injured child swallows large amounts of air, which can result in significant gastric distention. Decompression of the stomach facilitates physical examination of the abdomen, helps minimize the risk of aspiration, and helps prevent hypoventilation.

Hollow Organ Injuries

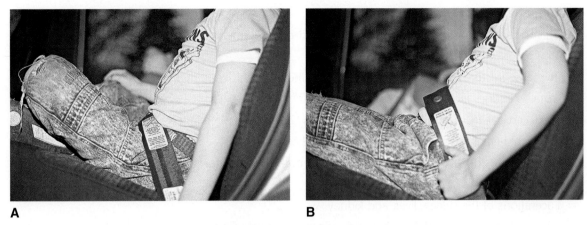

Figure 9-30 Lap-belt position. Correct (**A**) and incorrect (**B**) positions for lap belts on children.

PEDS Pearl

A child who is wearing a lap belt with no shoulder harness during a motor vehicle collision may sustain a Chance fracture and abdominal injuries involving the pancreas, duodenum, or intestines, with the potential for hematomas and bowel	rupture. A Chance fracture (also called a seat belt fracture) is a horizontal fracture of the thoracic or lumbar spine caused by a hyperflexion injury with little or no compression of the vertebral body.

- Most often injured as a result of blunt trauma
- Recognition often delayed
- Bladder
  - Most often injured as a result of blunt trauma due to automobile or auto-pedestrian collisions
  - Full bladder before incident or inappropriate use of lap belts may increase risk of bladder injury
  - Penetrating injuries may be caused by guns, knives, or fractured pelvic bones

Abdominal Wall Injuries

Evisceration
- Do not touch or try to replace the exposed organ.
- Carefully remove clothing from around the wound.
- Cover exposed organs and wound.
  - Apply a large sterile dressing, moistened with sterile water or saline, over the organs and wound.
  - Secure the dressing in place with a large bandage to retain moisture and prevent heat loss.

- Fractures of the pelvis in children are uncommon.
- Associated soft-tissue injuries may be severe and require emergency treatment.
- Many pelvic fractures occur in children struck by moving vehicles.
- Associated injuries include the following:
  - Skull, cervical, facial, and long bone fractures
  - Subdural hematomas, cerebral contusions, and concussions
  - Lung contusions, hemothorax, hemopneumothorax, ruptured diaphragm
  - Lacerations of the spleen, liver, and kidney
- Injuries that may be associated with and adjacent to pelvic fractures include damage to major blood vessels, retroperitoneal bleeding, rectal tears, and rupture or laceration of the urethra or bladder.
- Treatment of a pelvic fracture depends on the type of fracture. Some areas recommend application of the pneumatic antishock garment (PASG) for a child who has an unstable pelvis and shows signs of shock. Follow local protocol.

Pelvic Fractures

Because the pelvis contains major blood vessels, the patient with a pelvic fracture is at significant risk for serious hemorrhage.

Extremity Trauma

- Fractures are among the most frequently missed injuries in children with multiple trauma.
- Bilateral femur fractures can cause significant blood loss, resulting in hypovolemic shock.
- Be alert for evidence of possible child abuse:
  - Fractures of differing ages
  - Spiral fracture
  - Discrepancy between history and injury
  - Prolonged and/or unexplained delay in treatment
  - Different stories at different times
  - Poor health and hygiene
- Extremity immobilization
  - Immobilize the joint above and below the fracture site.
  - Assess and document pulses, motor function, and sensation in the affected extremity before and after immobilization.
  - Do not attempt to realign a fracture or dislocation, or straighten any angulation, unless obvious vascular compromise necessitates a position change.
- Amputated part
  - If a complete amputation has occurred:
    - Apply a sterile dressing soaked in NS to the stump, then splint and elevate it.

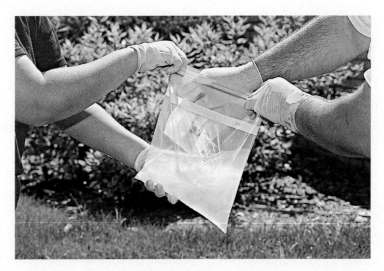

Figure 9-31   Care of an amputated part. Put the amputated part in a plastic bag or waterproof container. Place the plastic bag or waterproof container in water that contains a few ice cubes. Never place ice in direct contact with the amputated part.

- If profuse bleeding is present, apply direct pressure with a soft dressing and elevate the extremity.
- Immobilize the limb to prevent further injury.
- Gently rinse dirt and debris from the amputated part with sterile saline or RL solution.
  - Do not scrub.
  - Clean water is an acceptable alternative if sterile isotonic solution is not available.
- Put the amputated part in a plastic bag or waterproof container.
- Place the plastic bag or waterproof container in water that contains a few ice cubes (Figure 9-31). Never place ice in direct contact with the amputated part.
- Transport the amputated part with the patient.
  - Do not use dry ice.
  - Do not allow the part to freeze. Freezing renders tissues non-replantable.
  - Do not place the amputated part directly on ice or in water.
  - Do not complete partial amputations.
- Immobilize suspected fractures and dislocations and administer an analgesic before obtaining radiograph films.
- Consult an orthopedic surgeon to evaluate a child with a compartment syndrome, other causes of neurovascular compromise, or an open fracture.

Burns

- Thermal injury (see following section)
- Inhalation injury
  - Serious injury in the infant and child, particularly if preexisting pulmonary conditions are present
  - Present in 30% of victims of major flame burns
  - Consider when there is evidence of fire in enclosed space, singed nares, facial burns, charred lips, carbonaceous secretions, posterior pharynx edema, hoarseness, cough, or wheezing
  - Initial treatment guidelines
  - Ensure adequate airway, oxygenation, and ventilation
  - Draw arterial blood gases
  - Check carbon monoxide level
  - Have intubation/tracheostomy equipment available
- Chemical injury
  - Occurs when a child handles or swallows a caustic substance
  - In children, chemical burns usually involve household products
  - Alkaline agents cause liquefaction necrosis
    - Turns tissue fats and proteins to soap, damaging all tissue layers
    - Ingestion can cause esophageal stenosis
    - Alkalis (bases) used at home that can cause chemical burns include ammonia and phosphates, used in detergents and cleaners; silicates, used in detergents; sodium and calcium hypochlorite, used in pool chlorinating agents and household bleach; sodium carbonate, used in detergents; sodium hydroxide and potassium hydroxide, used in drain cleaners, oven cleaners, and denture cleaners
  - Acid agents cause coagulation necrosis
    - Damages superficial layers of tissue
    - Ingestions of corrosive substances can result in esophageal perforation
    - Acids used at home that can cause chemical burns include acetic acid, used in dyes, hair wave neutralizers, and disinfectants; hydrochloric acid, used in toilet bowl cleaners, metal cleaners; hydrofluoric acid, used in rust removers, tile cleaners; phosphoric acid, used in rustproofing, disinfectants, and detergents; sulfuric acid, used in drain cleaners, metal cleaners, and automobile battery fluid
  - Initial treatment guidelines
    - Contact a poison control center for advice before treating the patient, particularly if the substance was ingested.

Types of Burn Injuries

Inhalation injury increases mortality.

If the burn covers a large area, put the child in the shower.

- Wearing protective clothing, brush dry chemicals from the child's skin, using towels, sheets, or gloved hands. Remove any of the child's clothing that has come into contact with the chemical.
- DO NOT waste time trying to obtain specific neutralizing chemicals.
- Flush external chemical burns with copious amounts of room temperature/cool water, except for sodium burns. Cover metallic sodium burns with an oil-based dressing, such as petrolatum gel.
  - Flush most acid burns with water for 30 to 60 minutes.
  - Alkali injuries may require hours of flushing to remove the compound from the skin.
- Some chemicals (e.g., lye) can continue to burn tissue even after initial washing. Begin washing at the scene and continue for at least 20 minutes or until patient care has been transferred.
- Cover the patient with blankets to preserve body warmth.
- Electrical injury, lightning
  - External burns from an electrical injury may appear minor; extent of damage may not be initially apparent.
    - Injury is often extensive; deep tissues such as muscle, nerves, blood vessels, and bone can be destroyed even though the skin appears normal.
    - Tissues that have the least resistance are the most heat sensitive.
      - Bone has the greatest resistance, nerve tissue the least.
      - Cardiac arrest may occur from passage of the current through the heart.
  - Minor electrical burns usually occur as a result of an infant or toddler biting on an extension cord, resulting in localized burns to the mouth that usually involve the upper and lower lip that come in contact with the extension cord.
  - High-tension electrical wire burns
    - Result from high voltage
      - May occur at high-voltage installations (e.g., electric power stations)
        - Child touches an electric box or accidentally touches a high-tension electric wire
    - Most entrance wounds involve the upper extremity, with small exit wounds in the lower extremity.
    - Electrical path through the body may produce injury in any organ or tissue in the path of the current.
    - Cardiac dysrhythmias including ventricular fibrillation are common; renal damage is another complication.
    - Requires hospital admission for observation regardless of the extent of the surface area burn; mortality rate 3% to 15%.

- ○ Lightning burns
  - ▪ Occur when high-voltage current directly strikes a person (most dangerous) or when the current strikes the ground or an adjacent (in-contact) object.
  - ▪ Extent of burn depends on current path, the type of clothing, the presence of metal, and cutaneous moisture.
  - ▪ Entry, exit, and path lesions are possible; prognosis poorest for lesions of the head or legs.
  - ▪ Initial treatment guidelines
    - • Cervical spine precautions if injury was associated with fall.
    - • Protect and maintain airway; mechanical ventilation if indicated.
    - • Initial care is to preserve intravascular volume.
    - • Initiate cardiac monitoring.
    - • Check distal pulses of involved extremities every 15 minutes.
- • Radiation exposure: in children, usually caused by overexposure to sun.
- • Thermal burns are caused by exposure to some form of heat (e.g., flames, hot liquids, or hot solid objects).

Thermal Burns

- • Depth classification of a burn injury
  - ○ It is often days before depth can be determined accurately.
  - ○ Superficial burn (first degree) (Figure 9-32)
    - ▪ Example: sunburn
    - ▪ Only epidermis involved
    - ▪ Dry, no blisters
    - ▪ Minimal or no edema

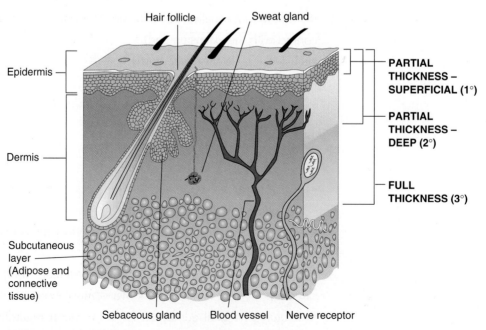

Figure 9-32 Depth classification of a burn injury.

- Painful and erythematous
- Heal in 2 to 5 days with no scarring

Any blistering qualifies as a second-degree burn.

- Partial-thickness burn (second degree)
  - Often caused by scalds
  - Epidermis and dermis involved, but dermal appendages spared
  - Superficial second-degree burns are blistered and painful
  - Deep second-degree burns may be white and painless
  - Healing
    - Superficial: 5 to 21 days with no grafting
    - Deep partial: 21 to 35 days with no infection. If infected, converts to full thickness.
- Full-thickness burn (third degree)
  - Typically result from flame or contact injuries
  - Epidermis and dermis involved; may include fat, subcutaneous tissue, fascia, muscle, and bone
  - Color may vary from yellow or pallid to black and charred, with a dry, waxy, or leathery appearance
  - Often insensate to pinprick because nerve endings have been destroyed
  - Large areas require grafting. Small areas may heal from the edges after weeks.

When determining the extent of a burn, include only partial- and full-thickness burns in the estimate.

- Methods for determining BSA percentage of a burn injury
  - The extent of a burn is classified as a percentage of the total BSA.
  - "Rule of nines" (Figure 9-33)
    - The adult body is divided into anatomic regions that have surface area percentages that are all multiples of 9%.
    - Less accurate for children who tend to have proportionally larger heads and smaller legs—pediatric version developed.
    - Calculations with the rule of nines tend to overestimate burn size
  - "Rule of palms"
    - May be used to estimate burns under 10% of BSA
    - The area from the wrist crease to finger crease (the palm) in the child equals 1% of the child's BSA
    - For example, if the child's palm would fit over the burned area five times, the extent of the burn is 5% of the total BSA
- Initial treatment guidelines
  - Remove all clothing and jewelry.
  - Assess for associated injuries or shock; be sure to assess the posterior surface of the patient for burn injury.
  - Keep burned extremities elevated above the level of the heart.
  - Do not place ice or wet sheets on the burn; if burns are more than 10% of BSA, apply clean, **dry** towels to burn to avoid hypothermia.

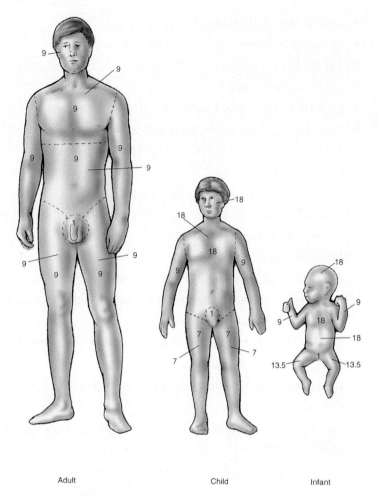

Adult   Child   Infant

Figure 9-33   The Rule of Nines for an adult, child, and infant.

- Keep the burned patient warm.
- Monitor vital signs at least every 15 to 30 minutes.
- Establish vascular access with LR solution.
  - Fluid resuscitation estimated at 3 to 4 mL × total BSA × patient weight in kilogram, not including fluids for insensible losses or other maintenance fluid requirements. Administer as with adults (one half of total in first 8 hours calculated from time of injury).
  - Desired response in a child is urine output of 0.5 to 1.0 mL/kg per hour.
- Urinary catheter insertion for fluid resuscitation or as indicated.
- Keep patient NPO.
- Insert nasogastric tube for all air transport patients as well as those with burns more than 20% total BSA or those who are intoxicated, intubated, or as indicated.
- Give intramuscular tetanus toxoid if patient has not been immunized in preceding 5 years
- Pain management: IV analgesia is often necessary to treat pain. Do

Burns Best Treated in a Burn Center	
• Second-degree burns involving more than 10% total BSA in adults or 5% total BSA in children • Chemical burns • All burns involving hands, face, eyes, ears, feet, perineum, or circumferential burns of torso or extremities • Any third-degree burns in a child • All inhalation injuries	• Electrical burns, including lightning injury • All burns complicated by fractures or other trauma • All burns in high-risk patients including elderly, very young, and those with preexisting diseases such as diabetes, asthma, and epilepsy

not attribute combativeness or anxiety to pain until adequate perfusion, oxygenation, and ventilation are established. Consider narcotic therapy for pain management.[16]

- Give pain medication IV in small increments, titrated to level of comfort.
- Provide emotional support to patient and family.

Case Study Resolution

After performing a primary survey to ensure there are no immediate life-threatening injuries, perform a thorough physical examination to determine the extent of known injuries and locate any other injuries. Try to obtain a thorough history. Administer oxygen, establish vascular access, and evaluate the patient's vital signs. The patient's respiratory rate is 18 breaths per minute, heart rate is 96 beats per minute, blood pressure is 140/80 mm Hg, and her skin is pink, warm, and dry. SpO_2 on room air is 98%. Clean and dress the abrasion over the left eye and cover the left ear with a sterile dressing. Place the patient on a cardiac monitor and obtain a bedside glucose test. Obtain necessary radiographs and laboratory studies, and perform additional interventions on the basis of your assessment findings and test results.

References

1. Templeton Jr. JM. Mechanism of injury: biomechanics. In: Eichelberger MR, ed. *Pediatric trauma: prevention, acute care, rehabilitation.* St. Louis: Mosby–Year Book, 1993:20–36.
2. Stafford PW, Blinman TA, Nance ML. Practical points in evaluation and resuscitation of the injured child. *Surg Clin North Am* 2002;82:273–301.
3. Rivara FP, Grossman D. Injury control. In: Behrman RE, Kliegman RM, Jenson HB, eds. *Nelson textbook of pediatrics,* 16th ed. Philadelphia: WB Saunders, 2000:231–236.
4. Committee on Injury and Poison Prevention. American Academy of Pediatrics: Falls from heights: windows, roofs, and balconies. *Pediatrics* 2001;107:1188–1191.

5. Meller JL, Shermeta DW. Falls in urban children: a problem revisited. *Am J Dis Child* 1987;141:1271–1275.

6. Barlow B, Niemirska M, Gandhi R, et al. Ten years of experience with falls from a height in children. *J Pediatr Surg* 1983;18:509–511.

7. Committee on Injury and Poison Prevention. American Academy of Pediatrics: bicycle helmets. *Pediatrics* 2001;108:1030–1032.

8. Gerardi MJ. Evaluation and management of the multiple trauma patient. In: Strange GR, Ahrens WR, Lelyveld S, et al., eds. *Pediatric emergency medicine: a comprehensive study guide,* 2nd ed. New York: McGraw-Hill, 2002:55–73.

9. Carruthers GN. Spinal immobilization. In: Dieckmann RA, Fiser DH, Selbst SM, eds. *Illustrated textbook of pediatric emergency & critical care procedures.* St. Louis: Mosby–Year Book, 1997:55–73.

10. Davis HW, Carrasco MM. Child abuse and neglect. In: Zitelli BJ, Davis HW, eds. *Atlas of pediatric physical diagnosis.* 4th ed. St. Louis: Mosby, 2002:55–73.

11. Evans RW, Wilberger JE. Traumatic disorders. In: Goetz CM, ed. *Textbook of clinical neurology,* 2nd ed. St. Louis: Elsevier, 2003:1129–1151.

12. Cantor RM, Leaming JM. Pediatric trauma. In: Marx JA, Hockberger RS, Walls RM, eds. *Rosen's emergency medicine: concepts and clinical practice,* 5th ed. St. Louis: Mosby, 2002:267–281.

13. Behrman RE, Kliegman RM, Jenson HB. Head and neck injuries. In: Behrman RE, Kliegman RM, Jenson HB, eds. *Nelson textbook of pediatrics,* 16th ed. Philadelphia: WB Saunders, 2000:2107.

14. Dickman CA, Rekate HL. Spinal trauma. In: Eichelberger MR, ed. *Pediatric trauma: prevention, acute care, rehabilitation.* St. Louis: Mosby–Year Book, 1993:362–377.

15. Proctor MR. Spinal cord injury. *Crit Care Med* 2002;30[Suppl]:S489–S499.

16. Kassis K, Grady M. *Trauma and burns in Johns Hopkins. In:* Gunn VL, Nechyba C, eds. *The Harriet Lane handbook: a manual for pediatric house officers,* 16th ed., St. Louis: Mosby, 2002:79–94.

17. Lucid WA, Taylor TB. Thoracic trauma. In: Strange GR, Ahrens WR, Lelyveld S, et al., eds. *Pediatric emergency medicine: a comprehensive study guide,* 2nd ed. New York: McGraw-Hill, 2002:92–100.

18. Woods WA, Mellick LB. Pediatric cervical spine injuries: avoiding potential disaster. Trauma Reports, July-August, 2003; http://www.findarticles.com/cf_dls/m0KHW/4_4/105044638/print.jhtml Accessed 12/7/2003.

19. Reuter D, Brownstein D. Common emergent pediatric neurologic problems. *Emerg Med Clin North Am* 2002;20:155–176.

20. Barkin RM, Marx JA. Abdominal trauma. In: Barkin RM, Rosen P. *Emergency pediatrics: a guide to ambulatory care,* 5th ed. St. Louis: Mosby, 1999:476–487.

Chapter Quiz

1. True or False: Penetrating trauma is the most common mechanism of serious injury in the pediatric patient.

2. The single most common cause of injury in children is:
   A) Motor vehicle crash.
   B) Falls.
   C) Pedestrian injuries.
   D) Firearm-related injuries.

3. What is the earliest clinical manifestation of compensated shock in children?
   A) Restlessness.
   B) Hypotension.
   C) Tachycardia.
   D) Diminished peripheral pulses.

4. A 10-year-old child presents with a knife impaled in his skull. Your best course of action regarding the impaled object will be to:
   A) Secure the object in place.
   B) Apply an occlusive dressing over the object.
   C) Remove the object immediately and apply direct pressure to the wound to minimize bleeding.
   D) Complete the primary survey and then remove the object to assess the length of the blade.

5. Which of the following is a manifestation of Cushing's triad?
   A) Hypotension.
   B) Tachycardia.
   C) Hypoglycemia.
   D) Bradycardia.

6. With which type of injury is a Chance fracture most commonly associated?
   A) Gunshot wound.
   B) Child abuse.
   C) Lapbelt use.
   D) Bicycle handlebars.

7. Which of the following is the most common type of skull fracture in the pediatric patient?
   A) Basilar.
   B) Linear.
   C) Depressed.
   D) Open.

8. Which of the following is an immediately life-threatening chest injury that must be identified and treated during the primary survey?
   A) Tension pneumothorax.
   B) Pulmonary contusion.
   C) Myocardial contusion.
   D) Aortic disruption.

9. When performing spinal stabilization, which of the following body areas should be secured to the backboard last?
   A) Head.
   B) Chest.
   C) Pelvis.
   D) Legs.

10. Under what conditions can an infant or child found in a safety seat be used to transport the child to the hospital?

Chapter Answers

1. False. Blunt trauma is the most common mechanism of serious injury in the pediatric patient.

2. B. Falls are the single most common cause of injury in children.

3. C. Tachycardia is the earliest clinical manifestation of compensated shock in children. Hypotension is a late sign of shock.

4. A. Leave the impaled object in place. The only indications for nonsurgical removal of an impaled object are: 1) It is not possible to ventilate the child without removing the foreign body (e.g., the object is impaled in the patient's cheek), 2) the presence of the object would interfere with chest compressions, or 3) the presence of the object interferes with patient transport. Manually secure the object, expose the wound area, control bleeding if present, and use a bulky dressing to help stabilize the object in place.

5. D. Increases in intracranial pressure cause characteristic changes in vital signs including hypertension, bradycardia, and an irregular breathing pattern (Cushing's triad). Cushing's triad is a LATE sign of increased ICP.

6. C. A Chance fracture is a horizontal fracture of the thoracic or lumbar spine caused by hyperflexion injuries with little or no compression of the vertebral body. Chance fractures are also called seatbelt fractures, since they are commonly associated with the wearing of lap-type seatbelts.

7. B. Linear skull fractures make up approximately 60% to 90% of skull fractures in children.

8. A. Immediately life-threatening injuries that must be identified and managed in the primary survey include airway obstruction, open pneumothorax, tension pneumothorax, massive hemothorax, flail chest, and cardiac tamponade. Potentially life-threatening injuries that must be identified and for which treatment must begin in the secondary survey include pulmonary contusion, myocardial contusion, aortic disruption, traumatic diaphragmatic rupture, tracheobronchial disruption, and esophageal disruption.

9. A. When performing spinal stabilization, secure the child's torso to the board first, the legs next, and the head last.

10. If the child's condition is stable, a child safety seat can be used for stabilization only after a brief inspection to ensure the seat has not sustained any major structural damage and only if the safety seat can be secured appropriately in the ambulance. If a child is critically injured or the child's condition has the potential to worsen, a safety seat should NOT be used for stabilization. Instead, the child should be removed from the seat onto a rigid backboard and immobilized.

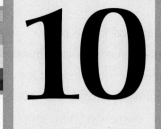

10 Selected Childhood Illnesses

Case Study

A 15-year-old boy presents with a fever, sore throat, fatigue, and aching joints. The boy's father says these symptoms were present when he awoke his son this morning. On questioning, the patient states he has been feeling "tired and achy for about a week." Physical examination reveals a temperature of 101.8° F and swollen lymph nodes. Upon review of his test results, the patient is diagnosed with infectious mononucleosis (IM).

How is this disease spread? What pathogen causes this disease? What precautions should be taken when providing care to this patient?

Objectives

1. Describe assessment findings, high-risk factors for infection, and appropriate interventions for a child with fever.
2. Discuss the characteristics of common childhood infectious diseases.
3. Describe the primary etiologies and general management of altered mental status in children.
4. Discuss the common types, causes, and management of pediatric seizures.
5. Discuss assessment findings that differentiate hypoglycemia from diabetic ketoacidosis (DKA).
6. Recognize the signs and symptoms of patients with hypoglycemia or DKA and formulate a treatment plan for each condition.
7. Identify two common pediatric psychiatric emergencies.
8. Explain the difference between a suicide attempt and a suicide gesture.

Fever

Anatomic and Physiologic Considerations

1. Newborns and neonates are unable to shiver to maintain body temperature.
2. A neonate is less able to dissipate excess heat than an older infant. A warm or hot environment can elevate the neonate's body temperature.
3. Infants in the first 3 months of life have an immature immunologic system and are more susceptible to severe infections and to infections by unusual organisms than an older infant or child.
4. The young child is particularly prone to temperature extremes because thermoregulatory controls are not completely developed.
5. Fever increases metabolic rate 7% for every degree of temperature elevation. Heart rate and respiratory rates also increase to meet the increased metabolic demand.
6. Infants and children have limited glycogen and glucose stores.

Description

Fever (pyrexia) in children is defined by a rectal temperature of 100.4° F (38° C) or higher. A prolonged fever can seriously weaken an infant or child because of exhausted energy stores and increased work of breathing. Increased metabolism places the child at risk for dehydration because of evaporative heat loss and a reduction in oral intake. A child can become quickly dehydrated because they rapidly lose large amounts of fluid in proportion to their body weight.

A child with serious disease may have a normal temperature.

The risk of bacteremia in infants increases as the degree of fever increases. Each degree elevation above 102.2° F (39° C) increases the risk. Children with a temperature of 103.1° F (39.5° C) to 103.8° F (39.9° C) have about a 3% incidence of bacteremia. Those with a temperature of 104° F (40° C) to 105.6° F (40.9° C) have a 4% risk, and those with a temperature greater than 105.8° F (41° C) have a 10% risk.[1] The limit of physiologic thermoregulation is 106° F (41.1° C). Fevers in this range and higher indicate not only bacteremia but also possible central nervous system (CNS) infection, pneumonia, or pathologic hyperthermia.[2]

Etiology

Increased body temperature in an infant may be caused by external factors such as excessive ambient heat. More commonly, bacteria, viruses, fungi, and certain antigens cause the release of stored protein substances called pyrogens. Pyrogens promote increased production of prostaglandins. Prostaglandins raise the thermostatic "set point" maintained by the hypothalamus (usually 98.6° F) to a higher level.

Causes of fever include the following:

- Infection caused by bacteria, viruses, or fungi

- CNS disorders involving injury to the hypothalamus
- Increased intracranial pressure caused by inflammation or bleeding
- Side effect of, or overdose of, some medications (e.g., salicylates, amphetamines)
- Hyperthermia from prolonged heat exposure
- Systemic infection and septic shock
- Pyrogenic reaction caused by contaminated intravenous (IV) fluid or medication administration
- Tissue destruction (e.g., severe injury)

- When did the fever begin and how high was it?
- What remedies have been used to reduce the fever (e.g., sponging with tepid water, administration of acetaminophen or ibuprofen)? What was the child's response to the measures taken?
- Recent immunizations? Exposure to other ill children or adults?
- What is the pattern of the fever?
  - Sustained
    - Fever remains consistently elevated with minimal variation during the day
    - Possible causes include CNS problems, scarlet fever
  - Intermittent
    - Wide temperature variations with return to normal at least once daily
    - Possible causes include bacterial or viral infection
  - Remittent
    - Fever is present each day although the degree fluctuates; temperature does not return to normal
    - Possible causes include pneumonia
- Are there any associated symptoms (e.g., chills, headache, malaise, earache, sore throat, cough, flank pain, painful or frequent urination, poor feeding, irritability, vomiting, diarrhea, altered mental status, bulging/sunken fontanelles, rash, or stiff neck)?
- Preexisting medical conditions (e.g., sickle cell disease, respiratory, cardiac, or renal disease)?

- Tachypnea and tachycardia are common with fever.
  - Normal respiratory rate for the child's age increases by approximately four to five breaths per minute for each degree Fahrenheit of fever.
  - Normal heart rate for the child's age increases by approximately 10 to 12 beats per minute for each degree Fahrenheit of fever.
  - Heart rates exceeding 160 beats per minute are not uncommon in infants with a high fever.

Additional History

Detailed initial assessment information and interventions were presented in Chapter 3 and are not repeated here. Additional history, signs and symptoms, and interventions specific to each condition discussed in this chapter are listed.

Physical Examination

Fever, tachycardia, and vasodilation are common in children with benign infections. Suspect septic shock when a child with this inflammatory triad experiences a change in mental status evidenced by inconsolable irritability, lack of interaction with parents, or inability to be aroused.

High-Risk Factors for Infection in Children with Fever

Sickle cell anemia
HIV/AIDS
Recent cancer therapy
Systemic lupus erythematosus
Nephrotic syndrome
Diabetics
Transplant recipients
Children who have undergone splenectomy
Infants younger than 3 months of age

Therapeutic Interventions

The site used for temperature measurement affects the accuracy of the reading obtained. A rectal temperature is the most accurate reflection of core temperature and should be the technique used in infants younger than 3 months. An axillary temperature may be used when accuracy is not essential. Oral temperature measurement requires correct placement of the thermometer under the child's tongue. This method is useful if the child is older than 5 years, is cooperative, does not have a rapid respiratory rate, and has not recently ingested hot or cold liquids. Tympanic thermometers are less invasive than rectal measurement and have good reported accuracy. Heat-sensing strips placed on the forehead identify fever less than 25% of the time.

- Low-grade fever is 100° F to 102.5° F; high-grade fever is more than 102.5° F.
- Altered mental status may accompany high-grade fever.
- Assess for possible causes of the fever:
  - Nuchal rigidity in a child or a bulging fontanelle in a quiet infant in a sitting position are possible signs of meningitis
  - Focal neurologic findings, such as unequal pupils or decreased unilateral movement, possibly indicating meningitis or a ventriculo-peritoneal (VP) shunt infection
  - Sunken eyes, lack of tears, dry mucous membranes, decreased skin turgor, and other signs of dehydration
  - Petechiae, purpuric lesions, or any rapidly spreading skin rash

- Fevers with temperatures less than 102.2° F (39° C) in healthy children generally do not require treatment.
- Administration of antipyretics often makes patients feel better and is beneficial in high-risk patients who have chronic cardiopulmonary diseases, metabolic disorders, or neurologic diseases and in those who are at risk for febrile seizures.
- Temperatures above 105.8° F (above 41° C) should be treated with antipyretics. Acetaminophen (Tylenol) and ibuprofen (Motrin, Advil) are equally effective antipyretic agents.
  - Aspirin has been associated with Reye syndrome in children and adolescents and is not recommended for the treatment of fever in children.
- Tepid sponge bathing in warm water may be used to reduce fever.
  - Do **not** use ice or cold-water baths to reduce fever. These methods cause shivering and constriction of the skin blood vessels, which then increases the core temperature.

- ◦ Do **not** give an infant or child an alcohol bath because the alcohol can be absorbed through the skin and cause excessively rapid cooling.
- If signs of dehydration or shock are present, establish IV access and administer a 20-mL/kg fluid bolus of normal saline or Ringer's lactate. Reassess.
- If a rash is present, document the pattern of distribution, appearance of the lesions, presence or absence of fever, history related to the development of the rash (i.e., chronic versus acute).

Selected Childhood Communicable Diseases

Rubeola (also called measles, red measles, 9-day measles, or "first disease" because it was the first of similar childhood rash infections to be described) is a highly contagious viral disease characterized by fever, cough, runny nose, conjunctivitis, and a characteristic rash.

Rubeola

Etiology

- The measles virus is a paramyxovirus, genus *Morbillivirus*.
- The virus has a short survival time (less than 2 hours) in the air or on objects and surfaces.

Epidemiology and Demographics

- In 1996, the largest measles outbreak in the United States affected primarily those who had not received a second dose of measles-mumps-rubella (MMR) vaccine. A record low annual total of 44 cases was reported in 2002. Most cases are now imported from other countries or linked to imported cases. Most imported cases originate in Asia and Europe.
- Transmission of the measles virus is primarily via respiratory droplets.
- Incubation period from exposure to early symptoms averages 10 to 12 days.
- Exposure to rash onset averages 14 days (range, 7 to 18 days).
- Measles may be transmitted from 4 days before to 4 days after rash onset.
- Patients with measles are most contagious from the onset of the prodromal period through the first 3 to 4 days of the rash.

Airborne transmission via aerosolized droplet nuclei has been documented in closed areas (e.g., examination room) for up to 2 hours after a person with measles occupied the area.

History

- History of exposure to someone with active measles
- Malaise, high fever
- Upper respiratory symptoms
- Tearing, red or itching eyes, photophobia
- Vomiting, diarrhea, abdominal pain

Physical Examination

- Typical presentation begins with 3 days of high fever and malaise.

- A cough, runny nose, and conjunctivitis follow within 24 hours. These symptoms gradually increase in severity, reaching a peak with the appearance of a rash on the fourth day.

- Approximately 2 days before the development of the rash, Koplik spots (tiny bluish-white dots surrounded by red halos) appear on the mucous membranes of the mouth (Figure 10-1A). These spots increase in number over a 3-day period and spread to involve the entire mucous membrane. They disappear by the end of the second day of the rash.

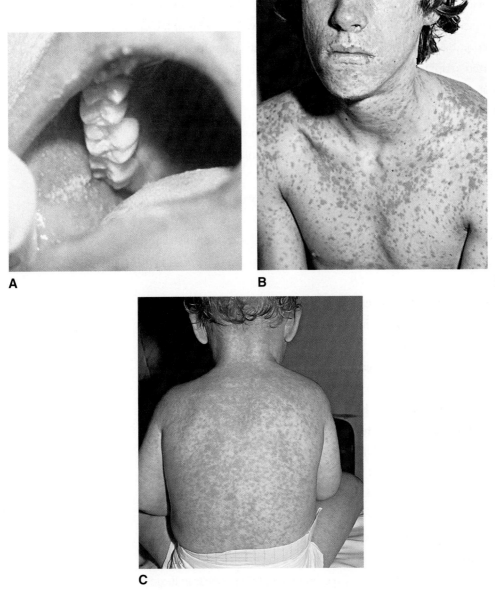

A   B   C

Figure 10-1   **Rubeola/measles. A,** Koplik spots, tiny bluish-white dots surrounded by red halos, appear on the mucous membranes of the mouth a day or two before the onset of the measles rash. **B,C,** The rash appears first at the hairline and then spreads from head to feet over about 3 days.

- The rash appears first at the hairline and then spreads from head to feet over about 3 days (Figure 10-1B,C). During this stage, a high fever, lymphadenopathy, and pharyngitis are typically present. The duration of the rash rarely exceeds 5 to 6 days. Fever that persists beyond the third day of the rash is usually caused by a complication.

Complications

Approximately 30% of reported measles cases have one or more complications. Complications of measles are more common among children younger than 5 years and adults older than 20 years. Reported complications, in order of frequency, include diarrhea, otitis media (occurring almost exclusively in children), pneumonia (most common cause of measles-related death in children), and acute encephalitis (most common cause of measles-related death in adults). Seizures (with or without fever) are reported in 0.6% to 0.7% of reported cases. Death from measles has been reported in approximately one to two per 1000 reported cases in the United States in recent years. Pneumonia accounts for about 60% of deaths.

Measles illness during pregnancy results in a higher risk of premature labor, spontaneous abortion, and low-birth-weight infants.

Therapeutic Interventions

- Use personal protective equipment. Initiate respiratory isolation (droplet) precautions.
- Treatment is primarily supportive. Care usually includes administration of antipyretics and ensuring adequate fluid balance.

Scarlet Fever

Scarlet fever is a rash that sometimes appears in people who have strep throat, and is usually seen in children under the age of 18.

Etiology

Scarlet fever is the result of infection by group A streptococci, the same bacteria that causes strep throat.

Epidemiology and Demographics

- Most common in children 1 to 10 years of age.
- Incubation period is 2 to 4 days.

History

- Sudden onset of sore throat and fever, followed shortly by nausea, vomiting, headache, and abdominal pain.
- Diffuse lymphadenopathy may appear just before the onset of the rash.

Physical Examination

- Rash looks like a sunburn with tiny red bumps that first appear in flexion areas and then becomes generalized (Figure 10-2A); most intense on the neck, axillae, and groin (Figure 10-2B); has the appearance and feel of a rough piece of sandpaper.

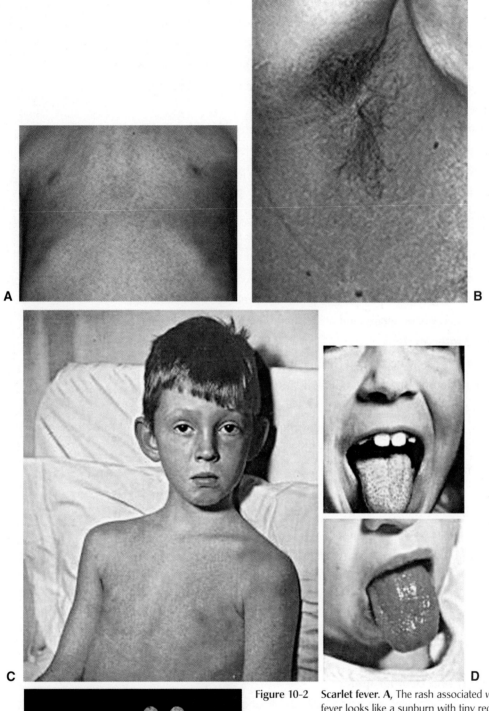

Figure 10-2   Scarlet fever. A, The rash associated with scarlet fever looks like a sunburn with tiny red bumps that first appear in flexion areas and then becomes generalized. **B,** The rash is most intense on the neck, axillae, and groin and has the appearance and feel of a rough piece of sandpaper. **C,** The tongue may be edematous and is initially reddened, with a white coating through which red papillae protrude (strawberry tongue). **D,** After several days, the white coat peels, leaving a red tongue studded with prominent papillae (red strawberry tongue, raspberry tongue). **E,** After the rash is gone, the skin on the tips of the fingers and toes often begins to peel.

- Petechiae may be present, especially on the distal extremities.
- Cheeks appear flushed, with a pale area around the lips (i.e., circumoral pallor).
- Pharynx appears inflamed, tonsils are edematous and may be covered with a gray–white exudate, and palate and uvula may be reddened and covered with petechiae.
- Tongue may be edematous and is initially reddened, with a white coating through which red papillae protrude (strawberry tongue) (Figure 10-2C); after several days the white coat peels, leaving a red tongue studded with prominent papillae (red strawberry tongue, raspberry tongue) (Figure 10-2D).
- Rash lasts about 2 to 5 days. After the rash is gone, the skin on the tips of the fingers and toes often begins to peel (Figure 10-2E).

Complications

Complications are rare but may include peritonsillar abscess, mastoiditis, otitis media, pneumonia, sepsis, and acute rheumatic fever.

Therapeutic Interventions

Hospitalization is rarely necessary. Treatment is primarily supportive and usually includes administration of antibiotics and antipyretics.

Rubella

Rubella (also called German measles, 3–day measles, or third disease) is a mild illness caused by the rubella virus that is characterized by a rash, fever, and lymphadenopathy.

Etiology

Rubella is caused by a togavirus, genus *Rubivirus*.
- Acquired rubella
  - Viral portal of entry is upper respiratory tract.
  - Replication is thought to occur in the nasopharynx and regional lymph nodes.
- Congenital rubella
  - Fetus is infected via placenta during maternal-acquired infection (Figure 10-3A).

Epidemiology and Demographics

- Incidence has decreased since introduction of rubella vaccine in 1969.
- Acquired rubella is transmitted by respiratory droplet secretions; incubation period is 14 days with a range of 12 to 23 days.
- Peak incidence in late winter and early spring.
- Rubella is most contagious when the rash is erupting, but virus may be shed from 7 days before to 5 to 7 days or more after rash onset.
- Infants with congenital rubella shed large quantities of virus from body secretions for up to 1 year and can therefore transmit rubella to persons caring for them who are susceptible to the disease.

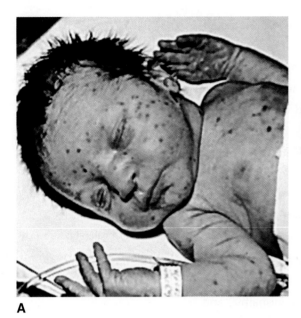

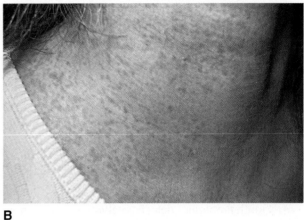

A   B

Figure 10-3   **A**, A 3-day-old infant with generalized macular lesions characteristic of neonatal purpura resulting from congenital rubella. His jaundice is caused by rubella hepatitis. **B**, Rubella/German measles.

History
- Variable low-grade fever
- Malaise

Physical Examination
- Acquired rubella
  - Symptoms are often mild.
  - In young children, appearance of a rash is typically the first sign of infection.
    - Blotchy rash appears first on the face and neck and then spreads from head to foot (Figure 10-3B).
    - Rash lasts about 3 to 5 days (thus the description "3-day measles"), is occasionally pruritic, and is more prominent after a hot shower or bath.
    - Rubella rash is fainter than measles rash.
  - In 65% to 95% of adolescents and adults, the rash is preceded by 1 to 5 days of complaints such as sore throat, headache, low-grade fever, anorexia, malaise, cough, and lymphadenopathy, typically of the cervical, postauricular, and suboccipital nodes.
  - Older children often complain of transient joint pain, particularly of the fingers, wrists, and knees.

Complications
Up to 85% of infants infected in the first trimester of pregnancy will be found to be affected if followed after birth.
- The most significant complications of rubella are birth defects if acquired during pregnancy. Fetal infection may result in spontaneous abortion, stillbirth, or malformations.
- The severity of the effects of rubella virus on the fetus depends largely

on the time of gestation at which infection occurs. The highest risk of developing long-term complications of congenital infection exists during the first trimester of gestation. The risk of congenital infection and long-term complications decreases during the second trimester. Birth defects may include deafness, cataracts, heart defects, mental retardation, and liver and spleen damage.

- Complications of acquired rubella include arthritis, arthralgia, encephalitis, thrombocytopenia, myocarditis (rare), and pericarditis (rare).

- Congenital infection with rubella virus can affect virtually all organ systems. Manifestations may be delayed from 2 to 4 years.

  Rubella deafness may be unilateral or bilateral and varies considerably in severity.

  - Deafness is the most common manifestation of congenital rubella infection.
  - Ophthalmologic defects: cataracts, glaucoma, retinopathy, and microphthalmia.
  - Cardiac defects: patent ductus arteriosus, ventricular septal defect, pulmonic stenosis, coarctation of the aorta.
  - Neurologic abnormalities: microcephaly, mental retardation, and behavioral problems.
  - Other abnormalities: bone lesions, splenomegaly, and hepatitis.

Therapeutic Interventions

Hospitalization is rarely necessary.

- Use personal protective equipment. Initiate respiratory isolation (droplet) precautions.
- Treatment is primarily supportive. Care usually includes administration of antipyretics and ensuring adequate fluid balance.

Fifth Disease

Fifth disease is a mild rash illness that is relatively common and mildly contagious. It occurs most often in children.

Etiology

Fifth disease is caused by infection with human parvovirus B19.

Epidemiology and Demographics

- Peak attack rates occur in children between 5 and 14 years of age.
- Transmitted by direct contact with respiratory secretions (e.g., saliva, sputum, or nasal mucus) of infected persons before the onset of the rash.
- Incubation period is 13 to 18 days.
- Occurs year-round, with a peak incidence in late winter and early spring.
- The infected child is contagious during the early part of the illness, before the rash appears. By the time the rash appears, he or she is probably no longer contagious.

History
- Low-grade fever, malaise, or a "cold" a few days before the rash appears.
- Asymptomatic infection is common.

Physical Examination
Fifth disease appears in stages:
- A rash appears on the face with large, bright red patches appearing over both cheeks (Figure 10-4A)
- The facial rash begins to fade on the following day and is replaced by a lacy red rash on the extremities (Figure 10-4B). The rash spreads to the buttocks and trunk over the next day or so.
- The rash may itch and usually resolves within 7 to 10 days of onset.
- The rash may fade and then reappear in previously affected sites on the face and body during the next 2 to 3 weeks. Recurrences may be stimulated by temperature changes, emotional upsets, and sunlight.

Complications
Fifth disease may cause an acute, severe anemia in persons with sickle cell disease or similar types of chronic anemia.

Therapeutic Interventions
Treatment is primarily supportive. Care usually includes administration of antipyretics, analgesics, and antipruritics as needed for comfort.

Roseola

Roseola is a viral illness that is also called "sixth disease"; *roseola infantum* because it occurs mostly in infants; *exanthem subitum*, which means "sudden rash"; rose rash of infants; and 3-day fever.

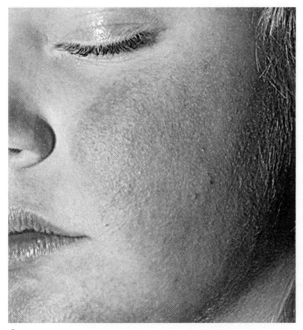

A

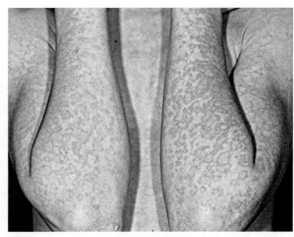

B

Figure 10-4   Fifth disease. **A**, A rash appears on the face with large, bright red patches appearing over both cheeks. **B**, The facial rash fades and is replaced by a lacy red rash on the extremities.

Etiology

Roseola is caused by human herpesvirus 6 (HHV-6) or occasionally by human herpesvirus 7 (HHV-7).

Epidemiology and Demographics

- Most cases occur between the ages of 6 months and 4 years, with more than one half of cases occurring in the second 6 months of life (9 months is the most common).
- Nearly one third of all infants develop roseola before the age of 2 years.
- More than 90% of children older than 2 years of age are seropositive for the virus causing roseola.
- Transmitted by saliva.
- Incubation period is 12 days with a range of 5 and 15 days.

History

- Most cases are asymptomatic or present with fever of unknown origin and occur without a rash.
- High fever (103° F to 106° F) lasting 3 to 5 days.
- Febrile seizures, irritability, or anorexia.

Physical Examination

After the fever resolves, a discrete rash begins on the chest and spreads over the next few hours or days to involve the face and extremities (Figure 10-5); rash fades quickly.

Complications

Although rare, complications of roseola may include febrile seizures, meningitis, encephalitis, pneumonitis, and hepatitis.

Therapeutic Interventions

Most cases of roseola are relatively mild and do not require hospitalization. Provide supportive care; fever control with antipyretics.

Chickenpox

Etiology

Chickenpox (Figure 10-6A) is the primary infection caused by the varicella-zoster virus (VZV), which is a member of the herpesvirus family. Herpes zoster (shingles) occurs when the dormant VZV reactivates and causes recurrent disease. Factors associated with recurrent disease include aging, immunosuppression, intrauterine exposure to VZV, and varicella at a young age (younger than 18 months).

Epidemiology and Demographics

- Spread by direct contact or airborne droplets from virus found in skin lesions or respiratory secretions; enters the body through the respiratory tract and conjunctiva.
- Peak incidence is in the spring.
- Predominant age is 5 to 10 years.

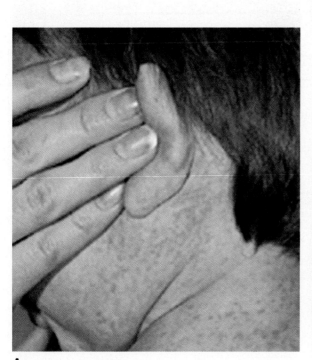
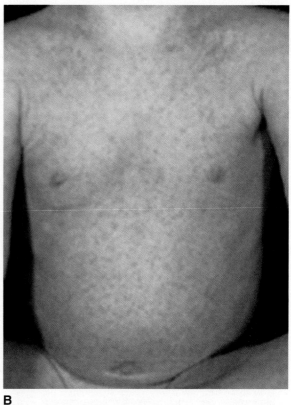

A   B

Figure 10-5   Roseola. A,B, After the fever resolves, a discrete rash appears on the chest and spreads to involve the face and extremities.

- Incubation period is from 14 to 16 days from exposure, with a range of 10 to 21 days.
  - Incubation period may be prolonged in immunocompromised patients.
- Infectious period begins 2 days before onset of clinical symptoms and lasts until all lesions have crusted.

History

- Chickenpox
  - Fever up to 102° F for 2 to 3 days
  - Malaise; itchy rash starting on the head and face and spreading to other parts of the body
  - Exposure to VZV 10 days to 3 weeks before the onset of illness
- Shingles: painful, localized rash that reflects the distribution of one to three dermatomes

Physical Examination

- Chickenpox
  - Generalized rash of papules, pustules, vesicles, and crusted lesions (Figure 10-6B).
  - Fever, cough, abdominal pain; fever is usually highest during the eruption of the vesicles; temperature generally returns to normal following disappearance of vesicles.

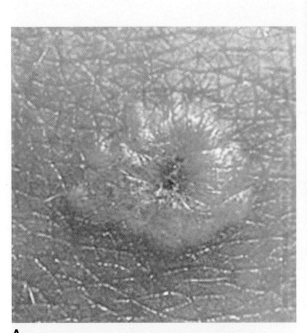

A

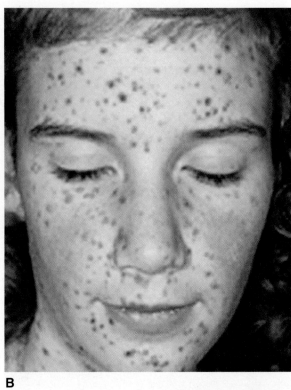

B

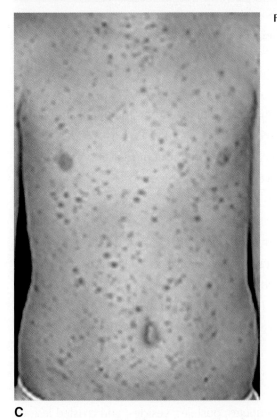

C

Figure 10-6   A, Chickenpox. **B,** Chickenpox consists of a generalized rash of papules, pustules, vesicles, and crusted lesions. **C,** Patients generally present with lesions at different stages at the same time.

- In mild cases, healthy children usually develop fewer than 50 lesions. In severe cases, a healthy child may develop 200 to 500 lesions. Patients generally present with lesions at different stages at the same time (Figure 10-6C).
  - Crusts generally fall off within 5 to 14 days.
  - Adolescents and adults at greater risk of complications.
- Shingles
  - Papular to vesicular rash limited to one to three dermatomes
  - Uncomplicated cases in persons younger than 50 years usually resolve in 2 to 3 weeks

Complications

Although most cases of acute varicella are mild and self-limited, complications may occur including bacterial infections of skin lesions, dehydration, pneumonia, and CNS manifestations ranging from aseptic meningitis to encephalitis. Complications are infrequent among healthy children; higher in persons older than 15 years and infants younger than 1 year.

Reye syndrome is an unusual complication of varicella (and influenza) that occurs almost exclusively in children who take aspirin during the acute illness. The etiology of Reye syndrome is unknown.

Congenital varicella syndrome results from maternal infection during pregnancy. The period of risk may extend through the first 20 weeks of gestation. The risk of congenital abnormalities from primary maternal varicella infection during the first trimester appears to be low (less than 2%). Abnormalities in the newborn may include low birth weight, hypoplasia of an extremity, skin scarring, localized muscular atrophy, encephalitis, cortical atrophy, and microcephaly.

Therapeutic Interventions

- Chickenpox: supportive care, cool or warm bath with oatmeal; calamine lotion/antihistamines for pruritus, antipyretics
- Shingles: supportive care, cool compresses to painful areas, analgesics

Infectious Mononucleosis

Infectious Mononucleosis is an acute multisystem illness most often associated with a primary infection by the Epstein-Barr virus (EBV). EBV is one of the most common human viruses.

Etiology

The EBV, a member of the herpesvirus family, causes more than 90% of IM cases.

Epidemiology and Demographics

- Occurs most commonly between the ages of 15 and 24 years.
- EBV is transmitted via saliva.
- EBV is shed in oral secretions for more than 6 months after acute infection and then intermittently for life.

- Incubation period in adolescents ranges from 30 to 50 days and may be shorter in children.
- No seasonal pattern.

History

- Most cases of primary EBV infection in infants and young children are asymptomatic or indistinguishable from other childhood infections.
- Fatigue, malaise, muscle aches, headache may last 7 to 14 days.
- May have a history of several days of a fever or sore throat.
- Cough, abdominal pain, or chest pain may be present.

Physical Examination

- Fever and lymphadenopathy are present in more than 90% of cases (Figure 10-7).
- Sore throat is often accompanied by moderate to severe pharyngitis with marked enlargement of the tonsils; more than 50% develop exudate.
- Splenic enlargement is present in 50% of cases and may occur rapidly enough to cause left upper quadrant abdominal discomfort and tenderness.
- Hepatomegaly is present in 10% of cases.

Complications

Complications are uncommon; however, one of the most worrisome is splenic hemorrhage or splenic rupture. Because minor trauma to the splenic area or sudden increases in intraabdominal pressure may precipitate rupture, contact sports should be avoided during the first month of illness.

Swelling of the tonsils and oropharyngeal lymphoid tissue may be substantial and cause airway obstruction manifested by stridor and interference with breathing. Airway impairment with progressive symptoms occurs in fewer than 5% of cases and is one of the most common indications for hospitalization with IM. It may be treated by administration of head-of-bed elevation, IV hydration, humidified air, and systemic corticosteroids.[3]

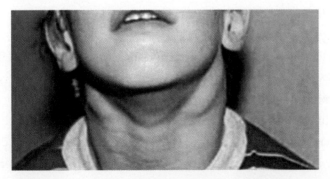

Figure 10-7   Adenopathy associated with the Epstein-Barr virus.

Therapeutic Interventions

- No isolation procedures other than hand washing and careful handling of oral secretions are recommended because the virus is also found frequently in the saliva of healthy people.

- Provide supportive care. Rest, fluids, analgesics, and antipyretics should be provided as needed for comfort.

- Short-term therapy with corticosteroids may be ordered for severe tonsillitis and prevention of airway compromise due to pharyngeal or laryngeal edema.

- Rash is uncommon with IM, but will occur in nearly 80% of patients who receive ampicillin or amoxicillin ("ampicillin rash"). The rash resolves without specific treatment.

Meningitis

Meningitis is an inflammation of the meninges, the membranes covering the brain and spinal cord. Viral or aseptic meningitis, which is the most common type, refers to a clinical syndrome of meningeal inflammation in which common bacterial agents cannot be identified in the cerebrospinal fluid (CSF).[4] Meningitis can also be caused by infections with several types of bacteria or fungi.

These organisms are present in the mucosa of the nasopharynx in 5% to 40% of young children at any given time.

Bacterial meningitis in children 2 months to 12 years of age is usually caused by *Streptococcus pneumoniae*, *Neisseria meningitidis*, or *Haemophilus influenzae* type b (Hib). In newborns, bacterial meningitis is usually acquired by contact and aspiration of maternal intestinal and genital tract secretions shortly before or during delivery. Maternal factors that increase the risk of meningitis in a neonate include premature rupture of the membranes, maternal infection during the last week of pregnancy, and prolonged labor.[5] Neonates with longer nursery stays can also be exposed to pathogens from newborn nursery staff.

In these patients, the infection that causes meningitis is usually secondary to another bacterial infection, such as an upper respiratory infection, pneumonia, sinusitis, or otitis media.

In older infants and children, most cases of bacterial meningitis involve the spread of one of the three common meningeal pathogens. The blood supply of the meninges lies adjacent to the venous system of the nasopharynx, mastoid process, and middle ear. The organism eludes the immune system, penetrates vulnerable sites of the blood–brain barrier (e.g., choroid plexus and cerebral capillaries), and spreads throughout the subarachnoid space. Because the meninges are continuous around the CNS and CSF flows in the arachnoid space, infection spreads quickly through the coverings of the brain. The inflammatory response causes the brain to become edematous and covered with a layer of purulent exudate (Figure 10-8).

Bacterial meningitis may also occur because of direct invasion of the CNS by bacteria. Examples of situations in which this may occur include skull fracture (CSF leak), penetrating injuries of the skull (toys, teeth),

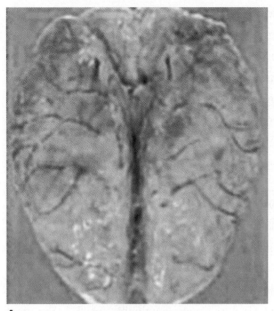
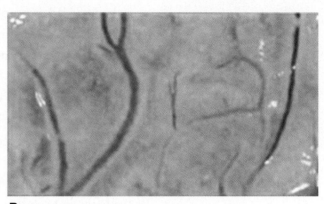

A   **B**

Figure 10-8   **A.** Brain with inflammatory exudate covering the cerebral hemispheres in purulent meningitis. **B,** Arachnoid membrane in purulent meningitis. Close-up view of the arachnoid membrane covering the purulent subarachnoid space, with penetrating blood vessels exhibiting inflammatory vasculitis and thrombosis.

congenital malformations, or a complication of neurosurgery, lumbar puncture, spinal anesthesia, or placement of a VP shunt.

Etiology

- About 90% of cases of viral meningitis are caused by enteroviruses, such as coxsackieviruses and echoviruses. Herpes viruses and the mumps virus can also cause viral meningitis.

- Before the 1990s, approximately 70% of cases of bacterial meningitis among children younger than 5 years were due to Hib. Vaccines now given to all children as part of their routine immunizations (beginning at about 2 months of age) have reduced the occurrence of Hib meningitis. In surveillance studies conducted by the Centers for Disease Control and Prevention (CDC), the incidence of Hib disease declined by 95% from 1987 to 1993 in children younger than 5 years.[7] *S. pneumoniae* and *N. meningitidis* are now the leading causes of bacterial meningitis.

> The median age of bacterial meningitis in the United States increased from age 15 months in 1986 to 25 years in 1995.[6]

Epidemiology and Demographics

- Enteroviruses, the most common cause of viral meningitis, are most often spread through direct contact with respiratory secretions (e.g., saliva, sputum, or nasal mucus) of an infected person. The incubation period for enteroviruses is usually between 3 and 7 days.

- Meningitis caused by *S. pneumoniae* (also called pneumococcal meningitis)
  - Most commonly occurs in infants younger than 8 months and after head injury.
  - Higher incidence in African Americans than in whites.

> *S. pneumoniae* is a common cause of bacteremia, sepsis, meningitis, pneumonia, sinusitis, and acute otitis media in children.

- ◦ Incidence of antibiotic resistance to penicillin and third-generation cephalosporins is increasing.
- Meningitis caused by *N. meningitidis* (also called meningococcal meningitis)
  - ◦ Two percent to 15% of healthy individuals (particularly adults) are asymptomatic carriers of the organism in their nasopharynx.
  - ◦ Most often occurs in children younger than 5 years; peak attack at 6 to 12 months of age; another peak attack occurs in adolescence.
  - ◦ Persons in the same household or daycare center, or anyone with direct contact with a patient's oral secretions are at increased risk of acquiring the infection. Close contacts should receive antibiotic prophylaxis.

History

The onset of acute meningitis has two predominant patterns.[6]

- Sudden onset (less common presentation)
  - ◦ Rapidly progressive manifestations of shock, purpura, disseminated intravascular coagulopathy (DIC), and reduced levels of responsiveness frequently resulting in death within 24 hours.
- Gradual onset (more common presentation)
  - ◦ Preceded by several days of fever accompanied by upper respiratory tract or gastrointestinal symptoms, followed by nonspecific signs of CNS infection such as increasing lethargy and irritability.
- Recent ear or upper respiratory infection
- History of fever may or may not be present in the neonate
- Apnea, respiratory distress in neonates
- Vomiting, headache, poor feeding, photophobia
- Altered mental status; excessive lethargy or irritability in infants (does not quiet when comforted by caregiver)

Physical Examination

Signs and symptoms vary depending on the child's age, underlying medical condition, and causative organism (Table 10-1).

- High fever, headache, and stiff neck are common symptoms of meningitis in patients older than 2 years. Symptoms can develop over several hours, or they may take 1 to 2 days.
- In newborns and infants younger than 2 to 3 months, fever, headache, and neck stiffness may be absent or difficult to detect. Newborns and young infants may initially present with subtle signs such as poor feeding, decreased activity, and irritability. A bulging fontanelle or high-pitched cry may be evident.
- Signs of meningeal irritation are usually present in older children, but may not be present (or present late in the course of the disease) in infants.

TABLE 10-1 *Bacterial Meningitis: Presentation By Age*

Assessment Findings	Younger than 2 to 3 mo	2 to 3 mo to 2 y	Older than 2 y
Apnea/cyanosis	Common	Rare	Rare
Fever	Common	Common	Common
Hypothermia	Common	Rare	Rare
Altered mental status	Common	Common	Common
Headache	Rare	Rare	Common
Seizures	Early finding	Early finding	Late finding
Ataxia	Rare	Variable	Early finding
Jitteriness	Common	Common	Rare
Vomiting	Common	Common	Variable
Stiff neck	Rare	Late finding	Common
Bulging fontanelle	Common	Common	Closed

Adapted from Barkin RM, Rosen P. Neurologic disorders. In: *Emergency pediatrics: a guide to ambulatory care,* 5th ed. St. Louis: Mosby, 1999:726.

- ○ Nuchal rigidity (stiff neck) (Figure 10-9A,B).
- ○ Positive Kernig's sign: The patient's leg is flexed 90-degrees at the hip and then extended; the inability to extend the patient's knees beyond 135-degrees without causing pain constitutes a positive test.
- ○ Positive Brudzinski's sign: Involuntary flexion of the patient's lower extremities (hips and knees) when the neck is flexed constitutes a positive sign.
- As the disease progresses, patients of any age may have seizures.
  - ○ Focal or generalized seizures occur in 20% to 30% of patients with meningitis.
- Rash (petechiae and/or purpura) may or may not be present in meningococcal meningitis.

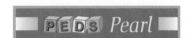

PEDS Pearl

Meningococcemia is a potentially life-threatening emergency in which *N. meningitidis*, the causative agent of meningitis, enters the bloodstream. A petechial rash (Figure 10-9C,D) is present in 50% to 60% of patients. Severe cases of meningococcemia may include purpura.

Complications

The mortality rate for bacterial meningitis after the neonatal period is less than 10%. Outcome depends on the patient's age, duration of the illness before initiating effective antibiotic therapy, the type of causative organism, the intensity of the patient's inflammatory response, the number of bacteria or the quantity of active bacterial products in CSF at the time of diagnosis, and the time needed to sterilize CSF cultures.[8]

Severe neurologic sequelae may occur in 10% to 20% of patients. The most common long-term neurologic sequelae include hearing loss, mental retardation, seizures, delay in acquisition of language, visual impairment, and behavioral problems. Hearing loss occurs in approximately 20% to 30% of patients after meningitis caused by *S. pneumoniae* and in 5% to

Behavioral and academic problems may not be apparent for several years after infection.

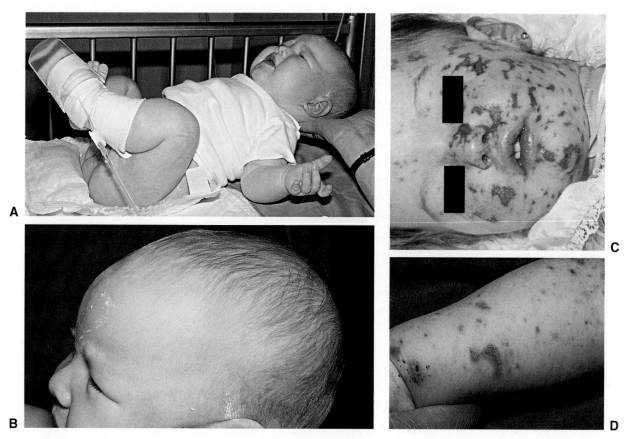

Figure 10-9   **Meningitis. A,** Nuchal rigidity and a positive Brudzinski's sign are demonstrated. On attempted passive flexion of the neck, the infant grimaces with pain, neck stiffness limits flexion, and the knees and hips are flexed to reduce traction on the meninges. **B,** This infant was also found to have a bulging anterior fontanelle when sitting quietly, reflecting increased intracranial pressure. **C,** Meningococcemia. This child manifests the purpuric and petechial rash characteristic of acute meningococcemia. **D,** Meningococcemia. Petechiae are more apparent in this close-up of an infant.

10% of patients after meningitis caused by Hib or *N. meningitidis*. Balance disturbances are common in these children because the vestibular portion of the inner ear is also affected. [8]

Therapeutic Interventions

- Use personal protective equipment. Initiate respiratory isolation (droplet) precautions.
- Viral meningitis
  - Treatment is primarily supportive. Care usually includes pain management, administration of antipyretics, attention to fluid balance, and monitoring for seizures.
- Bacterial meningitis
  - Establish and maintain a patent airway; suction as necessary.
  - Administer oxygen, place the child on a cardiac monitor and pulse oximeter.
  - Establish vascular access. If signs of shock or dehydration are present, administer a 20-mL/kg fluid bolus of normal saline or Ringer's lactate. Reassess. Do not overhydrate.

PEDs Pearl

Kernig's sign, Brudzinski's sign, and nuchal rigidity have been used as bedside diagnostic signs to assess a patient's risk for meningitis for almost a century. In a recent study,[30] researchers evaluated the diagnostic accuracy of these signs in 297 adults with suspected meningitis. The patients were prospectively evaluated for the presence of these meningeal signs before lumbar puncture was done. Kernig's sign (sensitivity, 5%; likelihood ratio for a positive test result [LR+], 0.97), Brudzinski's sign (sensitivity, 5%; LR+, 0.97), and nuchal rigidity (sensitivity, 30%; LR+, 0.94) did not accurately discriminate between patients with meningitis and patients without meningitis. The diagnostic accuracy of these signs was not significantly better in the subsets of patients with moderate meningeal inflammation or microbiologic evidence of CSF infection. Nuchal rigidity showed diagnostic value for only four patients with severe meningeal inflammation.

- Monitor intake and output closely.
- Monitor the head circumference of infants daily.
- Determine serum glucose level.
- Administer medications as ordered: antibiotics, antipyretics, vasopressors (if needed).
- Assess mental status, neurologic signs, and vital signs every 15 minutes to 1 hour depending on patient stability. Monitor for seizures.
- Facilitate presence of family during treatment.
- Obtain laboratory and radiographic studies.
  - Anticipate lumbar puncture, blood cultures, and other studies.

Common Pediatric Neurologic Emergencies

Normal brain function requires intact brain anatomy and a continuous supply of glucose and oxygen. Many conditions can interfere with brain activity and result in abnormal mental status including metabolic problems, infectious diseases, intracranial structural abnormalities, trauma, hypoxia, and poisonings. Possible causes of altered mental status are listed in Table 10-2.

A child with altered mental status will display changes in personality, behavior, or responsiveness that are inappropriate for his or her age. The child may appear agitated, combative, sleepy, withdrawn, slow to respond, or completely unresponsive. The most common causes of altered mental

TABLE 10-2 *Possible Causes of Altered Mental Status (AEIOUTIPPS)*

A	Alcohol, Abuse
E	Epilepsy, Electrolyte disorders, Encephalopathy, Endocrine
I	Insulin, Intussusception, Intoxication
O	Overdose (opiates, lead, sedatives, aspirin, carbon monoxide)
U	Uremia (kidney failure) and other metabolic causes, Underdosage
T	Trauma, Temperature, Tumor
I	Infection (encephalitis, meningitis, Reye syndrome, sepsis)
P	Psychological ("fake," "hysterical," or pseudoseizures)
P	Poisoning
S	Shock, Sickle cell disease, Subarachnoid hemorrhage, Space-occupying lesion, Shunt-related problems

status in the pediatric patient are hypoxia, head trauma, seizures, infection, hypoglycemia, and drug or alcohol ingestion.

First-impression findings that indicate altered mental status include unusual agitation, irritability, or confusion; reduced responsiveness; moaning or a weak cry. Other first-impression findings associated with altered mental status may include abnormal muscle tone or body position for the child's age, abnormal work of breathing, and pallor. During the primary survey, determine the patient's level of responsiveness using the AVPU scale. A more detailed neurologic assessment should be performed during the focused physical examination.

In addition to the SAMPLE or CIAMPEDS history, consider the following questions when obtaining a focused history for a patient with an altered mental status. This list will require modification on the basis of the patient's age and chief complaint.

- If the child's caregiver is available, ask him or her if the child's behavior appears unusual.
- When did the patient's symptoms begin?
  ◦ Was the onset of symptoms gradual or sudden?
  ◦ What was the child doing when it started/occurred?
  ◦ How rapidly have the patient's symptoms progressed?
  ◦ Any history of a similar episode?
- Any history of head trauma, seizures, poisoning, infection with fever (suggesting sepsis), meningitis, a VP shunt, or brain tumor?
- Any history of toxic exposure to alcohol, sedatives, or hypnotic agents?
- Any history of exposure to extremes of temperature (hot or cold)?
- What medication is the patient currently taking? Dosages? Compliance with medication regimen?

- Any history of diabetes or anorexia (potential causes of hypoglycemia)?
  - If the patient is a diabetic:
    - Does the child take insulin injections or oral diabetic medication?
    - When did the child last eat?
    - Any unusual exercise, recent illness?
- If the patient is a newborn:
  - Has the infant been ill?
  - When was the infant last fed?
  - Did the mother receive prenatal care?
  - Does the mother have diabetes?
  - Is the mother breast feeding? Has she taken any medications recently?
    - Sedative or hypnotic medications may be excreted in breast milk.
- If the child has had a seizure:
  - What was the child doing at the time of the seizure?
  - Did the child cry out or attract your attention in any way?
  - What did the seizure look like? When did the seizure start? How long did the seizure last?
  - Did the seizure begin in one area of the body and progress to others?
  - Did the patient lose bowel or bladder control?
  - When the child awoke, was there any change in speech or ability to move his or her extremities?
  - Did the child hit his or her head or fall?
  - Has the child recently had a fever, headache, or complained of a stiff neck?

Hypoglycemia can result from taking too much insulin or oral diabetic medication, missing a meal, or engaging in unusually energetic exercise.

A child can experience hypoglycemia after just a few hours of not eating or drinking.

Infants of diabetic mothers can develop severe hypoglycemia soon after birth.

The physical examination can provide important clues regarding the cause of the patient's altered mental status. Assessment of the patient with an altered mental status includes the following objective measurements and clinical parameters:

- Airway
  - Note the presence of any odors that may help determine the cause of the patient's altered mental status.
    - Fruity odor: possible DKA
    - Musty odor: possible hepatic coma
    - Urinelike smell: possible uremic encephalopathy
  - If cervical spine injury is suspected (by examination, history, or mechanism of injury), manually stabilize the head and neck in a neutral, in-line position or maintain spinal immobilization if already completed.
  - Use positioning or airway adjuncts as necessary to maintain patency. Suction as needed. Avoid the use of an oropharyngeal

Focused Physical Examination

Regardless of the cause of the patient's altered mental status, the priorities of care remain the same—airway, breathing, and circulation.

Difficulty with secretions, vomiting, and inadequate tidal volume are common and significant problems in the patient with an altered mental status.

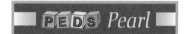

The airway of a child with an altered mental status is vulnerable to airway obstruction because of decreased muscle tone and depressed gag and cough reflexes. This may lead to airway obstruction, resulting in hypoxemia and respiratory failure or respiratory arrest. Repeat the primary survey at frequent intervals throughout your management of these patients and revise your treatment plan on the basis of the patient's response to your interventions.

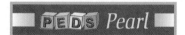

When assessing a child's level of orientation, remember to ask age-appropriate questions. For example, ask the child to tell you about his or her favorite cartoon character, sports personality, toy, or television show.

AEIOUTIPPS = TIPPS over Vowels

Headache

airway unless the patient is unresponsive. Use in a semiresponsive child may cause vomiting if a gag reflex is present.

- ◦ Perform tracheal intubation if the airway cannot be maintained by positioning or if prolonged assisted ventilation is anticipated. Consider the use of pharmacologic adjuncts to aid in intubation.
- Breathing
  - ◦ Patients with an altered mental status may breathe shallowly, even when skin color and respiratory rate appear normal.
  - ◦ Close observation is necessary to ensure adequate ventilation.
    - ▪ Initiate positive-pressure ventilation as necessary.
    - ▪ Intubation may be necessary to ensure a patent airway and adequate ventilation.
  - ◦ Pulse oximetry and continuous cardiac monitoring should be routinely performed for any infant or child who displays an altered mental status.
- Circulation and perfusion
  - ◦ Initiate cardiac monitoring and establish vascular access.
    - ▪ Infuse normal saline or lactated Ringer's at a to keep open (TKO) rate unless signs of shock are present.
    - ▪ If signs of shock are observed or if there is a history of dehydration, give a fluid bolus of normal saline at 20 mL/kg over a period of less than 20 minutes. Reassess. The bolus may be repeated up to two times if signs of shock persist.
  - ◦ Determine the blood glucose level. If the blood glucose level is low, treat with dextrose or glucagon.
  - ◦ Examine the skin for bruises (may suggest trauma or child abuse) or rashes (may suggest sepsis, meningitis).
- Disability
  - ◦ Assess pupil size and reactivity to light, and calculate a Glasgow Coma Scale score using the modified scale for the pediatric patient.
  - ◦ Administer naloxone if the child has an altered mental status and signs suggestive of an opioid overdose (e.g., pinpoint pupils, respiratory depression, and altered mental status).

Headache is a common complaint in the pediatric patient. Structural headaches are associated with underlying CNS pathology. Benign headaches will be discussed here.

Etiology

- Migraines are recurrent headaches that are categorized as vascular headaches because they involve changes in the diameter or size and chemistry of blood vessels that supply the brain.

- A tension headache is a benign headache also known as a muscle contraction or stress headache.
- Cluster headaches are attacks of severe pain, primarily localized to the eye, temple, forehead, or cheek region. The exact mechanism of cluster headache remains uncertain.

Epidemiology and Demographics

- Headache occurs in 37% of children by age 7 years and in 69% of children by age 14 years.
- Migraine headaches
  - Affect children of all ages but difficult to diagnose before age 4 years.
  - Family history is positive for vascular migraine headaches in 75% of patients.
  - Migraine without aura (common migraine) is the most common type of headache in the pediatric population.
  - Migraine with an aura (classic migraine) occurs in 14% to 30% of children with migraine.
- Tension headaches
  - Benign.
  - Can occur at any age, but onset during adolescence or young adulthood is common.
- Cluster headaches
  - Uncommon in children.

History

- Migraine headache
  - Defined as a recurrent headache with symptom-free intervals and at least three of the following:
    - Abdominal pain, nausea or vomiting
    - Throbbing or pulsatile character of the pain
    - Unilateral location
    - Associated aura (visual, sensory, motor)
    - Relief following rest or sleep
    - Positive family history
  - Headache triggers include minor head injuries, sleep deprivation, emotional stress, bright lights or noise, irregular eating patterns, substance abuse or withdrawal, or specific foods and chemicals such as monosodium glutamate (MSG), nuts, chocolate, cola drinks, hot dogs, or spicy meats. Often no trigger can be identified.
  - Rarely awakens patient from sleep.
  - Pain generally lasts from 1 to 3 hours, but may last as long as 24 hours.
    - May be accompanied by intense nausea and vomiting.

- May be preceded for hours or days by pallor, decreased or increased appetite, mood changes, dizziness, or tinnitus.
- Tension headaches
  - Pain of mild to moderate intensity described as a bandlike sensation around the head.
  - History of anxiety, stress.
  - No aura.
  - May be accompanied by photophobia.
  - Not aggravated by physical activity.
  - Often associated with muscle spasms of the neck and shoulder.
- Cluster headaches
  - Pain begins without warning, and reaches a peak within 10 to 15 minutes; each episode lasts 10 minutes to 3 hours.
  - Cluster episodes may occur several times a day and recur for 1 to 4 months.
  - Pain is often described as an excruciating boring pain behind one eye, as if the eye is being pushed out.
  - Facial swelling and tearing of the eye on the affected side is typically present; cheek may be flushed and warm.
  - Episodes often occur during sleep and awaken the patient.

Physical Examination

Be suspicious for another cause of the headache if signs/symptoms are accompanied by any of the following:

- Seizures
- Altered mental status
- Loss of responsiveness
- Fever
- Nuchal rigidity
- Petechiae
- Abnormal visual fields
- Intense irritability
- Bulging fontanelle
- Progressive headache lasting for days
- Isolated pain location that patient can point to with one finger
- Pain that is relieved with vomiting
- Trauma
- Change in the characteristics of the headache
- Rapid onset of the "worst headache of my life" or "thunder clap" headache
- Pain that awakens child from sleep
- Headache associated with Valsalva maneuver
- Headache associated with vomiting

- Simple partial seizures (also called "focal" or "focal motor") produce focal symptoms.
  - Average seizure lasts 10 to 20 seconds.
  - Patient remains conscious.
  - May verbalize during the seizure.
  - No postictal event following the seizure.
  - Characterized by motor or sensory symptoms without impairment of consciousness.
    - Motor: forceful turning of the head and eyes to one side, unilateral clonic movements beginning in the face or extremities
    - Sensory: paresthesias or pain localized to a specific area
- Complex partial seizures
  - Most common type of seizure in children and adults.
  - Consciousness is always impaired.
  - May begin as a simple partial seizure and progress or may begin as a complex seizure.
  - Average duration is 1 to 2 minutes.
  - Often preceded by a sensory aura (visual, auditory, or olfactory).
  - Often includes automatisms (purposeless repetitive movements such as picking at clothes, lip smacking, chewing, eye blinking, rubbing or caressing objects, walking or running in a nondirective, repetitive fashion).
  - Postictal confusion or sleep may follow the seizure.

Generalized Seizures

- All generalized seizures have an abrupt onset and involve an alteration of consciousness.
- Begin with abnormal discharges in both cerebral hemispheres simultaneously.
- Widespread firing of neurons.
- Absence seizures (petit mal) (Figure 10-10)
  - Transient loss of awareness of surroundings without loss of motor tone
  - May have automatisms
  - Uncommon before age 5 years; more prevalent in girls
  - Never associated with an aura
  - Rarely last longer than 30 seconds
  - No postictal state
- Tonic-clonic seizures (also called generalized motor seizures or grand mal seizures)
  - Very common
  - Typical phases:
    - Aura (a peculiar sensation that precedes a seizure)

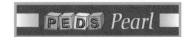
PEDS Pearl

Simple partial seizures may be confused with tics; however, tics are characterized by shoulder shrugging, eye blinking, and facial grimacing and primarily involve the face and shoulders. Tics can be briefly suppressed, but partial seizures cannot be controlled.[9]

Complex partial seizures are also called temporal lobe seizures because they are associated with focal lesions of the temporal lobe.

The older the child, the greater the frequency of automatisms. Automatisms are not remembered by the child.

The most common auras experienced by a child are epigastric discomfort/pain and a feeling of fear.

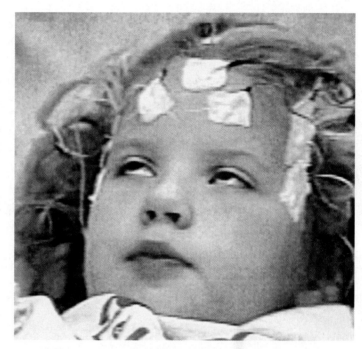

Figure 10-10 Absence seizure. This 8-year-old had a history of brief staring spells reported by teachers and family. Typical absence seizures were recorded during a video electroencephalogram with staring and ocular supraversion lasting under 10 seconds, activated by hyperventilation.

- • Auras include an unusual taste, a dreamy feeling, a visual disturbance (e.g., flashing light, floating light), an unpleasant odor, or a rising or sinking feeling in the stomach
- ▪ Loss of consciousness
- ▪ Tonic phase
  - • Continuous motor tension or rigidity
  - • May be heralded by a high-pitched cry
  - • Lasts 15 to 20 seconds
- ▪ Clonic phase
  - • Rhythmic contractions alternating with relaxation of all muscle groups
  - • Longest phase of the seizure; may last several minutes
  - • Sphincter control lost, particularly the bladder (urinary incontinence)
  - • Patient unable to take a deep breath due to contractions in chest and intercostal muscles; may become hypoxic
  - • May bite tongue or cheek
  - • Clonic phase slows toward the end of the seizure
  - • Patient often sighs as the seizure comes to an abrupt stop
- ▪ Postictal state (also known as "quiet phase"): The period of gradual awakening following a seizure characterized by confusion, disorientation, and fatigue.

- Any or all of the following may last minutes to hours:
  - Change from unresponsive to drowsy, confused, combative
  - Deep, Kussmaul-type respirations
  - Salivation, tachycardia, headache, partial paralysis (Todd paralysis); usually transient
  - Amnesia for seizure
- Vomiting and intense frontal headache common
- Myoclonic seizures
  - **Myoclonus** is a shocklike contraction of a muscle.
  - Characterized by sudden but short contractions of either single muscles or muscle groups.
  - May occur in isolation or repetitively.
    - Not associated with loss of consciousness or postictal state
- Atonic seizures: abrupt loss of muscle tone, usually causing the child to collapse
- Infantile spasms
  - Head nodding with flexion or extension of the trunk and extremities, often in clusters during drowsiness or immediately on awakening
  - May be triggered by unexpected stimuli
  - Usual onset after 2 months, peak onset 4 to 6 months
  - Symptomatic (67%): CNS malformation, any acquired infantile brain injury, tuberous sclerosis, inborn errors of metabolism
  - Cryptogenic (33%): associated with better outcome, less mental retardation

Febrile Seizures

- Generalized seizures occurring with fever in childhood; occur in 2% to 3% of children

  Recurrent febrile seizures occur in 30% to 50% of cases.

- Criteria:
  - Ages 3 months to 5 years (most occur between ages 6 and 18 months)
  - Fever greater than 38.8° C (101.8° F)
  - No CNS infection
- Simple febrile seizure
  - Usually associated with a core temperature that increases rapidly to 38.8° C (101.8° F) or greater.

  Ninety percent of febrile seizures are simple febrile seizures.

  - Seizure is usually generalized, tonic-clonic, lasts a few seconds to 15 minutes.
  - Followed by a brief postictal period of drowsiness.
- Complicated (also known as atypical) febrile seizure
  - Duration is longer than 15 minutes, may have repeated seizures within the same day, focal seizure activity or focal findings are present during the postictal period.

- Febrile seizures lasting longer than 30 minutes are called febrile status epilepticus.
- Strong family history of febrile seizures in siblings and parents suggests a genetic predisposition.
- Extracranial sources of infection include acute respiratory illnesses (common), acute gastroenteritis, urinary tract infections, roseola, and otitis media.
  - One study implicated viral causes in 86% of cases.
  - Immunizations may be a cause.
- Risk of epilepsy after febrile seizures is low.

Status Epilepticus

- **Status epilepticus** is a single seizure lasting longer than 30 minutes or repeated seizures without full recovery of responsiveness between seizures and lasting longer than 30 minutes.
- Multiple causes including hyperglycemia or hypoglycemia, electrolyte imbalance, trauma (e.g., concussion, contusion, subdural, epidural, parenchymal hemorrhage), infection (e.g., meningitis or abscess), tumor, poor compliance with antiepileptic medications, and difficult-to-control epilepsy.
- Potentially life-threatening; requires immediate treatment.

Pseudoseizures

- Diagnosis should be made only after a thorough history and physical examination and exclusion of "true" seizures.
- Pseudoseizures occur typically between 10 and 18 years of age; more frequent among girls.
- Occur in many patients with a history of epilepsy and in some with ongoing true seizures.
- May appear realistic but frequently are bizarre, with unusual postures, verbalizations, and uncharacteristic tonic or clonic movements.
- Several distinguishing features of a pseudoseizure:
  - Lack of cyanosis
  - Normal reaction of the pupils to light
  - No loss of sphincter control
  - Absence of tongue biting or injury during the attack
- Many patients moan or cry during a pseudoseizure.
- Some patients can be persuaded to have an attack on request.

Therapeutic Interventions

- Use personal protective equipment.
- Protect the patient against self-injury and aspiration of vomitus.
  - If the patient is sitting or standing, help him or her to the floor. Move furniture and other objects away from the patient as necessary.
  - Loosen restrictive clothing; remove eyeglasses.

- Open and maintain the airway as needed. Suction the airway as needed. Avoid stimulation of the posterior pharynx during suctioning because this may stimulate vomiting.
- Give high-concentration oxygen and provide assisted ventilation if necessary.
    - If the patient's breathing is adequate, apply oxygen by non-rebreather mask at 15 L/min.
    - Provide positive-pressure ventilation with 100% oxygen if the seizure is prolonged or if the child is cyanotic, has shallow chest rise with bradypnea, or has an oxygen saturation reading below 90% despite high-concentration oxygen. Assess the adequacy of the ventilations delivered.

- Consider electrocardiogram (ECG) monitoring. ECG monitoring is generally indicated for any infant or child who displays an abnormal respiratory rate or effort, heart rate, perfusion, blood pressure, or mental status. However, do not delay lifesaving interventions to set up a monitor.
- Check glucose and administer dextrose IV if serum glucose level is below 60 mg/dL.
- Diagnostic tests
    - Depends on clinical scenario. Consider assessment of electrolytes, calcium, magnesium, blood urea nitrogen (BUN), creatinine, and liver function tests, complete blood count (CBC), toxicology screen and anticonvulsant levels if indicated, blood culture (if infection is suspected).
    - Consider a computed tomography (CT) scan and lumbar puncture if indicated.
- Anticonvulsant therapy
    - Most pediatric neurologists delay treatment until a second seizure occurs, unless the first episode was status epilepticus. All patients with status epilepticus require treatment.
    - If the child has persistent/repetitive tonic-clonic seizures, consider anticonvulsant administration.
        - A benzodiazepine (diazepam, lorazepam, or midazolam) may be used initially for termination of persistent/repetitive seizures because they are effective for immediate control of prolonged tonic-clonic seizures in most children.
            - Rectal diazepam (Valium) or lorazepam (Ativan) or intramuscular midazolam (Versed) are acceptable alternatives if vascular access cannot be readily obtained.
        - Typically, a longer acting anticonvulsant is administered simultaneously because benzodiazepines have a relatively short half-life.

Do **not** insert your fingers, an oropharyngeal airway, a padded tongue blade, or a bite block into the patient's mouth during an active seizure. Do not try to restrain body movements during the seizure.

Treat hypoglycemia if present. Correct any metabolic imbalances.

- If the seizure activity ceases after benzodiazepine therapy or if the seizure persists, phenytoin is usually given immediately.
  - Fosphenytoin (Cerebyx) has advantages over the older formulation of phenytoin because it is water soluble, less irritating after IV injection, and well absorbed after intramuscular injection.
  - The older preparation of phenytoin may be used and can be safely added to normal saline but not to glucose-containing solutions.
- After the seizure
  - If there is no possibility of cervical spine injury, place the patient in lateral recumbent position to aid drainage of secretions.
  - If the patient's spine has been stabilized due to suspected trauma and vomits, the patient and backboard should be turned as a unit and the patient's airway cleared with suctioning.
  - Administer antipyretics if indicated.
  - Evaluate neurologic status and vital signs for signs of increased intracranial pressure.

Unacceptable Interventions
- Failure to use personal protective equipment
- Failure to protect the child from injury
- Failure to administer supplemental oxygen
- Failure to measure oxygen saturation
- Failure to assist ventilation with a bag-valve-mask device and 100% oxygen if the seizure is prolonged or if the child is cyanotic, has shallow chest rise with bradypnea, or has an oxygen saturation reading below 90% despite high-concentration oxygen
- Failure to reassess respiratory status after initiating assisted ventilations
- Failure to recognize signs of deterioration to respiratory failure or arrest and the need for more aggressive interventions
- Failure to monitor the cardiac rhythm in any infant or child who displays an abnormal respiratory rate or effort, abnormal heart rate, perfusion, blood pressure, or mental status
- If suctioning is required, failure to limit suctioning to 10 seconds or less per attempt
- Failure to assess serum glucose level
- Failure to administer dextrose for documented hypoglycemia
- Attempting tracheal intubation while the child is having a seizure

Conditions that Mimic Seizures
- Syncope
  - Syncope (fainting) is frequently confused with seizures. Some children experiencing syncope may have associated myoclonic movements.

○ With syncope, the patient regains consciousness almost immediately (no postictal phase).
- Breath-holding spells
  ○ Two types: cyanotic and pallid
  ○ Cyanotic
    ▪ Usually predictable and provoked by upsetting or scolding an infant or young child.
    ▪ Rare before 6 months of age, peak at about 2 years of age, and subside by 5 years of age.
    ▪ Onset of the episode is signaled by a brief, shrill cry followed by forced expiration and apnea.
    ▪ Rapid onset of generalized cyanosis and a loss of consciousness that may be associated with repeated generalized clonic jerks, and bradycardia.
    ▪ A spell can occur repeatedly within a few hours or it can recur sporadically, but it is always stereotyped.
  ○ Pallid
    ▪ Much less common than cyanotic breath-holding spells.
    ▪ Typically precipitated by a painful experience, such as falling and striking the head or a sudden startle.
    ▪ Child stops breathing, rapidly loses consciousness, becomes pale and hypotonic; may have a tonic seizure.
    ▪ Bradycardia with periods of asystole of longer than 2 seconds may be recorded.
- Tics
  ○ Present with head shaking, blinking, twitching, or other movement disorders and may include vocalizations.
  ○ Occur during periods of anxiety or stress.
  ○ Child may be able to suppress the movement, which is usually nonrhythmic (different from seizures).
  ○ Not associated with a loss of consciousness, but may mimic simple partial seizures.
- Hereditary chin trembling
  ○ May be confused with seizures due to repeated episodes of rapid (three per second) chin-trembling movements.
  ○ Brief attacks; precipitated by stress, anger, and frustration.
  ○ Inherited trait; findings on the neurologic examination and EEG are normal.
- Night terrors and somnambulism
  ○ Night terrors
    ▪ Common, particularly in boys between 5 and 7 years of age.
    ▪ Occur in 1% to 3% of children and are usually short-lived.

The average breath-holding spell lasts approximately 40 seconds. Breath-holding spells should be assumed to be respiratory emergencies until proven otherwise. Place the child in a lateral recumbent position to protect against aspiration.

PEDS Pearl

Breath-holding spells are frequently misdiagnosed as seizures, and a careful history may allow differentiation between the two conditions. In a seizure, there is a change in muscle tone and posture before the development of cyanosis, whereas in a breath-holding spell, cyanosis precedes changes in muscle tone. Furthermore, the lack of postictal symptoms in breath-holding spells may help to differentiate the two conditions.[31]

- Sudden onset; commonly occurs within 2 hours after falling asleep.
- Child may sit up in bed screaming, thrashing about, and exhibiting rapid breathing, tachycardia, dilated pupils, and sweating.
- Child often has a glazed look in his or her eyes, is incoherent, unresponsive to comforting; unaware of caregiver or surroundings.
- Event may last up to 30 minutes, after which the child goes back to sleep and has no memory of the event the next day.
  - Somnambulism
    - Approximately one third of children with night terrors experience somnambulism (sleepwalking).
    - Occur in school-aged children, who "wake up and walk around" during the nondreaming phase of sleep.
- Benign paroxysmal vertigo (BPV)
  - Typically develops in toddlers and is relatively rare beyond 3 years of age.
  - Attacks develop suddenly and are associated with ataxia, causing the child to fall or refuse to walk or sit.
  - Horizontal nystagmus may be evident during the duration of the attack; child appears frightened and pale.
  - Consciousness and ability to verbalize are not disturbed; lethargy or drowsiness does not follow completion of the episode.
  - Attacks vary in duration (seconds to minutes), frequency (daily to monthly), and intensity.
  - Vertigo is verbalized by older children.
  - Susceptible to motion sickness and may develop migraine headaches several years later.
- Sandifer syndrome
  - Infants with gastroesophageal reflux can present with back arching or head turning (Sandifer syndrome).

Gastrointestinal Disorders

Gastroenteritis

Gastroenteritis is an inflammation of the stomach and small and large intestines. The primary manifestation of the illness is diarrhea, but it may be accompanied by nausea, vomiting, and abdominal pain. Gastroenteritis may be caused by pathogens acquired as a result of exposure to child-care settings or hospitals, food-borne or water-borne disease, exposure to antimicrobial agents, travel, or exposure to animals (e.g., pets).

Etiology (Partial List)
Although at least 25 different bacteria and parasites can cause gastro-

enteritis, viruses are responsible for 70% to 80% of infectious diarrhea cases in the developed world. Bacterial pathogens account for another 10% to 20% of cases, and parasitic organisms cause fewer than 10% of cases.[10]

- Viral: rotavirus (most common), enteric adenovirus, noroviruses (Norwalk-like viruses), calicivirus, astrovirus, parvovirus
  - Rotavirus infection most common cause of diarrhea in infants and young children younger than 5 years; tends to produce severe diarrhea
  - Adenoviruses and astroviruses cause diarrhea mostly in young children, but older children and adults can also be affected.
  - Noroviruses are more likely to cause diarrhea in older children and adults.
- Bacterial: *Salmonella* species, *Shigella* species, *Campylobacter jejuni*, *Yersinia enterocolitica, Escherichia coli, Clostridium difficile*
- Parasitic: *Giardia lamblia, Cryptosporidium* species
- 40% of gastroenteritis cases are idiopathic.

Epidemiology and Demographics

Gastroenteritis in children is most often contracted by poor hygiene, contamination through the fecal-oral route, and poor food-handling practices. Handling diapers, fecal-oral transmission, and cleaning toys remain sources of concern in daycare centers.[11]

- Viruses are suspected when vomiting is prominent, the incubation period is longer than 14 hours, and the entire illness is over in less than 72 hours. Viral pathogens are likely when there are no warning signs of bacterial infection (i.e., high fever, bloody diarrhea, severe abdominal pain, more than six stools per 24 hours) and there are no epidemiologic clues from the history (i.e., travel, antibiotic use) that suggest an alternative diagnosis.[12]
  - Noroviruses are very contagious and can spread easily from person to person. Both stool and vomit are infectious. Persons infected with norovirus are contagious from the moment they begin feeling ill to at least 3 days after recovery.
  - In the United States, rotavirus and astrovirus infections occur from October to April; adenovirus infections occur throughout the year.
  - Outbreaks can occur in settings such as schools, child-care facilities, banquet halls, cruise ships, dormitories, and campgrounds.
- Highest incidence of shigellae is in children 1 to 4 years old, particularly during the warm season; illness uncommon in infants younger than 6 months.
- Most cases of campylobacteriosis are associated with handling raw poultry or eating raw or undercooked poultry meat.

Viral gastroenteritis is often called the "stomach flu," although it is not caused by the influenza viruses.

- Estimated 2 million cases of salmonella gastroenteritis per year in the United States; rates of infection are highest in infants and young children.
- *Giardia* is one of the most common causes of water-borne disease (drinking and recreational water [such as water in swimming pools, hot tubs, fountains, lakes, rivers, springs, ponds]) in humans in the United States. The parasite is found in every region of the United States and throughout the world.

History

When obtaining a history, attempt to determine the following[13]:

- When and how the illness began (e.g., abrupt or gradual onset and duration of symptoms)
- Stool characteristics (watery, bloody, mucous, greasy, etc.)
- Frequency of bowel movements
- Presence of fever, blood, and/or pus in the stool
- Signs/symptoms of volume depletion (thirst, tachycardia, decreased urination, lethargy, decreased skin turgor)
- Associated symptoms and their frequency and intensity (nausea, vomiting, abdominal pain, cramps, headache, altered mental status)
- Risk factors for particular diarrheal diseases or for their spread:
  - Travel to a developing area
  - Day-care center attendance
  - Consumption of unsafe foods (e.g., raw meats, eggs, or shellfish; unpasteurized milk or juices) or swimming in or drinking untreated fresh surface water from, for example, a lake or stream
  - Visiting a farm or petting zoo or having contact with reptiles or with pets with diarrhea

Physical Examination

- Signs and symptoms include diarrhea (may be watery or bloody depending on causative organism), vomiting, headache, and fever.
- Signs of dehydration are often present including sunken eyes, sunken fontanelle, decreased tearing, poor skin turgor, unusual drowsiness or fussiness, decreased urine output, and dry mucous membranes.
- Increased dehydration risk in children with a history of prematurity, poor prenatal care, teen-aged parents, or poverty.

Therapeutic Interventions

Treatment is primarily supportive and is directed at preventing or treating dehydration.

- If there are no signs, or signs of mild to moderate dehydration, initiate rehydration and electrolyte replacement by the oral route. Colas, fruit juice, and sports drinks are not recommended for use in oral rehydration therapy because they may cause osmotic worsening of diarrhea and their low sodium content may contribute to the development of hyponatremia.[14,15]

- If signs of moderate to severe dehydration exist, establish vascular access and administer an IV bolus of normal saline or Ringer's lactate at 10 to 20 mL/kg. Reevaluate. Repeat if needed based on the patient's clinical presentation.

- If the child has abdominal pain, use an age-appropriate pain assessment tool to monitor the child's degree of discomfort.

- Administer antipyretics as needed. Antiemetic and antidiarrheal medications are generally not indicated.

- Monitor stools for amount, frequency, color, and consistency.

Diabetic Emergencies

- Glucose is the basic fuel for body cells. The brain must constantly be supplied with glucose because it cannot store it. The level of glucose in the blood must remain constant to ensure proper functioning of the brain and body cells.

- Insulin and glucagon are hormones secreted by the pancreas (Figure 10-11). Because glucose is a large molecule, insulin helps glucose enter the body's cells to be used for energy. Without insulin, glucose remains outside the cell. Glucose may not get into cells because of inadequate food intake or a lack of insulin.

- As blood glucose levels increase, the pancreas secretes insulin. Insulin decreases the blood glucose toward normal. If blood glucose levels fall below normal, the pancreas secretes glucagon, which increases blood glucose toward normal.

- Diabetes mellitus is a disease involving the pancreas. The pancreas produces either too little insulin or stops producing it completely. There are two major types of diabetes:

- Type I (insulin-dependent) diabetes
  - Usually begins during childhood (juvenile diabetes)
  - In this type of diabetes
    - Little or no insulin is produced by the pancreas
    - Insulin receptors are available but, without insulin, glucose is unable to enter most body cells
  - Requires treatment with insulin

- Type II (noninsulin-dependent) diabetes
  - Usually affects people older than 40 years, especially those who are overweight

Pathophysiology of Diabetes

The brain is the only tissue that does not require insulin for glucose transport. Glucose can enter brain cells without insulin.

Ten percent of the diabetic population has type I diabetes.

Ninety percent of the diabetic population has type II diabetes.

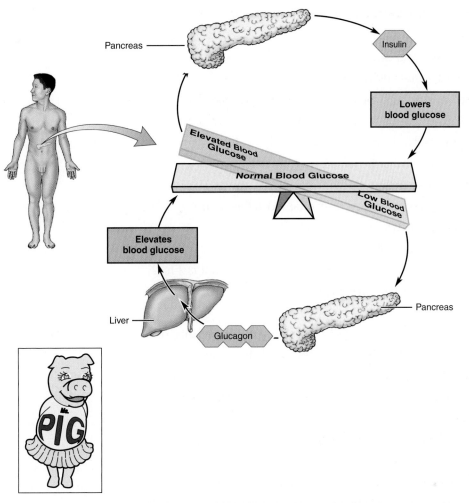

Figure 10-11 Regulation of blood glucose by the pancreas. As blood glucose levels increase, the pancreas secretes insulin. Insulin decreases the blood glucose toward normal. If blood glucose levels fall below normal, the pancreas secretes glucagon, which increases blood glucose toward normal. Ms. PIG reminds you that the **P**ancreas secretes **I**nsulin and **G**lucagon.

- Type II diabetes is rare in younger children, but may occur in adolescents. The incidence of type II diabetes in children is on the rise due to increased pediatric obesity.
- In this type of diabetes
  - The amount of insulin produced by the pancreas may be adequate or may be insufficient to meet the body's needs.
  - Insulin receptors on the body's cells may be decreased, or insulin may be unable to attach to them, impairing insulin's action.
- Noninsulin-dependent diabetes can often be managed by diet, exercise, and oral medications. Some require insulin.

Focused History

- Any history of diabetes?
- Does the child take insulin injections or oral diabetic medication?
- Does the child take his or her medications regularly?

- When did the child last take his or her medication?
- If the patient takes insulin
  - Did you take your insulin today?
  - How much insulin did you take?
  - Any recent change in medications (additions, deletions, or change in dosages)?
  - Has your insulin dosage changed recently?
  - When did you last eat?
  - Any unusual exercise or recent illness?
  - Has this happened before? How often does this occur?
- If the patient is a newborn
  - Has the infant been ill?
  - What is the newborn being fed? When was the infant last fed?
  - Does the mother have diabetes?

Hypoglycemia

Hypoglycemia (low blood sugar) may occur in diabetic patients, often as a result of treatment with insulin or oral hypoglycemic agents. Hypoglycemia is precipitated by an excess of insulin (Figure 10-12). Sugar rapidly leaves the blood, quickly affecting the nervous system because neurons cannot use fats or proteins as an energy source. This results in poor concentration, lack of coordination, and related symptoms. Hypoglycemia stimulates the sympathetic nervous system, resulting in tachycardia, anxiety, tremors, and pale, moist skin. Because these signs mimic those of compensated shock, hypoglycemia is often called insulin shock.

Hypoglycemia is common in metabolically stressed children because a child is unable to store large quantities of glucose and mobilize what he or she can store. Prolonged hypoglycemia can lead to irreversible brain damage.

In children, alcohol intoxication increases susceptibility to hypoglycemia and altered mental status because alcohol suppresses the ability of the liver to make glucose.

Etiology

The blood sugar level may become too low if the diabetic patient

- Has taken too much insulin
- Has not eaten enough food

PEDS *Pearl*			
Signs and Symptoms of Hypoglycemia			
History: Rapid onset, took too much insulin, ate less than usual, increased exercise			
Hunger	Irritability	Weakness	Agitation
Headache	Nausea	Diaphoresis	Blurred vision
Fatigue	Dizziness	Tachycardia	Tremors
Staring	Inability to concentrate	Incoordination	Seizures

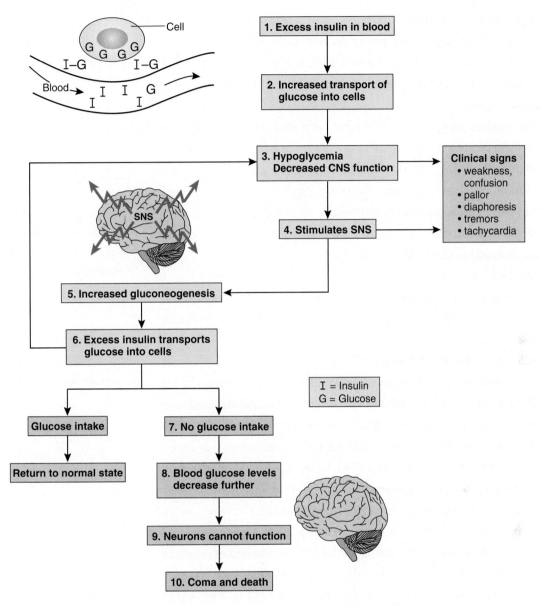

Figure 10-12 Hypoglycemia (insulin shock). *CNS,* central nervous system; *SNS,* sympathetic nervous system; *I,* insulin; *G,* glucose.

- Has overexercised and burned off sugar faster than normal
- Experiences significant physical (e.g., infection) or emotional stress

Physical Examination

- Signs and symptoms of hypoglycemia are very nonspecific.
    - Early signs: headache, hunger, nausea, weakness, irritability, agitation
    - Later signs: cool, pale, clammy skin; tachycardia, tachypnea, abdominal pain (stomach ache), dizziness, sweating, pallor, confusion, tremors, seizures, coma
- Signs and symptoms of hypoglycemia in a neonate include poor muscle tone, tremors, jitteriness, increased work of breathing, apnea, lethargy, seizures, acidosis, and coma.

Therapeutic Interventions

- Use personal protective equipment. In addition to appropriate interventions to ensure a patent airway, adequate breathing, and effective circulation, consider the following actions if the patient shows signs of hypoglycemia.

- Infuse normal saline or lactated Ringer's at a TKO rate unless signs of shock are present. If signs of shock are observed or if there is a history of dehydration, give a fluid bolus of normal saline at 20 mL/kg over a period of less than 20 minutes. Reassess. The bolus may be repeated up to two times if signs of shock persist.

- Determine blood glucose level. If the blood glucose level is low, treat with dextrose or glucagon.

- Alert child.
  - Oral glucose gel should be given **only** if the patient can swallow without choking, has a gag reflex, and has an AVPU of "A" or can be roused to alertness.

- Child with altered mental status
  - If the child has an altered mental status and the blood glucose level is less than 60 mg/dL, establish IV access and administer dextrose. If the patient is a newborn and the blood glucose level is less than 40 mg/dL, establish IV access and administer dextrose.
  - Newborn: Give 0.5 to 1 g/kg (5 to 10 mL/kg) of 10% dextrose in water ($D_{10}W$) over 20 minutes. Mix one part 50% dextrose in water ($D_{50}W$) to four parts sterile water or normal saline.
  - For the patient 1 month to 2 years old: Give 0.5 to 1 g/kg (2 to 4 mL/kg) of 25% dextrose in water ($D_{25}W$) over 5 to 10 minutes. Mix one part $D_{50}W$ to one part sterile water or normal saline.
  - For children older than 2 years: Give 0.5 to 1 g/kg (1 to 2 mL/kg) of $D_{50}W$ over 5 to 10 minutes.

- If IV access cannot be established, give intraosseous (IO) dextrose. If IV and IO access cannot be obtained, give 1 mg glucagon intramuscularly.
  - Glucagon mobilizes glycogen stores from the liver and raises blood glucose levels. However, glucagon will be ineffective in young infants (younger than 3 months old) and children with inadequate glycogen stores due to poor nutrition or starvation.
  - If glucagon is given, place the child on his or her side after administration (unless contraindicated) because glucagon may cause nausea.

- Monitor the child's clinical response closely.
  - Obtain and document vital signs at least every 30 minutes.
  - Recheck the blood glucose level within 10 minutes and frequently thereafter until the level stabilizes.

If the patient's condition is critical, do not delay treatment to obtain a glucose measurement.

The dextrose concentration and dosage are age-dependent.

PEDS Pearl

If the child with hypoglycemia shows improvement in his or her mental status with treatment and subsequently shows deterioration in his or her level of consciousness, continued hypoglycemia may be present or a coexisting problem with neurologic manifestations.

Hyperglycemia

Diabetic ketoacidosis is also called diabetic coma.

Excess glucose in the blood is called hyperglycemia (Figure 10-13). This condition is due to two factors. The first is the inability of glucose to enter the cells, where it can be burned for energy. Failure to move the glucose into the cells causes the glucose to accumulate in the blood. The second is the making of additional glucose. In the absence of insulin, the body makes glucose from protein. The excess glucose accumulates in the blood because it cannot be used by the cells. The kidneys cannot reabsorb the excess glucose and excrete it in the urine (glycosuria). When the kidney excretes a lot of glucose, it must also excrete a lot of water. Glycosuria causes polyuria (excretion of a large volume of urine). Loss of water in the urine causes dehydration and thirst (polydipsia).

Because the cells cannot burn glucose as fuel, they burn fatty acids instead. The rapid, incomplete breakdown of fatty acids produces strong acids called ketoacids. This produces DKA.[16]

Deep, rapid breathing (Kussmaul respirations) partially compensates for the increasing acid level through exhalation of carbon dioxide. Acidosis causes abdominal pain and emesis. Emesis further contributes to dehydration. Another ketone produced by fatty acid breakdown is acetone. Acetone smells fruity and results in a fruity breath odor. High levels of glucose and ketones in the blood cause altered mental status. Unless sufficient fluid is consumed, severe dehydration leading to shock and lactic acidosis can occur.

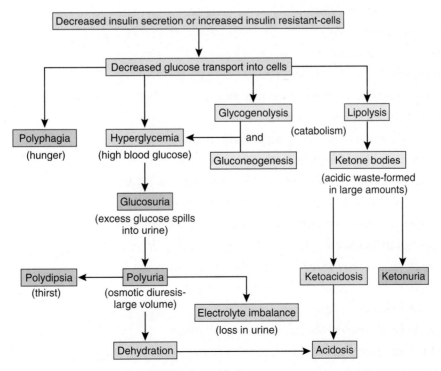

Figure 10-13 Development of diabetic ketoacidosis.

PEDS *Pearl*

Signs and Symptoms of Hyperglycemia

History: Gradual onset (hours to days); excessive food intake containing sugar, insufficient insulin dosage

Altered mental status (varies from drowsiness to coma)

Rapid, deep breathing (Kussmaul respirations)

Sweet or fruity (acetone) breath odor

Loss of appetite	Thirst
Dry skin	Abdominal pain
Nausea and/or vomiting	Tachycardia
Normal or slightly decreased blood pressure	Weakness

Etiology

The blood sugar level may become too high when the diabetic patient

- Has not taken his or her insulin
- Has eaten too much food that contains or produces sugar
- Experiences physical (e.g., infection, surgery) or emotional stress

History

- Excessive food intake containing sugar
- Insufficient insulin dosage
- Infection, surgery, emotional stress
- Common presenting symptoms of new-onset or worsening diabetes
  - Polydipsia (excessive thirst)
  - Polyuria (frequent urination)
  - Polyphagia (excessive eating)

Physical Examination

- Many diabetic patients wear medical identification insignia that can provide diagnostic clues in unresponsive patients.
- A slight increase in respiratory rate is seen early in DKA. Kussmaul respirations (deep, rapid, and intense respirations) may develop later.
- Tachycardia is common in hypoglycemic patients and those in DKA.
- Blood pressure may be decreased secondary to dehydration.
- Poor skin turgor, dry mucous membranes, sunken fontanelle may be evident because of dehydration.
- Abdominal examination may reveal nonspecific pain, tenderness, or distention.

Therapeutic Interventions

- Establish and maintain a patent airway; suction as necessary.
- Administer 100% oxygen.
- Place the child on a cardiac monitor and pulse oximeter.

- Determine serum glucose level.
- Assess mucous membranes, skin turgor, and (in children younger than 6 years) capillary refill.

Do **not** give dextrose-containing solutions.

- If signs of dehydration or shock are present, establish IV access and administer a 20-mL/kg fluid bolus of normal saline. Reassess. Multiple boluses (up to 60 mL/kg) may be required to restore adequate circulation in the severely ill child.
- Monitor the child's clinical response closely.
  - Electrolyte imbalances (particularly of potassium) may lead to ECG abnormalities and dysrhythmias. Monitor the ECG closely.
  - Obtain and document vital signs at least every 30 minutes.
  - Recheck the blood glucose level hourly.
- Additional therapy includes insulin therapy, fluid replacement, and electrolyte and bicarbonate balance.

TABLE 10-3 *Assessment and Management of Pediatric Diabetic Emergencies*

Assessment	Hypoglycemia	Hyperglycemia
First impression	Normal or decreased responsiveness Pale, diaphoretic	Normal or decreased responsiveness Face flushed
Breathing	Normal to increased rate	Initial respirations deep, rapid Late: Kussmaul respirations
Circulation	Tachycardia Normal or delayed capillary refill Normal or cool, pale, clammy skin	Normal heart rate or tachycardia Skin dry, warm, flushed
Focused history	Rapid onset (minutes to hours) Took too much insulin Ate less food than usual Increased exercise Headache, dizziness, seizures	Gradual onset (hours to days) Excessive food intake containing sugar Insufficient insulin dosage Polyuria, polydipsia, polyphagia
Focused physical examination	Normal breath odor Tremors, staring, inability to concentrate, incoordination, irritability	Possible fruity breath odor Abdominal pain Signs of dehydration Nausea and/or vomiting
Initial management	ABCs, oxygen, IV, dextrose IV or glucagon IM	ABCs, oxygen, IV, fluid challenge for signs of dehydration or shock

ABC, airway, breathing, circulation; IM, intramuscular; IV, intravenous.

Hematologic Disorders

Sickle cell disease is an inherited disorder. Its principal features include chronic hemolytic anemia and recurrent painful episodes. These and other elements of the disease are the result of mutant sickle cell hemoglobin (Hb S) within the red blood cells.

The syndromes that make up sickle cell disease are mainly sickle cell anemia (Hb SS), sickle cell-β° thalassemia, Hb SC disease (Hb SC), and sickle cell-β+ thalassemia. Sickle cell trait (Hb AS) lacks anemia and recurrent pain, which distinguishes it from the disease.[17] Hemolytic anemia gradually develops in affected newborns over the first 2 to 4 months, paralleling the replacement of much of the fetal hemoglobin by Hb S.

Vasoocclusive pain is the most common of the sickle cell crises and occurs when distorted ("sickled") red blood cells obstruct blood flow and cause tissue ischemia. Sites most often affected by the vasoocclusive process are bones, abdominal viscera, pulmonary parenchyma, and the CNS. Children often begin to have more frequent vasoocclusive episodes from 5 to 10 years of age, and the episodes sometimes become more severe.

Epidemiology and Demographics

- In the United States, African Americans and Hispanics are most commonly affected.
- Disease severity is variable.
- Predictors of a severe course of sickle cell disease are anemia, painful episodes, and dactylitis ("hand-foot syndrome") before the age of 24 months.

History

- Known presence of sickle cell disease or trait.
- Pain, swelling, or warmth of joints or extremities.
- Pain is frequently described as throbbing, usually without physical findings.
- Children younger than 5 years may experience hand-foot syndrome with swelling and tenderness of hands and/or feet (Figure 10-14).
  - Often the earliest presentation of sickle cell anemia
  - Common in infants
- Older patients typically experience pain in the long bones, back, joints, and abdomen.
- Bedwetting is a common sequela of sickle renal disease.

Physical Examination

- Short stature, impaired growth, and delayed puberty are common.
- Priapism (vasoocclusive crisis) is relatively frequent.

Sickle Cell Anemia

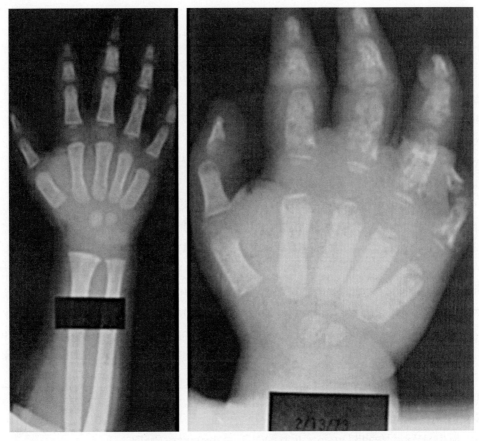

Figure 10-14 Radiographs of an infant with sickle cell anemia and acute dactylitis. Left, The bones appear normal at the onset of the episode. **Right,** Destructive changes and periosteal reaction are evident 2 weeks later.

- Tachycardia, tachypnea.
- Chest pain, hypoxia, dyspnea, fever, and infiltrates on chest radiograph = acute chest syndrome.
- Distortion of bones secondary to bone marrow expansion.
- Pain with weight bearing or with rotation of hip or arm.
- Signs/symptoms of stroke
  - Strokes caused by cerebrovascular occlusion are a frequent cause of hemiplegia. As many as 10% of children with sickle cell anemia, mainly preadolescent and older patients, exhibit sequelae of cerebrovascular occlusion.
  - Stroke is more common after the age of 5 years, with the peak being between 6 and 9 years. There may be subtle, sickle cell–related brain injury in young children with sickle cell disease, with 25% to 30% of children suffering occult strokes. [18]

Therapeutic Interventions

- Establish and maintain a patent airway; suction as necessary.
- Administer oxygen; place the child on a cardiac monitor and pulse oximeter.

- Determine serum glucose level.
- Establish IV access and administer analgesics titrated to pain relief.
- Maintain normovolemia through oral or IV therapy.
- Transfusion may be necessary in patients with severe anemia or hypoxia.
- Antibiotics and antipyretics may be ordered.
- Facilitate presence of family during treatment.
- Monitor intake and output closely.
- Obtain laboratory and radiographic studies.

Immunologic Disorders

Acquired immunodeficiency syndrome (AIDS) is caused by the human immunodeficiency virus (HIV). HIV progressively destroys the body's ability to fight infection and certain cancers by killing or damaging cells of the body's immune system.

Acquired Immunodeficiency Syndrome and Human Immunodeficiency Virus Infection

Etiology

HIV–1, a human retrovirus.

Epidemiology and Demographics

- According to the World Health Organization (WHO), at the end of 2003 there were 2.5 million children younger than 15 years living with HIV/AIDS worldwide, 700,000 new infections, and 500,000 child deaths due to HIV/AIDS in that year.
- The estimated number of diagnoses of AIDS through 2002 in the United States was 886,575. Adult and adolescent AIDS cases totaled 877,275 with 718,002 cases in males and 159,271 cases in females. Through the same period, 9300 AIDS cases were estimated in children younger than age 13.
- Most HIV infection in children is acquired via transmission from mother to child. HIV transmission occurs in utero by the virus entering the fetal circulation from maternal blood, by exposure to infected blood or secretions during labor and delivery, or by ingestion of breast milk.
- HIV in children because of transfusion of contaminated blood or clotting factor components (e.g., during treatment of hemophilia or other coagulation disorders) is now rarely observed in the United States.
- Transmission may also occur by sexual exposure, either sexual abuse in younger children or consensual sex in older adolescents and young adults.
- Half of all new cases of HIV infection are in children and young adults younger than 25 years.[19]

- Although researchers have found HIV in the saliva of infected people, there is no evidence that the virus is spread by contact with saliva. Laboratory studies reveal that saliva has natural properties that limit the power of HIV to infect. Scientists also have found no evidence that HIV is spread through sweat, tears, urine, or feces.[20]
- Immaturity of the neonatal immune response may be responsible for the more rapid progression of HIV infection in children than adults.[21]

History

- Infant born to HIV-infected mother
- High-risk behaviors
- Persistent weight loss
- Frequent or recurrent infections
- Maternal history of blood transfusion before 1985

Physical Examination

- Failure to thrive and abnormalities of the CNS with microcephaly and developmental delay are the most important primary manifestations of HIV infection in children.[22]
- Cardiac abnormalities are common. Children with HIV infection have a faster heart rate, higher left ventricular mass, and lower left ventricular function than uninfected children.[23]
- Children with rapid disease progression have a higher resting heart rate and respiratory rate than other infants with perinatally acquired HIV, and chronic heart disease was found in 53% of 34 children with HIV who died before 5 years of age.[24]
- Of 81 children with HIV infection evaluated in one study, arrhythmias occurred in 35%, unexpected cardiac arrest in 9%, transient congestive heart failure in 10%, and chronic congestive heart failure in 10%.[25]
- Nephropathy affects 3% to 40% of children with HIV infection, is more common in African Americans, and occurs late in the course of disease. Although renal disease may be associated with renal failure, it is not usually the cause of death in children with HIV infection.[26]
- In children, *Pneumocystis carinii* pneumonia occurs at an early age, with peak age of onset at 3 to 6 months of age.
- General lymphadenopathy.
- Oral thrush.
- Scars from recurrent herpes simplex virus or herpes zoster infections.

Therapeutic Interventions

- Use personal protective equipment. Initiate appropriate isolation precautions.
- Administer antiretroviral therapy as ordered.
- Obtain laboratory and radiographic studies as necessary. Obtain consent per policy when HIV antibody tests are performed.

- When possible, encourage enrollment of the HIV-infected child into available clinical trials.
- Provide patient/caregiver education and psychological support.

Psychiatric Disorders

Synonyms

- Major depressive disorder: biologic or psychotic depression
- Dysthymia: neurotic depression, chronic depression (at least 1 year in youths)
- Depressive disorder not otherwise specified: minor, recurrent, brief depression

Etiology

- Genetic: positive family history
- Environment: stressors, losses, abuse, emotional trauma
- Organic (biologic): biochemical imbalances in CNS neurotransmitters from drugs, infection, chronic medical illnesses

Epidemiology and Demographics

- Studies regarding depression report childhood report rates of 0.4% to 2.5% and 0.4% to 8.3% in adolescence.
- At least twice as many girls as boys meet criteria for depression during adolescence.
- Family history of mood disorders, anxiety, or substance abuse is common.
- Depression is associated with 80% of suicides.
- Within 2 years of the first depressive episode, 40% of children who have had a first major depressive episode will have a recurrence.
- Twenty percent to 50% of depressed children have two or more diagnoses, including an anxiety disorder (30% to 80%), a disruptive behavior disorder (10% to 80%), dysthymic disorder (30% to 80%), or substance abuse disorder (20% to 30%).[27]
- Untreated dysthymic disorder is generally chronic and is associated with increased risk for the subsequent development of major depression (70%), bipolar disorder (13%), and substance abuse disorder (15%).[27]
- Twenty percent of adolescents presenting with major depressive symptoms develop manic episodes later.[27]
- Eighty percent of patients respond to antidepressant therapy, psychotherapy, or both, when treated by qualified professionals.

History

- Feelings of hopelessness or pessimism
- Feelings of guilt, worthlessness, or helplessness

- Loss of interest or pleasure in activities once enjoyed
- Decreased energy, a feeling of fatigue or of being "slowed down"
- Difficulty concentrating, remembering, making decisions
- Restlessness or irritability
- Sleeping too much or cannot sleep
- Chronic pain or persistent headaches or stomachaches that are not caused by physical illness or injury
- Feelings of rejection, particularly by peers/classmates
- Social isolation or "running with a bad crowd"
- Frequent absences from school, poor performance in school, deterioration in schoolwork
- Significant change in eating and/or sleeping patterns
  - Failure to gain rather than weight loss
  - Impressive gain seen in atypical depression
- Talk of or efforts to run away from home
- Thoughts or expressions of suicide or self-destructive behavior

Physical Examination

Symptoms vary according to age and developmental level.

Therapeutic Interventions

- After ensuring that you and your co-workers are safe, ensure the safety of the child. Do not leave the patient alone.
- Determine the risk of danger to self or others. If the patient is a danger to himself or others, restraints may be necessary. Mobilize necessary resources.
- Assess the patient for the presence of trauma or a medical condition and treat accordingly.
- Remove objects that may cause harm to the patient or others.
- Administer medications as ordered.

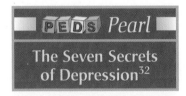

PEDS Pearl

The Seven Secrets of Depression[32]

Depression is (a) common, (b) often missed, (c) not hard to diagnose if you look for it, (d) often severe, (e) often recurrent, (f) costly, and (g) highly treatable. These facts are "secrets" in the sense that they are not well understood by the American public or by many physicians.

ABCD's of Physically Restraining a Child

A: Assistance in applying restraints. At least four healthcare or law enforcement personnel are needed (at least one for each extremity).

B: Body substance isolation precautions. Be careful to avoid contact with bodily fluids.

C: Communicate with the patient and family. Constantly monitor the patient.

D: Document the reason for restraints, type of restraint used, time placed, status of the patient's airway, breathing, and circulation before and after restraints were applied, reassessments of the patient, and the time removed.

Adapted from Prendergast HM, Anderson TR. Psychiatric emergencies. In: Strange GR, Ahrens WR, Lelyeld S, et al., eds. *Pediatric emergency medicine: a comprehensive study guide*, 2nd ed. New York: McGraw-Hill, 2002:762–771.

- If the patient is discharged home, discuss plan for follow-up mental health appointment. Ask the caregiver to make the appointment while in the emergency department.

Bipolar Disorder

Bipolar disorder (previously known as manic-depressive disorder) is a brain disorder that causes unusual shifts in a person's mood, energy, and ability to function.

Bipolar disorder causes dramatic mood swings that alternate from overly "high" and/or irritable (the manic phase) to sad and hopeless (the depression phase), and back again. When manic, the patient appears restless, is easily distracted, requires less sleep and food than usual, is extremely irritable, has racing thoughts and talks very fast, jumping from one idea to another; has increased activity and gestures (e.g., pacing, tapping feet), and believes he or she possesses special powers and/or abilities. Mood changes can occur over minutes, hours, days, or there may be lengthy periods of normal mood between episodes. This form of the illness is called bipolar I disorder. However, some people never develop severe mania but instead experience milder episodes of mania (hypomania), alternating with depression. This form of the illness is called bipolar II disorder.

Severe episodes of mania or depression include psychotic symptoms such as hallucinations and delusions and aggressive or violent behavior. People with bipolar disorder who have psychotic symptoms are sometimes incorrectly diagnosed with schizophrenia.

Etiology
- Exact cause has not been discovered, but there are significant genetic components.
- Most people never know why they develop bipolar disorder.

Epidemiology and Demographics
- Tends to run in families.
- Onset before puberty is thought to be infrequent.
- Approximately 20% of adults with bipolar disorder had symptoms before age 20 years.
- Episodes of mood swings tend to become closer together with age.

History
- Mood instability and problems with conduct and impulse control.
- Anxiety disorders, such as posttraumatic stress disorder and obsessive-compulsive disorder, may simultaneously present in patients with bipolar disorder.

Physical Examination
- Depression is the first symptom of bipolar disorder in about 70% of patients.

- Signs of mania may be evident (previously described).
- Psychotic symptoms, such as delusions (false beliefs), hallucinations (seeing or hearing things that are not real), or aggressive behavior may be present.

Therapeutic Interventions

- After ensuring that you and your co-workers are safe, ensure the safety of the child. Do not leave the patient alone.
- Determine the risk of danger to self or others. If the patient is a danger to self or others, restraints may be necessary. Mobilize necessary resources.
- Assess the patient for the presence of trauma or a medical condition and treat accordingly.
- Administer medications as ordered. Children and adolescents with bipolar disorder are often treated with mood stabilizers, such as lithium. Some anticonvulsant medications may be used because they also possess mood-stabilizing effects. Psychological treatment with pharmacologic treatment is more effective than either form of treatment alone.

Drug Pearl: Lithium

- Lithium is an antipsychotic medication used in the treatment of manic episodes of bipolar disorder. The ability to tolerate lithium is greater during the acute manic phase and decreases when manic symptoms subside.
- Lithium should generally not be given to patients with significant renal or cardiovascular disease, severe debilitation or dehydration, or sodium depletion, since the risk of lithium toxicity is very high in such patients.
- Lithium toxicity typically occurs at blood levels of 2.0 mEq/L. Some patients may experience toxicity at lower doses. Lithium toxicity is closely related to serum lithium levels and can occur at doses close to therapeutic levels.
- Early signs of lithium toxicity include diarrhea, vomiting, drowsiness, muscular weakness, and clumsiness. At more toxic levels, physical examination findings may include nystagmus, increased deep-tendon reflexes, ataxia, giddiness, marked tremulousness, tinnitus, confusion, and blurred vision. Such manifestations may progress to include seizures, coma, and cardiac dysrhythmias. This progression is more likely to occur in patients with lithium levels above 2.5 mEq/L. Permanent CNS damage may ensue.
- **Lithium toxicity is a medical emergency** and should be managed in an intensive care setting. Fluid and electrolyte monitoring, treatment of dysrhythmias and respiratory compromise, and prevention of further gastrointestinal absorption may be required.

Schizophrenia is a group of psychotic disorders characterized by disturbances in thought, mood, behavior, sense of self, and interaction with others. **Schizoaffective disorder** is a disorder similar to schizophrenia. Individuals with this illness experience symptoms of both schizophrenia and affective disorders (either bipolar disorder or depression).

Etiology

- There is no known single cause of schizophrenia; may result from a combination of genetic, environmental, and behavioral factors.
- Strong family predisposition, although a genetic cause for childhood schizophrenia has not been as well established as it has for adult schizophrenia.
  - An identical twin of a person with schizophrenia has the highest risk (40% to 50%) of developing the illness. A child whose parent has schizophrenia has about a 10% chance.
- Some researchers believe that schizophrenia results from a chemical imbalance in the brain, and are investigating the involvement of multiple neurotransmitters, such as dopamine, serotonin, glutamate, and γ-aminobutyric acid (GABA).
- Research funded by the National Institute of Mental Health (NIMH) has found that schizophrenia may be a developmental disorder resulting when neurons form inappropriate connections during fetal development. These errors may lie dormant until puberty, when changes in the brain that occur normally during this critical stage of maturation interact adversely with the faulty connections.

Epidemiology and Demographics

Childhood-onset schizophrenia (onset of psychotic symptoms before age 12) is rare. Age of onset may be 5 or 6 years, although the psychotic symptoms of schizophrenia (hallucinations and delusions) are extremely uncommon before adolescence.

History

- Difficulty with school work and peer relationships
- Disorganized speech/thinking

Physical Examination

Signs and symptoms may include the following:

- Hallucinations (visual hallucinations are more common in children than in adults)
- Delusions (less common in children than in adults)
- Possible abnormal motor movements
- Combative behavior
- Unusual mannerisms
- Flight of ideas (rapid succession of thoughts)
- Word salad (unrelated combination of words)

- Echolalia (repeating words)
- Neologisms (newly invented words)
- Clang associations (speaking in rhyming words)

Therapeutic Interventions

Safety is a priority when dealing with a psychotic child.

- After ensuring that you and your co-workers are safe, ensure the safety of the child. Do not leave the patient alone.
- Determine the risk of danger to self or others. If the patient is a danger to self or others, restraints may be necessary. Mobilize necessary resources.
- A child who presents with new-onset psychotic symptoms needs a thorough evaluation to rule out a possible medical cause (e.g., toxic exposure, seizure disorder, tumor, infectious or metabolic cause).
- Provide a quiet environment. When communicating with the child, do not argue with the child. Provide specific instructions and repeat them as needed.
- Schizophrenia is usually treated with antipsychotic medication. Antipsychotic medications do not cure the disorder, but they can reduce symptoms and help prevent relapses. Antidepressant medications and mood-stabilizing medications are also used to treat affective symptoms (depressive or manic symptoms) in schizoaffective disorder.
- Once acute symptoms have lessened, a combination of medicine and psychosocial/rehabilitation interventions can be beneficial.
- Obtain laboratory, radiographic, and imaging studies as ordered.

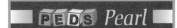
PEDS *Pearl*

When applying physical restraints, do not inflict unnecessary pain or use unreasonable force. ***Never leave a restrained patient unattended.*** This caution applies to the use of physical and chemical restraints.

Neuroleptic Malignant Syndrome

Neuroleptic malignant syndrome (NMS) is a rare, but life-threatening, reaction to a neuroleptic (antipsychotic) medication. Prompt diagnosis and discontinuation of neuroleptics are essential.

NMS is thought to be caused by an acute reduction in dopamine activity because of drug-induced dopamine blockade. Signs of NMS usually appear within 2 weeks after therapy with antipsychotics is begun or the dosage of the medication is increased, but may occur after months of stable-dose treatment.

The four hallmarks of NMS are hyperthermia in the absence of infection, severe generalized muscular rigidity ("lead pipe"), autonomic instability, and changing levels of consciousness. Other signs of NMS include ratcheting movement of the joints ("cog wheeling"), diaphoresis, tachycardia, hypertension or hypotension, tremor, and incontinence.

NMS evolves over 24 to 72 hours and lasts 5 to 10 days with oral medications or much longer with depot intramuscular medications. NMS has an estimated mortality rate of 10% to 20%. Death usually results from respiratory failure, cardiovascular collapse, myoglobinuric renal failure, dysrhythmias, or diffuse intravascular coagulation.

Attention deficit/hyperactivity disorder (ADHD) is a behavioral syndrome characterized by a persistent pattern of inattention/easy distractibility, behavioral and emotional impulsivity, and *sometimes* hyperactivity or severe restlessness. Inattention, impulsivity, and restlessness must cause significant impairment in at least two areas of function (school, peer relationships, family relationships, and work, mood regulation, and self-esteem) and must have been continuously present for at least 6 months. For example, a child who misbehaves in the classroom and is disruptive, but does not exhibit similar problems on the playground or at home, does not meet diagnostic criteria.[28]

Etiology

- Family studies suggest there is a genetic component to ADHD.

Epidemiology and Demographics

- Most common significant behavioral disorder in childhood, affecting 3% to 7% of children between the ages of 7 and 17 years.
- Male-to-female ratio is approximately 3:1.
- Persists into adolescence and adulthood in 30% to 50% of patients.
- More than 50% of individuals with ADHD have at least one comorbid condition, which include learning disorder, restless legs syndrome, ophthalmic convergence insufficiency, depression, anxiety disorder, antisocial personality disorder, substance abuse disorder, conduct disorder, and obsessive-compulsive behavior.

History

- Thirty percent to 50% of persons with ADHD have coexisting psychiatric conditions.
- Inquire about a family history of ADHD.

Physical Examination

- Fewer than half of persons with ADHD are hyperactive.
- Presentation varies depending on the age and developmental level of the patient (Table 10-4).
- Physical examination is usually normal; symptoms may not be evident in a medical setting.

Therapeutic Interventions

- Once diagnosed, ADHD is usually treated with stimulant-class medications.
- If the child is disturbed or agitated, maintain a calm, objective demeanor and provide a safe environment in which to assess the child. Limit the number of people in the area to those who are essential to the care of the patient.
- When talking with the child, convey respect and an expectation of good behavior. Keep questions simple and explain your reasons for questions.

TABLE 10-4 *Behavioral Signs of Attention Deficit/Hyperactivity Disorder*

Preschool (3 to 5 y)	School-Age (6 to 12 y)	Adolescent (13 to 18 y)	Adult
"Always on the go"	Easily distracted, hard to stay on task	Restless, rather than hyperactive	Multiple jobs, relationships
Aggressive (hits or pushes others)	Homework poorly organized, incomplete, and contains careless errors	School work disorganized and incomplete	Misjudges time available, frequently late
Dangerously daring	Impatient, blurts out answers, fails to wait turn in games	Procrastination on most tasks	Mood lability and flash anger outbursts
Noisy, interrupts	Often out of seat	Engages in risky behavior (speeding, drug experimentation)	Many projects started but few completed
Excessive temper tantrums	Perceived as immature	Poor peer relationships	
Insatiable curiosity		Poor self-esteem	
Low levels of compliance		Difficulty with authority figures	

From Dodson WW. Attention deficit–hyperactivity disorder. In: Jacobson JL, ed. *Psychiatric secrets*, 2nd ed. Philadelphia: Hanley and Belfus, 2001:302–309.

- If warranted, laboratory and/or radiographic studies should be obtained to rule out organic disease, trauma, or concomitant illness.

Suicide in Children and Adolescents

Suicidal behavior is often divided into attempts and gestures. A **suicide attempt** involves lethal self-destructive behavior for the purpose of ending one's life. A **suicide *gesture*** involves nonlethal self-destructive behavior performed with the conscious or subconscious intent of obtaining attention, rather than ending life.

Etiology

Possible factors associated with suicide or a suicide attempt may include the following:

- Family history of emotional disorder, especially with suicide attempt.
- Availability of lethal means such as firearms.
- Substance use and abuse.
- Sexual and other abuse.
- Low or below-average levels of serotonin (may be associated with poor impulse control and linked to suicide and violent behavior).
- Parent-child conflict.
- Extreme anxiety, agitation, or rage.
- Situational stresses caused by events such as debilitating illness, physical abuse, or pregnancy.

- Gay and bisexual youth may be at greater risk because of gender identity issues, increased use of substances, or the effects of victimization.

Epidemiology and Demographics

- Each year, approximately 25% of high school students seriously consider suicide, 15% make a plan, 8% make some type of attempt, and 2% come to medical attention because of a suicide attempt.[29]
- Suicide is virtually nonexistent in children younger than 5 years and rare in children from 5 to 9 years of age.
- Suicide is the third-leading cause of death for young adults 15 to 24 years old, after injuries and homicides; it is the fourth-leading cause of death in 10- to 14-year-olds.
- Although suicide rates are highest for white males, the suicide rate for African American males aged 10 to 19 years doubled from 1981 to 1998.
- Although data on the rate of suicide attempts in the United States are not available, estimates range from five to 45 attempts per successful suicide.
  - Adolescent females are three times more likely to attempt suicide than males, usually by toxic ingestion or superficial cutting.
  - Males are five times more likely to complete suicide because they are more likely to use violent means—firearms, hanging, wrist-slashing, jumping from heights, or placing themselves in front of moving vehicles.
  - Preadolescents attempt suicide most commonly by jumping from heights; self-poisoning, hanging, stabbing, and running into traffic are less common.
  - Firearms are the most commonly used method in successful suicides, accounting for 40% to 60% of cases; hanging, carbon monoxide poisoning, and drug overdoses each account for approximately 10% to 15%.[29]

History

Attempt to determine the following:

- Details of the current situation
- Any apparent triggers during the 48 to 72 hours preceding the gesture or attempt
  - Recent suicide attempt by friend or family member
  - Media attention to suicide
  - Academic failure, disciplinary action in school, public humiliation
  - Encounter with law enforcement personnel (arrest)
  - Family stress (illness or loss)
  - Anniversary of a loss
  - Rejection by boyfriend or girlfriend
  - Increased alcohol or drug use

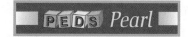

PEDS Pearl

Episodes of self-poisoning that occur after 6 years of age are less likely to be accidental and should be treated as if the behavior had suicidal potential or as a possible case of child abuse and neglect.[27]

Most children or adolescents who commit suicide give some clue to their distress or their plan to commit suicide.

"There is no evidence that discussing suicide with individuals increases their likelihood of harming themselves. On the other hand, there is evidence that suicidal persons who seek medical care do not discuss suicidal thoughts, symptoms of depression, or patterns of drug use unless specifically asked. Given that suicide is a leading cause of death in adolescence, the physician will prevent more deaths by asking about suicide than by auscultating the lungs."

From Boris NW, Dalton R. Suicide and attempted suicide. In: Behrman RE, Kliegman RM, Jenson HB, eds. *Nelson textbook of pediatrics*, 17th ed. Philadelphia: WB Saunders, 2004:87.

TABLE 10-5 *Developmental Concepts of Death*

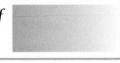

Concept of Death	Perception
Up to age 5 y	Death viewed as a reversible process
Ages 5 to 9 y	Death tends to be internalized; begins to understand the concept of irreversibility
Age 9 y and older	Death viewed as irreversible, final

From Prendergast HM, Anderson TR. Psychiatric emergencies. In: Strange GR, Ahrens WR, Lelyeld S, et al., eds. *Pediatric emergency medicine: a comprehensive study guide*, 2nd ed. New York: McGraw-Hill, 2002:762–771.

- Current talk of suicide or making a plan
  - More than 50% of young people who commit suicide make comments such as "I wish I were dead" or "I just can't deal with this any longer" within the 24 hours before death.
- Access to firearms, knives, or medication
- History of suicide attempts (methods, places, circumstances, and consequences of prior suicide attempts)
- Presence or absence of a psychiatric history
- Strong wish to die, preoccupation with death, understanding of the permanence of death (Table 10-5)
- Exposure to suicidal behavior in the family

Physical Examination

- Injuries caused by risk-taking behavior
- Intentional cutting or scarring, especially of the wrists

Therapeutic Interventions

- Your first concern must be your own safety. After ensuring that you and your co-workers are safe, ensure the safety of the child. Do not leave the patient alone.

Avoid sarcasm, joking, daring, or ridiculing an individual who divulges thoughts of suicide.

- Determine the risk of danger to self or others. If the patient is a danger to self or others, restraints may be necessary. Mobilize necessary resources.
- Assess the patient for the presence of trauma or a medical condition and treat accordingly.
- Any statements regarding suicide attempts or suicidal ideation should be taken seriously, regardless of the patient's age and developmental level, documented, and followed up on.
  - When communicating with the patient and his or her family, show understanding of the situation and convey a desire to help.
  - Listen carefully to the patient's problems and perceptions.

- Be aware of your own emotional reactions to dealing with potentially suicidal patients and their families.
- After the patient has been evaluated in the emergency department, a decision should be made regarding the need for hospitalization, removal from the patient's current environment, or discharge home. Indications for hospitalization or removal from the current environment include the following:
  - Danger to self or others
  - Active suicidal ideation (plan and intent)
  - High intent or lethality of attempt
  - Severely depressed or intoxicated
  - Family is unable to care for the child
  - Outpatient treatment has been unsuccessful
  - Physical or sexual abuse
  - Unable to maintain no-suicide contract
  - Previous history of suicide attempts
  - Patient requires stabilization on or adjustment of medication
  - Practical limitations exist on providing patient supervision, support, or the ability to ensure the patient's safety
- If the decision is made to discharge the patient home, a safety plan must be agreed to. Components of the plan include the following:
  - Assurance of the family's ability to provide 24-hour supervision
  - Removal of all weapons from the home
  - Lock up of alcohol, medications, matches, lighters, toxic chemicals, and sharp objects (e.g., razors, knives)
  - Develop a "no suicide" contract
  - Patient and family must be committed to a plan for mental health treatment. The caregiver should make the appointment while in the emergency department.

> A mental health expert should be consulted before making the decision to send the patient home without hospitalization.

Case Study Resolution

IM is an acute multisystem illness most often associated with a primary infection by the EBV. EBV is one of the most common human viruses and causes more than 90% of IM cases. IM is transmitted via saliva. The incubation period in adolescents ranges from 30 to 50 days.

No isolation procedures other than hand washing and careful handling of oral secretions are recommended because the virus is also found frequently in the saliva of healthy people. Rest, fluids, analgesics, and antipyretics should be provided as needed for comfort.

Web Resources

www.nimh.nih.gov (National Institute of Mental Health)

www.i-h-s.org (International Headache Society)

www.ahsnet.org (American Headache Society)

www.w-h-a.org (World Headache Alliance (WHA))

www.chadd.org (Children and Adults with Attention-Deficit/Hyperactivity Disorder)

www.narsad.org (National Alliance for Research on Schizophrenia and Depression (NARSAD))

References

1. Barkin RM, Rosen P. Fever in children. In: *Emergency pediatrics: a guide to ambulatory care,* 5th ed. St. Louis: Mosby, 1999:240–249.

2. Powell KR. Fever. In: Behrman RE, Kliegman RM, Jenson HB, eds. *Nelson textbook of pediatrics,* 17th ed. Philadelphia: WB Saunders, 2004:839–841.

3. Jenson HB. Epstein-Barr virus. In: Behrman RE, Kliegman RM, Jenson HB, eds. *Nelson textbook of pediatrics,* 17th ed. Philadelphia: WB Saunders, 2004:1062–1066.

4. Rotbart HA. Aseptic and viral meningitis. In: Long SS, ed. *Principles and practice of pediatric infectious diseases,* 2nd ed., St. Louis: Elsevier, 2003:284–291.

5. Reynolds E, Kelley SJ. Infectious disease emergencies. In: Kelly SJ, ed. *Pediatric emergency nursing,* 2nd ed. Norwalk, CT: Appleton & Lange, 1994:423–452.

6. Prober CJ. Central nervous system infections. In: Behrman RE, Kliegman RM, Jenson HB, eds. *Nelson textbook of pediatrics,* 17th ed. Philadelphia: WB Saunders, 2004:2039–2047.

7. Centers for Disease Control and Prevention. Progress toward elimination of *Haemophilus influenzae* type b disease among infants and children-United States, 1983-1994. *MMWR* 1995; 44:545.

8. Sáez-Llorens X, McCracken Jr. GH. Meningitis. In: Gershon AA, Hotez PJ, and Katz SL, eds. *Krugman's infectious diseases of children,* 11th ed., St. Louis: Mosby, 2004:373–388.

9. Johnston MV. Seizures in childhood. In: Behrman RE, Kliegman RM, Jenson HB, eds. *Nelson textbook of pediatrics,* 17th ed. Philadelphia: WB Saunders, 2004:1994–2009.

10. Merrick N, Davidson B, Fox S. Treatment of acute gastroenteritis: too much and too little care. *Clin Pediatr [Phila]* 1996;35:429–435.

11. Barkin RM, Ward DG. Infectious diarrheal disease and dehydration. In: Marx JA, ed. *Rosen's emergency medicine concepts and clinical practice,* 5th ed. St. Louis: Mosby, 2002:2315–2326.

12. Goodgame RW. Viral causes of diarrhea. *Gastroenterol Clin North Am* 2001;30:779–795.

13. Guerrant RL. Practice guidelines for the management of infectious diarrhea. *Clin Infect Dis* 2001; 32:331–351.

14. Burkhart DM. Management of acute gastroenteritis in children [erratum appears in *Am Fam Physician* 2000;61:2614]. *Am Fam Physician* 1999;60:2555–2563, 2565–6.

15. American Academy of Pediatrics, Provisional Committee on Quality Improvement, Subcommittee on Acute Gastroenteritis. Practice parameter: the management of acute gastroenteritis in young children. *Pediatrics* 1996;97:424–436.

16. Herlihy B, Maebius NK. *The human body in health and illness.* Philadelphia: WB Saunders, 2000.

17. Embury SH, Vichinsky EP. Sickle cell disease. In: Hoffman R, ed. *Hematology: basic principles and practice,* 3rd ed. New York: Churchill Livingstone, 2000:510–543.

18. Quirolo K, Vichinsky E. Hemoglobin disorders. In: Behrman RE, Kliegman RM, Jenson HB, eds. *Nelson textbook of pediatrics,* 17th ed. Philadelphia: WB Saunders, 2004:1624–1633.

19. World Health Organization. *HIV/AIDS and young people: Hope for tomorrow.* http://www.unaids.org/publications/documents/children/children/JC656-Child&Aids-E.pdf.

20. National Institute of Allergy and Infectious Diseases (NIAID). *HIV infection and AIDS: an overview (October 2003).* http://www.niaid.nih.gov/factsheets/hivinf.htm (Accessed 5/29/04).

21. Luzuriaga K, Sullivan JL. Viral and immunopathogenesis of vertical HIV-1 infection. In: Pizzo PA, Wilfert CM, eds. *Pediatric AIDS: the challenge of HIV infection in infants, children, and adolescents,* 3e. Baltimore: Williams & Wilkins, 1998:89–104.

22. Havens PL. Pediatric HIV infection. In: Cohen J, Powderly WG, Berkley SF, et al, eds. *Infectious diseases,* 2nd ed. St. Louis:Elsevier, 2004:1343–1356.

23. Lipshultz SE, Easley KA, Orav EJ, et al. Cardiovascular status of infants and children of women infected with HIV-1 (P2 C2 HIV): a cohort study. *Lancet* 2002;360:368–373.

24. Shearer WT, Lipshultz SE, Easley KA, et al. Alterations in cardiac and pulmonary function in pediatric human immunodeficiency virus type 1 disease progressors. *Pediatrics* 2000;105:e9.

25. Luginbuhl LM, Orav EJ, McIntosh K, et al. Cardiac morbidity and related mortality in children with HIV infection. *JAMA* 1993;269:2869–2875.

26. Boris NW, Dalton R, Forman MA. Mood disorders. In: Behrman RE, Kliegman RM, Jenson HB, eds. *Nelson textbook of pediatrics,* 17th ed. Philadelphia: WB Saunders, 2004:84–86.

27. Dodson WW. Attention deficit-hyperactivity disorder. In: Jacobson JL, ed. *Psychiatric secrets,* 2nd ed. Philadelphia: Hanley and Belfus, 2001:302–309.

28. Bechtold DW. Psychosocial aspects of pediatrics and child and adolescent psychiatric disorders. In: Hay Jr WW, Hayward AR, Levin MJ, et al., eds. *Current pediatric diagnosis and treatment.* New York: McGraw-Hill/Appleton & Lange, 2003.

29. Thomas KE, Hasbun R, Jekel J, et al. The diagnostic accuracy of Kernig's sign, Brudzinski's sign, and nuchal rigidity in adults with suspected meningitis. *Clin Infect Dis* 2002;35:46–52.

30. Rubin DH, Conway Jr. EE, Caplen SM, et al. Neurologic Disorders. In: Marx JA, ed. *Rosen's emergency medicine concepts and clinical practice,* 5th ed. St. Louis: Mosby, 2002:1433–1542.

31. Wulsin LR. Depressive disorders. In: Jacobson JL, ed. *Psychiatric secrets,* 2nd ed. Philadelphia: Hanley and Belfus, 2001:72–76.

Chapter Quiz

1. Which of the following best describes the characteristics of a simple febrile seizure?
   A) Lasts longer than 15 minutes.
   B) Only one occurs per 24 hour period.
   C) Usually caused by a central nervous system infection.
   D) Associated with a core temperature that increases rapidly to 104°F or greater.

2. During the clonic phase of a tonic-clonic seizure:
   A) The child experiences an unusual taste, visual disturbance, or an unpleasant odor.
   B) The child experiences continuous motor tension or rigidity.
   C) The child experiences rhythmic contractions alternating with relaxation of all muscle groups.
   D) The child gradually awakens but is tired and confused.

3. Which of the following are typically used first in the management of prolonged/repetitive seizures?
   A) Barbiturates
   B) Benzodiazepines
   C) Phenothiazines
   D) Phenytoin

4. Select the **correct** statement regarding absence seizures.
   A) Absence seizures are also known as grand mal seizures.
   B) Absence seizures are associated with a transient loss of awareness of surroundings without loss of motor tone.
   C) Absence seizures typically last 30 seconds to 2 minutes.
   D) Absence seizures are associated with a postictal state.

5. Febrile seizures are most common in children _____ .
   A) 3 months to 5 years of age
   B) 1 to 8 years of age
   C) 6 months to 6 years of age
   D) 10 to 14 years of age

6. Select the correct statement regarding syncope.
   A) Syncope due to orthostatic hypotension produces signs and symptoms including lightheadedness and loss of consciousness.
   B) Syncope that occurs when a patient is lying down is almost always metabolic in origin.
   C) Syncope is uncommon before age 10 and is most prevalent in adolescent boys.
   D) The syncopal child's family history is usually positive for similar episodes in most patients.

7. Which of the following organs is responsible for secretion of insulin and glucagon?
   A) Liver
   B) Spleen
   C) Pancreas
   D) Gallbladder

8. It is 0830. A 7-year-old girl has reported to the school nurse's office complaining of a headache, hunger, nausea, and weakness. There is no evidence of trauma. The patient is wearing a bracelet that indicates she is a diabetic. You suspect this child is experiencing:
   A) An absence seizure.
   B) Hypoglycemia.
   C) Hyperglycemia.
   D) Salicylate poisoning.

9. In some situations, it may be difficult to distinguish hypoglycemia from diabetic ketoacidosis. When in doubt as to which condition your patient may be experiencing you should assume that any diabetic patient with an altered mental status has:
   A) Hyperglycemia
   B) Hypoglycemia

10. Select the **correct** statement:
    A) Hyperglycemia should be treated with IV glucagon.
    B) Hypoglycemia should be treated with IV dextrose.
    C) Hypoglycemia should be treated with insulin therapy.
    D) Hyperglycemia should be treated with IM glucagon.

11. Select the **incorrect** statement concerning diabetic ketoacidosis:
    A) The onset of symptoms is gradual.
    B) The patient's symptoms are usually due to taking too much insulin.
    C) The patient's skin is usually flushed and warm.
    D) The patient often complains of excessive thirst and frequent urination.

12. Which of the following signs and symptoms is a possible indication of hypoglycemia in an infant?
    A) Irritability.
    B) Thirst.
    C) Increased urine output.
    D) Increased feeding.

13. Initial treatment of a symptomatic 4-month-old infant with hypoglycemia would include
    _____ .

    A) 2 mL/kg of $D_{10}W$ IV
    B) 5 to 10 mL/kg of $D_{10}W$ IV
    C) 1 to 2 mL/kg of $D_{50}W$ IV
    D) 2 to 4 mL/kg of $D_{25}W$ IV

14. What is the most common manifestation of congenital rubella infection?
    A) Cataracts.
    B) Deafness.
    C) Patent ductus arteriosus.
    D) Mental retardation.

15. List three of the most common causes of altered mental status in the pediatric patient.
    A)
    B)
    C)

16. The most common type of headache in the pediatric population is:
    A) Migraine with an aura.
    B) Migraine without an aura.
    C) Cluster headache.
    D) Tension headache.

Chapter Quiz Answers

1. C. A simple febrile seizure is usually associated with a core temperature that increases rapidly to 38.8°C or greater; usually generalized, tonic-clonic; lasts a few seconds to 15 minutes and is followed by a brief postictal period of drowsiness. With a complicated (atypical) febrile seizure, the seizure lasts longer than 15 minutes, may have repeated seizures within the same day, and focal findings may be present during the postictal period.

2. C. During a tonic-clonic seizure the child experiences an unusual taste, visual disturbance, or an unpleasant odor (aura), continuous motor tension or rigidity (tonic phase), rhythmic contractions alternating with relaxation of all muscle groups (clonic phase), and gradually awakens but is tired and confused (postictal phase).

3. B. A benzodiazepine (diazepam, lorazepam, or midazolam) is typically used initially for termination of persistent/repetitive seizures because they are effective for the immediate control of prolonged tonic-clonic seizures in most children.

4. B. Absence seizures, also called petit mal seizures, are associated with a transient loss of awareness of surroundings without loss of motor tone. Absence seizures are uncommon before age 5 years, are

more prevalent in girls, are never associated with an aura, and rarely last longer than 30 seconds. There is no postictal state associated with an absence seizure.

5. A. Febrile seizures are most common in children 3 months to 5 years (most occur between ages 6 and 18 months) of age.

6. D. The syncopal child's family history is usually positive for similar episodes in most (90%) patients. Syncope due to orthostatic hypotension produces lightheadedness, but no loss of consciousness. Syncope that occurs when a patient is lying down is almost always cardiac (not metabolic) in origin. Syncope is uncommon before age 10 and is most prevalent in adolescent girls (not boys).

7. C. The pancreas is responsible for secretion of insulin and glucagon.

8. B. This child's presentation is consistent with early signs and symptoms of hypoglycemia. If untreated, the patient may experience tremors, tachycardia (increased heart rate), and cool, pale skin.

9. B. In some situations, it may be difficult to distinguish hypoglycemia from diabetic ketoacidosis. When in doubt as to which condition your patient may be experiencing you should assume that any diabetic patient with an altered mental status has hypoglycemia.

10. B. Hypoglycemia can be easily reversed with glucose. If vascular access is unavailable, hypoglycemia can be reversed with IM glucagon.

11. B. Diabetic ketoacidosis is associated with a gradual onset of symptoms. The patient's skin is usually flushed and warm and the patient often complains of excessive thirst and frequent urination. Symptoms are often the result of failure to take insulin, eating more food than usual that contains sugar, or a recent illness or infection.

12. A. Signs and symptoms of hypoglycemia in an infant include irritability, jitteriness, poor feeding, high-pitched cry, hypotonia, hypothermia, diaphoresis, tachypnea, pallor, cyanosis, apnea, and arrest. Increased urine output and thirst are associated with hyperglycemia.

13. D. Newly born: 200 mg/kg (2 mL/kg of a $D_{10}W$ solution) slow IV push. Newborn: 0.5 to 1 g/kg (5 to 10 mL/kg) of $D_{10}W$ over 20 minutes. For one month to two years of age: 0.5 to 1 g/kg (2 to 4 mL/kg) of $D_{25}W$ over 5 to 10 minutes. For children older than 2 years: 0.5 to 1 g/kg (1 to 2 mL/kg) of $D_{50}W$ over 5 to 10 minutes.

14. B. Congenital infection with rubella virus can affect virtually all organ systems. Deafness is the most common and often the sole manifestation of congenital rubella infection, especially after the 4th month of gestation.

15. The most common causes of altered mental status in the pediatric patient are hypoxia, head trauma, seizures, infection, hypoglycemia, and drug or alcohol ingestion.

16. B. Migraine without aura (common migraine) is the most common type of headache in the pediatric population.

Environmental Emergencies

11

Case Study

You are a paramedic called to the parking lot of a shopping mall. A crowd has gathered around a vehicle in which an 18-month-old girl appears to be sleeping in her car seat. The ambient temperature is 108° F. A passerby noticed the child in the vehicle and called 9-1-1. All windows in the vehicle are rolled up and you can see that the child's skin appears flushed through the window. While gaining access to the child, her mother arrives and states she has been inside the mall for approximately 2 hours with her other two children. You estimate the temperature inside the vehicle to be 130° F.

After removing the child from the vehicle, you find her unresponsive. She is breathing shallowly at a rate of 12 breaths per minute. A weak pulse is present.

What should be done for this child?

Objectives

1. Discuss the etiology, history, assessment findings, and management of hypothermia.
2. Discuss the etiology, history, assessment findings, and management of heat-related illnesses.
3. Define near-drowning.
4. Discuss the etiology, history, assessment findings, and management of near-drowning.

Anatomic and Physiologic Considerations

- Temperature control is less predictable in children.
- Infants and young children have a slightly higher core temperature than adults. They become hypothermic at a slightly higher temperature.

- A child's core temperature will decrease faster than an adult's will because the body surface area is proportionately larger.
- Heat loss occurs more quickly because of the child's higher ratio of body surface area (skin) to body volume.
- The head of an infant or young child accounts for approximately 20% of the total body surface.
- Infants and young children have less subcutaneous fat, thus, less insulation.
- Underdeveloped compensatory mechanisms (e.g., shivering) produce insufficient heat and quickly deplete their limited energy reserves. The newly born are at the highest risk for hypothermia.

Temperature Regulation

- Body temperature is maintained by balancing heat loss and heat production.
- Heat production occurs during the transformation of food into energy (metabolism) and during physical exercise.
- Most heat loss occurs through the skin, primarily by radiation from exposed areas and evaporation of sweat. Heat loss may be accelerated by convection (wind blowing across exposed skin) or conduction (direct transfer of heat to another substance, such as water) (Figure 11-1).
- Hypothalamus
  - Brain's primary control center for body temperature and heat regulation
  - Receives body temperature messages directly from circulating blood and from peripheral skin receptors
  - Acts as a thermostat, maintaining temperature very near 98.6° F (37° C)

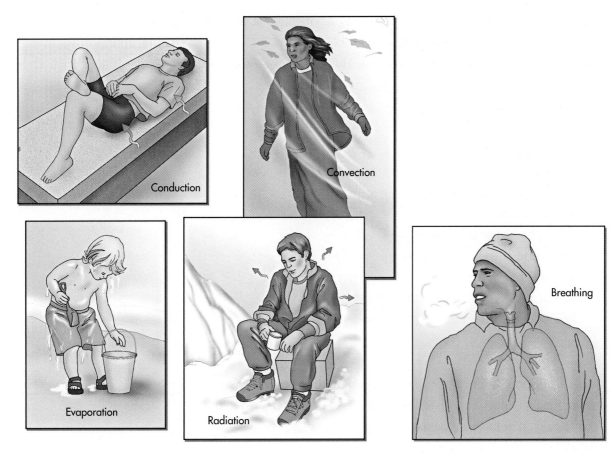

Figure 11-1 Mechanisms of heat dissipation.

Cold-Related Emergencies

Hypothermia (core body temperature below 95° F [35° C]) may result from a decrease in heat production, an increase in heat loss, or a combination of these factors. Hypothermia may be divided into three categories: mild (93.2° F to 96.8° F [34° C to 36° C]), moderate (86° F to 93° F [30° C to 34° C]), and severe (below 86° F [30° C]).

Etiology

Hypothermia is frequently associated with cold-water submersion incidents.

- Hypothermia is a result of exposure to conditions resulting in excessive heat loss. Exposure may include a body of water.
- Hypothermia may also be the result of abnormal control of body temperature as seen in conditions such as sepsis, metabolic derangements, ingestions, central nervous system (CNS) disorders, and endocrinopathies.
- Hypothermia can also result from child abuse (e.g., punishment by cold exposure, neglect).

- Neonates, trauma victims, intoxicated patients, the mentally ill, and the chronically disabled are particularly at risk for hypothermia.
- Factors that can increase susceptibility to hypothermia include the following:
  - ○ Inadequate or wet clothing
  - ○ Dehydration
  - ○ Poor caloric intake
  - ○ Low body weight
  - ○ Poor physical condition
  - ○ Hypoglycemia
  - ○ Recent trauma or burn injury
  - ○ Cold, windy weather conditions
  - ○ Immersion in water
  - ○ Use of alcohol, barbiturates, or antipsychotic medications
  - ○ Preexisting illness, including hypothyroidism, hepatic failure, or sepsis

Epidemiology and Demographics

- Usually obvious: exposure to cold environment
- Hypothermia may be missed, especially in association with other injuries, such as multiple trauma.

History

See Table 11-1.
- Shivering ceases below 86° F to 89.6° F as glycogen stores are depleted or insulin is no longer available for glucose transfer
- In severe hypothermia, the skin is pale or cyanotic, pupils may be fixed and dilated, muscles are rigid, and there may be no palpable pulses.

Physical Examination

Management depends on the degree of heat loss (Table 11-1).
- Handle patient gently; avoid jostling
- Assess responsiveness, breathing (assess for 30 to 45 seconds), and pulse (assess for 30 to 45 seconds)
- Administer warmed and humidified 100% oxygen. Perform tracheal intubation if the hypothermic child is unconscious or if ventilation is inadequate.
- Monitor core temperature, heart and respiratory rates, and blood pressure continuously. Use low-reading thermometers to measure core temperature at 5-minute intervals.
- Rewarming
  - ○ Passive external rewarming is appropriate for all hypothermic patients. If there is a possibility that the patient will become hypothermic again, no other rewarming measures should be undertaken.

Therapeutic Interventions

TABLE 11-1 *Signs/Symptoms and Management of Hypothermia*

Assesment	Mild (Core Temp 93.2° F to 96.8° F [34° C to 36° C])	Moderate (Core Temp 86° F to 93° F [30° C to 34° C])	Severe (Core Temp Below 86° F [30° C])
Airway	Patent	Patent	Compromised
Breathing	Normal	Decreased respiratory rate	Slow, shallow, or absent respirations
Circulation	Normal heart rate Normal BP Pale, dry, or wet skin	Normal heart rate, bradycardia, atrial fibrillation Normal BP or hypotension Pale, cyanotic, or mottled skin	Osborne waves on ECG Cyanotic or mottled skin Body appears lifeless Spontaneous VF
Mental status	AVPU = A Slurred speech	AVPU = V Decreased responsiveness	AVPU = P or U Extreme disorientation
Other signs/symptoms	Shivering Uncoordinated movement	Stiffening muscles Shivering ceases below 86° F to 89.6° F	Loss of deep tendon reflexes Stiff, rigid muscles
Initial management	Remove to warm environment Apply warm, dry clothing, and blankets Apply radiant heat, warm air, or heat packs	Remove to warm environment Apply warm, dry clothing, and blankets Apply radiant heat, warm air, or heat packs to thorax only	Warm, humidified oxygen Warm IV fluids Continue rewarming until core temperature above 95° F (35° C) or return of spontaneous circulation, or resuscitation efforts cease

BP, blood pressure; ECG, electrocardiogram; VF, ventricular fibrillation.

- If sustained warmth can be ensured, provide active external rewarming for mildly hypothermic patients; active external rewarming *to the torso only* for moderately hypothermic patients; and active internal rewarming for severely hypothermic patients. Initiate cardiopulmonary resuscitation (CPR) before internal rewarming for severely hypothermic patients with apnea and pulselessness.
- Warming methods
  - Passive external rewarming (appropriate for all types of hypothermia) includes moving the patient to a warm environment and application of warm, dry clothing and blankets.
  - Active external rewarming includes application of radiant heat, warm air, or heat packs.
  - Active internal rewarming includes warm IV fluids (normal saline [NS]); warm, humidified oxygen, peritoneal lavage, extracorporeal rewarming through partial cardiopulmonary bypass; and esophageal rewarming tubes.

Avoid intravenous (IV) fluids containing lactate because lactate is poorly metabolized by a hypothermic liver.

- If the child is in cardiac arrest and ventricular tachycardia (VT) or ventricular fibrillation (VF) is present, attempt defibrillation.
  - ○ Deliver up to three shocks to determine fibrillation responsiveness. If the patient fails to respond to three initial defibrillation attempts or initial drug therapy, subsequent defibrillation attempts or additional boluses of medication should be deferred until the core temperature rises above 86° F (30° C). Begin CPR and rewarming. Successful conversion to normal sinus rhythm may not be possible until rewarming is accomplished.
    - ▪ Drug metabolism is reduced and medications can accumulate to toxic levels in the peripheral circulation if they are administered repeatedly in the severely hypothermic patient. IV medications are often withheld if the child's core body temperature is below 86° F (30° C).
  - ○ If core temperature rises above 86° F (30° C), continue CPR. Give IV medications as indicated, but space at longer than standard intervals. Repeat defibrillation for VF/VT as core temperature rises. Begin active internal rewarming.
- During rewarming, patients who have been hypothermic for more than 45 to 60 minutes may require volume administration because their vascular space expands with vasodilation.

Rewarming shock may occur during rapid external rewarming of moderate or severely hypothermic patients due to peripheral vasodilation and relative hypovolemia.

- During rewarming, significant hyperkalemia may develop. Monitor the electrocardiogram (ECG) and laboratory values closely. Management of hyperkalemia may include administration of calcium chloride, sodium bicarbonate, glucose plus insulin, and Kayexalate.
- Laboratory studies: complete blood count and platelets, serum electrolytes, glucose, creatinine, amylase, prothrombin time, partial thromboplastin time, arterial blood gases
- Consider toxicology screen, cervical spine radiograph, chest radiograph
- Resuscitation efforts should generally be continued until the child's core temperature is at least 86° F to 89.6° F (30° C to 32° C).

Heat-Related Emergencies

- Heat cramps occur because of inadequate perfusion secondary to dehydration and sodium depletion. Cramps occur primarily in those skeletal muscles subjected to intense exercise, usually the hamstring and calf muscles.

Etiology

- Heat exhaustion is caused by exposure to a high-temperature environment, with continuous sweating and lack of appropriate replenishment of water or salt.

Heat exhaustion is a more severe level of dehydration.

- Blood volume and sweat production fall as dehydration begins, reducing the body's ability to cool.
- Elevated core temperature increases metabolic demand. The cardiovascular system may not be able to respond proportionately due to reduced preload.
- Heat stroke is severe hypovolemic shock.
  - Core temperature may rise above 107.6° F (42° C)
  - Cellular injury occurs from shock as well as severe temperature elevation
  - Lactic acidosis, neuronal injury, and rhabdomyolysis result
  - Mortality is estimated to be 50% to 80%; aggressive therapy may lower mortality to 15% to 20%

Epidemiology and Demographics

- Incidence of heat-related illnesses increase during seasonal heat waves.
- Infants and child athletes are prone to heat stress.
  - Higher rate of heat transfer from the environment.
  - Higher baseline metabolic rate.
  - Sweating capacity is not as great in children as adults.
  - Adolescent and child athletes may exercise poor judgment and ignore (or be unaware of) the warning signs of heat-related illness.
- Accidental deaths occur with infants and children locked in automobiles.
  - Interior and trunk temperature of automobiles can reach higher than 150° F (65° C) in 15 minutes or less.

History

- Reported symptoms may include headache, nausea, extreme fatigue, and lightheadedness or dizziness.

Additional History

- Determine description of and duration of exercise and environmental conditions to which the child has been exposed.
- Ascertain if the child has a chronic illness (e.g., cystic fibrosis), recent activity, or takes medications (e.g., anticholinergics, diuretics) that may increase the risk of fluid and electrolyte imbalance.
- Reported symptoms may include headache, nausea, extreme fatigue, lightheadedness, or dizziness.

Physical Examination

See Table 11-2 for signs/ symptoms and management of heat-related illnesses.

- Shaking chills, leg cramps, tachycardia, elevated temperature
- Skin condition varies depending on extent of heat illness ranging from dry to excessive perspiration
- Confusion, combativeness, aggressiveness

TABLE 11-2 *Signs/Symptoms and Management of Heat-Related Illnesses*

Assessment	Heat Cramps (Core Temperature Normal or Slightly Elevated)	Heat Exhaustion (Core Temperature Slightly Elevated; 100.4° F [38° C] to 104° F [40° C])	Heat Stroke (Core Temperature Above 104° F [40° C])
Airway	Patent	Patent; possible compromise	Compromised
Breathing	Normal	Normal	Varies
Circulation	Normal heart rate or tachycardia Diaphoretic	Tachycardia Diaphoretic Hypotension	Hot, dry, flushed skin; pale as condition worsens Weak peripheral pulses with signs of shock
Mental status	AVPU = A	AVPU = V	AVPU = P or U
Other signs/ symptoms	Painful cramping of abdomen or any extremity	Decreased urine output Headache, body aches Thirst	Muscle stiffness and cramps Seizures Coma
Initial management	Remove from hot environment Rest Give diluted oral electrolyte solution	Remove from hot environment Remove clothing Ensure patent airway; oxygen, assist ventilations as needed If alert, rehydrate with oral fluids If necessary, establish IV/IO access and give an IV fluid bolus 20 mL/kg normal saline or Ringer's lactate Monitor blood glucose levels; treat hypoglycemia	Remove from hot environment; remove clothing; cover child in sheets soaked in saline or cold water Apply cold packs to head, neck, axillae, groin Ensure patent airway; oxygen, assist ventilations as needed Monitor body temperature; discontinue active cooling when child's temperature reaches about 102° F (39° C) Cardiac monitor Establish IV/IO access IV fluid bolus 20 mL/kg normal saline or Ringer's lactate

IO, intraosseous; IV, intravenous.

- Progressive deterioration in level of responsiveness to unresponsiveness

Management of heat stroke:

- Ensure patent airway; administer oxygen and assist ventilations as needed.
- Remove from hot environment; remove clothing.
  - Cover child in sheets soaked in saline or cold water.
  - Apply cold packs to head, neck, axilla, and groin.

Therapeutic Interventions

- ◦ Monitor body temperature; discontinue active cooling when child's temperature reaches about 102° F (39° C).
- Apply a cardiac monitor.
- Establish IV/intraosseous (IO) access.
    - ◦ Give a 20-mL/kg fluid bolus of NS or lactated Ringer's (LR) solution. Repeat the primary survey to assess response.
    - ◦ If no improvement, give another 20-mL/kg NS or LR fluid bolus and assess response.
    - ◦ If the child continues to demonstrate signs of inadequate perfusion, give a third 20-mL/kg fluid bolus of NS or LR.
    - ◦ Monitor rectal temperature continuously.
    - ◦ Place urinary catheter and nasogastric tube. Monitor urine output to assess efficacy of fluid resuscitation.
- Check serum glucose. Administer dextrose IV if glucose level is below 60 mg/dL.
- Treat seizures if they occur.
- Obtain laboratory tests: Complete blood count, electrolytes, glucose, creatinine, prothrombin and partial thromboplastin times, creatine kinase, liver function tests, arterial blood gases, urinalysis, and serum calcium, magnesium, and phosphate.
- Heat stroke, shock, and rhabdomyolysis can lead to acute renal failure, which may cause electrolyte abnormalities, including hyperkalemia.
    - ◦ ECG signs of hyperkalemia may include peaked T waves, a wide QRS complex, bradycardia, or ventricular dysrhythmias.
    - ◦ If hyperkalemia is present, possible interventions include IV or IO administration of sodium bicarbonate, calcium, and insulin followed by glucose.

Submersion Incidents

Terminology

- Drowning: death from suffocation in a liquid
- Near-drowning: survival, at least temporarily, after suffocation in a liquid
- Secondary drowning: death occurring longer than 24 hours after submersion secondary to severe respiratory decompensation (e.g., acute respiratory distress syndrome [ARDS], pulmonary edema)
- Immersion syndrome: death following submersion in extremely cold water

Etiology[1]

- Approximately 90% of near-drownings involve aspiration of fluid into the lungs, usually less than 20 mL/kg

- About 10% involve "dry drowning"; laryngospasm occurs, preventing aspiration of fluid
- Fresh water inactivates surfactant, leading to alveolar collapse and pulmonary dysfunction. Salt water dilutes surfactant, leading to alveolar collapse and pulmonary dysfunction (Figure 11-2). Both salt and fresh water damage the basement membrane, leading to fluid shifts, ARDS, and pulmonary edema.
- The steps to death progress from aspiration of fluid to pulmonary dysfunction to hypoxemia to anoxic brain injury and cardiac decompensation to death.

The type of water aspirated ultimately has little clinical significance.

- Drowning is the second most common cause of death by unintentional injury among children.
- Drowning may occur in lakes, rivers, streams, swimming pools, hot tubs, bathtubs, toilets, buckets, and washing machines.
- Toddlers most commonly drown in pools and bathtubs, occasionally toilets or buckets of water.
- Adolescents most commonly drown in larger bodies of water (e.g., lakes, rivers, or ocean).
- Approximately 90% of drownings occur in fresh water. About 50% occur in swimming pools.
- Prognosis is poor if the patient is comatose or CPR is in progress on arrival in the emergency department.

Epidemiology and Demographics

Risk factors include epilepsy, alcohol, intentional trauma, and lack of supervision.

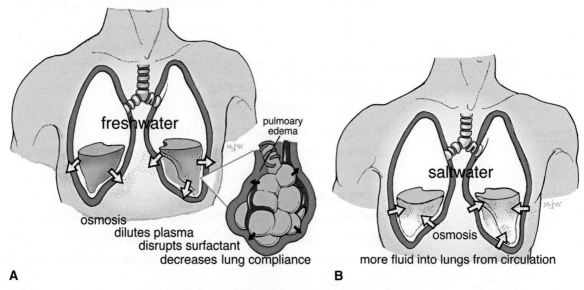

A

B

Figure 11-2   The effects of fresh water (**A**) and salt water (**B**) on the lungs.

History

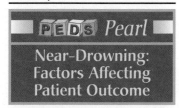

Near-Drowning: Factors Affecting Patient Outcome

- Duration of the submersion
- Duration and severity of hypoxia
- Water temperature
- Duration and degree of hypothermia
- Diving reflex
- Age of the victim
- Water contamination
- Duration of cardiac arrest
- Promptness of initial treatment
- Response to initial treatment
- Associated injuries (particularly head and cervical spine trauma)

- When was the child last seen?
- Estimated length of submersion?
- How much time elapsed before CPR was started?
- Did the child lose consciousness?
- Any possibility of trauma (e.g., diving injury)?
- Approximate water temperature (warm, tepid, cold, icy)?
- Did the victim use alcohol or other drugs before the incident?
- Was the water clean or contaminated, salt or fresh?
- Does the patient have any medical history that may have contributed to the incident (e.g., seizures, asthma)?
- Were barriers present around the body of water (e.g., pool fence)?
- Was the child supervised by a responsible adult?
- Was the child using a flotation device?
- Appearance when pulled from the water (e.g., limp, blue, apneic, pulseless)?
- Consider possible abuse or neglect (the mechanism proposed in the history should match actual physical findings)

Physical Examination

Carefully assess breath sounds, pulse oximetry, respiratory effort, pulses, and mental status. Frequent reassessment is necessary because the child can decompensate quickly.

Depending on the type and duration of submersion, the patient's presentation may vary from asymptomatic to cardiac arrest.

- Mental status
- Airway and breathing
  - Many patients will be tachypneic.
  - Wheezing and crackles are common following aspiration; can indicate the presence of pulmonary edema.
- Circulation
  - If a pulse is present, determine the rate and strength.
  - Assess capillary refill.
- Disability
  - Pay particular attention to level of responsiveness, pupillary response, motor and sensory function.
  - If possible, determine a Glasgow Coma Scale score.

Therapeutic Interventions

Any patient rescued from a submersion incident requires airway management in conjunction with cervical spine precautions.

- If there is any mechanism of injury that could damage the neck or spine (e.g., diving incident), or if the patient has an altered mental status and spinal injury cannot be ruled out, maintain manual in-line c-spine stabilization throughout the assessment and management of the patient until the patient has been properly secured to a backboard.
- If possible, open the child's airway as soon as his head is above water. If the child is apneic, immediately begin mouth-to-mask or bag-mask ventilation. Suction the mouth, nose, and pharynx as soon as possible. Administer 100% oxygen.

- Intubate if the child is apneic or unresponsive.
  - Improves oxygenation and ventilation
  - Allows direct removal of foreign material from the airway
  - Allows application of continuous positive airway pressure (CPAP) or positive end-expiratory pressure (PEEP). Provide PEEP if there is increased resistance to ventilation, crackles on pulmonary auscultation, or continuing hypoxia despite assisted ventilation. Place a PEEP valve on the exhalation port of the bag-mask device and adjust it to a pressure level of 3 to 5 mm Hg.[2]

    Higher pressures should not be used due to the risk of barotrauma.

- If available, use pulse oximetry to monitor oxygenation.
- Monitor the patient's cardiac rhythm.
  - Begin CPR immediately if no pulse is present.
  - Treat dysrhythmias according to resuscitation guidelines.
    - If indicated, deliver up to three shocks and then assess the child's core body temperature. If the child's core body temperature is below 86° F (30° C) and a shockable rhythm (VF/VT) is present, withhold further shocks until the child's temperature is above 86° F (30° C).
    - If moderate hypothermia is present, IV medications should be administered at longer than standard intervals.
- Establish IV access with NS or LR. In patients with signs of shock, administer a bolus of NS or LR solution at 20 mL/kg, then reassess circulatory status.
- Remove wet clothing, dry the patient, and apply blankets to reduce further heat loss and hypothermia.
  - Submersion victims are at risk from immersion hypothermia.
  - Decompress the stomach if there is significant distention due to swallowed water or air.
- After the initial assessment and warming, assess the child's blood glucose level.
- Shivering and vigorous struggling can lower blood glucose levels.
- Assess for hypoglycemia and administer dextrose if indicated.

Table 11-3 lists a grading system that can help predict the likelihood of mortality.

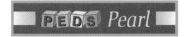

PEDS Pearl

All submersion victims should be transported to the hospital for evaluation and observation, even those who appear to have recovered fully. Signs of pulmonary infection may appear many hours after the submersion event.

TABLE 11-3 *Classification for Submersion Events According to Severity*

Clinical Findings	Severity	Mortality (%)
Normal lung auscultation with coughing	1	0
Abnormal lung auscultation with crackles in some lung fields	2	0.6
Abnormal lung auscultation with crackles in all lung fields (acute pulmonary edema) without arterial hypotension	3	5.2
Abnormal lung auscultation with crackles in all lung fields (acute pulmonary edema) with arterial hypotension	4	19.4
Isolated respiratory arrest	5	44
Cardiopulmonary arrest	6	93

From Szpilman D. Near-drowning and drowning classification: a proposal to stratify mortality based on the analysis of 1,831 cases. *Chest* 1997;112:660–665.

Human and Selected Animal Bites

Human Bites

There is a greater risk of tissue damage and infection with human bites than for those produced by animal exposures.

Etiology

- More than 40 organisms have been identified in the human mouth.

Epidemiology and Demographics

- There are an estimated 250,000 human bites every year.
- Infection rates as high as 50% have been reported after human bites; probably reflects the susceptibility for these wounds to be inflicted on the hands.

History

- Child abuse
- Fight with another child

Physical Examination

- Deep injury may be present, particularly with clenched-fist injuries (the fist of an individual strikes the teeth of another).
  - Reposition the hand to the clenched and neutral positions to examine soft tissues and tendons.

Therapeutic Interventions

- Irrigate the wound copiously with sterile NS by high-pressure syringe irrigation, with care taken not to inject into the tissue or inflict additional trauma.
- Wounds at high risk of infection include puncture wounds, minor hand or foot wounds, wounds with care delayed beyond 12 hours, cat or

human bite wounds, and wounds in asplenic or immunosuppressed patients. In general, these wounds should not be sutured. Wounds that involve tendons, joints, deep fascial layers, or major vasculature should be evaluated by a plastic or hand surgeon and, if indicated, closed in the operating room.[3]

- Prophylactic antibiotics are only indicated for wounds at risk for infection, as listed above. Antibiotics of choice include amoxicillin/clavulanic acid or trimethoprim-sulfamethoxazole in combination with clindamycin for the penicillin-allergic patient. Initial doses should be given in the emergency department and continued for 3 to 5 days.[3]
- Plastic surgery may be needed for cosmetically challenging injuries.
- Tetanus immunization is recommended if the child has not had a booster within the last 5 years.
- Consider radiographs for deep bite wounds in which there is the possibility of foreign body, bone disruption, or fracture, especially when involving the scalp or hand.

Epidemiology and Demographics

- Fifteen percent to 20% of animal bites become infected; pathogenic organisms can be cultured from most wounds.
- Most dog-related attacks occur in children between the ages of 6 and 11 years of age.
  - Boys are attacked more often than girls are.
  - Approximately two thirds of the attacks occur around the home.
  - Seventy-five percent of the biting animals are known by the child.
  - Seventy-five percent of the injuries occur to the face, head, and neck.
  - Almost one half of the attacks are unprovoked.
  - Dog bites usually cause abrasions, puncture wounds, and lacerations with or without an associated avulsion of tissue.
  - Estimates for the rate of clinical infection range from 2% to 30%.
- In the past 30 years, there have been approximately 20 deaths per year in the United States from dog-inflicted injuries.
  - Sixty-five percent of these deaths occurred in children younger than 11 years.
  - Rottweilers, pit bulls, and German shepherds accounted for more than 50% of all fatal bite–related injuries.
- There are an estimated 450,000 reported cat bites per year.
  - Occur primarily in girls.
  - Almost all are inflicted by known household animals.
  - Cats typically leave a deep puncture wound.
    - Wound care is difficult; increased risk of infection.

Dog and Cat Bites

Dog bite injuries alone accounted for about 0.4% of all emergency department visits in a national study.[4]

With puncture wounds, the bacteria are deeper and more difficult to cleanse. As a result, they are associated with a higher rate of infection than lacerations.

- Estimates for the rate of clinical infection range from 16% to 50%.
  - Cat scratch disease, an illness caused by *Bartonella henselae*, may occur after a cat bite. It usually presents with regional adenopathy about 14 days (range, 3 to 50 days) after the scratch.
    - Cats younger than 1 year are more likely to be involved.
    - Fifty percent of cases involve children younger than 15 years.

History

- Type of animal
- Provoked or unprovoked attack
- Location of the attack
- Time elapsed since the injury (important factor in infection control and wound closure)
- History of drug allergies
- Immunization status of the child and animal

Physical Examination

- Determine the location, type, size, and depth of the wound.
- Assess for foreign material in the wound and the condition of the underlying structures. If the bite occurred on an extremity, evaluate the range of motion of the affected area.
  - Look closely at the web spaces between the fingers for evidence of a bite or scratch in a patient with lymphadenopathy of an upper extremity.
- Consider the possibility of a fracture or penetrating injury of the skull in patients, particularly infants, who have sustained dog bite injuries to the face and head.
- Assess the wound for internal injury with the body part in the same position in which it was bitten (i.e., a hand laceration inflicted with the digits flexed may hide a tendon injury if examined only in the extended position).[5]
- Patients with *Pasteurella multocida* infection typically develop symptoms rapidly.
  - *P. multocida* is carried in the mouths of most dogs and is found in 25% of dog bites. The same pathogen is found in the mouths of 80% of cats and is the most common organism cultured from cat bite wounds (including lion, cougar, and tiger bites).[6] Infection may develop rapidly with erythema, swelling, and intense pain, often within 12 to 24 hours of the injury.
  - *Staphylococcus aureus* and *P. multocida* are isolated together in 20% to 30% of dog and cat exposures.

Therapeutic Interventions

- Irrigation and care are similar to that specified for human bites.
- Wounds that involve tendons, joints, deep fascial layers, or major

vasculature should be evaluated by a plastic or hand surgeon and, if indicated, closed in the operating room.[3]

- Plastic surgery may be needed for cosmetically challenging injuries.
- Tetanus immunization is recommended if the child has not had a booster within the last 5 years.
- Consider the need for rabies prophylaxis.
- Consider radiographs for deep bite wounds in which there is the possibility of foreign body, bone disruption, or fracture, especially when involving the scalp or hand.

Case Study Resolution

This child's presentation is consistent with heat stroke. Remove the child from the hot environment and remove her clothing. Cover the child in sheets soaked in saline or cold water. Apply cold packs to the child's head, neck, axillae, and groin. Ensure a patent airway and administer oxygen. Begin rapid transport to the closest appropriate facility as soon as possible. Monitor the child's body temperature and discontinue active cooling measure when the child's temperature reaches about 102° F (39° C). Attach a cardiac monitor, establish vascular access, and assess the child's serum glucose level. Give a fluid bolus of 20 mL/kg NS or LR. Reassess.

References

1. Hostetler MA. Near-drowning. In: Garfunkel LC, Kaczorowski J, Christy C, eds. *Mosby's pediatric clinical advisor: instant diagnosis and treatment.* St. Louis: Mosby, 2002:536–537.
2. Foltin GL, Tunik MG, Cooper A, et al. *Teaching resource for instructors in prehospital pediatrics for paramedics.* New York: Center for Pediatric Emergency Medicine, 2002.
3. Fleisher GR, Ludwig S, eds. *Textbook of pediatric emergency medicine,* 4th ed. Philadelphia: Lippincott, Williams & Wilkins; 2000.
4. Weiss HB, Friedman DI, Cohen JH. Incidence of dog bite injuries treated in emergency departments. *JAMA* 1998;279:51–53.
5. Frieshtat R. Animal bites. In: Garfunkel LC, Kaczorowski J, Christy C, eds. *Mosby's pediatric clinical advisor: instant diagnosis and treatment.* St. Louis: Mosby, 2002:151.
6. Finberg R. Animal exposures. In: Finberg L, Kleinman RE, eds. *Saunder's manual of pediatric practice,* 2nd ed. Philadelphia: WB Saunders, 2002:426–428.

Chapter Quiz

1. Which of the following statements is true regarding heat exhaustion?
   A) Heat exhaustion can be distinguished from other heat-related illness by its altered mental status and a rectal temperature exceeding 104°F (40°C).
   B) Heat exhaustion poses an immediate threat to life.
   C) Heat exhaustion is treated by removing the patient to a cool area and providing rest along with either oral or IV rehydration.
   D) Treatment for heat exhaustion includes removing the child's clothing and applying ice-water soaked sheets.

2. The IV fluid of choice in a child with severe hypothermia is:
   A) Lactated Ringer's solution.
   B) 50% dextrose in water.
   C) 5% dextrose in water.
   D) Normal saline.

3. Submersion with at least temporary survival is called:
   A) Drowning.
   B) Near-drowning.
   C) Secondary drowning.
   D) Asphyxiation.

4. The body's thermoregulatory center is found in the:
   A) Pituitary.
   B) Hypothalamus.
   C) Thyroid.
   D) Cerebellum.

5. True or False: A 6-year-old boy is suffering from hypothermia. He is unresponsive and breathing shallowly at a rate of 4 to 6 breaths per minute. A carotid pulse is barely palpable at 50 beats/minute. Management of this child's airway should be limited to bag-valve-mask ventilation because insertion of a tracheal tube is likely to precipitate ventricular fibrillation.

6. List four factors that can increase the pediatric patient's susceptibility to hypothermia:
   A)
   B)
   C)
   D)

7. True or False: There is a greater risk of tissue damage and infection with human bites than those produced by animal exposures.

8. A 2-year-old was found submerged in a backyard pool. The child is unresponsive with a respiratory rate of 6 breaths/minute and a heart rate of 76 beats/minute. Your first intervention should be to:
   A) Establish vascular access.
   B) Assist breathing with a bag-valve-mask device.
   C) Assess the child's serum glucose level.
   D) Apply the cardiac monitor.

9. Select the **correct** statement regarding mild hypothermia:
   A) Muscle stiffening/rigidity is common with mild hypothermia.
   B) Management of mild hypothermia should include administration of warm, humidified oxygen and warm IV fluids.
   C) An infant or child with mild hypothermia usually has an age-appropriate heart rate.
   D) Extreme disorientation is common with mild hypothermia.

10. True or False: A 14-month-old was found submersed in a 5-gallon paint bucket that had been filled with water. Mom found the child and pulled her from the water. A neighbor heard the mother's cries for help and called 9-1-1. Mom states she found the child was not breathing but did have a pulse. Her face was blue. Mom began mouth-to-mouth breathing. After approximately 2 minutes of rescue breathing, the child began breathing spontaneously. When the paramedics arrive on the scene, the child is alert and acting appropriately for her age. Mom does not wish to have the child transported to the hospital for evaluation. Based on this information, it is reasonable to leave the child in the care of the mother with instructions to see her pediatrician with 48 hours.

Chapter Quiz Answers

1. C. Heat exhaustion is treated by removing the patient to a cool area and providing rest along with either oral or IV rehydration. Heat stroke poses an immediate threat to life and can be distinguished from other heat-related illness by its altered mental status and a rectal temperature exceeding 104°F (40°C). Heat stroke treatment (not heat exhaustion) includes removing the child's clothing and covering the child in sheets soaked in saline or cold water.

2. D. Normal saline is the IV fluid of choice in a child with severe hypothermia. IV fluids containing lactate should be avoided because lactate is poorly metabolized by a hypothermic liver.

3. B. Drowning is death from suffocation in a liquid. Near-drowning is survival, at least temporarily, after suffocation in a liquid. Secondary drowning is death occurring longer than 24 hours after submersion secondary to severe respiratory decompensation.

4. B. The body's thermoregulatory center is found in the hypothalamus.

5. False. This child is not ventilating adequately. Ventilate him with 100% oxygen with a bag-valve-mask device and prepare to intubate. Tracheal intubation enables provision of effective ventilation with warm, humidified oxygen, and it can isolate the airway to reduce the likelihood of aspiration.

6. Factors that can increase susceptibility to hypothermia include inadequate or wet clothing, dehydration, poor caloric intake, low body weight, poor physical condition, hypoglycemia, recent trauma or burn injury, cold, windy weather conditions; immersion in water, use of alcohol, barbiturates, or antipsychotic medications; preexisting illness, including hypothyroidism, hepatic failure, or sepsis.

7. True. There is a greater risk of tissue damage and infection with human bites than those produced by animal exposures. More than 40 organisms (potential pathogens) have been identified in the human mouth.

8. B. Your first priorities are management of the patient's airway, breathing, and circulation. Because the patient's respiratory rate is slow, assist breathing with a bag-valve-mask. After ensuring adequate ventilation, apply the cardiac monitor, establish vascular access, and assess the patient's serum glucose level.

9. C. An infant or child with mild hypothermia usually has an age-appropriate heart rate. Muscle stiffening/rigidity and extreme disorientation are findings seen with severe hypothermia. Warm, humidified oxygen and warm IV fluids are recommended for the severely hypothermic patient.

10. False. All submersion victims should be transported to the hospital for evaluation and observation, even those who appear to have recovered fully.

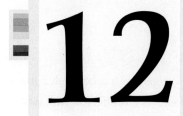

12 Toxicological Emergencies

Case Study

An 18-month-old boy was found holding a bottle of bleach. When his mother yelled, the child dropped the bottle and some bleach spilled onto the front of him. It is unknown if the child actually drank any of the bleach. You find the child crying. His color is pink and he does not show any obvious signs of respiratory distress.

What should you do next?

Objectives

1. Define poison.
2. Explain the role of a Poison Control Center (PCC).
3. Describe the routes of entry of toxic substances into the body.
4. Explain why children are at risk for toxic exposures.
5. Identify the pediatric age group at the greatest risk for unintentional poisoning.
6. Define toxidrome.
7. List five common toxidromes and typical signs and symptoms associated with each.
8. Describe the general management principles for a toxic exposure by ingestion.
9. List the principles of gastric decontamination.
10. Identify the types of ingestions for which activated charcoal should be used.
11. Describe the use of specific therapies for poisonings caused by acetaminophen, β-blockers, calcium channel blockers, iron, opiates, salicylates, and tricyclic antidepressants.

Introduction

A **poison** is a substance that, on ingestion, inhalation, absorption, application, injection, or development within the body in relatively small amounts, may cause structural damage or functional disturbance.

- Poisons can be found in four forms: solid, liquid, spray, or gas.
  - Solid poisons include medicines, plants, powders (e.g., laundry detergent, automatic dishwasher detergent), granular pesticides, and fertilizers.
  - Liquid poisons include lotions, liquid laundry soap, furniture polish, lighter fluid, and syrup medicines.
  - Poisons in spray form include insecticides, spray paint, and some cleaning products.
  - Gases or vapors that are poisonous (invisible poisons) include carbon monoxide from hot water heaters and furnaces, exhaust fumes from automobiles, and fumes from gas or oil-burning stoves.

Poisoning by ingestion is the focus of this chapter.

- Poisons may enter the body through ingestion, inhalation, injection, or absorption (Figure 12-1).

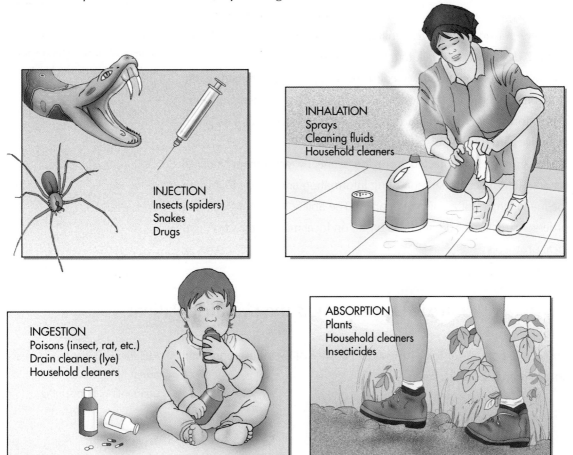

INJECTION
Insects (spiders)
Snakes
Drugs

INHALATION
Sprays
Cleaning fluids
Household cleaners

INGESTION
Poisons (insect, rat, etc.)
Drain cleaners (lye)
Household cleaners

ABSORPTION
Plants
Household cleaners
Insecticides

Figure 12-1 Poisons may enter the body through ingestion, inhalation, injection, and absorption.

- Most poisons enter the body by means of the gastrointestinal (GI) tract.
- Carbon monoxide is the most commonly inhaled toxin. Examples of other toxic gases include cyanide, phosgene, and nitrous dioxides. Glue sniffing and smoking crack are other examples of poisoning by inhalation.
- Injected poisons include self-administered medications (e.g., insulin overdose), intravenous (IV) drug abuse, and venomous bites and stings.
- Poisoning by absorption may occur with the use of insecticides, cleaners, and drugs snorted through the nose.
- Poisonings may be unintentional or intentional.
  - Most poisonings are unintentional (accidental) and may occur because of dosage errors, idiosyncratic reactions, environmental exposure, occupational exposure, or childhood poisoning.
  - Intentional poisonings may result from acts of terrorism, suicide (self-poisoning), or homicide (murder).

Poison Control Centers

In the United States, poison centers are information sources and do not provide direct patient treatment.

- PCCs provide free, 24-hour emergency telephone service for the public and medical professionals. The telephone number is 1-800-222-1222 for every poison center in the United States. Call this number 24 hours a day, 7 days a week to talk to a poison expert.[1]
- The telephone is staffed by medical personnel highly trained in the recognition and assessment of poisonings, first-aid treatment, and drug information, reducing the time required to diagnose and establish definitive care for the poisoned patient.
- The PCC is often contacted from the scene by emergency medical services (EMS) personnel requesting information and advice regarding the management of a poisoned patient. The ability to accept treatment orders/instructions from a PCC is based on local medical direction and local protocols.

Toxic Exposure and the Pediatric Patient

- Children are at risk for toxic exposures because of their developmental and environmental characteristics.
  - Developmental
    - Curious by nature
    - Mobile
    - Explore their environment by putting most things in their mouths
    - Imitate the behavior of others

Children younger than 6 years are at the greatest risk for unintentional poisoning.

Many poisonings take place during mealtime or when the family routine is disrupted.

Poisonings in older children and adolescents usually represent manipulative behavior, chemical or drug abuse, or genuine suicide attempts.[2]

- ▪ Inability to discriminate a toxic substance from a nontoxic one
- ▪ Drawn to attractive packaging and smell of many products found around the home
- ◦ Environmental
  - ▪ Toxic substances (e.g., household cleaning agents, gardening chemicals, plants) are often accessible to a child (Figure 12-2)
    - • Improper storage
    - • Availability of substances in their immediate environment
  - ▪ Inattentiveness of caregiver/inadequate supervision
- • Of the more than 2 million human poisoning exposures reported to the Toxic Exposure Surveillance System (TESS) of the American Association of Poison Control Centers (AAPCC) in 2002
  - ◦ More than 50% (51.6%) occurred in children younger than 6 years
  - ◦ More than 30% occurred in children younger than 3 years
- • Most cases of pediatric toxic exposure
  - ◦ Are unintentional
  - ◦ Occur in the home
  - ◦ Involve only a single substance
- • Death due to unintentional poisoning in young children is uncommon for the following reasons:
  - ◦ Increased product safety measures (e.g., child-resistant packaging)
  - ◦ Increased poison prevention education
  - ◦ Early recognition of exposure
  - ◦ Improvements in medical management

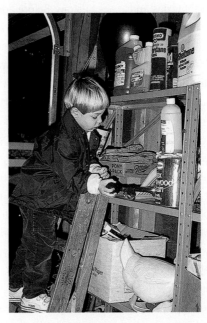

Figure 12-2 Toxic substances such as household cleaning agents and gardening chemicals are often within reach of a curious child.

Substances Most Frequently Involved in Pediatric Exposures[3] (Children Younger than 6 Y)

Substance	%*
Cosmetics and personal care products	13.3
Cleaning substances	10.3
Analgesics	7.4
Foreign bodies	7.1
Topicals	7.0
Plants	5.1
Cough and cold preparations	5.1
Pesticides	4.1
Vitamins	3.7
GI tract preparations	3.2
Antimicrobials	2.8
Antihistamines	2.6
Arts/crafts/office supplies	2.6
Hormones and hormone antagonists	2.3
Hydrocarbons	1.8

*Percentages are based on total number of exposures in children younger than 6 years (1,227,381) rather than the total number of substances.

Drug Pearl
Activated Charcoal

- Activated charcoal is a fine, black, tasteless powder produced from organic materials that effectively adsorbs (binds with) toxins and prevents their systemic absorption. Charcoal can only bind a drug that is *not yet absorbed* from the GI tract.
- The usual pediatric dose of activated charcoal is 1 g/kg of body weight by mouth or nasogastric tube.
- Activated charcoal should *never* be administered to a patient who has a depressed gag reflex or altered mental status unless it is administered by nasogastric tube and the airway is protected by a tracheal tube. Aspiration of charcoal may cause a severe and potentially fatal pneumonitis.
- Activated charcoal looks like mud. The patient may be more willing to drink it if he or she cannot see it.

Consider placing the medication in a covered opaque container and have the child drink through a straw. Before administering activated charcoal, shake the container thoroughly. If it is too thick to shake well, remove the cap and stir it until well mixed.
- Be prepared for vomiting. (Charcoal stains any clothing it contacts.) Have suction readily available.
- Activated charcoal is contraindicated in poisonings involving ingestion of caustics (e.g., hydrochloric acid, bleach, ammonia) or hydrocarbons (e.g., gasoline, kerosene).
- Activated charcoal is ineffective for iron, lithium, heavy metals, and most solvents and is not recommended for poisonings involving these substances.

Assessment of the Child with a Possible Toxic Exposure

Scene Safety

Consider the possibility of a toxic exposure in any situation involving a patient with an altered mental status.

Upon arrival at a scene, perform a scene size-up to determine the nature of the incident and request additional support, if necessary. Ensure the scene is safe before proceeding with patient assessment.

If the caller identified the nature of the incident at the time of dispatch (e.g., ingestion of a relative's medication, swallowed bleach, or acetaminophen overdose), contact with your poison center may be advisable to determine the toxicity of the substance and identify an appropriate treatment plan. However, you may not be aware that the situation involves a toxic exposure until arrival at the scene. The environment may reveal fire, smoke, spilled liquids, open containers, or a chemical odor indicating a toxic exposure. In such situations, determine the need for special protective equipment (and additional resources) before attempting patient assessment.

Detailed initial assessment information and interventions were presented in Chapter 3 and are not repeated here. Additional history, signs and symptoms, and interventions specific to each disorder are listed.

Additional History

Critical questions to ask in a toxic exposure situation include what, when, where, why, and how.

The history provides critical information in the assessment of the patient with a suspected toxic exposure. In addition to the SAMPLE or CIAMPEDS history, consider the following questions when obtaining a focused history for a patient with a toxic exposure. This list will require modification on the basis of the patient's age and chief complaint.

- What is the poison?
  - Determine the exact name of the product, if possible (Figure 12-3).
  - Obtain histories from different family members to help confirm the type and dose of exposure.
  - Are there any pill bottles, commercial products, or plants to support the history?
- How was it taken (i.e., ingested, inhaled, absorbed, or injected)?
- When was it taken?
- Where was the child found? How long was the child alone? Any witnesses? Any other children around?
- How much was taken?
  - Number of pills, amount of liquid
  - How many/amount available before ingestion?
  - How many/much now in the container?
  - Where is the substance stored?
- What is the child's age? Weight?
- Has the child vomited? How many times?

Knowing the time of ingestion is critical when considering gastric emptying and antidote administration.

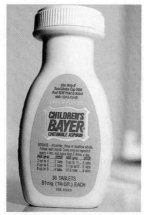

Figure 12-3 If the toxic exposure involves ingestion, obtain the bottle or container of the ingestant. If the specific substance is unknown or if there is any doubt as to the agent ingested, obtain all medicines from the home and transport them to the hospital with the child.

- What home remedies have been attempted (ask specifically about herbal or folk remedies)?
- Has a PCC been contacted? If so, what instructions were received? What treatment has already been given?
- Has the child been depressed or experienced recent emotional stress?
  - Divorce, death in the family
  - Possible suicide attempt in older school–aged child or adolescent

Focused Physical Examination

When performing a physical examination on a patient with a known or suspected toxic exposure, be vigilant in your search for information regarding the severity and cause of the exposure. Changes in the patient's mental status, vital signs, skin temperature and moisture, and pupil size may provide a constellation of physical findings that are typical of a specific toxin. Characteristic findings that are useful in recognizing a specific class of poisoning is called a **toxidrome** (Tables 12-1 and 12-2). Your physical examination findings may provide the only clues to the presence of a toxin if the patient is unresponsive. Familiarity with common toxidromes will enable you to recognize the diagnostic significance of your history and physical examination findings and implement an appropriate treatment plan.

TABLE 12-1 *Clinical Presentations of Specific Toxidromes*

		Toxidrome
Anticholinergic	Signs/symptoms	Agitation or reduced responsiveness, tachypnea, tachycardia, slightly elevated temperature, blurred vision, dilated pupils, urinary retention, decreased bowel sounds; dry, flushed skin
	Typical agents	Atropine, diphenhydramine, scopolamine
	Primary antidote	Physostigmine
Cholinergic	Signs/symptoms	Altered mental status, tachypnea, bronchospasm, bradycardia or tachycardia, salivation, constricted pupils, polyuria, defecation, emesis, fever, lacrimation, seizures, diaphoresis
	Typical agents	Organophosphate insecticides (malathion), carbamate insecticides (carbaryl), some mushrooms, nerve agents
	Primary antidote	Atropine
Opioid	Signs/symptoms	Altered mental status, bradypnea or apnea, bradycardia, hypotension, pinpoint pupils, hypothermia
	Typical agents	Codeine, fentanyl, heroin, meperidine, methadone, oxycodone, dextromethorphan, propoxyphene
	Primary antidote	Naloxone
Sedative/hypnotic	Signs/symptoms	Slurred speech, confusion, hypotension, tachycardia, pupil dilation or constriction, dry mouth, respiratory depression, decreased temperature, delirium, hallucinations, coma, paresthesias, blurred vision, ataxia, nystagmus
	Typical agents	Ethanol, anticonvulsants, barbiturates, benzodiazepines
	Primary antidote	Benzodiazepines: flumazenil
Sympathomimetic	Signs/symptoms	Agitation, tachypnea, tachycardia, hypertension, excessive speech and motor activity, tremor, dilated pupils, disorientation, insomnia, psychosis, fever, seizures, diaphoresis
	Typical agents	Albuterol, amphetamines (e.g., "ecstasy"), caffeine, cocaine, epinephrine, ephedrine, methamphetamine, phencyclidine, pseudoephedrine
	Primary antidote	Benzodiazepines

PEDS Pearl

It is important to note that a patient may not present with all of the signs and symptoms associated with a single toxidrome and, when multiple substances are involved, it may be impossible to identify a specific toxidrome.

TABLE 12-2 *Toxicology Memory Aids*

Anticholinergic syndrome (antihistamines, tricyclic antidepressants)	Mad as a hatter—confused delirium Red as a beet—flushed skin Dry as a bone—dry mouth Hot as Hades—hyperthermia Blind as a bat—dilated pupils
Cholinergic syndrome ("SLUDGE" or "DUMBELS")	Salivation, Lacrimation, Urination, Defecation, Gastrointestinal distress, Emesis Diarrhea, Urination, Miosis (pinpoint pupils), Bronchospasm/Bronchorrhea/Bradycardia, Emesis, Lacrimation, Salivation

Assessment of the patient with a possible toxic exposure includes the following objective measurements and clinical parameters:

Airway

- Look for signs of airway edema, burns, excessive crying, stridor, and drooling. If the child has any of these signs or refuses to eat or drink, suspect a significant airway injury.
- As you assess the patient's airway, note the presence of any odors that may help determine the cause of the patient's condition (Table 12-3).
- Use positioning or airway adjuncts as necessary to maintain patency and suction as needed.
- Perform tracheal intubation if the airway cannot be maintained by positioning or if prolonged assisted ventilation is anticipated. Consider the use of pharmacologic adjuncts to aid in intubation.
  - Severe upper airway injury following a caustic ingestion may prevent routine endotracheal intubation.
  - The use of succinylcholine for rapid sequence intubation can result in prolonged paralysis in patients with organophosphate toxicity.

Breathing

- An increased respiratory rate may result from theophylline or hydrocarbon ingestion or agents that cause metabolic acidosis such as ethylene glycol, methanol, and salicylates (the increased respiratory rate is a compensatory mechanism for acidosis).

Because poisoned patients can deteriorate rapidly, frequent reassessment of the primary survey is necessary.

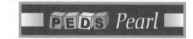

PEDS Pearl

The effects of toxins may result in altered mental status, emesis, or seizures, increasing the patient's risk of airway obstruction, aspiration, and lung damage. Be alert to potential airway problems and ensure suction is readily available.

TABLE 12-3 Odors and Toxins

Odor	Toxin
Acetone	Acetone, isopropyl alcohol, salicylates
Alcohol	Ethanol, isopropyl alcohol
Bitter almonds	Cyanide
Carrots	Water hemlock
Fishy	Zinc or aluminum phosphide
Fruity	Isopropyl alcohol, chlorinated hydrocarbons (e.g., chloroform)
Garlic	Arsenic, organophosphates, dimethyl sulfoxide (DMSO), phosphorus, thallium
Glue	Toluene
Mothballs	Camphor
Pears	Chloral hydrate, paraldehyde
Rotten eggs	Sulfur dioxide, hydrogen sulfide
Shoe polish	Nitrobenzene
Vinyl	Ethchlorvynol
Wintergreen	Methyl salicylates

Consider the possibility of a toxic exposure in an otherwise healthy patient with pulmonary edema.

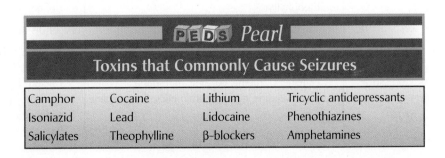

PEDS Pearl

- Acute poisoning can result from toad toxins or the licking of toads. Some aphrodisiacs intended for topical application contain toad venoms that cause vomiting, bradycardia, and other dysrhythmias when ingested.
- The recreational licking of live toads in order to achieve a hallucinogenic effect is most prevalent in the southeastern United States and is primarily a practice of teenagers.[4]
- Significant toxicity has been reported after licking or ingesting cane or marine and Colorado River toads.

Mental status is frequently affected by drugs and toxins.

- Noncardiogenic pulmonary edema is possible with any overdose that has led to apnea and has been associated with the following:
  - Heroin, meperidine, methadone, barbiturates, cocaine, and salicylates
  - After aspiration of chemicals such as kerosene and gasoline
  - After exposure to toxic gases such as chlorine, phosgene, and carbon monoxide
- Bradypnea may result from exposure to sedative/hypnotics, barbiturates, opioids, clonidine, alcohol, organophosphates, carbamates, strychnine, venom from the Mojave rattlesnake, and botulinum toxin.
- If ventilation is adequate, provide 100% supplemental oxygen as necessary. Use a nonrebreather mask or blow-by as tolerated. If breathing is inadequate, assist ventilation using a bag-valve-mask device with 100% oxygen. If abdominal distention occurs, consider placing a nasogastric tube (if not contraindicated) to release air from stomach.

Circulation

- Place the child on a cardiac monitor.
- Sedative/hypnotics, opioids, β-blockers, calcium channel blockers, digoxin, clonidine, organophosphates and carbamate insecticides, and some eye drops (e.g., Visine) cause bradycardia. Plants that contain cardiac glycosides such as lily of the valley, foxglove, and oleander also cause bradycardia.
- Examples of substances associated with an increased heart rate include amphetamines, caffeine, cocaine, ephedrine, phencyclidine, and theophylline.

Disability (Mental Status)

- Anticholinergic agents, cocaine, amphetamines, ethanol, sedative-hypnotic withdrawal, and hypoglycemic agents frequently cause central nervous system (CNS) stimulation, which is manifested as agitation and delirium.
- Benzodiazepines, sedative-hypnotics, barbiturates, and alcohols cause CNS depression. Agents such as ethanol and salicylates induce hypoglycemia, which may contribute to CNS depression. Some agents, such

PEDS Pearl

Toxins that Commonly Cause Seizures

Camphor	Cocaine	Lithium	Tricyclic antidepressants
Isoniazid	Lead	Lidocaine	Phenothiazines
Salicylates	Theophylline	β-blockers	Amphetamines

as tricyclic antidepressants, cause dose-related CNS excitation and depression.

Vital Signs

- Many toxins can produce changes in the patient's blood pressure, heart rate, respiratory rate, and temperature (Table 12-4). The patient's mental status, skin temperature and moisture, and pupil size should also be assessed and documented. Frequent reassessment is important to note any trends or changes in the patient's condition.
- When assessing the patient's oxygen saturation, remember that
  - Any condition that reduces the strength of the arterial pulse may interfere with the measurement of the SpO_2. This includes hypotension, hypothermia, vasoconstrictive drugs, or placement of the oximeter sensor distal to a blood pressure cuff.
  - Pulse oximeters may record falsely elevated amounts of oxyhemoglobin in patients with abnormal forms of hemoglobin, such as carboxyhemoglobin or methemoglobin.

Pupils

- Assessment of pupil size is important in the evaluation of a toxic patient.
- Agents such as opioids, clonidine, phencyclidine, and some sedative-hypnotics may cause constricted pupils (miosis).
- Meperidine (Demerol) is an opioid that may cause pupil *dilation*.
- Pupil dilation may result from sympathomimetics, anticholinergics, antihistamines, and hypoxia.

Pupil dilation is a less specific physical finding than pupil constriction.

TABLE 12-4 *Toxins and Vital Sign Changes*

Vital Sign	Increased	Decreased
Temperature	Amphetamines, anticholinergics, antihistamines, antipsychotic agents, cocaine, monoamine oxidase inhibitors, nicotine, phenothiazines, salicylates, sympathomimetics, theophylline, tricyclic antidepressants, serotonin reuptake inhibitors	Barbiturates, carbon monoxide, clonidine, ethanol, insulin, opiates, oral hypoglycemic agents, phenothiazines, sedative/hypnotics
Pulse	Amphetamines, anticholinergics, antihistamines, cocaine, phencyclidine, sympathomimetics, theophylline	Alcohol, β-blockers, calcium channel blockers, carbamates, clonidine, digoxin, opiates, organophosphates
Respirations	Amphetamines, barbiturates (early), caffeine, cocaine, ethylene glycol, methanol, salicylates	Alcohols and ethanol, barbiturates (late), clonidine, opiates, sedative/hypnotics
Blood pressure	Amphetamines, anticholinergics, antihistamines, caffeine, clonidine, cocaine, marijuana, phencyclidine, sympathomimetics, theophylline	Antihypertensives, barbiturates, β-blockers, calcium channel blockers, clonidine, cyanide, opiates, phenothiazines, sedative/hypnotics tricyclic antidepressants (late)

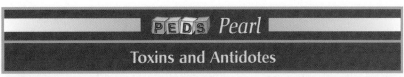

Toxins and Antidotes

Toxin	Antidote
Acetaminophen	N-Acetylcysteine (NAC, Mucomyst)
Arsenic, mercury, other metals	British Anti-Lewisite (BAL) in oil (dimercaprol)
Benzodiazepines	Flumazenil (Romazicon)
β-blockers	Glucagon
Calcium channel blockers	Calcium chloride, calcium gluconate, glucagon
Carbon monoxide	Oxygen, hyperbaric oxygen
Coumadin	Vitamin K
Cyanide	Amyl nitrite, sodium nitrite, sodium thiosulfate
Digitalis glycosides	Digoxin-specific Fab antibodies (Digibind)
Iron	Deferoxamine (Desferal)
Isoniazid	Pyridoxine (vitamin B_6)
Lead	Ethylenediaminetetraacetic Acid (EDTA), BAL,
Methanol, ethylene glycol	Dimercaptosuccinic Acid (DMSA)
Methemoglobinemia	Ethanol (ethyl alcohol), Fomepizole (4-MP)
Opiates	Methylene blue
Organophosphate/carbamate pesticides	Naloxone (Narcan) Atropine, pralidoxime (2-PAM, Protopam)
Tricyclic antidepressants	Sodium bicarbonate

- Nystagmus (rapid, jerky eye movement) may be seen with exposure to anticonvulsants (especially carbamazepine and phenytoin), lithium, ethanol, barbiturates, sedative-hypnotics, monoamine oxidase inhibitors, isoniazid, and phencyclidine.

General Guidelines for Managing the Poisoned Patient

Most poisoned patients require only supportive therapy. Table 12-5 provides a list of commonly ingested substances, associated signs and symptoms, and possible interventions. Table 12-6 provides a list of substances that are particularly toxic, even in small doses.

The poisoned patient can often be appropriately managed using the following general guidelines:

- Use personal protective equipment.
- Ensure adequate airway, ventilation, and circulation.
- If cervical spine trauma is suspected, manually stabilize the spine until the patient has been fully stabilized to a backboard or the cervical spine has been cleared.
- Obtain a thorough history and perform a focused physical examination.

- Consider hypoglycemia in an unresponsive or seizing patient. Check serum glucose level.
- Initiate cardiac monitoring and obtain vascular access as indicated.
- Consult with a PCC as needed for specific treatment to prevent further absorption of the toxin (or antidotal therapy).
  - Decontamination procedures as indicated
  - Opioid overdose: naloxone
  - Organophosphates: high-dose atropine
  - Tricyclic antidepressants: sodium bicarbonate
  - β-blockers: glucagon
  - Dystonic reactions: diphenhydramine.
- Frequently monitor vital signs and electrocardiogram (ECG) findings.
- Safely obtain any substance or substance container of a suspected poison and transport it with the patient.

Decontamination methods used will depend on the toxin and type of exposure.

- Skin
  - If the toxic exposure involved absorption of the substance through the patient's skin, protect yourself by donning appropriate personal protective equipment. This may include specific clothing and respiratory gear designed to protect you while caring for the patient.
  - Remove the child's clothing and place it in plastic bags.
  - Flood exposed areas of the skin with water to remove residual material from the skin. Try to avoid contaminating uninvolved areas of skin on the patient.
  - Wash exposed areas with soap and water for 10 to 15 minutes with gentle sponging.
- Eyes
  - If the toxin has had direct contact with the eye, protect yourself by donning appropriate personal protective equipment.
  - Remove any contaminated clothing from the patient and place it in plastic bags.
  - Irrigate the exposed eye with saline or lukewarm water for at least 20 minutes, except in alkali exposures, which require 30 to 60 minutes of irrigation.
  - To minimize the risk of contaminating the unaffected eye, attach IV tubing to a bag of normal saline and use the end of the IV tubing to flush the eye. Make sure the eyes are open.
  - If a sink is used to decontaminate the eyes, do not use the full force of a faucet to irrigate the affected eye. Instead, use a pitcher or similar container to pour water into the eye.

Decontamination

Gentle sponging should be used to avoid abrasions that would permit greater absorption of the toxin.

Airway protection is the primary concern during GI tract decontamination procedures.

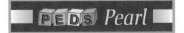

Many studies have failed to show a clear benefit of treatment with ipecac or lavage plus activated charcoal over treatment with charcoal administered alone.

- GI tract decontamination
  - The purpose of gastric decontamination is to prevent further absorption of the toxin by removing it from the GI tract or by binding it to a nonabsorbable agent.
  - Activated charcoal
    - Treatment of choice for GI tract decontamination for substances that can adsorb onto charcoal (Figure 12-4).
    - Insertion of a tracheal tube is **essential** in a patient with a depressed gag reflex or altered mental status, especially in those undergoing gastric lavage.
    - Repeat-dose charcoal is useful in the management of theophylline, phenobarbital, phenytoin, salicylates, and carbamazepine ingestions.
    - Cathartics are no longer recommended as a method of GI tract decontamination.
- Gastric lavage
  - Indications
    - Orogastric lavage with a large-bore tube may be useful in patients who arrive within 1 hour after a life-threatening ingestion and/or those who are obtunded.
    - Decision to lavage should be made in consultation with a toxicologist or PCC.

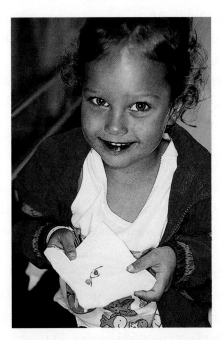

Figure 12-4 This young girl has brought a sample of the mushrooms she ate to the hospital to help identify them. She has been given activated charcoal.

- ◦ Contraindications
  - ▪ Caustic or hydrocarbon ingestions
  - ▪ Coingestion of sharp objects
- ◦ Insertion of a tracheal tube before gastric lavage should be performed in the patient with altered mental status or a depressed gag reflex to protect against aspiration of gastric contents.
- ◦ Procedure
  - ▪ Position child on left side with the head slightly lower than the body.
  - ▪ Insert a large-bore orogastric tube (18 to 20 French).
  - ▪ Instill normal saline until gastric contents are clear.
  - ▪ Save initial return for toxicological examination.
- ◦ Complications may include aspiration, esophageal rupture, tracheal intubation, GI tract perforation, hypothermia, and electrolyte imbalances.
- • Whole-bowel irrigation
  - ◦ Involves the administration, orally or via a gastric tube, of polyethylene glycol solution (Golytely, Colyte) in large volumes and at rapid rates to mechanically cleanse the GI tract.
    - ▪ Has been shown to be useful in certain ingestions when charcoal is not effective such as ingestion of toxic iron or lithium, lead chips, or a large volume of toxic substance (cocaine swallowed in packages)
    - ▪ May also be useful in delayed therapy of enteric-coated or sustained-release preparations such as salicylates, calcium channel blockers, and β-blockers
  - ◦ Contraindications: GI tract hemorrhage or obstruction, ileus, unresponsive patient, or patient with an altered mental status who is not intubated

- • pH alteration: urinary alkalinization
  - ◦ Urinary alkalinization may be used to facilitate elimination of weak acids such as salicylates, barbiturates, and methotrexate from the body
  - ◦ Sodium bicarbonate is given IV bolus and followed by a continuous infusion
  - ◦ Goal is urinary pH of 7 to 8
  - ◦ Monitor closely for electrolyte disturbances (e.g., hypocalcemia)

Hemodialysis is useful for low-molecular-weight substances that have a low volume of distribution and low binding to plasma proteins, such as aspirin, theophylline, lithium, and alcohols.

Watch the child closely for the development of gastric distention, which may interfere with ventilation.

Enhanced Elimination

TABLE 12-5 *Specific Drug Ingestions*

Aspirin (Acetylsalicylic Acid)

Description	Common antipyretic, analgesic, anti-inflammatory agent More than 200 products contain aspirin Metabolic acidosis common in children Common products: Pepto-Bismol, Excedrin, Alka-Seltzer
Signs/symptoms	Early signs and symptoms include tachypnea, diaphoresis, hyperpyrexia, vomiting, and tinnitus or deafness Mild: nausea/vomiting Moderate: tachypnea, tinnitus, dehydration, confusion, fever, metabolic acidosis, respiratory alkalosis Severe: severe metabolic acidosis, coma, seizures, renal failure
Interventions	ABCs, oxygen Activated charcoal appropriate for stable patients, but should not be given to moderately or severely ill patients; start IV line for moderate to severe ingestion; fluid resuscitation if shock present Alkalinization of urine with sodium bicarbonate; alkalinization is important in increasing the elimination of salicylate and decreasing the entry of salicylate into the CNS Severe poisonings require hemodialysis Serum salicylate level on arrival and 6 h after ingestion (toxicity of salicylates correlates poorly with serum levels), CBC, electrolytes, glucose, ABGs to assess for acidosis, coagulation studies, chest radiograph, monitor

Acetaminophen

Description	Common analgesic with antipyretic properties One of the five most common drugs ingested by children Rapidly absorbed from GI tract and metabolized by liver Common products: Nyquil, Percogesic, Comtrex
Signs/symptoms	Initially, mild nausea or no symptoms Does not usually present with altered mental status in the first 24 h; mental status changes suggest polydrug overdose Over several days, vomiting, abdominal pain, and jaundice occur caused by potentially fatal injury to the liver Increased liver enzymes
Interventions	ABCs, oxygen, IV fluids, activated charcoal Draw liver enzymes, acetaminophen/paracetamol level Specific antidote is N-acetylcysteine (NAC or Mucomyst): very effective; give within 8 h of ingestion Serum acetaminophen level 4 h after ingestion, liver function tests, CBC, electrolytes, coagulation panel, serum/urine toxicology screen

Barbiturates

Description	Highly toxic agents that depress the CNS; anticonvulsant properties High abuse potential; alcohol enhances toxicity Common products: pentobarbital, phenobarbital, secobarbital, amobarbital
Signs/symptoms	Dysrhythmias, hypotension, hypothermia; "Barb blisters"—hemorrhagic blisters over areas of pressure that develop about 4 h after ingestion Ataxia, slurred speech, flaccid muscle tone Infants born to addicted mothers will be physically dependent on the drug and will show signs of withdrawal within 72 h of birth (e.g., high-pitched cry, tremors, vomiting, seizures)

Continued

TABLE 12-5 *Specific Drug Ingestions—cont'd*

Interventions	ABCs, oxygen, IV, monitor Activated charcoal; intubate if needed Urine alkalinization with sodium bicarbonate can increase phenobarbital excretion; consider hemodialysis or peritoneal dialysis Treat barb blisters as second-degree burns Possible fluid challenges and vasopressors to maintain blood pressure Serum/urine toxicology screen, glucose level
β-Blockers	
Description	Small ingestions may cause serious toxicity in infant Slow-release forms may lead to delayed and prolonged toxicity Common products: propranolol, metoprolol, atenolol
Signs/symptoms	Bradycardia with variable degrees of AV block and hypotension Possible altered mental status; possible bronchospasm in asthmatics Seizures, coma
Interventions	ABCs, oxygen, IV, cardiac monitor Treat bradycardia per resuscitation guidelines; have pacer at bedside Possible glucose plus insulin or glucagon Possible fluid challenges and vasopressors to maintain blood pressure CBC, electrolytes, glucose
Calcium Channel Blockers	
Description	Small ingestions may cause serious toxicity in infant Slow-release forms may lead to delayed and prolonged toxicity Common products: diltiazem (Cardizem), verapamil (Isoptin, Calan)
Signs/symptoms	Bradycardia with variable degrees of AV block and hypotension Possible altered mental status Hyperglycemia (secondary to blockage of insulin release); seizures, coma
Interventions	ABCs, oxygen, IV, cardiac monitor Treat bradycardia per resuscitation guidelines; have pacer at bedside Possible calcium chloride or calcium gluconate Possible glucose plus insulin or glucagon Possible fluid challenges and vasopressors to maintain blood pressure CBC, electrolytes, glucose
Carbamate Insecticides	
Description	Less toxic than organophosphates, although effects are similar Toxicity is usually limited to muscarinic effects; nicotinic effects uncommon Common products: flea and tick powders, ant killers
Signs/symptoms	Muscarinic effects: vomiting, diarrhea, abdominal cramping, bradycardia, excessive salivation and sweating
Interventions	Protective equipment, remove contaminated clothing, ABCs, oxygen, IV, cardiac monitor Remove affected clothing Administer charcoal Atropine is given until signs of muscarinic toxicity (e.g., symptomatic bradycardia, bronchorrhea, or wheezing) are reversed Treat coma and seizures if they occur

TABLE 12-5 *Specific Drug Ingestions—cont'd*

Caustics (Acids, Alkalis)

Description	Alkaline agents cause liquefaction necrosis, a deep penetration injury that turns tissue, fats, and proteins to soap, damaging all tissue layers. Tissue destruction continues until the substance is significantly neutralized by tissue or the concentration is greatly reduced. Acids cause an immediate coagulation-type necrosis, which damages superficial layers of tissue and denatures protein, altering its structure in a process similar to cooking an egg white. This process creates an eschar, which tends to self-limit further damage. An acid injury may continue to evolve for up to 90 min after the ingestion. Common alkaline products: bleach, ammonia, dishwasher detergent, laundry detergent, drain and oven cleaners Common acid products: sulfuric, hydrochloric, or hydrofluoric acid
Signs/symptoms	Severe burns to the stomach or esophagus may be present with little external evidence of the severity of the injury Upper airway obstruction with difficulty breathing, speaking, or swallowing Gastrointestinal hemorrhage, esophageal or gastric perforation Vomiting, stridor, drooling: If two of these three symptoms are present, likelihood of GI burns is high. Of these signs, vomiting is the most powerful predictor of severe esophageal injury. Severity of injury due to caustics depends on nature, concentration, and volume of the caustic solution; duration of exposure, presence or absence of stomach contents, esophageal reflux after the ingestion, tone of pyloric sphincter
Interventions	Protective equipment, ABCs, oxygen, IV Priority = airway management; flexible fiberoptic intubation over an endoscope is preferable to standard orotracheal intubation. Intubation may further traumatize damaged areas or perforate the pharynx; therefore, blind nasotracheal intubation is contraindicated. Emergent cricothyrotomy may be necessary. Do NOT induce vomiting: Increased tissue damage as esophagus is reexposed to the substance. Activated charcoal is contraindicated because caustics are poorly adsorbed by charcoal; creates a problem with visualization during endoscopy Controversy exists regarding whether attempts should be made to neutralize the caustic substance with water or milk. If a history of significant ingestion with oral lesions or if child is otherwise symptomatic, perform endoscopy to determine extent of injury.

Clonidine

Description	Used for the treatment of hypertension and sometimes used to alleviate opioid and nicotine withdrawal symptoms Available in pills and sustained-release transdermal patches Several pediatric cases of clonidine toxicity have followed ingestion, mouthing, or inadvertent dermal application of clonidine transdermal patches; severe toxicity has been reported after ingestion of as little as 0.1 mg (1 tablet) by a child
Signs/symptoms	Altered mental status, pupil constriction, respiratory depression (Note: these symptoms can appear exactly like opiate toxicity making it difficult to distinguish clonidine ingestion from opiate overdose.) Hypotension, bradycardia (may be initially hypertensive)

Continued

TABLE 12-5 *Specific Drug Ingestions—cont'd*

Interventions	ABCs, oxygen, IV, cardiac monitor Treat coma, hypotension, bradycardia, and hypothermia (usually resolve with supportive measures such as fluids, atropine, dopamine, and warming) Naloxone may be helpful in reversing effects (conflicting evidence) Gastric decontamination (lavage preferred)
Digoxin	
Description	Used for treatment of congestive heart failure and supraventricular dysrhythmias Several plants contain cardiac glycosides (digoxin-like substances) including foxglove, oleander, and lily of the valley
Signs/symptoms	Altered mental status, nausea and vomiting, abdominal pain, headache Almost any cardiac dysrhythmia may occur
Interventions	ABCs, oxygen, IV, cardiac monitor Activated charcoal Treat symptomatic or unstable dysrhythmias per resuscitation guidelines Gastric aspiration or lavage may increase vagal tone and precipitate bradydysrhythmias Administer antidote (digoxin immune Fab [Digibind]) for life-threatening dysrhythmias caused by digoxin overdose Avoid calcium chloride and potassium when treating digoxin toxicity Serum digoxin level, electrolytes (especially potassium, calcium, magnesium), renal panel, liver function tests, continuous ECG
Ethanol (Ethyl Alcohol, Alcohol)	
Description	In young children, alcohol suppresses the liver's ability to manufacture glucose; alcohol intoxication increases susceptibility to hypoglycemia and altered mental status As little as 30 to 60 mL of 40% ethanol can cause altered mental status and hypoglycemia in toddlers Common products: Ethanol level often more than 50% in mouthwashes, colognes, and after shave; cough syrup, flavorings
Signs/symptoms	Characteristic breath odor Hypothermia, hypoglycemia in younger children Respiratory depression, altered mental status, slurred speech, sedation Gastric irritation, vomiting Myocardial depression, hypotension due to vasodilation
Interventions	ABCs, oxygen Treatment is primarily supportive Administer glucose if hypoglycemia present Ethanol level, glucose level, basic metabolic profile, serum osmolality
Ethylene Glycol (Antifreeze), Methanol (Methyl Alcohol, Wood Alcohol)	
Description	Ethylene glycol is metabolized to oxalic and glycolic acids, leading to profound metabolic acidosis and coma; as little as 5 mL may be toxic to an infant Methanol, found in window-washer fluid or gas-line antifreeze, is metabolized to formic acid, with the same effect as ethylene glycol; as little as 15 mL may be toxic to an infant

TABLE 12-5 *Specific Drug Ingestions—cont'd*

Signs/symptoms	Altered mental status with appearance of inebriation or reduced responsiveness, or coma Tachypnea, tachycardia, nausea and emesis; abdominal pain, muscle incoordination, seizures; blurred vision possible with methanol
Interventions	ABCs, oxygen, IV Administer glucose if hypoglycemia present Fomepizole is an antidote for methanol and ethylene glycol poisoning, indications for use are levels 20 mg/dL or higher or high anion gap metabolic acidosis Ethanol may be used when fomepizole is not available Consider hemodialysis in severe cases (renal failure, blindness, and severe metabolic acidosis refractory to bicarbonate therapy) Methanol level, ABG, glucose, basic metabolic profile, serum osmolality

Heavy Metal Poisoning (Zinc, Lead, Mercury, Arsenic)

Description	Poisoning may affect every body system including CNS, heart, lungs, liver, kidney The metals deposit themselves in the body and are excreted slowly 85% of arsenic exposures involve children younger than 6 y[5]
Signs/symptoms	Irritability, headaches, confusion, paresthesias around lips and mouth Nausea/vomiting, metallic taste, palpitations, ECG changes Watery ricelike diarrhea with arsenic; garlic odor to breath or feces with arsenic Burns, corneal changes with zinc Metal fume fever: inhaling metal oxides causes fever, chills, vomiting Lead poisoning: headaches, anorexia, abdominal pain, seizures
Interventions	Protective equipment ABCs, oxygen, IV Arsenic—chelation therapy; mercury—chelation therapy, treat seizures; zinc—chelation therapy, antipyretics, analgesics; lead—chelation therapy, treat seizures CBC, electrolytes, urinalysis; arsenic—serum arsenic, 24-h urine, liver function tests, renal panel; mercury—serum mercury, 24-h urine; zinc—no specific laboratory tests; lead—serum lead, 24-h urine, erythrocyte protoporphyrin level, serum iron and iron-binding capacity, abdominal radiographs

Hydrocarbons (Petroleum Distillates)

Description	Toxic dose varies depending on agent involved and whether it was aspirated, ingested, or inhaled Common products: lamp oil, gasoline, lighter fluid, kerosene, furniture polish, turpentine, pine oil, phenol
Signs/symptoms	Coughing and choking on initial ingestion; gradual increase in work of breathing Odor of hydrocarbon on breath Dry, persistent cough; crackles, wheezes, diminished breath sounds, tachypnea Nausea/vomiting Dizziness, altered mental status Dysrhythmias possible May cause skin surface burns

Continued

TABLE 12-5 *Specific Drug Ingestions—cont'd*

Interventions	Protective equipment, remove contaminated clothing and wash skin with soap and water ABCs, oxygen, assist ventilations as necessary, anticipate need for intubation Activated charcoal contraindicated; consult Poison Control
Iron	
Description	In an infant, ingestion of 600 to 900 mg supplemental iron (generally 2 to 3 tablets) can cause severe toxicity In survivors, severe scarring and obstruction of GI tract may develop Common products: multivitamins, prenatal vitamins
Signs/symptoms	Nausea (initial symptoms may appear flulike), emesis and diarrhea, possibly with blood; abdominal pain; severely poisoned child may present with lethargy or coma and signs of shock
Interventions	ABCs, oxygen, IV (aggressive IV fluids) NOT bound to activated charcoal Antidote: deferoxamine (child's urine will turn pink, salmon, or rose in color) Obtain abdominal radiograph because most iron tablets are radiopaque (except chewable vitamins and children's liquid). Whole-bowel irrigation if positive radiograph findings. Serum iron levels, coagulation studies, electrolytes, CBC, serum glucose, stool for occult blood, type and crossmatch
Isoniazid (INH)	
Description	Used in the treatment of tuberculosis; depletes vitamin B_6, which is required for synthesis of GABA, an inhibitory neurotransmitter. Reduced GABA concentration can lead to seizures. Initial signs of poisoning typically appear within 30 min to $2^1/_2$ h of ingestion
Signs/symptoms	Slurred speech, dizziness, ataxia, vomiting, and tachycardia may progress to seizures or coma; metabolic acidosis, altered mental status, tachypnea, hypotension
Interventions	ABCs, oxygen, IV Activated charcoal Treat coma, seizures, and metabolic acidosis if they occur Pyridoxine (vitamin B_6) is specific antidote and usually terminates diazepam-resistant seizures
Isopropyl Alcohol (Rubbing Alcohol)	
Description	Isopropyl alcohol is a potent CNS depressant (twice as potent as ethanol) and is metabolized to acetone, which may contribute to and prolong CNS depression Adsorbs poorly to activated charcoal (approximately 1 g of charcoal will bind 1 mL of 70% alcohol) Widely used as a disinfectant and antiseptic
Signs/symptoms	Altered mental status with the appearance of inebriation, slurred speech, reduced responsiveness, coma; tachycardia, hypotension, nausea and emesis, abdominal pain due to gastric irritation; hypoglycemia and hemorrhagic gastritis are possible Distinct breath odor of acetone (because isopropyl alcohol is metabolized to acetone)

TABLE 12-5 *Specific Drug Ingestions—cont'd*

Interventions	ABCs, oxygen, IV, monitor; monitor airway closely Treatment is primarily supportive—observe for at least 6 to 12 h Administer glucose if hypoglycemia present Do NOT induce vomiting (risk of rapidly developing coma) Glucose level, serum isopropyl alcohol levels, basic metabolic profile, serum osmolality Large ingestion may require dialysis if coma or myocardial depression occurs

Opiates

Description	Common products: Codeine, fentanyl, heroin, meperidine, methadone, oxycodone, dextromethorphan, propoxyphene
Signs/symptoms	Altered mental status, bradypnea or apnea, bradycardia, hypotension, pinpoint pupils, hypothermia Suspect opioid toxicity when the clinical triad of CNS depression, respiratory depression, and miosis (pinpoint pupils) are present
Interventions	ABCs, oxygen, IV, cardiac monitor; cervical spine immobilization if trauma is suspected Tracheal intubation is indicated in patients who cannot protect their airway. Obtain serum glucose level; give dextrose if indicated Administer naloxone for significant CNS and/or respiratory depression. Assist respirations with a bag-valve mask as necessary. If an IV cannot be established, administer naloxone IM. Larger than usual doses of naloxone may be required for diphenoxylate/atropine (Lomotil), methadone, propoxyphene, pentazocine, and the fentanyl derivatives.

Organophosphates

Description	Widely used pesticides; signs and symptoms usually occur within 30 min to 2 h of exposure but may be delayed up to several hours Chemical pneumonitis may occur if a product containing a hydrocarbon solvent is aspirated In the acute phase, there is no test that can identify organophosphate toxicity; initial management based on clinical findings Common products: No-Pest Strips, roach killers, diazinon, malathion, and parathion
Signs/symptoms	Early signs are muscarinic: nausea, vomiting, abdominal cramps, urinary and fecal incontinence, increased bronchial secretions, cough, wheezing, dyspnea, sweating, salivation, miosis, blurred vision, lacrimation Nicotinic effects include twitching, fasciculations, weakness, hypertension, tachycardia, and in severe cases paralysis and respiratory failure; death is usually caused by respiratory muscle paralysis There is frequently a solvent odor and some describe a garliclike odor of the organophosphate Pay careful attention to respiratory muscle weakness; sudden respiratory arrest may occur
Interventions	Protective equipment, remove contaminated clothing, decontamination procedures; ABCs, oxygen, IV, cardiac monitor Administer activated charcoal Atropine is antidote for muscarinic effects; goal is drying of airway secretions to maintain oxygenation and ventilation—tachycardia is NOT a contraindication to its use; treatment must usually continue for at least 24 h

Continued

TABLE 12-5 *Specific Drug Ingestions—cont'd*

	Pralidoxime is antidote for nicotinic effects; treatment is generally necessary for at least 48 h If intubation is required, note potential interactions between neuromuscular blockers and organophosphates
Sedative/Hypnotics	
Description	CNS depressants with primary effect of respiratory depression Category includes barbiturates, benzodiazepines (e.g., alprazolam, clorazepate, chlordiazepoxide, clonazepam, diazepam, flurazepam, lorazepam, midazolam, oxazepam, temazepam, triazolam), and antihistamines
Signs/symptoms	Slurred speech, confusion, hypotension, tachycardia, pupil dilation or constriction, decreased temperature Overdose in children tends to cause excitation rather than CNS depression
Interventions	ABCs, oxygen Activated charcoal Benzodiazepine antidote (flumazenil) as directed; flumazenil should not be used routinely in setting of overdose—may be used as a diagnostic tool in pure benzodiazepine toxicity; contraindicated in patients with seizure disorders, chronic use of benzodiazepines, coingestion of substances that can cause seizures (includes tricyclic antidepressants, theophylline, chloral hydrate, isoniazid, and carbamazepine); may precipitate seizures that are difficult to control. Serum/urine toxicology screen; investigate reason for toxicity
Theophylline	
Description	Widely used; narrow therapeutic index; many dosage forms Many drug-drug, drug-disease, and drug-food interactions Increased mortality associated with children younger than 2 y in acute overdoses
Signs/symptoms	Agitation, tachycardia, nausea and emesis, depressed mental status Hypotension possible, electrolyte disturbances common Sinus tachycardia common, but SVT and other dysrhythmias possible Seizures, status epilepticus
Interventions	ABCs, oxygen, IV, cardiac monitor Well bound to activated charcoal; give if asymptomatic or minimally symptomatic Dysrhythmias may respond to a short-acting β-adrenergic antagonist, such as esmolol Seizures minimally responsive to conventional anticonvulsant agents Serum theophylline level, electrolytes, glucose, ABG, 12-lead ECG
Tricyclic Antidepressants (TCAs)	
Description	Cause intraventricular conduction delays and serious dysrhythmias; also have anticholinergic effects Progression from early to late symptoms may be rapid Common products: amitriptyline, desipramine, doxepin, trazodone, nortriptyline
Signs/symptoms	Early signs: tachycardia, restlessness, anxiety, increased temperature Late signs (Three C's): Coma, Convulsions, Cardiac dysrhythmias (with widening of QRS complex, prolonged QT interval) Hypotension, dilated pupils, slurred speech, dry mouth, urinary retention

TABLE 12-5 *Specific Drug Ingestions—cont'd*

Interventions	ABCs, oxygen, IV, cardiac monitor
	Treat seizures, prevent injury
	Continuous ECG monitoring, even in the patient who is asymptomatic at presentation
	Treat symptomatic or unstable dysrhythmias per resuscitation guidelines; sodium bicarbonate for ventricular dysrhythmias
	If hypotension present, IV fluid bolus of 10 mL/kg; monitor for pulmonary edema; vasopressors for persistent hypotension
	Serum/urine toxicology screen, cardiac enzymes, electrolytes; serum drug levels do not necessarily predict outcome and are not helpful in acute management

ABC, airway, breathing, and circulation; ABG, arterial blood gas; AV, atrioventricular; CBC, complete blood count; CNS, central nervous system; ECG, electrocardiogram, GI, gastrointestinal; GABA, γ-aminobutyric acid; IM, intramuscular; IV, intravenous; SVT, supraventricular tachycardia.

TABLE 12-6 *Toxicity in Small Doses*

Benzocaine

Description	Found in many first-aid ointments and infant teething formulas
	Benzocaine is metabolized to aniline and nitrosobenzene, which can cause methemoglobinemia (especially in infants younger than 4 mo). Methemoglobinemia has occurred in an infant after ingestion of 100 mg of benzocaine (amount in 1/4 tsp of Baby Orajel).
	Common products: Americaine Topical Anesthetic First Aid Ointment (20% benzocaine), Baby Orajel (7.5%), Baby Orajel Nighttime Formula (10%)
Signs/symptoms	Symptoms begin 30 min to 6 h after ingestion
	Tachycardia, tachypnea, and cyanosis that do not respond to oxygen
	Agitation, hypoxia, metabolic acidosis, coma, seizures with more severe exposures
	Note: Pulse oximetry is unreliable for saturations less than 85%
Interventions	Gastric lavage if patient presents within 30 min of ingestion and has ingested less than 1/4 tsp of benzocaine-containing substance, followed by activated charcoal
	Antidote is methylene blue. Indications for use are methemoglobin levels above 30% and symptoms of respiratory distress or altered mental status

Camphor

Description	Found in over-the-counter liniments and cold preparations
	Rapid acting neurotoxin that produces CNS excitation and depression
	Pediatric toxic dose: 1 g (equivalent to 10 mL of Campho-Phenique or 5 mL of camphorated oil)
	Rapid onset of symptoms 5 to 120 min after ingestion
	Common products: Campho-Phenique (10.8% camphor), Vicks VapoRub (4.18%), camphorated oil (20% camphor), Mentholatum (9% camphor), BENGAY Children's Rub (5%)
Signs/symptoms	Initial feeling of generalized warmth that may be followed by altered mental status (confusion, delirium, restlessness, hallucinations)
	Muscle twitching and fasciculations may precede seizures, but seizures may occur without preceding symptoms

Continued

TABLE 12-6 *Toxicity in Small Doses—cont'd*

Interventions	GI decontamination if it can be accomplished within 1 h of ingestion followed by activated charcoal, seizures are managed with benzodiazepines, supportive care
Chloroquine	
Description	Used for treatment and prophylaxis of malaria and specific connective tissue diseases Powerful rapidly acting cardiotoxin capable of causing sudden cardiorespiratory collapse One 300-mg tablet resulted in the death of a 3-year-old and 750 mg caused ventricular fibrillation in a 13-year-old
Signs/symptoms	Bradycardia, ventricular tachycardia/fibrillation, torsades de pointes, profound hypotension, shock; drowsiness followed by excitability; dyspnea, sudden apnea; dysphagia, facial paresthesias, tremor, slurred speech, hyporeflexia, seizures, coma
Interventions	Diazepam appears to have a cardioprotective effect in chloroquine poisoning IV fluids and vasopressors as needed to manage hypotension, sodium bicarbonate for wide QRS complex dysrhythmias
Lomotil	
Description	Antidiarrheal that is a combination opiate/anticholinergic preparation Onset is biphasic: early anticholinergic toxicity, opiate toxicity delayed 8 to 30 h Respiratory depression can occur as late as 24 h after ingestion and does not appear to be correlated with the dose ingested and severity of symptoms
Signs/symptoms	Signs and symptoms vary and depend on the time since the ingestion: Manifestations may represent either anticholinergic or opioid intoxication; opioid effects often predominate Opioid: constricted pupils, respiratory depression, respiratory arrest Anticholinergic: dilated pupils; warm, dry skin; tachycardia, flushed face
Interventions	Naloxone: repeated doses may be necessary because duration of effect is much shorter than that of Lomotil; anticholinergic symptoms may appear when naloxone is given Because of the risk of sudden respiratory arrest, admit and observe all children with Lomotil ingestion for at least 24 h
Methyl Salicylate	
Description	Mechanism: salicylate toxicity Oil of wintergreen contains 98% methyl salicylate; 1 tsp contains 7 g of salicylate (equivalent to 21 adult aspirin tablets). Less than 1 tsp has resulted in a child's death. Common products: topical liniments (e.g., BENGAY, Icy Hot Balm), oil of wintergreen food flavoring
Signs/symptoms	Onset of symptoms typically within 2 h of ingestion Tachypnea, diaphoresis, hyperpyrexia, vomiting, tinnitus, hyperthermia, seizures, coma
Interventions	Activated charcoal, urine alkalinization, hemodialysis, serum salicylate level (toxicity of salicylates correlates poorly with serum levels)
Tetrahydrozoline (Imidazoline)	
Description	Structurally similar to clonidine Toxicity: 1 to 2 drops of 0.1% solution in infants Onset of symptoms delayed 2 to 6 h after ingestion Common products: Visine (tetrahydrozoline), Afrin (oxymetolazine)
Signs/symptoms	Initial hypertension followed by hypotension, bradycardia, seizures, coma
Interventions	GI decontamination If initial hypertension severe, consider titratable medication (e.g., esmolol, nitroprusside) Fluids, vasopressors may be necessary for treatment of hypotension

CNS, central nervous system; GI, gastrointestinal; IV, intravenous.

TABLE 12-7 *Selected Poisonous Plants*

Plant Name	Toxin	Remarks
Black henbane	Hyoscyamine, scopolamine	Anticholinergic
Castor bean	Ricin toxalbumin	Mimics septic shock; ricin (obtained from castor beans) is used in chemical warfare
Deadly nightshade	Atropine	Gastric irritation, fever, diarrhea
Dieffenbachia (dumb cane, mother-in-law's tongue, dumb plant, tuft root)	Calcium oxylate crystals	Mucous membranes of mouth typically affected with severe pain, swelling, and sensation of biting into glass
Foxglove	Digitoxin	Cardiovascular toxin
Holly	Five toxins	Nausea, vomiting, abdominal cramping, diarrhea
Jimsonweed	Hyoscyamine, scopolamine	Anticholinergic; 50 to 100 seeds = 3 to 6 mg atropine
Lily of the valley	Cardiac glycosides	Cardiovascular toxin
Mandrake	Hyoscyamine, scopolamine	Anticholinergic; ripe fruit nontoxic
Oleander	Cardiac glycosides	Cardiovascular toxin
Philodendron	Calcium oxalate crystals	More than 200 varieties of this popular houseplant; mild oral mucosal irritation, GI upset
Poison hemlock	Coniine	Nicotine-like toxin; professed to be used in the execution of Socrates
Pokeweed (unripe berries)	Phytolaccine	Berries edible when cooked correctly: "poke salad"; nausea, GI cramps, diaphoresis, emesis, diarrhea
Pothos	Calcium oxylate crystals	Pothos ivy, devil's ivy, hunter's robe, golden pothos
Rhododendron	Grayanotoxin, rhodojaponin, asebotoxin	Includes over 1000 species of azaleas and rhododendrons, including mountain laurel, dwarf laurel, rose bay, western Labrador tea, and Japanese pieris; cardiovascular toxin; bradycardia, hypotension, nausea, vomiting, abdominal pain
Rhubarb	Soluble calcium oxylate crystals	Renal toxin; stalks are edible
Tobacco plants	Nicotine	Nicotine-like toxin
Water hemlock	Circutoxin	Neurotoxin; seizures = severe toxicity and a common cause of death
Yellow oleander	Digoxin, digitoxin	Cardiovascular toxin
Yew	Taxine; similar to cardiac glycosides	Cardiovascular toxin; dizziness, dry mouth, nausea, emesis, rash, cyanosis, coma, bradycardia, dysrhythmias
Pitted fruits (e.g., apricot seeds, bitter almonds, peach kernels) – chewed pits	Cyanogenic glycosides*	Cyanosis, difficulty breathing, vomiting, weakness, coma, seizures, cardiovascular collapse

GI, gastrointestinal.
*Contain amygdalin—a plant compound that contains sugar and produces cyanide.

Case Study Resolution

Quickly and carefully, assess the child to determine the patency of his airway. You find the child is acting normally for his age. Examination of the child's mouth reveals no signs of an exposure. His respiratory rate is 26 breaths per minute, heart rate is 114 beats per minute, and the child has no signs of difficulty breathing, speaking, or swallowing. Wash off the bleach from the child's body. Contact a PCC if additional advice is needed.

Web Resources

• atsdr1.atsdr.cdc.gov/child/ochchildhlth.html (Agency for Toxic Substances and Disease Registry)

References

1. American Association of Poison Centers. http://www.1-800-222-1222.info/1800/home.asp (Accessed 5/9/04).

2. Dart RC, Rumack BH. Poisoning. In: Hay Jr WW, Hayward AR, Levin MJ, et al., eds. *Current pediatric diagnosis and treatment,* 15th ed. location: publisher, 2000.

3. Watson WA, Litovitz TL, Rodgers Jr GC, et al. 2002 Annual report of the American Association of Poison Control Centers Toxic Exposure Surveillance System. *Am J Emerg Med* 2003;21:353–421.

4. Linden CH. Digitalis glycosides. In: Ford MD, Delaney KA, Ling LJ, et al., eds. *Clinical toxicology.* Philadelphia: WB Saunders, 2001:379–390.

5. Leikin JB. Arsenic. In: Strange GR, Ahrens WR, Lelyveld S, et al. *Pediatric emergency medicine: a comprehensive study guide,* 2nd ed. New York: McGraw-Hill, 2002:586–588.

Chapter Quiz

1. List five common toxidromes and provide an example of a typical agent in each category:

   A) Toxidrome _____ ; example _____

   B) Toxidrome _____ ; example _____

   C) Toxidrome _____ ; example _____

   D) Toxidrome _____ ; example _____

   E) Toxidrome _____ ; example _____

Questions 2 through 8 refer to the following scenario.

A 3-year-old is found barely responsive by her babysitter. The babysitter was distracted "for just a minute" by a telephone call and lost track of the child. The child was located on the ground just outside the garage door. The patient's skin looks flushed and she is laboring to breathe. You note secretions are draining from the patient's mouth and she has been incontinent of urine. The child is unaware of your presence.

2. From the information provided, complete the following documentation regarding the Pediatric Assessment Triangle:

   Appearance:

   Breathing:

   Circulation:

3. Based on the information provided, your FIRST intervention should be to:
   A) Establish vascular access.
   B) Suction the airway.
   C) Perform a secondary (head-to-toes) survey.
   D) Perform tracheal intubation.

4. For each of the following, record the estimated values for a 3-year-old child:
   A) Weight:
   B) Respiratory rate:
   C) Heart rate:
   D) Blood pressure:

5. Your assessment reveals the child will open her eyes and withdraw in response to a painful stimulus but makes incomprehensible sounds. Her Glasgow Coma Scale score is:
   A) 6
   B) 8
   C) 10
   D) 12

6. The child's respiratory rate is 44/min, heart rate is 158/min, and blood pressure is 80/60. Her skin is warm and moist. Her pupils are equal and reactive at 2 mm. Auscultation of her lungs reveals bilateral diffuse wheezes. Excessive oral secretions are present. These findings are most consistent with the _____ toxidrome.

7. Further questioning of the babysitter reveals that the child may have been out of sight for 20 to 30 minutes before she was found. The babysitter recalls having seen an open bottle of white liquid on the floor of the garage. As you continue interviewing the babysitter, a coworker tells you that he smells garlic on the child's breath. This child was most likely exposed to:
A) An organophosphate.
B) Camphor.
C) A narcotic.
D) A beta-blocker.

8. You are instructed to administer atropine to this patient. Which of the following statements is **correct**?
A) Question the order. Atropine is indicated for symptomatic bradycardias. This patient is not bradycardic.
B) Administer the atropine as instructed. Atropine is being ordered in this situation to increase the patient's blood pressure.
C) Question the order. Although atropine may be used in situations such as this, the patient is tachycardic. Atropine is contraindicated if a tachycardia is present.
D) Administer the atropine as instructed. In this situation, atropine is being given to dry the patient's airway of secretions.

Chapter Quiz Answers

1. Toxidromes are a group of signs and symptoms useful for recognizing a specific class of poisoning. Common toxidromes include anticholinergic, cholinergic, opiate, sedative/hypnotic, and sympathomimetic.
A) Toxidrome anticholinergic; example atropine, diphenhydramine, scopolamine
B) Toxidrome cholinergic; example organophosphates, carbamate insecticides, some mushrooms, nerve agents
C) Toxidrome opioid; example codeine, fentanyl, heroin, meperidine, methadone, oxycodone, dextromethorphan, propoxyphene
D) Toxidrome sedative/hypnotic; example ethanol, anticonvulsants, barbiturates, benzodiazepines
E) Toxidrome sympathomimetic; example albuterol, amphetamines, caffeine, cocaine, epinephrine, ephedrine, methamphetamine, phencyclidine, pseudoephedrine

2. Pediatric Assessment Triangle (first impression) findings:
Appearance: barely responsive, incontinent of urine, unaware of your presence
Breathing: increased work of breathing evident
Circulation: skin is flushed; no evidence of bleeding

3. B. The presence of secretions draining from the mouth of a child that is unaware of your presence requires immediate intervention. Clear the airway with suctioning.

4. "Normal" values for a 3-year-old child:
   A) Weight: 14 kg (31 lb.)
   B) Respiratory rate: 24 to 40
   C) Heart rate: 90 to 150
   D) Blood pressure: BP > 70
   Refer to the tables and formulas in Chapter 3 if you need to review this information.

5. B. The patient's Glasgow Coma Scale score is 8.
Eyes:	To pain	2
Verbal:	Incomprehensible sounds	2
Motor:	Withdraws from pain	4

6. This patient's physical findings are most consistent with the cholinergic toxidrome.

7. A. The patient's physical findings and additional information regarding the events surrounding the exposure strongly suggest organophosphate exposure.

8. D. Atropine is the antidote for the muscarinic effects of organophosphate exposure. The goal of atropine administration in this situation is drying of airway secretions to maintain oxygenation and ventilation. Tachycardia is NOT a contraindication to its use.

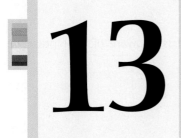

13 Child Maltreatment

Case Study

On her return home after work, a 4-month-old infant is found unresponsive by her 22-year-old mother. The infant was left in the care of mom's 24-year-old boyfriend. The boyfriend states the infant has been fussy, crying most of the day. He says he placed the infant on the sofa for a nap 2 hours ago and thought he was still sleeping when the mother arrived home.

Your examination reveals the infant is unresponsive with shallow, irregular breathing at a rate of eight to 14 breaths per minute. A weak pulse is present at 44 beats per minute. The infant's skin is pale and cool. You notice bruising on both sides of the infant's neck.

How should you proceed?

Objectives

1. Define child maltreatment and child neglect.
2. Describe indicators of possible child abuse or neglect.
3. Describe documentation and reporting requirements for situations involving suspected abuse or neglect.

Child Maltreatment

Child maltreatment includes intentional physical abuse or neglect, emotional abuse or neglect, and sexual abuse of children, usually by adults. The National Center on Child Abuse and Neglect has established definitions of the various types of abuse. State law defines specific acts that constitute the various forms of abuse, and they vary from state to state.

- Neglect is the failure to provide for the child's basic needs. Neglect can be physical, educational, or emotional.
  - Physical neglect can include not providing adequate food or

Terminology

There are four types of abuse: neglect, physical abuse, sexual abuse, and psychological abuse.

clothing, appropriate medical care, supervision, or proper weather protection (heat or coats).

- Educational neglect includes failure to provide appropriate schooling, special educational needs, or allowing excessive truancies.
- Psychological neglect includes the lack of any emotional support and love, chronic inattention to the child, and exposure to spouse abuse or drug and alcohol abuse.
- Physical abuse is the inflicting of a nonaccidental physical injury upon a child.
  - This may include burning, hitting, punching, shaking, kicking, beating, or otherwise harming a child.
  - It may, however, have been the result of overdiscipline or physical punishment that is inappropriate to the child's age.
- Sexual abuse is inappropriate adolescent or adult sexual behavior with a child.
  - It includes fondling a child's genitals, making the child fondle the adult's genitals, intercourse, incest, rape, sodomy, exhibitionism, sexual exploitation, or exposure to pornography.
  - To be considered child abuse, these acts have to be committed by a person responsible for the care of a child (for example a baby-sitter, parent, or daycare provider) or related to the child. If a stranger commits these acts, it would be considered sexual assault and handled solely by the police and criminal courts.
- Psychological maltreatment is a pattern of caregiver behavior or extreme incidents that convey to children that they are worthless, flawed, unloved, unwanted, endangered, or only of value to meeting another's needs.
  - This can include parents or caretakers using extreme or bizarre forms of punishment or threatening or terrorizing a child.
  - The term *psychological maltreatment* is also known as emotional abuse or neglect, verbal abuse, or mental abuse.

Risk Factors for Child Maltreatment

Child Risk Factors

- Premature birth or neonatal separation
- Congenital defect
- Developmental disability
- Physical disability
- Chronic illness
- Multiple birth

Caregiver Risk Factors

- Often abused as a child
- Young maternal age

- History of mental illness or criminal activity
- Financial stress, unemployment
- Physical illness of parent or child
- Marital or relationship stress
- Low self-esteem, depressed
- Substance abuse

Characteristics of the Child Abuser

- Shows little concern for the child's injury, treatment, or prognosis
- Denies the existence of (or blames the child for) the child's problems in school or at home
- Seldom touches or looks at the child
- Has little perception of how a child could feel, physically or emotionally
- Asks teachers or other caregivers to use harsh physical discipline if the child misbehaves
- Sees the child as entirely bad, worthless, or burdensome
- Demands a level of physical or academic performance the child cannot achieve
- Looks primarily to the child for care, attention, and satisfaction of emotional needs

Characteristics of the Abused or Neglected Child

- Accidental versus intentional injury
  - Children are often injured; however, not all children with injuries are abused.
  - Child abuse is unlikely if the child's story is volunteered without hesitation, and matches that of the caregiver.
  - Distinguishing between an intentional injury and an accident is a challenge.
- The following signs may signal the presence of child abuse or neglect:
  - Cries hopelessly during treatment or cries very little in general
  - Shows sudden changes in behavior or school performance
  - May constantly seek favors, food, or things
  - Has not received help for physical or medical problems brought to the parents' attention
  - Does not look at caregiver for reassurance
  - Has learning problems (or difficulty concentrating) that cannot be attributed to specific physical or psychological causes
  - Is always watchful, as though preparing for something bad to happen
  - Lacks adult supervision
  - Is overly compliant, passive, or withdrawn
  - Comes to school or other activities early, stays late, and does not want to go home

History and Physical Examination

- Gathering the history
  - Obtain the history in a nonaccusatory manner
  - Do not accuse the caregiver(s)
- When performing the physical examination, consider the following:
  - Where is the injury?
  - Is the injury/condition compatible with the history given?
  - Is this type of injury consistent with what you would expect for the child's age?
  - How did the injury occur?
  - Are there any other unexplained injuries on the child's body?
  - What is the size and shape of the injury (if applicable)?
  - Does the child appear clean and well cared for?
  - Does there appear to have been a delay in seeking medical attention?
- Red flags
  - Historical factors
    - No history of injury, but injury is found.
    - History incompatible with type or degree of injury.
    - History of the way in which the injury occurred is vague.
      - Or caregiver has no idea how it happened
    - Inconsistent history
      - History changes each time it is told to another healthcare professional.
      - When interviewed separately, caregivers give contradictory histories.
    - History that does not match the developmental stage of the child.
  - Behavioral factors
    - Significant delay between time of injury and time of presentation.
    - Caregiver does not show degree of concern appropriate to severity of child's injury.
  - High-risk presentations
    - Unexplained or poorly explained death of an infant
    - Unexplained apnea
    - Ingestion or toxin exposure with suspicious history
    - Repeated drug or toxin exposure
- Interacting with the caregiver
  - No matter how difficult the situation, you must maintain a professional and nonjudgmental attitude.
  - Do not display anger or use an accusatory approach during your interaction with the caregiver. Confrontation and accusation delay treatment and are counterproductive.

- Physical
  - ◦ Nonspecific symptoms suggestive of sexual abuse
    - ▪ Genital or anal pain or discomfort
    - ▪ Pain on urination or defecation
    - ▪ Urinary frequency
    - ▪ Constipation or bowel withholding
    - ▪ Irritation or inflammation of genital or perianal area
    - ▪ Recurrent urinary tract infection without anatomic or hygiene explanation
  - ◦ Specific signs (must be differentiated from physical signs of alternative causes)
    - ▪ Acute evidence of genital or anal trauma (e.g., bleeding, laceration, bruising)
    - ▪ Scarring of anus, hymen, or vagina
    - ▪ Evidence of sexually transmitted disease
    - ▪ Presence of sperm and/or seminal fluid
    - ▪ Pregnancy
- Behavioral
  - ◦ Symptoms may include behavior or physical manifestations
  - ◦ Nightmares, restlessness, difficulty concentrating, appetite disturbance, phobic fears related to the offender or certain situations, withdrawal tendencies, hostility, regression (e.g., baby talk, infantile behavior, bed wetting), truancy

Signs and Symptoms of Sexual Abuse

Psychological Abuse

- Belittling, threatening, rejecting, isolating, exploiting acts by caregiver
- Lack of self esteem
- Over or under achievers
- Excessively passive or aggressive behavior
- Hyperactivity
- Speech disorders
- Failure to thrive
- Sleep or feeding disorders
- Depressed or suicidal behavior
- Developmental delays

Indicators of Psychological Abuse

Psychological abuse is often difficult to detect.

Munchausen Syndrome by Proxy

Munchausen syndrome by proxy (MSBP) is a form of mental illness in which the parent or caregiver is responsible for producing a faked illness in a child to obtain attention from medical professionals.

- The child may be nearly suffocated, given toxic substances to ingest, or be drugged, resulting in multiple medical procedures and hospitalizations.
- Caregiver denies knowledge as to the cause of the child's illness.
- Child's symptoms subside when separated from caregiver.
- Frequent visits to multiple physicians and hospitals with normal findings.
- Frequent hospitalizations at many different hospitals.
- Common presentations include bleeding, seizures, apnea, diarrhea, vomiting, fever, and rash.
- Mother often found to be perpetrator.[1]
  - Often has knowledge of healthcare system from her own illness or employment.
  - Mother and child appear closely bonded but father often distant.
  - Mother often appears as "ideal" parent—very helpful and bonded to staff, but resists attempts to get to know her.
  - Level of denial high. Often refuses to acknowledge actions, even when confronted with direct proof. Often good at convincing even skilled interviewers that they are normal ("sick but slick" syndrome).
- These children are at high risk for death and serious long-term disability.

Reporting Requirements and Documentation

Each state and U.S. Territory designates individuals, typically by professional group, who are mandated by law to report child maltreatment. Any person, however, may report incidents of abuse or neglect.

Individuals Typically Mandated to Report

Individuals typically designated as mandatory reporters have frequent contact with children. Such individuals include the following:

- Healthcare workers
- School personnel
- Child care providers
- Social workers
- Law enforcement officers
- Mental health professionals

Some states also mandate animal control officers, veterinarians, commercial film or photograph processors, substance abuse counselors, and firefighters to report abuse or neglect. Four states (Alaska, Arkansas, Connecticut, and South Dakota) include domestic violence workers on the list of mandated reporters. Approximately 18 states require all citizens to report suspected abuse or neglect regardless of profession.

- In the prehospital setting, notify the receiving facility staff (preferably a physician or charge nurse) of your suspicions.
- In the emergency department, notify law enforcement personnel and Child Protective Services. After ensuring that security or law enforcement personnel are available (to prevent possible removal of the child from the facility), explain the following to the caregiver:
  - Why an inflicted injury is suspected.
  - Legal reporting obligations.
  - Law enforcement personnel and Child Protective Services have been (or will be) contacted.

Reporting Penalties

Many cases of child abuse or neglect are not reported or investigated even when suspected by professionals. Almost every state and U.S. Territory imposes penalties, in the form of a fine or imprisonment, on those who "knowingly" and/or "willfully" fail to report. To prevent malicious or intentional reporting of cases that are not founded, several states and Territories impose additional penalties for false reports of child abuse or neglect.

Documentation

Documentation should include the following:

- Description of the scene
  - General appearance of the home and other children
  - Appearance of the room where the injury occurred
  - Any unusual, unsafe, or unsanitary conditions
  - Behavior of those present at the scene
- History of the injury or illness
  - Document the when, where, and how regarding the injury
  - Document who was present
  - Indicate any discrepancies in statements in the record
    - Statements made by the caregivers should be documented exactly as stated and noted in quotation marks
- Findings from the physical examination
  - Objectively document physical examination findings including the type, number, size, and location of injuries
  - Document any pattern of injury, if observed

Document the caregiver's comments exactly as stated and enclose in quotation marks.

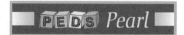

Current information regarding guidelines and laws for reporting child abuse and neglect can be obtained from the National Clearinghouse on Child Abuse and Neglect Information at *http://nccanch. acf.hhs.gov/topics/reporting/ guidelines.cfm.*

Case Study Resolution

On the basis of the information provided, you should be suspicious of SBS. Begin positive-pressure ventilation with 100% oxygen and a bag-valve-mask device. The infant's heart rate is less than 60 beats per minute with obvious signs of hypoperfusion. Begin cardiopulmonary resuscitation and provide additional resuscitative measures as necessary.

Remember that no matter how difficult the situation, you must maintain a professional and nonjudgmental attitude. Do not confront or accuse the infant's caregivers. Objectively document your physical examination findings and all pertinent information including the type, number, size, and location of injuries; when, where, and how the injury occurred; who was present; and any discrepancies in their statements. In the prehospital setting, notify the receiving facility staff (preferably a physician or charge nurse) of your suspicions. In the emergency department, notify law enforcement personnel and Child Protective Services. After ensuring that security or law enforcement personnel are available, explain to the mother why an inflicted injury is suspected, your obligation to report the incident to protect the infant, and that law enforcement personnel and Child Protective Services have been contacted.

References

1. Walker AR, Wissow LS. Child abuse. In: Nichols DG, Yaster M, Lappe DG, et al., eds. *Golden hour: the handbook of advanced pediatric life support*, 2nd ed. St. Louis: Mosby, 1996:469–486.
2. Kelly SJ. Child abuse and neglect. In: *Pediatric emergency nursing*, 2nd ed. Norwalk, CT: Appleton & Lange, 1994:89–107.

Chapter Quiz

1. Which of the following statements about Munchausen Syndrome by Proxy (MSBP) is correct?
   A) The child's father is most often the perpetrator.
   B) The child typically has a history of a congenital defect or chronic illness.
   C) The caregiver denies knowledge as to the cause of the child's illness.
   D) The father and child have usually established a close bond, but the mother is distant.

2. List two conditions that may produce skin findings that appear to be bruises:
   A)
   B)

3. Select the **incorrect** statement concerning Shaken Baby Syndrome (SBS):
   A) Women are most likely to shake a child.
   B) Crying is the most common trigger, usually due to parental/caregiver anger and frustration.
   C) Male babies are more likely to be shaken.
   D) Shaking just 2 to 3 seconds can cause bleeding in and around the brain.

4. List three child risk factors for child maltreatment:
   A)
   B)
   C)

5. True or False: Strangers pose the greatest risk of sexual abuse to children.

Chapter Quiz Answers

1. C. Munchausen Syndrome by Proxy (MSBP) is a form of mental illness in which the parent or caregiver is responsible for producing a faked illness in a child to obtain attention from medical professionals. The caregiver denies knowledge as to the cause of the child's illness. The mother and child appear closely bonded but the father is often distant. The mother is often found to be the perpetrator. These children are at high risk for death and serious long-term disability.

2. Skin findings that may appear to be bruises may actually be Mongolian spots, or bruises due to Ehlers–Danlos Syndrome (EDS) or coagulation disorders such as hemophilia, von Willebrand's disease, thrombocytopenic purpura, or leukemia.

3. A. Men are most likely to shake a child. Crying is the most common trigger, usually due to parental/caregiver anger and frustration. Male babies are more likely to be shaken. Shaking just 2 to 3 seconds can cause bleeding in and around the brain. Most shaking probably lasts 20 seconds or less, with perhaps as many as 40 to 50 shakes.

4. Child risk factors for child maltreatment include premature birth or neonatal separation, congenital defect, developmental disability, physical disability, chronic illness, and multiple birth.

5. False. Children who are sexually assaulted usually have frequent contact with their assailant. Contact often occurs in a trusted person's home and usually involves a male assailant and a female victim. Male victims involved in heterosexual relationships are unlikely to report an incident.

Death of an Infant or Child

14

Case Study

The mother of a 3-month-old infant has called you to her home. She says that she was laying her son down for a nap and noticed that his lips were blue and he was not breathing. She thinks the episode lasted about 10 seconds. The infant has been sick with an upper respiratory infection and was seen by his pediatrician several days ago. The baby is acting normally now. The infant's father appears shortly after your arrival and says he will watch his son. He insists that his child not receive further care.

What would you do next?

Objectives

1. Define sudden infant death syndrome (SIDS).
2. Discuss the typical assessment findings associated with SIDS.
3. Define apparent life-threatening event (ALTE).
4. Identify common grief reactions demonstrated by parents immediately after the death of an infant or child.

Sudden Infant Death Syndrome

Description

SIDS is also called crib death or cot death.

SIDS is the sudden and unexpected death of an infant that remains unexplained after a thorough case investigation, including performance of a complete autopsy, examination of the death scene, and review of the clinical history.[1]

Etiology[2]

- Respiratory tract infections appear to play an important role as a trigger for SIDS.
- Most SIDS victims have suffered tissue hypoxia for some time before death or have an increased reactivity of their pulmonary airways and vessels.

- The final pathway leading to death apparently involves large intrapulmonary pressure swings, but whether these are caused by upper airway obstruction, lower airway occlusion, or asphyxic gasping is unknown.

- SIDS is the third-leading cause of infant mortality in the United States and the most common cause of postneonatal infant mortality (1 month to 1 year of age).[3]

- Approximately 90% of all SIDS deaths occur during the first 6 months of life, most between the ages of 2 and 4 months.

- Most of these infants die at home, usually during the night after a period of sleep.

- In the northern hemisphere, up to 95% of deaths occur between October and April.[4]

- SIDS occurs more often in infant boys than in girls (approximately a 60% to 40% male-to-female ratio).

- African American and Native American infants are two to three times more likely to die from SIDS as other infants. A lower incidence is seen among Hispanic and Asian infants.

- Although rarely observed, when SIDS has been seen, reports indicate the apparently healthy infant suddenly turns blue, stops breathing, and becomes limp without making a cry or struggling.

- The SIDS rate has declined by 42% since 1992, when the recommendation was issued to have infants sleep on their backs and sides rather than their stomachs (Table 14-1).[5]

"Infants who have suffered such a near-miss death event (ALTE) show striking epidemiologic similarities to those who have died of SIDS. They are therefore widely regarded as a living model for SIDS and have hence been extensively studied. However, there are some problems with this approach.

- First, as is probably the case with SIDS, a large number of treatable disease entities can cause ALTE. These cannot always be identified from investigations performed after an event has occurred. A proportion of apparently idiopathic ALTE is caused by an identifiable mechanism (such as pneumonia or meningitis) that is temporary and, if identified, can be treated and therefore does not bear any relationship to SIDS itself.

- Second, it will always be impossible to say whether an infant who was resuscitated by his or her parents would indeed have died without this intervention.

- Third, certain "abnormalities" identified after ALTE (such as gastro-esophageal reflux [GER]) may be coincidental and irrelevant to the ALTE themselves.

Epidemiology and Demographics

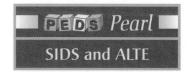
PEDS Pearl
SIDS and ALTE

The term *near-SIDS* or *near-miss SIDS* (now called an apparent life-threatening event or ALTE) has been applied to those infants who were about to die, but were found early enough for successful resuscitation.

TABLE 14-1 *Risk Factors for Sudden Infant Death Syndrome*

Maternal Risk Factors	Infant Risk Factors
• Young age	• Male gender
• Multiparity	• Low birth weight
• Smoking during pregnancy	• Low birth length
• Maternal drug abuse	• Premature birth
• Previous fetal deaths	• Blood type B
• Anemia during pregnancy	• Low Apgar scores
• Low social class	• Low hematocrit at 48 hours
• Low family income	• Prone sleeping position
• Short interpregnancy interval	• Overheating
• Unmarried mother	• Not breast fed
• Late attendance of antenatal clinic	• Previous cyanotic episode
• Postnatal depression	• Previous sudden infant death syndrome in family
• Attendance to psychiatrist	

From Poets CF, Southhall DP. Sudden infant death syndrome and apparent life-threatening events. In: Taussig LM, Landau LI, eds. *Pediatric respiratory medicine*. Philadelphia: Mosby, 1999:1079–1099.

Therefore there are some inherent ambiguities in the relationship between SIDS and ALTE, and this must be borne in mind if one draws conclusions from studies performed in infants with ALTE to the pathophysiology of SIDS."[2]

Autopsy Findings

Some SIDS victims will not have these findings.

- Infant typically appears well nourished and well cared for.
- Rigor mortis and postmortem lividity are generally present.
- Intrathoracic serosal petechiae are often found on the surfaces of lungs, pericardium, and intrathoracic portion of the thymus.
  - It is possible that the petechiae observed in SIDS are indicative of a period of prolonged asphyxia (during which gasping occurred) rather than of a specific disease mechanism (such as upper airway obstruction) that has led to death.[2,6,7]
- Blood-stained frothy secretions in the airway and lungs
  - Found in approximately 60% of SIDS victims.[8]
  - May be caused by a combination of pulmonary edema and high transpulmonary pressures (as with vigorous breathing movements) immediately before death.[2]
- Most SIDS victims (56% to 79%) show histologic evidence of an upper respiratory tract infection, and infectious agents, mostly viruses, have been isolated in 40% to 80% of SIDS cases.[2]

An ALTE has been defined as "an episode that is frightening to the observer and that is characterized by some combination of apnea (central or occasionally obstructive), color change (usually cyanotic or pallid but occasionally erythematous or plethoric), marked change in muscle tone (usually marked limpness), choking, or gagging."[9] In clinical practice, the term *ALTE* has been restricted to events that fulfill these criteria, but also involve vigorous stimulation or resuscitation.[2]

"Most idiopathic ALTEs appear to be caused by the progressive development of hypoxemia, which may progress until it becomes life-threatening or even fatal because of a failure of these infants to resuscitate themselves by arousal or gasping. This hypoxemia apparently does not, in most instances, result from a primary cessation of respiratory efforts, but is more likely to be caused by some form of upper or lower airway closure (such as obstructive apnea) and may also involve the sudden development of an intrapulmonary right-to-left shunt. The triggers eliciting these airway closures remain unknown."[2]

A wide spectrum of diseases and disorders has been found to precipitate an ALTE. The most frequent are digestive (about 50%), neurologic (30%), respiratory (20%), cardiovascular (5%), metabolic, endocrine (under 5%), or diverse other problems, including abusive head injury. Fifty percent of ALTEs remain unexplained (Table 14–2).[10,11]

- From a distance, use the Pediatric Assessment Triangle to form your first impression of the patient. Evaluate the child's appearance, work of breathing, and circulation to determine the severity of the child's illness or injury and assist you in determining the urgency for care.
- Perform a primary survey.
  - Assess the ABCs and determine the need for initiation/continuation of cardiopulmonary resuscitation (CPR).
  - Begin resuscitation using standard resuscitation guidelines if your assessment does not **clearly** indicate death, as in cases when the infant is still warm and flexible.
    - Rigor mortis is an obvious sign of death.
    - Dependent lividity is considered an obvious sign of death only when there are extensive areas of reddish-purple discoloration of the skin in dependent areas of an unresponsive, breathless, and pulseless patient.
    - In some areas, both lividity and rigor mortis must be present to be considered signs of obvious death.
  - If resuscitation is provided
    - Calmly explain what you are doing. Explain the roles of each member of the resuscitation team. Keeping your explanations

Apparent Life-Threatening Event

Interventions for SIDS

If sufficient personnel are on the scene, assign one emergency medical services (EMS) professional to remain with the caregiver and provide comfort during the resuscitation effort.

TABLE 14-2 *Possible Underlying Diagnoses in Patients Presenting with Apparent Life-Threatening Event*

Respiratory Tract Disorders	Gastrointestinal Disorders
Bronchiolitis	Gastroesophageal reflux
Pneumonia	Toxic shock syndrome caused by gastroenteritis
Pertussis	Reye syndrome
Tracheoesophageal fistula	
Aspiration	
Laryngomalacia; tracheomalacia	
Pierre Robin syndrome	
Neurologic Disorders	**Metabolic Disorders**
Meningitis	Medium-chain acyl-CoA deficiency
Epileptic seizures	Biotinidase deficiency
Ondine curse syndrome (central hypoventilation)	Ornithine transcarbamylase deficiency
Spinal muscular atrophy (Werdnig Hoffmann)	Glutaric aciduria type II
Hyperekplexia (startle disease)	Systemic carnitine deficiency
Joubert syndrome	
Arnold Chiari malformation	
Myopathies	
Cardiovascular Disorders	**Others**
Long QT syndrome	Cyanotic breath-holding spells
Cardiac dysrhythmias	Anemia
Aortic stenosis	Intentional suffocation (smothering)
Vascular ring	Munchausen syndrome by proxy

From Poets CF, Southhall DP. Sudden infant death syndrome and apparent life-threatening events. In: Taussig LM, Landau LI, eds. *Pediatric respiratory medicine*. Philadelphia: Mosby, 1999:1079–1099.

simple, provide frequent updates about what is happening and the infant's status, even if there is no change.

- Permit the caregivers to remain within sight of the infant.
- If possible, allow a caregiver to accompany the infant during transport to the emergency department.
- If possible, allow caregivers to briefly touch the infant.

Do **not** express your own opinion about the cause of an infant's death in front of caregivers. Document your findings objectively.

- If the primary survey clearly indicates death or if the infant's response to resuscitation efforts was unsuccessful, follow local protocols regarding resuscitation and transport.
  - Some areas have an obvious death, field termination, death in the field, or similar protocol that is applicable to this type of situation.
  - In some areas, you may be required to leave the body at the scene pending the arrival of the medical examiner. In others, you may be asked to transport the body to a hospital or morgue.
  - If the body must remain at the scene
    - Inform the caregivers in a sensitive manner and explain why.

- Explain that the infant is dead. Do not use euphemisms such as "expired" or "passed away."
- Initiate grief support for the family as soon as possible.
- Remain with the family until law enforcement personnel assume responsibility for the body and grief support personnel are on the scene to assist the family.
- While awaiting the arrival of grief support, law enforcement personnel, or the medical examiner, obtain the names of neighbors, relatives, or friends that you can contact to help care for other children in the home.
  - If you are asked to transport the body to a hospital, encourage the caregivers to hold or touch the infant while you are on the scene.

    Allowing the caregivers to hold the body enables them to focus on the reality of the death and provides an opportunity for them to say goodbye.

    - Tell the caregivers the name and address of the hospital, and then write down the information for them. Do not assume they will remember.
    - If the caregivers cannot accompany you to the hospital, contact a family member or close friend who can arrive quickly and drive them.
    - En route to the hospital, allow the caregivers to touch and hold the infant.

History and Documentation

A focused history must be obtained and the incident must be carefully documented, whether or not resuscitation efforts are initiated. Elicit the necessary information as tactfully as possible. Begin by asking the infant's name. After obtaining this information, use the baby's name when asking questions about the incident. Do not refer to the infant as "the baby," "it," or use other nonspecific words. The information in Table 14-3 should be obtained, if time permits.

SIDS Prevention

- Place an infant supine for sleep.
  - "Back to sleep" or "face up to wake up" slogans.
  - Side sleeping is not recommended.
- Place an infant on a firm surface for sleep. Avoid placing the infant on soft or padded sleep surfaces (e.g., pillows, sheepskins, sofas, soft mattresses, waterbeds, beanbag cushions, quilts, comforters).
- Avoid the use of soft materials in the infant's sleep environment (over, under, or near the infant). This includes pillows, comforters, quilts, sheepskins, and stuffed toys. Blankets, if used, should be tucked in around the crib mattress.
- Do not overbundle the infant or dress the infant too warmly.
- Avoid exposure to cigarette smoke.

TABLE 14-3 *Sudden Infant Death Syndrome History and Documentation*

Questions	Observations of the Scene
What is the baby's name? What happened? What is baby's* age? What does baby weigh? What time was baby put to bed? When did baby fall asleep? Who last saw baby alive? Who found baby? What did that person do? What position was baby in when he/she was found? Was cardiopulmonary resuscitation attempted? Did baby share a bed with anyone else? What was the general health of baby? Had baby been ill recently? Was baby taking any medications?	Position and location of the infant on arrival General appearance of the home and other children, appearance of the room where the death occurred, condition and characteristics of the crib or sleep area Bedding (e.g., pillows, sheets, blankets, etc.), any objects in the crib (e.g., toys or bottles), or any unusual or dangerous items that could cause choking or suffocation Medications Electrical and mechanical devices in use in the room including vaporizers, space heaters, fans, and infant electronic monitors (e.g., apnea monitor or heart rate monitor) Behavior of those present at the scene

*Substitute the infant's name for "baby."

- Adults (other than parents) and children or other siblings should not share a bed with an infant. Parents who smoke or use substances such as drugs or alcohol that impair parental arousal should not share a bed with their infant.

Death of an Infant or Child

When communicating with the caregivers, be aware of your nonverbal communication.

Table 14-4 summarizes common caregiver reactions to the death of an infant or child.

- When communicating with caregivers about the death of an infant or child, speak slowly in a quiet, calm voice. Pause every few seconds and ask the caregivers if they understand what is being said.

Use the first name of the infant or child.

- Preface the bad news by saying, "This is hard to tell you, but..." Using simple terms (not medical jargon), explain that the infant or child is dead. Use the words "death," "dying," or "dead" instead of euphemisms such as "passed on," "no longer with us," or "has gone to a better place."

Be prepared for extremes in behavior ranging from screaming to no response.

- Assume nothing as to how the news is going to be received. The caregiver's reaction to the disclosure of bad news may be anger, shock, withdrawal, disbelief, extreme agitation, guilt, or sorrow. In some cases, there may be no observable response, or the response may seem inappropriate.
- Allow time for the shock to be absorbed and as much time as necessary for questions and discussion.

TABLE 14-4 *Coping with the Death of an Infant or Child*

Caregiver Reaction	Intervention/Response
Shock, denial ("This can't be happening.") • Suddenness of the death left no time for preparation or goodbyes • Difficult to comprehend the death of an infant who did not appear to be sick • Inability or refusal to believe the reality of the event • Numbness, repression of emotional response	• Allow the caregivers to express their grief • Refer to the infant by name and encourage the caregivers to talk about the baby • Provide an opportunity for the caregivers to see and hold the infant's body • Do **not** say, "Time heals …"
Guilt ("If only I had …" "If only I had checked on the baby sooner." "If only I had taken the baby to the doctor with that slight cold.") • Caregiver often feels guilty about not being with the infant at the time of the incident to prevent it from happening or that the infant's death was his or her fault	• Provide reassurance that the caregiver did not cause the infant's death • Encourage caregivers to ask questions • Keep answers to questions as brief as possible • Do **not** say, "This happened because …"
Anger ("Why my baby?") • Caregiver's anger is related to his or her inability to control or change the situation • Anger is displaced and projected to anything and everything	• Do not take anger or insults personally • Be tolerant and empathetic • Do not become defensive • Use good listening and communication skills • Do **not** say, "I know how you feel."
Helplessness, frustration ("What am I going to do?" "Why is this happening to me?") • Surfacing of painful feelings • Caregiver feels alone, disconnected, and alienated	• Ensure availability of a family friend, relative, or religious representative to provide further support • Encourage participation in local sudden infant death syndrome program support services • Do **not** say, "You can still have other children."

- Questions frequently asked include, "Was I to blame?" "Did my baby suffer?" "Why did my baby die?" "What will happen next?" In the case of a SIDS death, common questions include, "What causes SIDS?" "What can I do to prevent another child from dying of SIDS?" "Are there symptoms I should have known about that could have prevented the death?"
- It is important to provide adequate information to the caregivers. This may require repeating answers or explanations to make sure they are understood. Emphasize to the grieving caregivers that they were not responsible for the infant's death and the death could not be prevented.

• An empathic response, such as "You have my (our) sincere sympathy," may be used to convey your feelings. However, there are times that silence is appropriate. Silence respects the family's feelings and allows them to regain composure at their own pace.

• Allow the family the opportunity to see and hold the infant or child. If equipment is still connected to the infant or child, prepare the family for what they will see. A child should be gowned and an infant should be gowned and diapered before the family views the body. Accompany them if necessary and assist them in relinquishing the infant's body when they are ready to do so. Some caregivers may prefer not to view the body. If this is their preference, do not attempt to force them to do so.

- Arrange for follow-up and continued support for the family during the grieving period.

Help for the Healthcare Professional

Although difficult for the family, the death of a child is also emotionally draining for healthcare professionals. Reactions suggesting a need for assistance include persistent feelings of anger, self-doubt, sadness, depression, or a desire to withdraw from others, identification with the infant's caregiver, avoidance of the caregiver, or feelings of blame toward the caregiver. It may be helpful for the healthcare team to meet and discuss the feelings that normally follow a pediatric death.

In some organizations, critical incident stress management (CISM) is mandatory after every pediatric death. Although psychological debriefing is widely used throughout the world to prevent posttraumatic stress disorder (PTSD), the effectiveness of CISM has been questioned in recent journal articles.[12-14] There is no convincing evidence that it does so. Most studies show that individuals who receive debriefing fare no better than those who do not receive it. Some evidence suggests that it may be harmful. As a result, CISM should not be mandatory and should be used with caution.[15,16]

Case Study Resolution

This infant may have experienced an ALTE. Attempt to convince the father that a medical evaluation is important and the baby should be transported for evaluation by a physician. If the father continues to refuse further treatment or transport for his son, seek the advice of medical direction. It may be helpful to have the medical direction physician speak directly with the baby's father by phone.

Web Resources

- www.sidscenter.org (National SIDS/Infant Death Resource Center [NSIDRC])
- www.aap.org (American Academy of Pediatrics)
- www.cpsc.gov (U.S. Consumer Product Safety Commission)
- www.nichd.nih.gov (National Institute of Child Health and Human Development)
- www.sidsalliance.org (First Candle/SIDS Alliance)

References

1. Willinger M, James LS, Catz C. Defining the sudden infant death syndrome (SIDS): deliberations of an expert panel convened by the National Institute of Health and Human Development. *Pediatr Pathol* 1991;11:677–684.

2. Poets CF, Southhall DP. Sudden infant death syndrome and apparent life-threatening events. In: Taussig LM, Landau LI, eds. *Pediatric respiratory medicine.* Philadelphia: Mosby, 1999:1079–1099.

3. Hunt CE, Hauck FR. Sudden infant death syndrome. In: Behrman RE, Kliegman RM, Jenson HB, eds. *Nelson textbook of pediatrics,* 17th ed. Philadelphia: WB Saunders, 2004:1380–1385.

4. Guntheroth WG. *Crib death: the sudden infant death syndrome.* New York: Futura, 1989.

5. Singh GK, Yu SM. Infant mortality in the United States: trends, differentials, and projections, 1950 through 2010. *Am J Public Health* 1995;85:957–964.

6. Brouardel P. *La pendaison, la strongulation, la suffocation, la submersion.* Paris: J-B Bailliere et Fils, 1897:20.

7. Winn K. Similarities between lethal asphyxia in postneonatal rats and the terminal episode in SIDS. *Pediatr Pathol* 1986;5:325–335.

8. Beckwith JB. The sudden infant death syndrome. *Curr Probl Pediatr* 1973;3:3–35.

9. National Institutes of Health consensus development conference on infantile apnea and home monitoring, Sept 29-Oct 1, 1986. *Pediatrics* 1987;79:292–299.

10. Kahn A. Recommended clinical evaluation of infants with apparent life-threatening event: consensus document of the European Society for the Study and Prevention of Infant Death, 2003. *Eur J Pediatr* 2004;163:108–115.

11. Altman RI, Brand DA, Forman S, et al. Abusive head injury as a cause of apparent life-threatening events in infancy. *Arch Pediatr Adolesc Med* 2003;157:1011–1015.

12. Bledsoe BE. Critical incident stress management (CISM): benefit or risk for emergency services? *Prehosp Emerg Care* 2003;7:272–279.

13. Bledsoe BE, Barnes DE. Beyond the debriefing debates. *Emerg Med Serv* 2003;32:60–68.

14. Devilly GJ, Cotton P. Psychological debriefing and the workplace: defining a concept, controversies and guidelines for intervention. *Austral Psychol* 2003;38:144–150.

15. McNally RJ, Bryant RA, Ehlers A. Does early psychological intervention promote recovery from posttraumatic stress? *J Am Psychol Soc* 2003;4:421–445.

Chapter Quiz

You respond to a private residence for a 5-month-old male that is reportedly not breathing.

1. You are met by distraught parents who ask you to save their baby. You should first:
    A) Open the infant's airway.
    B) Perform a scene survey.
    C) Assess the infant's mental status.
    D) Ensure law enforcement personnel are en route to the scene.

2. Which of the following signs is consistent with sudden infant death syndrome (SIDS)?
    A) Bulging fontanelle.
    B) Blood leaking from the ears.
    C) Blood-tinged fluid in the mouth.
    D) Multiple bruises on the chest and abdomen.

3. Under which circumstances would you consider **NOT** beginning resuscitation efforts?
    A) The infant is cyanotic.
    B) Vomitus is present in the airway.
    C) The infant's torso is warm to the touch but his extremities are cool.
    D) The infant is cold to the touch and pooling of blood is evident where he was in contact with the bed.

4. SIDS is caused by:
    A) Malnutrition.
    B) Physical abuse.
    C) Airway obstruction.
    D) An unknown cause.

Chapter Quiz Answers

1. B. Rapidly survey the scene, examining the surroundings. Perform a primary survey. Then begin the initial assessment by first assessing the child's mental status, then airway, breathing, circulation, and life-threatening conditions. A brief history will need to be obtained from the parents, but do not allow this to interfere with your efforts to save this patient.

2. C. A SIDS victim often has cold skin, frothy or blood-tinged fluid in the mouth and nose, lividity or dark, reddish-blue mottling on the dependent side of the body. Rigor mortis may be present. The child typically appears well nourished and healthy. Never discuss or imply child maltreatment as a possible cause of the infant's death.

3. D. Pooling in dependent areas of the body (also referred to as dependent lividity) is indicative of a "prolonged down time" (dead for a significant period). Follow local protocols regarding resuscitation and transport.

4. D. Although there are many theories about the possible causes of SIDS (second-hand smoke, sleeping position, mattress construction, etc.), the exact cause is yet unknown. SIDS is determined as the cause of death only after an autopsy is performed and all other possible causes are ruled out.

Children with Special Healthcare Needs

15

Case Study

An 18-month-old is exhibiting signs of respiratory distress. The child has a tracheostomy and has been ventilator dependent since birth. Your first impression reveals a pale, anxious child on a ventilator. You observe pale skin with cyanosis around the child's lips, nasal flaring, and minimal chest rise with ventilated breaths. You hear the sound of the high-pressure alarm on the ventilator.

What should you do next?

Objectives

1. Define children with special healthcare needs.
2. Define technology-assisted children.
3. Discuss specific assessment and management considerations for children with special healthcare needs.

Overview

- Children with special healthcare needs are those who have or who are at risk for chronic physical, developmental, behavioral, or emotional conditions that necessitate use of health and related services of a type and amount not usually required by typically developing children.[1,2]
- Technology-assisted children are a subgroup of children with special healthcare needs who depend on medical devices for their survival.
  - *Assistive technology* is a term used to describe devices used by children and adults with a disability to compensate for functional limitations and to enhance and increase learning, independence, mobility, communication, environmental control, and choice.
- The number of children with special healthcare needs is increasing. Children with gastrostomy tubes, indwelling central lines, tracheosto-

PEDS *Pearl*

Examples of disorders and diseases of children with special healthcare needs	
• Deformities present at birth or acquired, such as club feet, dislocated hip, cleft palate, mal-united fractures, scoliosis, spina bifida, and congenital genitourinal tract and gastrointestinal tract anomalies • Heart conditions due to congenital deformities and those resulting from rheumatic fever	• Cancer • Cerebral palsy • Cystic fibrosis • Diabetes • Hemophilia • Hydrocephalus • Many muscle and nerve disorders • Neurofibromatosis • Premature infant • Rheumatoid arthritis • Sickle cell anemia • Some conditions of epilepsy

mies, pacemakers, and home ventilators are frequently encountered by healthcare professionals.

   ◦ These children are particularly susceptible to medical problems involving the airway, breathing, and circulation.

   ◦ Vital signs may be controlled by the child's medical device.

      ▪ Heart rate may be determined by a child's pacemaker.

      ▪ Ventilator settings may determine the respiratory rate for a child on a home ventilator.

   ◦ Equipment failure may result in a medical emergency.

• Many children with special healthcare needs

   ◦ Are small for age

      ▪ Weight or baseline vital signs may fall outside the typical range for the child's age

      ▪ May require equipment sizes that differ from those estimated by age

   ◦ Have sensory or motor deficits with or without normal cognitive function

      ▪ Physical and mental abilities may not be the same as those for other children of similar age.

   ◦ Have a sensitivity or allergy to latex because of their repeated exposure to supplies and products made from latex.

Treat each child with respect, compassion, and consideration when providing care.

Cognitive Disabilities

• Cognitive disabilities affect an individual's awareness, memory, and ability to learn, process information, communicate, and make decisions.

   ◦ Cognitive limitations of varying degrees may be found in children with mental retardation, autism, multiple disabilities, or traumatic brain injury.

- ○ Possible causes include inherited disorders, trauma, anoxia, infections, metabolic disorders, intracranial hemorrhage, or other conditions that may damage the brain.
- ○ A child with a cognitive disability may have associated deficits such as a motor impairment, behavioral/emotional disorder, medical complications, or seizure disorder.
- The physical examination of a child with a cognitive disability is no different from that of other children, but the child's ability to communicate and understand will be affected. The degree of impairment will vary depending on the child's age, the child's illness or injury, and the severity of his or her disability.

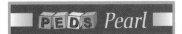

When communicating with a child in a wheelchair, keep in mind that the wheelchair is an extension of the child's personal space.

Physical Disabilities

Approximately half of emergency medical services (EMS) responses to children with special healthcare needs are unrelated to the child's special needs and include traditional causes of EMS calls such as injury.[3]

- A physical disability involves some type of mobility limitation.
- Conditions such as cerebral palsy, spinal bifida, and muscular dystrophy often involve mobility limitations.
- To enhance mobility, the child may use a corrective splint, wheelchair, braces, crutches, or other device.

A child with special healthcare needs who has any of the following conditions should be considered unstable or critical[10]: • Partial or total airway obstruction in children with tracheostomies • Respiratory difficulties in ventilator-dependent children • Bradycardia, irregular pulses, or signs of compensated shock in children with pacemakers	• Fever, nausea, vomiting, headache, or a change in mental status in children with CSF shunts • Signs of worsening illness despite appropriate home therapy in any child with a chronic health problem Since ventilator-dependent children always require assisted ventilation, critical status applies only if one or more additional signs are present.

Assessment and Management Considerations

Initial Assessment

- From a distance, use the Pediatric Assessment Triangle to form your first impression of the patient. Evaluate the child's appearance, work of breathing, and circulation to determine the severity of the child's illness or injury and assist you in determining the urgency for care.

- ◦ The child's caregiver is often the best resource regarding the child's special healthcare needs. The caregiver can usually tell you what is "normal" for the child regarding his or her mental status, vital signs, normal assessment findings and level of activity, ongoing health problems, medications, and medical devices currently in use.
- ◦ Look for a medical identification bracelet or necklace. A younger child may not have one because of the parent's fear that the child will pull it off, but an older child may wear one.
- ◦ Ask the child's caregiver if an EIF is available (Figure 15-1). The American Academy of Pediatrics (AAP) and the ACEP advocate the use of this form for children with special healthcare needs. When completed, the form contains important information for use by healthcare personnel.

The emergency information form (EIF) can be downloaded or printed from the Web site of the American College of Emergency Physicians (ACEP) at http://www.acep.org.

- If the child appears sick (unstable), proceed immediately with the primary survey and treat problems as you find them. If the child appears "not sick" (stable), complete the initial assessment.
- Perform a focused or detailed physical examination, based on the patient's presentation and chief complaint. Remember: Your patient's condition can change at any time. A patient who initially appears "not sick" may rapidly deteriorate and appear "sick." Reassess frequently.

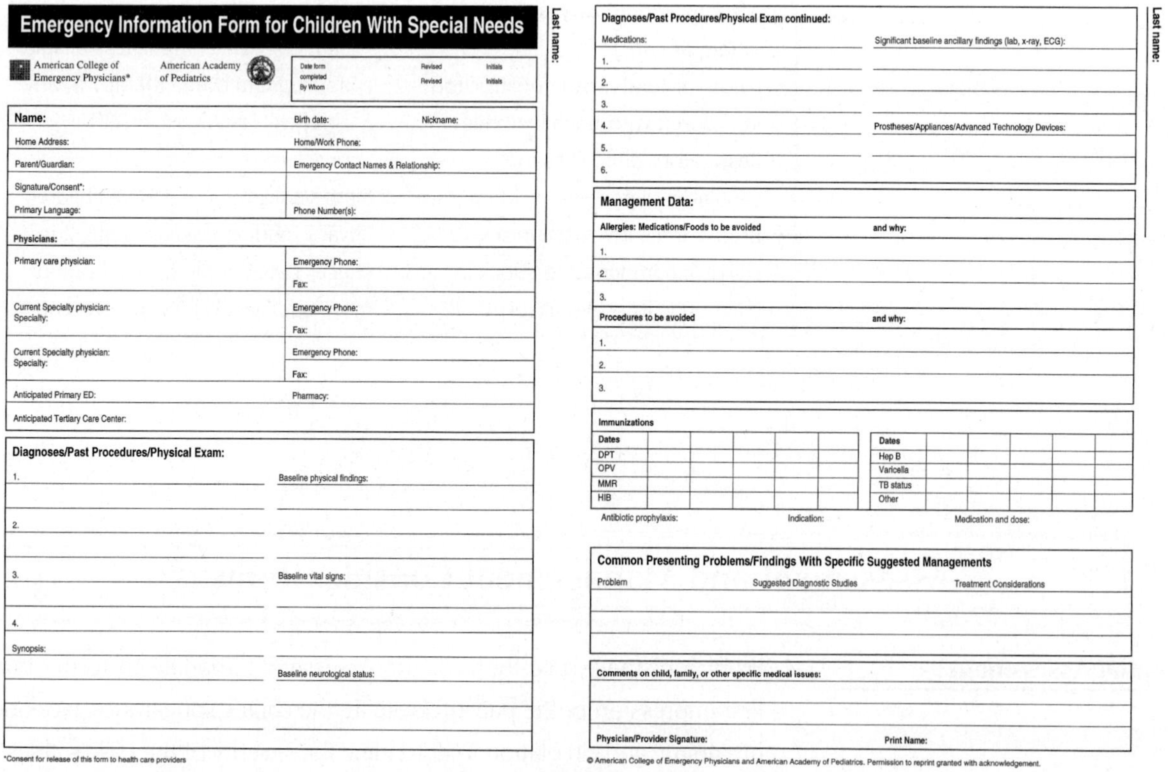

Emergency Information Form for Children With Special Needs

American College of Emergency Physicians* | American Academy of Pediatrics

Date form completed By Whom | Revised | Initials | Revised | Initials

Last name:

Name: | Birth date: | Nickname:
Home Address: | Home/Work Phone:
Parent/Guardian: | Emergency Contact Names & Relationship:
Signature/Consent*:
Primary Language: | Phone Number(s):

Physicians:
Primary care physician: | Emergency Phone: | Fax:
Current Specialty physician: Specialty: | Emergency Phone: | Fax:
Current Specialty physician: Specialty: | Emergency Phone: | Fax:
Anticipated Primary ED: | Pharmacy:
Anticipated Tertiary Care Center:

Diagnoses/Past Procedures/Physical Exam:
1. | Baseline physical findings:
2.
3. | Baseline vital signs:
4.
Synopsis:
Baseline neurological status:

*Consent for release of this form to health care providers

Diagnoses/Past Procedures/Physical Exam continued:
Medications: | Significant baseline ancillary findings (lab, x-ray, ECG):
1.
2.
3.
4. | Prostheses/Appliances/Advanced Technology Devices:
5.
6.

Management Data:
Allergies: Medications/Foods to be avoided | and why:
1.
2.
3.
Procedures to be avoided | and why:
1.
2.
3.

Immunizations

Dates						Dates					
DPT						Hep B					
OPV						Varicella					
MMR						TB status					
HIB						Other					

Antibiotic prophylaxis: | Indication: | Medication and dose:

Common Presenting Problems/Findings With Specific Suggested Managements
Problem | Suggested Diagnostic Studies | Treatment Considerations

Comments on child, family, or other specific medical issues:

Physician/Provider Signature: | Print Name:

© American College of Emergency Physicians and American Academy of Pediatrics. Permission to reprint granted with acknowledgement.

Figure 15-1 Emergency identification form for children with special healthcare needs.

Airway and Breathing Considerations

- Dyspnea is common in children with chronic illnesses because they have difficulty swallowing and handling their airway secretions. Excessive airway secretions and salivation may occur because of muscle weakness, brainstem injury, or other disease processes and increases the child's risk of aspiration.

- Children with tracheostomies or cerebrospinal fluid (CSF) shunts, children on home ventilators, and children with constant positive airway pressure (CPAP) or bilevel positive airway pressure (BiPAP) devices are vulnerable to airway obstruction.

- Some congenital syndromes or diseases are associated with limited cervical motion, making intubation difficult.

  ○ An infant or child with Klippel-Feil syndrome has congenital fusion of the cervical vertebrae and severe shortness of the neck (Figure 15-2). Intubation can be difficult because of their inability to flex or extend their necks.

  ○ The child with Down syndrome is often difficult to intubate because neck rigidity and a large tongue obscure visualization of the glottis. Use of a curved blade may be more effective in displacing the large tongue to the left, permitting better visualization and easier intubation.

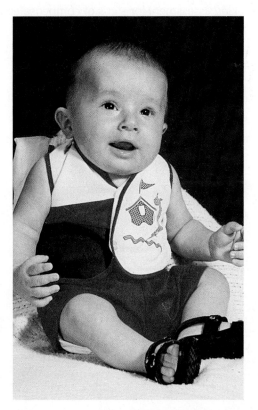

Figure 15-2   This infant with Klippel-Feil syndrome demonstrates a short neck because of fused cervical vertebrae.

- A child with juvenile-onset rheumatoid arthritis may have arthritis involving the temporomandibular joint, limiting mouth opening, and the cervical spine, limiting flexion and extension of the neck. It can be difficult or impossible to intubate these children because of their limited mouth opening and limited cervical flexion and extension.[4]
- The caregiver of an infant or child on a home apnea monitor may request evaluation of the patient after a monitor alarm. Evaluate each patient to determine life threats and the cause of the alarm.
  - When an apnea monitor is used, sensors are positioned on each side of the patient's chest (Figure 15-3). The monitor is intended to alarm primarily on the cessation of breathing timed from the last detected breath. Apnea monitors also use indirect methods to detect apnea, such as monitoring of heart rate. False alarms can occur because of a loose lead, low battery, or accidental shut off.
  - Because many apnea monitors contain a computer chip that can be downloaded to determine if the apnea or high/low heart rate alarms were accurate or caused by artifact, an apnea monitor should be transported with the patient.

Circulation Considerations

- Technology-assisted children may have a higher than normal resting heart rate, making assessment for signs of compensated shock difficult to detect.
- The infant or child with congenital heart disease (e.g., tetralogy of Fallot) may have chronic peripheral and/or central cyanosis. Consult the child's caregiver about the patient's baseline skin color.
- The infant or child with a vascular access device (VAC; i.e., central venous catheter [CVC], implanted port, or peripherally inserted central

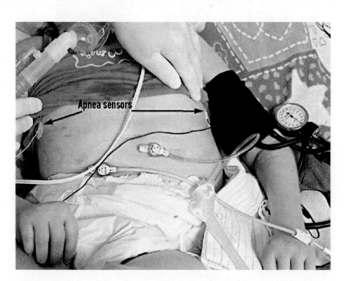

Figure 15-3   Apnea monitor sensors are positioned on each side of the patient's chest.

catheter [PICC]) may require assistance because of a dislodged or damaged catheter, catheter obstruction, leakage from the catheter, or complications associated with these devices, such as a pneumothorax.

Disability (Mental Status)

AVPU and the pediatric Glasgow Coma Scale may not be appropriate for these children.

Altered mental status and/or reduced responsiveness may be the normal baseline in a child with special healthcare needs. Compare your assessment findings with the information provided by the patient's caregiver about the child's baseline mental status, behavior, and level of functioning.

Cerebrospinal Fluid Shunts

Purpose and Components

- CSF is produced in the choroid plexus located in the ventricles of the brain. CSF circulates through the ventricular system and around the spinal cord and is then reabsorbed by vessels in the brain.
- Hydrocephalus ("water on the brain") develops when there is an interruption of this normal circulation due to an increase in CSF production, obstruction of CSF flow, or a decrease in CSF absorption (Figure 15-4).
  - Hydrocephalus often presents in infancy and coexists with many congenital and acquired brain disorders such as myelomeningocele, intraventricular hemorrhage, and CSF infection.
  - Signs and symptoms vary according to age. The young infant presents with a combination of irritability, lethargy, vomiting, a full fontanelle, and a head circumference that is larger than normal. After approximately 12 months of age, the head circumference changes more slowly, and the diagnosis becomes based on irritability, vomiting, lethargy, and ventriculomegaly detected by brain imaging. Older children usually complain of headache before other symptoms or signs of increased intracranial pressure (ICP).[5]

Shunts have a high complication rate.

- To drain excess CSF and reduce ICP, a shunting system is surgically implanted into the brain to drain (shunt) CSF from the ventricular

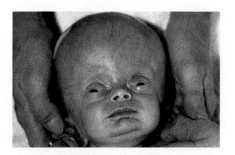

Figure 15-4   Hydrocephalus.

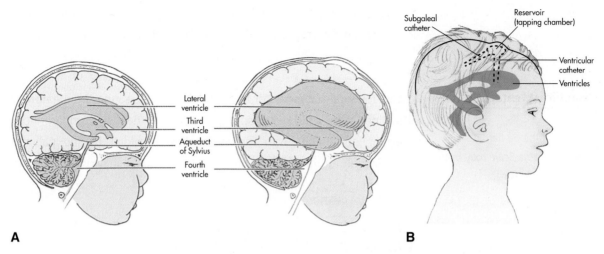

Figure 15-5   A, Untreated hydrocephalus. **B,** Cerebrospinal fluid shunt. The reservoir is usually palpable behind the ear.

system into another part of the body (Figure 15-5). A typical shunting system consists of a proximal catheter, a one-way valve system, and a distal catheter. On-off valves, antisiphon devices, and reservoirs may also be attached. The proximal catheter exits the skull through a surgically created hole ("burr hole"). The one-way valve usually contains a reservoir that is used to withdraw CSF or administer medications. The distal catheter is placed into a body cavity to allow drainage and absorption of CSF. The on-off valve is used for intermittent shunting and can be used to assess shunt function.

- Shunts are named for the position of their proximal and distal catheters. The proximal catheter is usually inserted into one of the ventricles of the brain. The distal catheter is tunneled under the skin and is most often placed in the peritoneal cavity (ventriculoperitoneal [VP] shunt). However, the catheter can also be placed in the right atrium (ventriculoatrial [VA] shunt) (Figure 15-6), pleural cavity (V-pleural shunt), gallbladder, ureter, urinary bladder, or thoracic duct, among others. In VP shunts, an extra length of the distal catheter is inserted into the peritoneal cavity to allow for growth.[6]

> Some patients have more than one shunt, which may or may not be connected, whereas others may also have old, nonfunctioning shunts that were not removed.[6]

- VP shunts are prone to complications. The overall failure rate is 40% at 1 year after insertion and 50% at 2 years.[7,8]
- The child with a malfunctioning shunt may present with irritability, headache, neck pain, vomiting, a bulging or full fontanelle in infants, new seizures or a change in the child's seizure pattern, behavioral changes, or "just not acting right." The child's caregiver is usually most familiar with the child's condition and can tell you if the shunt is the problem.
- In the first few months after surgery, misplacement, disconnection, or

Complications

These are signs of increased ICP, due to fluid accumulation within the brain.

Obstruction of the shunt system can occur at any time.

ROUTES OF DRAINAGE OF VP AND VA SHUNTS

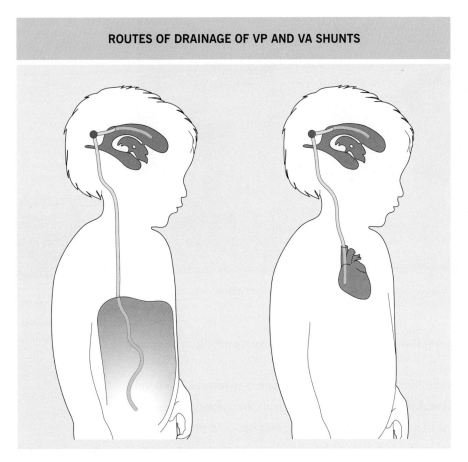

Figure 15-6   Routes of drainage of ventriculoperitoneal (VP) and ventriculoatrial (VA) shunts. Ventriculoperitoneal shunts drain cerebrospinal fluid (CSF) from the cerebral ventricles to the peritoneal cavity via catheter tubing implanted superficially over the rib cage. The lower end of the peritoneal catheter lies free in the abdomen. Ventriculoatrial shunts drain CSF via a convenient neck vein such as the jugular and the superior vena cava to the right atrium.

migration of the equipment can occur. These causes are identified in a "shunt series," which is a series of three radiographs including a skull film, chest film, and abdominal film.

- Infection usually occurs in the first few months after surgery and may be evidenced by obstruction, local wound problems, or unexplained fever (Figure 15-7).
  - Abdominal pain may be present because of infected CSF draining into the peritoneal cavity, causing peritoneal inflammation.
  - If infection is present, redness, edema, or tenderness may be observed along the path of the shunt tubing. A child with a shunt infection is usually, but not always, febrile.
- Shunt failure that occurs after several years most often results from fractured tubing, overdrainage, or erosion of the equipment through the skin or into an abdominal viscus.
  - Overdrainage of the shunt can occur as the child spends more time in an upright position. A siphoning effect on the distal tubing can

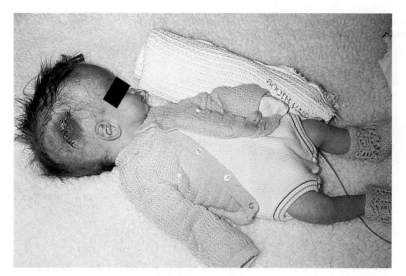

Figure 15-7   External shunt infection in a premature infant with poor nutritional status.

generate negative pressure across the valve, resulting in excessive drainage.

○ Perforation of the stomach or intestinal wall may result in peritonitis with signs and symptoms of shock. Surgical intervention is necessary.

• A pseudocyst may develop when bacteria and bacterial products enter the peritoneal cavity via the shunt catheter. This can cause an inflammatory response that involves a portion of the greater omentum, which wraps around the distal tip of the shunt catheter and seals off the catheter outlet. The resulting cyst fills with CSF, giving rise to abdominal pain and recurrence of the hydrocephalus (Figure 15-8).

• A child with signs of increasing ICP may vomit, increasing his or her risk of aspiration.

• Ensure suction equipment is readily available.

• Administer supplemental oxygen, assist ventilation as necessary, and be prepared to intubate.

• If the child shows signs of shock or if hypotension is present, begin aggressive volume resuscitation using isotonic fluids. If necessary, administer a catecholamine intravenous (IV) infusion to maintain blood pressure in the high-normal range.

• Check the child's blood sugar and administer IV dextrose if indicated.

• Treat seizures if indicated.

• Hospital management typically includes treatment of a CSF shunt infection with systemic antibiotics.

• Tapping the reservoir of the CSF shunt and aspirating fluid to temporarily lower ICP may be necessary and should be performed by a qualified and experienced healthcare professional.

PEDS Pearl

Causes of CSF Shunt Malfunction

D	Displacement (catheter migration), disconnection of shunt components, drainage—overdrainage or inadequate drainage
O	Obstructed or fractured catheter, kinking of distal catheter
P	Perforated abdominal viscus, peritonitis, pseudocyst
E	Erosion of the equipment through the skin

Management

Maintenance of an adequate blood volume and blood pressure is critical for brain perfusion. If the blood pressure is reduced, so is cerebral perfusion pressure.

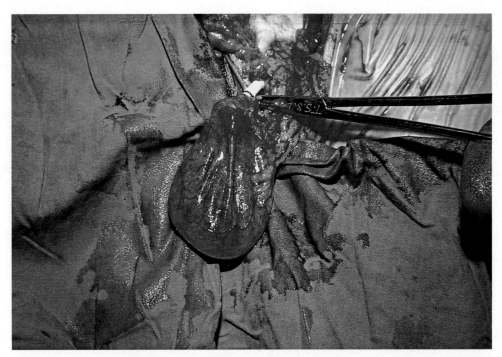

Figure 15-8   A pseudocyst may develop when bacteria and bacterial products enter the peritoneal cavity via the shunt catheter. This can cause an inflammatory response that involves a portion of the greater omentum, which wraps around the distal tip of the shunt catheter and seals off the catheter outlet. The resulting cyst fills with cerebrospinal fluid, giving rise to recurrence of the hydrocephalus.

Gastric Tubes and Gastrostomy Tubes

Gastric Tubes

Many children with these tubes can eat, but they are unable to ingest sufficient calories so a G-tube is placed to supplement their feedings.

Gastric tubes and gastrostomy tubes (G-tube) are used to provide nutrition to an infant or child who is unable to take food by mouth for an extended period. A gastric tube is a small tube passed through the nose (nasogastric) or mouth (orogastric) into the stomach (Figure 15-9). Although the diameter of the tube is small, it is uncomfortable for the patient and associated with irritation of the nasal and mucous membranes. Because of these limitations, a gastrostomy is performed when prolonged or permanent enteral nutrition is needed.

Gastrostomy Tubes

Feeding tube adapters are critical, expensive, and specific to the child's tube. Do not lose or throw away!

A gastrostomy feeding tube is either a tube or a button (skin-level device) that is surgically placed into the stomach through the abdominal wall (Figure 15-10). Initially, a full gastrostomy tube is placed (Figure 15-11) and later replaced with a button (Figure 15-12). If the child has a gastrostomy button, ask the caregiver for the feeding tube adapter for it if the patient requires evaluation in the emergency department. A jejunostomy tube (J-tube) is another type of feeding tube that passes through the abdomen into the small intestine, bypassing the stomach.

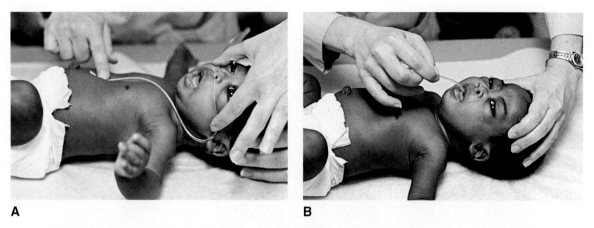

A   **B**

Figure 15-9   **A,** Measuring the tube for an orogastric feeding from the tip of the nose to the earlobe and to the midpoint between the end of the xiphoid process and umbilicus. **B,** Inserting the orogastric tube.

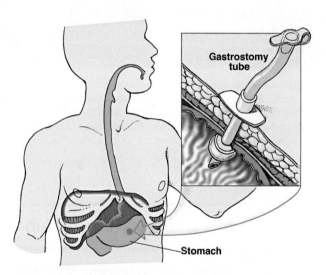

Gastrostomy tube

Stomach

Figure 15-10   A gastrostomy tube is surgically placed into the stomach through the abdominal wall.

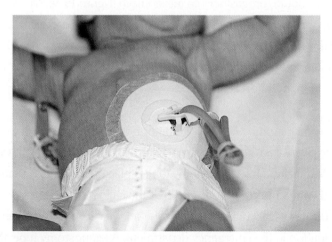

Figure 15-11   Gastrostomy tube.

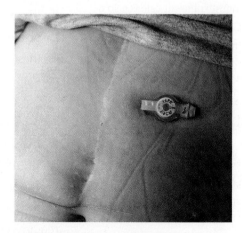

Figure 15-12   Gastrostomy button.

All tubes have a balloon or mushroom-shaped tip on the inside of the stomach and a disk, clamp, or crossbar on the outside to keep them in place. If the balloon or mushroom sinks into the stomach or if the outside disk or clamp is too loose, stomach contents may leak out around the tube. After healing is complete (usually 2 to 3 weeks), a natural tract (fistula) is formed between the stomach and skin, which helps hold the tube in place.

Complications

Common complications encountered with gastrostomy tubes include wound infection, obstruction of the tube, dislodgement of the tube, peritonitis, aspiration, leakage around the tube, bowel obstruction, electrolyte imbalance, dehydration, nausea, and diarrhea.

Management

Gastric Tube

- If the child has an orogastric or nasogastric feeding tube in place and shows signs of possible aspiration (e.g., choking, coughing, and/or cyanosis), suction the airway, and administer oxygen. Monitor the patient's oxygen saturation and cardiac rhythm, and repeat the primary survey frequently.

- If the tube has become partially dislodged, it can be removed without harming the child. The tape should be removed from the child's face and the tube gently pulled out through the nose or mouth. When transferring care of the child, be certain to inform the receiving health-care provider of your actions so the tube can be replaced.

PEDS Pearl

Conditions for Which Gastrostomy Tubes are Used

Swallowing dysfunction	Esophageal atresia
Severe gastroesophageal reflux	Esophageal burns or strictures
Craniofacial abnormalities	Chronic malabsorption
Severe failure to thrive	Severe facial injuries secondary to trauma

PEDS Pearl

Complications of Enteral Feeding Tubes

Wound infection	Pulmonary aspiration of formula
Dehydration	Electrolyte imbalance
Tube obstruction	Tube dislodgement
Peritonitis	Leakage around the tube
Bowel obstruction	Nausea, diarrhea

- If it is necessary to deliver positive-pressure ventilations to the child, the feeding tube can be used to decompress the stomach and relieve pressure on the diaphragm.

Gastrostomy Tube

- Look at the insertion site for signs of irritation, infection, or bleeding.
    - Skin irritation is not an emergent problem and can be evaluated by the child's physician.
    - If signs of infection are present, the child needs physician evaluation.
    - If bleeding is present, apply direct pressure with a sterile dressing.
- Inspect the insertion site to see if the tube has become dislodged.
    - If the tube is dislodged, you may observe a small amount of bleeding at the site and stomach contents may leak out of the hole. Cover the hole with a sterile dressing. Avoid using occlusive dressings because moisture accumulates under the dressing and can predispose the area to infection.
    - In the emergency department, assess the insertion site to determine if a temporary tube can be inserted.

Once the tube is out, the fistula will begin to close and may close completely within 4 to 6 hours.

Tracheostomy Tubes

Indications

A tracheostomy is a surgical opening into the trachea between the second through fourth tracheal rings (Figure 15-13). The opening (stoma) may be temporary or permanent. A child with an upper airway obstruction (e.g., subglottic stenosis, trauma, tumor, soft tissue swelling, foreign body, severe burns), impaired ability to effectively clear secretions (e.g., neuromuscular disorders), or those who require prolonged mechanical ventilation (e.g., bronchopulmonary dysplasia, chronic respiratory insufficiency, paralysis) may require a tracheostomy.

Equipment

Most tracheostomy tubes are made of polyvinyl chloride or silastic (silicone rubber) and have an angle more acute than an adult tube. The tube softens at body temperature, conforming to the shape of the trachea. These tubes are popular because they are lightweight and resist formation of crusted respiratory secretions. To decrease the possibility of an allergic reaction, some children require a metal tracheostomy tube, which is usually made of stainless steel or sterling silver. A metal tube contains an inner cannula.

Some tracheostomy tubes are custom-made to accommodate unusual anatomy or pathology.

Tracheostomy tubes have a neckplate (flange) that rests on the patient's neck over the stoma. Holes are present on each side of the neckplate through which soft tracheostomy tube ties are inserted and used to secure the tube in place.

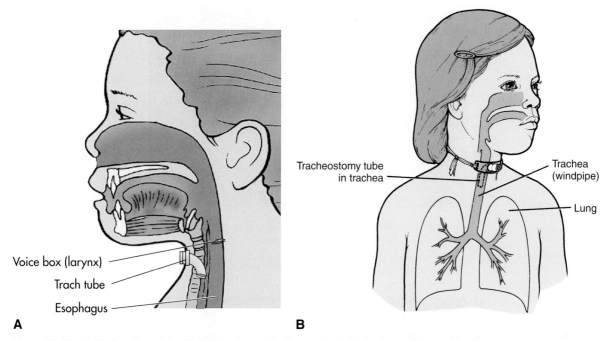

Voice box (larynx)
Trach tube
Esophagus

A

Tracheostomy tube in trachea

Trachea (windpipe)

Lung

B

Figure 15-13 **A**, Tracheostomy tube. **B**, Tracheostomy tube in position in the trachea and secured in place.

If it is necessary to replace a tracheostomy tube, try to use the same length and diameter tube as the one that is already in place.

All tracheostomy tubes have a standard-size opening or hub outside the patient's neck to enable attachment of a bag-valve-mask device. Metal tracheostomy tubes require an adapter to make this connection.

Tracheostomy tubes range in size from 000 (for neonates) to 10 (for older adolescents). The size of the tube is marked on the sterile packaging and on the flange of the tube. A pediatric tracheostomy tube may be cuffed or uncuffed. If a cuff is present, it can be inflated with air or sterile water, depending on the brand of tube used (Figure 15-14).

Types of Tracheostomy Tubes
- Single cannula
  - All neonatal tracheostomy tubes and most pediatric tubes are single-cannula tubes.
  - A single-cannula tracheostomy tube has one lumen that is used for airflow and suctioning of secretions (Figure 15-15). When it is necessary to change the tube, a new tube must be inserted quickly

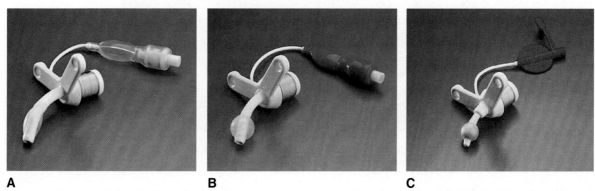

A   **B**   **C**

Figure 15-14 **A**, Cuffed TTS (tight-to-shaft) tracheostomy tube. When completely deflated, the cuff collapses tight to the shaft of the tube. **B**, Air-filled cuff. **C**, Foam cuff.

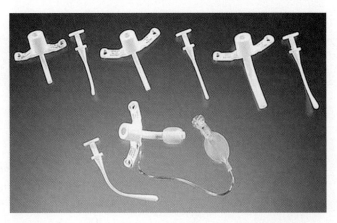

Figure 15-15 Neonatal and pediatric cuffed and uncuffed single-cannula tracheostomy tubes.

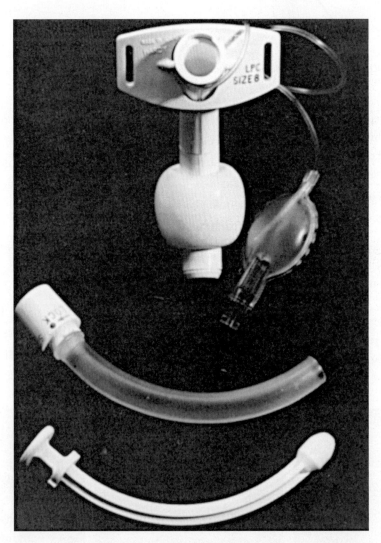

Figure 15-16 Double-cannula tracheostomy tube. Tracheostomy tube (*top*) with inner cannula (*middle*) and obturator (*bottom*).

because there is nothing to keep the stoma open once the old tube is removed. When a new tube is inserted, an obturator is placed inside the tube to keep the flexible tube from kinking. After the new tube is in position, the obturator is quickly removed to permit ventilation.

- Double cannula
  - Consists of an outer cannula (main shaft), inner cannula, and an obturator (stylet) (Figure 15-16)
  - The obturator is used only to guide the outer tube during insertion. When the outer cannula has been inserted, the obturator must be removed to permit ventilation.
  - Once the outer tube is in place, the inner cannula is inserted and locked in place. The inner cannula may be disposable or reusable. A reusable inner cannula must be periodically removed for brief periods for cleaning.
- Fenestrated
  - A fenestrated tracheostomy tube helps the child learn to breathe through the upper airway, to expel secretions, and to talk. A fenestrated tube has small holes (fenestrations) in the side of the tube (Figure 15-17). When a decannulation cap (plug) is attached to the tracheostomy tube, airflow through the stoma is blocked. Airflow is redirected through the holes in the tube, upward past the vocal cords, and out through the nose and mouth.
  - If the child cannot breathe through his or her nose or mouth, the decannulation cap **must** be removed to enable the child to breathe through the stoma.

When the inner tube is removed for cleaning, the outer tube keeps the child's airway open.

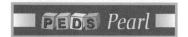

PEDS Pearl

Metal tubes and large plastic tubes typically have a removable inner cannula, which must be removed and cleaned several times each day. Because of the small diameter of the tubes used in infants and young children, most nonmetallic pediatric tracheostomy tubes do not have an inner cannula.[11]

Complications

Although the child's caregiver is taught how to replace a tracheostomy tube at home, emergency care will be sought if the child is away from home or if the caregiver is unable to replace the tube.

Assessment and Management

An infant or child with a tracheostomy is often connected to an apnea monitor or pulse oximeter during periods when his or her caregiver is not present to provide direct supervision (e.g., bedtime).

The most common complications encountered with tracheostomies are dislodgement of the tube, obstruction of the tube, and infection. Incorrect reinsertion of a tracheostomy tube may result in bleeding, formation of a false tract, or perforation of the trachea or esophagus, with resulting inability to ventilate and development of subcutaneous emphysema, pneumothorax, and pneumomediastinum.[9]

Assess the child for signs of respiratory distress. If signs of respiratory distress are present, the child's history may help identify the cause of the problem.

- Consider a lower airway obstruction if the child has a history of fever and gradual worsening of his or her respiratory status.
- Consider a mucus plug, if the child's onset of symptoms was sudden and associated with a change in the consistency of his or her tracheostomy tube secretions.

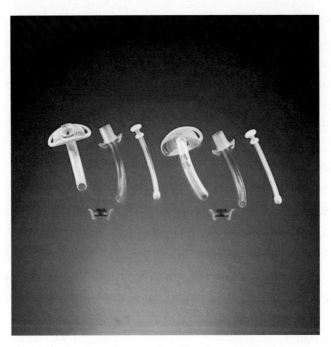

Figure 15-17   Disposable cannula cuffless fenestrated tracheostomy tubes with decannulation caps (shown in red).

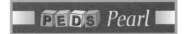

Assume that any infant or child with a tracheostomy and signs of respiratory distress has an obstructed tube. Possible causes of the obstruction include increased secretions, a mucus plug, an obturator that was inadvertently left in the tracheostomy tube, or equipment failure, among other causes.

- Consider a displaced or obstructed tracheostomy tube if the child has signs and symptoms consistent with a possible obstruction (see PEDS Pearl).
- In a ventilator-dependent child, a recent change in home ventilator settings or a ventilator malfunction may also cause worsening respiratory symptoms. Ask the child's caregiver about this possibility.

Clearing an Obstructed Tracheostomy Tube
- If a tracheostomy tube obstruction is suspected, attempt to ventilate through the tube with a bag-valve device to assess tube patency. If the child is on a home ventilator, disconnect the tracheostomy tube from the ventilator and attach the tube to the bag-valve device.
- If it is difficult to compress the bag, prepare to assess for tube obstruction.
  - Place the child in a supine position. Place a small towel roll beneath the shoulders to extend the neck and improve access to the tracheostomy tube.
  - Examine the tracheostomy tube. Ensure that the tube is properly positioned and the obturator has been removed. If the child has a fenestrated tube, make sure the decannulation cap has been removed from the tube.
- If the child's condition has not improved, consider instilling 1 mL of normal saline into the tracheostomy tube (see Sidebar).
- Select a suction catheter of appropriate size. The suction catheter

An infant or child with an obstructed tracheostomy tube will initially exhibit signs of respiratory distress that will progress to respiratory failure and arrest if the obstruction is not cleared.

In the field, ask the child's caregiver to provide you with suctioning equipment and supplies, because the items they use will be appropriate for the child's needs.

should be no more than one half the internal diameter of the tube being suctioned.

- ◦ To determine the correct size suction catheter, use a length-based resuscitation tape or multiply the external diameter of the tracheostomy tube (in millimeters) by two. For example, if the tracheostomy tube is 4 mm in diameter, use an 8-French suction catheter.

- ◦ It is important to use a suction catheter of appropriate size to allow the entry of air around the catheter during suctioning. A suction catheter that is too large can obstruct the airway.

- Set the suction pressure (portable or wall-mounted) to −100 mm Hg or less.

- If possible, preoxygenate the patient. Give blow-by oxygen by holding the oxygen tubing close to the opening of the tracheostomy tube. Set the oxygen flow rate to 10 to 15 L per minute. If necessary, ventilate the child with a bag-valve device by attaching the bag to the tracheostomy tube.

The upper airway filters and humidifies inspired air. Because a tracheostomy bypasses the upper airway, dried secretions can easily accumulate and occlude the tracheostomy, despite regular tracheostomy care.

- Gently insert the suction catheter into the tracheostomy tube (Figure 15-18).

- ◦ Do not use excessive force when inserting the suction catheter because this may damage the soft tissues of the trachea.

- ◦ The catheter should be inserted to 0.5 cm beyond or just to the end of the tracheostomy tube. Insertion of the suction catheter and suctioning should take no longer than 10 seconds per attempt.

  - ▪ Insert the catheter without applying suction. Once the catheter is in the tracheostomy tube, apply suction while slowly withdrawing the catheter, rolling it between your fingers to suction all sides of the tube.

- ◦ If suctioning equipment is not immediately available, attempt to clear the obstruction by quickly inserting and removing the obturator. This technique should *not* be used when suctioning equipment is available.

- Monitor the child's heart rate and color throughout the procedure. Stop suctioning immediately if the heart rate begins to slow or if the child becomes cyanotic.

- After suctioning, reassess the patient. Observe the child's rate and depth of breathing, skin color, heart rate, and mental status. Auscultate breath sounds and assess pulse oximetry, if available.

- ◦ If breathing is adequate, administer oxygen.

- ◦ If breathing is inadequate, suctioning must be repeated. Administer oxygen and allow the child to rest for 30 to 60 seconds (or provide assisted ventilation with high-concentration oxygen) before beginning another attempt (Figure 15-19).

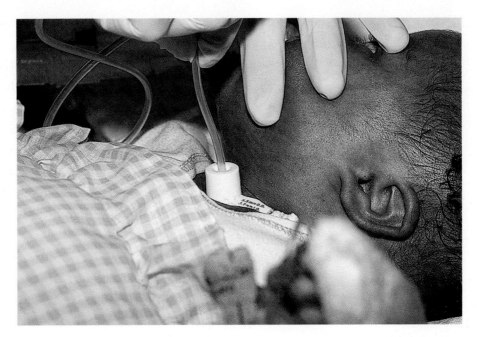

Figure 15-18   Suctioning a tracheostomy tube.

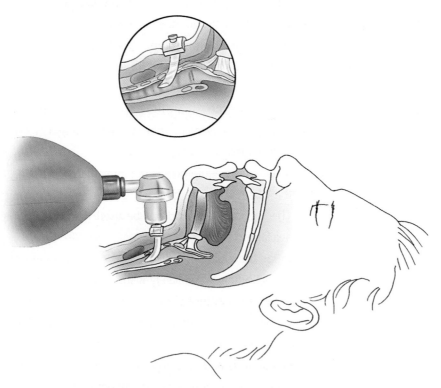

Figure 15-19   Ventilating through a stoma with a bag-valve device.

The lower airway is considered a "sterile" area. The upper airway is considered a "clean" area. The same suction catheter can be used to suction from a sterile to a clean area, but not from a clean to a sterile area.[12] In other words, suction the trachea first, then the mouth and nose. The suction catheter may *not* be used to first suction the mouth and nose and then the trachea.

Signs of Possible Tracheostomy Tube Obstruction

- Altered mental status with restlessness, agitation
- Increased work of breathing
- Raspy noises from tracheostomy tube during respiration
- Change in sounds during respiration
- Diminished breath sounds
- Nasal flaring, retractions
- Difficulty eating or sucking
- Decreased oxygen saturation
- Marked use of accessory muscles
- Poor peripheral perfusion; mottling
- Tachycardia (bradycardia is a late sign)
- Inadequate chest rise during spontaneous or assisted ventilation
- High peak pressure alarm on ventilator
- Difficulty ventilating when providing assisted ventilation
- Cyanosis, bradycardia, and unresponsiveness (late findings)

Removal of the tracheostomy tube is called **decannulation**.

  ◦ If there is no improvement, prepare to remove and replace the tracheostomy tube.

Removing and Replacing a Tracheostomy Tube

To remove a tracheostomy tube

- Assemble and prepare the equipment.
  ◦ Ensure oxygen, suction, and a bag-valve device with mask are immediately available.
  ◦ Ask the child's caregiver if a replacement tracheostomy tube is available. If the caregiver is not available, determine the size of the current tracheostomy tube by checking the wings (flanges) of the tube.
    ▪ Attempt to locate the same size and model tracheostomy tube. If a similar tube is not available, use a tube of similar size. Select a tube with the same outer diameter as the child's tube or one-half–size smaller.
    ▪ Inspect the new tube for cracks and tears. If the new tube has a cuff, inflate the cuff and check for leaks. Completely deflate the cuff. Avoid touching the portion of the tube that will be inserted into the trachea.
    ▪ Insert the obturator into the new tube and ensure that it slides in and out easily. The obturator serves as a stylet to guide the tube during insertion. Its blunt tip helps to protect the stoma from trauma during insertion.
    ▪ Moisten the new tracheostomy tube with normal saline or a small amount of water-soluble lubricant to ease insertion.

Suctioning and Normal Saline	
Instillation of normal saline before suctioning is controversial and has limited value. However, administration usually stimulates a cough that moves secretions from distal to proximal airways. "It has been common practice to instill a bolus of normal saline into the (endotracheal [ET] or tracheostomy) tube before suctioning. However, this technique may contribute to lower airway colonization and nosocomial pneumonia through repeated washing of organisms from the	tube's surface into the lower airway.[13,14] In this 1994 study, suction catheter insertion dislodged up to 60,000 viable bacterial colonies. A 5-mL saline instillation dislodged up to 310,000 viable bacterial colonies. "The use of saline has been shown to have an adverse effect on Sao_2 and should not be used routinely in patients receiving mechanical ventilation who have a pulmonary infection.[15] Although the pediatric research is scarce, routine use of normal saline with ET tube suctioning should be avoided."[14,16]

Indications for Tracheostomy Tube Suctioning

- Indication by the patient that suctioning is necessary
- Suspected aspiration of gastric or upper airway secretions
- Visible secretions in the airway; secretions bubbling in the tracheostomy tube
- Wheezes, crackles, or gurgling on inspiration or expiration audible to the patient and/or caregiver with or without auscultation
- More frequent or congested-sounding cough
- Patient unable to clear secretions by coughing
- Altered mental status, restlessness, or irritability
- Unexplained increase in work of breathing, respiratory rate, or heart rate
- Decrease in vital capacity and/or oxygen saturation
- Unilateral or bilateral absent or diminished breath sounds
- Cyanosis

- If time permits, cut tracheostomy ties to the appropriate length and thread the tracheostomy tie through the flange on one side of the new tube.
  - Some patients may use a tracheostomy tube holder that uses Velcro or nylon hooks to secure the tube in place instead of ties (Figure 15-20).
- If a tracheostomy tube is unavailable, an endotracheal tube with an *outer* diameter equivalent to the child's tracheostomy tube can be inserted though the stoma in an emergency.
  - An endotracheal tube and tracheostomy tube that are designated as the same size may not actually be equivalent.
- Using age-appropriate language, explain the procedure to the child.
- Suction the tracheostomy tube to minimize secretions.
- If the existing tube has a deflatable cuff, deflate the cuff by connecting a 5- to 10-mL syringe to the valve on the pilot balloon. With the syringe, aspirate air or water until the pilot balloon collapses.
- While holding onto the tracheostomy tube with one hand, cut or untie the cloth ties that hold the tube in place with the other.
- Removing the tube
  - If the child has a single-cannula tracheostomy tube, slowly withdraw the tube (Figure 15-21).
  - If the child has a double-cannula tracheostomy tube, remove the inner cannula. If the inner cannula is reusable, clean it, and reinsert it. If the inner cannula is disposable, remove and discard it, and insert a new inner cannula.

Cutting the pilot balloon will not reliably deflate the cuff.

Because a cough can dislodge the tracheostomy tube, be sure to hold on to the tube when the ties are not secure.

The inner cannula of a reusable tube is cleaned with hydrogen peroxide and rinsed with normal saline.

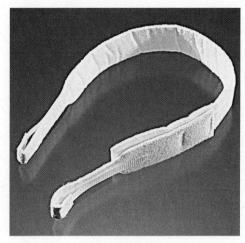

Figure 15-20   Tracheostomy tube holder with Velcro hooks that attach easily to the flanges on the tracheostomy tube.

In most patients with a tracheostomy, the upper airway connected to their trachea is patent, enabling bag-valve-mask ventilation and standard orotracheal intubation if necessary. If oxygen is administered through the mouth and nose, cover the stoma with sterile gauze.

- ◦ If replacing the inner cannula fails to clear the airway, remove the outer cannula as well, administer oxygen, and then replace both tubes at the same time.
- • Administer oxygen until the new tracheostomy tube is inserted.
  - ◦ Oxygen can be administered directly through the stoma.
  - ◦ If airflow can be heard and felt through the upper airway, oxygen can be administered by mask.
  - ◦ If there is a significant delay in replacing the tracheostomy tube, the child may require positive pressure ventilation. If the upper airway is obstructed, deliver positive pressure ventilation by ventilating the stoma with a bag-valve device using a neonatal mask.
- • With the obturator in place inside the new tube, gently insert the tube into the stoma using a downward and forward motion that follows the curve of the trachea (Figure 15-22).
  - ◦ If necessary, place gentle traction on the skin above or below the stoma to ease insertion.
  - ◦ If the tracheostomy tube cannot be inserted easily, withdraw the tube, administer oxygen, and begin again. If the second attempt is unsuccessful, try a smaller tube. **Never force the tube**. Forcing the tube can create a false tract.
- • After insertion, remove the obturator from the tracheostomy tube.
- • Connect a bag-valve device to the tracheostomy tube and ventilate the child. *Do not let go of the tracheostomy tube* until it has been secured with tracheostomy ties or a tracheostomy tube holder.

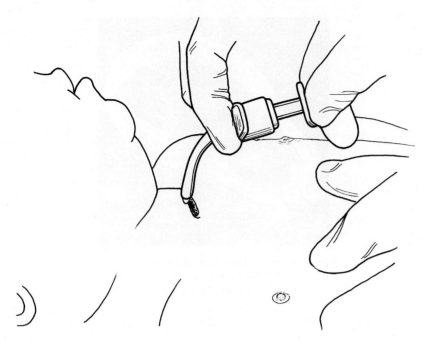

Figure 15-21   Slowly withdraw the tracheostomy tube.

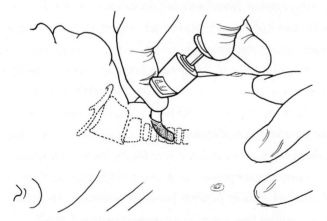

Figure 15-22   With the obturator in place inside the new tracheostomy tube, gently insert the tube into the stoma using a downward motion, following the curve of the trachea.

- Check for proper placement of the tracheostomy tube.
  - Signs of proper placement include equal bilateral chest rise, equal breath sounds (either spontaneous or with assisted ventilation), and improvement in mental status and heart rate and decreased work of breathing.
  - Signs of improper placement include resistance during insertion of the tube, bleeding from the stoma, lack of chest rise or poor compliance during assisted ventilation, or development of subcutaneous air in the tissues surrounding the stoma.

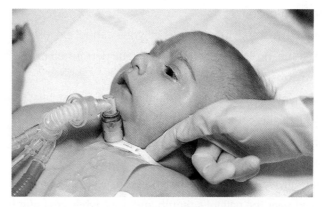

Figure 15-23 Tracheostomy ties or a tracheostomy tube holder should be snug enough that you can place only one finger between the fastening device and the patient's skin.

A suction catheter or feeding tube may be used as a guide to facilitate insertion of a new tracheostomy tube. Insert the suction catheter through the new tracheostomy tube, and then insert the suction catheter into the stoma without applying suction. Slide the tracheostomy tube along the suction catheter and into the stoma, until it is in the proper position. *Do not let go of the suction catheter at any time before removing it from the tracheostomy tube.* Withdraw the suction catheter from the tracheostomy tube. Assess the patient.

A child with a tracheostomy may have some airway narrowing, requiring a smaller tracheal tube than usual for his or her age and size.

Note the length of the original tracheostomy tube and use it as a guide for depth of insertion of the tracheal tube.

- After confirming proper placement of the tracheostomy tube, secure the tube using tracheostomy ties or a tracheostomy tube holder. The ties or holder should be snug enough that you can place only one finger between the fastening device and the patient's skin (Figure 15-23).

Placing a Tracheal Tube in a Tracheostomy

- If a new tracheostomy tube is not available or if replacement attempts are unsuccessful, try to insert a tracheal tube. Insertion of a tracheal tube is a temporizing measure until a tracheostomy tube of the proper size can be replaced.
- To place a tracheal tube through the stoma
  - Select a tracheal tube that is the same or slightly smaller size than the child's tracheostomy tube.
    - If the tracheal tube has a cuff, inflate the cuff and check for leaks. Completely deflate the cuff. Avoid touching the portion of the tube that will be inserted into the trachea.
    - Moisten the distal end of the tracheal tube with a saline or a small amount of water-soluble lubricant.
  - Place the child in a supine position. Place a small towel roll beneath the shoulders to extend the neck.
  - Oxygenate the patient if possible just before inserting the tracheal tube.
  - Gently slide the tracheal tube through the stoma and into the airway, directing the tip downward after passing it through the stoma.
    - The insertion depth of the tracheal tube should equal the distance between the flange and the distal tip of the tracheostomy tube.
  - If the tracheal tube is cuffed, inflate the cuff to stabilize the tube and minimize air leakage. Secure the tube in place.

- Tracheal intubation
  - If a tracheostomy tube or tracheal tube cannot be inserted through the stoma, orotracheal intubation can be performed unless an upper airway obstruction is present.
- If the patient's condition does not improve or if a tracheal tube cannot be inserted, attempt assisted ventilation through the stoma.
  - For best results, attach a neonatal mask to the bag-valve device and place the mask over the stoma.
  - Alternatively, deliver positive-pressure ventilation with a mask placed over the patient's mouth and nose while covering the stoma with a gloved hand to prevent the escape of air.

Home Ventilators

A child may require long-term mechanical ventilation for many reasons including the following:

- Inadequate respiratory drive secondary to a congenital brain abnormality or brainstem damage
- Weak respiratory muscles due to neuromuscular disease
- Cervical spinal cord injury or other conditions that impair the conduction of nerve impulses to respiratory muscles
- Severe chronic pulmonary disease, such as bronchopulmonary dysplasia or cystic fibrosis

Some children require continuous mechanical ventilation, others require intermittent ventilatory support (e.g., during sleep).

Ventilator Emergencies

If signs of respiratory distress are present in a child on a ventilator, identification and treatment of possible causes are important. The DOPE mnemonic can be used to recall possible reversible causes of acute deterioration in an intubated child.

- **D**isplaced tube (e.g., right mainstem or esophageal intubation) or **D**isconnection of the tube or ventilator circuit—reassess tube position, ventilator connections
- **O**bstructed tube (e.g., blood or secretions are obstructing airflow)—suction
- **P**neumothorax (tension)—needle thoracostomy
- **E**quipment problem/failure (e.g., empty oxygen source, inadvertent change in ventilator settings, low battery)—check equipment and oxygen source

If you suspect ventilator malfunction and you cannot quickly find and correct the problem

- Disconnect the ventilator tubing from the tracheostomy tube.
- Attach a bag-valve device to the tracheostomy tube and provide manual ventilation with supplemental oxygen.
- Watch for equal chest rise and listen for equal breath sounds.
- If the patient's chest rise is shallow, ensure that the bag-valve device is securely connected to the tracheostomy tube. If chest rise does not improve, assess the tracheostomy tube for obstruction as previously described.

Noninvasive Mechanical Ventilation

CPAP and BiPAP are noninvasive methods of ventilatory assistance used in spontaneously breathing patients. They do not require a tracheal tube or tracheostomy.

Continuous Positive Airway Pressure

CPAP is the delivery of slight positive pressure (like blowing through a straw) to prevent airway collapse and improve oxygenation and ventilation in spontaneously breathing patients. When using CPAP, the child wears a mask that covers the mouth and nose, providing continuous increased airway pressure throughout the respiratory cycle as the child breathes. CPAP may be used to assist ventilation in children with neuromuscular weakness, chronic pulmonary edema, tracheomalacia, or obstructive sleep apnea. Some children use the device continuously, whereas others require it only at night when airway obstruction is most likely.

Bilevel Positive Airway Pressure

Like CPAP, BiPAP is delivered through a tight-fitting mask that fits over either the patient's nose or the mouth and nose. In BiPAP therapy, two (bi) levels of positive pressure are delivered; one during inspiration (to keep the airway open as the patient inhales) and the other (lower) pressure during expiration to reduce the work of exhalation. The BiPAP device can be set to deliver pressure at a set rate or to sense when an inspiratory effort is being made by the patient and deliver a higher pressure during inspiration. BiPAP is used in the treatment of patients with chronic respiratory failure and may be helpful in the transition from invasive to noninvasive respiratory support.

Assessment and Management

A child who requires noninvasive mechanical ventilation has a higher-than-average risk for partial or total airway obstruction. The patient may be removed from a CPAP or BiPAP device if it interferes significantly with assessment and interventions. The child will be still able to breathe but may tire easily. If the patient exhibits signs of respiratory distress, administer supplemental oxygen or provide assisted ventilation as necessary.

Vascular Access Devices

VADs are catheters placed in children who require frequent blood withdrawal, prolonged or frequent IV fluid or drug administration, and/or nutritional support. The catheters are inserted into the central circulation for long-term use, usually for weeks or months. VADs have allowed many patients to be treated as outpatients rather than have prolonged hospital stays.

Although several types of VADs are available, they can be classified into three general categories.

- CVCs
- Implanted ports
- PICCs

- CVCs implanted for long-term use are typically referred to by the individual that created them (e.g., Broviac, Hickman).
- The catheter is surgically inserted into the external jugular, subclavian, or cephalic veins, with the catheter tip in the superior vena cava, just above the right atrium. The other end of the catheter is tunneled subcutaneously and exits the skin on the anterior chest wall.
- A small cuff is located around the catheter about one inch inside the point where the catheter enters the patient's skin. Fibrous tissue grows around the cuff, anchoring the catheter in place and creating a barrier against infection (Figure 15-24A).
- The external portion of a tunneled catheter may have a single, double, or triple lumen, depending on the patient's treatment needs. A small cap covers each lumen and is filled with heparin or saline solution to keep blood clots from occluding the catheter (Figure 15-24B).

- An implanted (or subcutaneous) port is surgically placed completely below the skin, with no parts external to the skin. Like the tunneled catheters, a silastic catheter is inserted into a central vein and advanced so that the tip lies at the junction of the superior vena cava and the right atrium. However, the other end is tunneled subcutaneously and is attached to a port (reservoir).
- The port can be palpated as a raised disk under the skin. To administer medications or draw blood, a needle is inserted through the skin overlying the port. The port has titanium or plastic housing and a hard silicone septum that is self-sealing. To extend the life of the septum, a special "Huber" needle is used to access it (Figure 15-25).

Central Venous Catheters

These catheters are also referred to as "tunneled catheters."

Implanted Ports

Implanted ports are known by their brand names (e.g., Portacath, Mediport, or Infusaport).

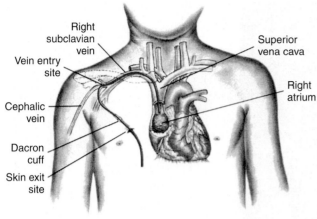

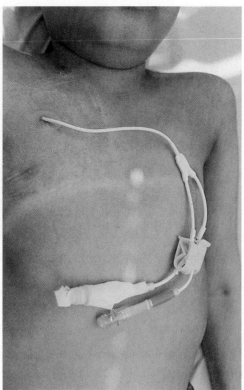

A

Figure 15-24   **A,** Central venous catheter insertion and exit site.
B, External venous catheter (note the redness from the dressing site).

B

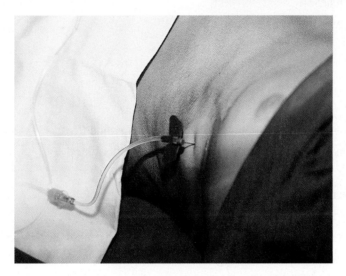

Figure 15-25   To administer medications or draw blood through an implanted port, a special Huber needle is used to access the septum of the device.

Peripherally Inserted Central Catheters

PICC lines are also called nontunneled catheters because they enter the skin near the point at which they enter the vein.

- PICCs are not inserted directly into a central vein. Instead, a PICC line is inserted into an antecubital vein and then advanced into the subclavian vein so that the tip lies in the superior vena cava or right atrium.
- PICC lines are small (23 to 16 gauge) single-lumen or double-lumen catheters. Their small size is advantageous for use in infants and small children (Figure 15-26).
- A PICC line does not require surgical placement; it can be inserted at the bedside, usually by a specially trained nurse.

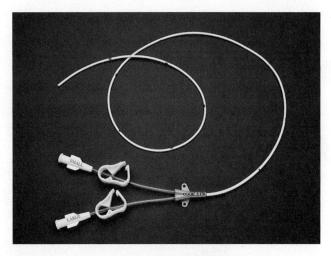

Figure 15-26   A peripherally inserted central catheter (PICC).

- PICC lines are less expensive and are associated with fewer complications than CVCs.

Emergencies from CVCs may result from local or systemic complications associated with their use:
- Infection or allergic reaction
- Breakage and leakage
- Air embolism
- Infusion errors
- Catheter migration
- Catheter obstruction

If a CVC is dislodged or damaged, apply direct pressure as needed to control hemorrhage. Clamp the exposed catheter to prevent further blood loss and treat for shock, if indicated.

Vascular Access Device Emergencies

Emergent Use of Vascular Access Devices

Do not administer medications or fluids through a CVC unless other methods of vascular access cannot be obtained (e.g., peripheral or central line access), you have received special training to access central catheters, and an emergent condition exists.

Case Study Resolution

This child is exhibiting clear signs of respiratory distress while on a ventilator. Use the DOPE mnemonic to recall the possible reversible causes of acute deterioration in an intubated child.
- **D**isplaced tube (e.g., right mainstem or esophageal intubation) or **D**isconnection of the tube or ventilator circuit–reassess tube position, ventilator connections
- **O**bstructed tube (e.g., blood or secretions are obstructing airflow)–suction
- **P**neumothorax (tension)–needle thoracostomy

- *E*quipment problem/failure (e.g., empty oxygen source, inadvertent change in ventilator settings, low battery)—check equipment and oxygen source

A high-pressure ventilator alarm often indicates a mechanical or medical problem that has increased airflow resistance, such as an obstructed tracheostomy tube or worsening pulmonary disease. If you suspect ventilator malfunction and cannot quickly find and correct the problem, disconnect the ventilator tubing from the tracheostomy tube. Attach a bag-valve device to the tracheostomy tube and provide manual ventilation with supplemental oxygen. Watch for equal chest rise and listen for equal breath sounds. If the patient's chest rise is shallow, ensure that the bag-valve device is securely connected to the tracheostomy tube. If chest rise does not improve, assess the tracheostomy tube for obstruction. Provide additional interventions as necessary.

Web Resources

- www.aap.org/advocacy/emergprep.htm (Emergency Preparedness for Children with Special Health Care Needs—American Academy of Pediatrics)
- www.ems-c.org (Emergency Medical Services for Children)
- www.ds-health.com (Down Syndrome: Health Issues)
- www.easterseals.com/site/PageServer (Easter Seals)
- www.nichcy.org/ (National Dissemination Center for Children with Disabilities)

References

1. McPherson M, Arango P, Fox H, et al. A new definition of children with special health care needs. *Pediatrics* 1998;102[Pt 1]:137–140.

2. Newacheck PW, Strickland B, Shonkoff JP, et al. An epidemiologic profile of children with special health care needs. *Pediatrics* 1998;102[Pt 1]:117–123.

3. Hazinski MF, Markenson M, Neish S, et al. Response to cardiac arrest and selected life-threatening medical emergencies: the medical emergency response plan for schools—a statement for healthcare providers, policymakers, school administrators, and community leaders. *Ann Emerg Med* 2004;43:83–99.

4. Infosino A. Pediatric upper airway and congenital anomalies. *Anesthesiol Clin North America* 2002;20:747–766.

5. Kestle JRW. Pediatric hydrocephalus: current management. *Neurol Clin* 2003;21:883–895.

6. Teoh DL. Tricks of the trade: assessment of high-tech gear in special needs children. *Clin Pediatr Emerg Med* 2002;3:62–75.

7. Drake JM, Kestle JR, Milner R, et al. Randomized trial of cerebrospinal fluid shunt valve design in pediatric hydrocephalus. *Neurosurgery* 1998;43:294–305.

8. Kestle JR, Drake JM, Cochrane DD, et al. Lack of benefit of endoscopic ventriculoperitoneal shunt insertion: a multicenter randomized trial. *J Neurosurg* 2003;98:284–290.

9. Bower CM. The surgical airway. In: Dieckmann RA, Fiser DH, Selbst SM, eds. *Illustrated textbook of pediatric emergency and critical care procedures.* St. Louis: Mosby, 1997:116–122.

10. Foltin GL, Tunik MG, Cooper A, et al. *Teaching resource for instructors in prehospital pediatrics for paramedics.* New York: Center for Pediatric Emergency Medicine, 2002.

11. Wood RD. Diagnostic and therapeutic procedures in pediatric pulmonary patients: general principles. In: Taussig LM, Landau LI, eds. *Pediatric Respiratory Medicine.* St. Louis: Mosby, 1999:244–262.

12. Perry AG, Potter PA. *Clinical nursing skills and techniques,* 3rd ed. St. Louis: Mosby, 1994.

13. Hagler DA. Endotracheal saline and suction catheters: sources of lower airway contamination. *Am J Crit Care* 1994;3:444–447.

14. Hockenberry MJ. *Wong's nursing care of infants and children.* 7th ed. St. Louis: Mosby, 2003.

15. Ackerman MH. Instillation of normal saline before suctioning in patients with pulmonary infections: a prospective randomized controlled trial. *Am J Crit Care* 1998;7:261–266.

16. Curley MAQ, Moloney-Harmon PA. *Critical care nursing of infants and children,* 2nd ed. Philadelphia: WB Saunders, 2001.

Chapter Quiz

1. List three categories of vascular access devices:

   A)

   B)

   C)

2. You are preparing to suction a child with a tracheostomy. You should set the suction pressure to
   _____ mm Hg.

   A) −30 to −70

   B) −60 to −100

   C) −90 to −120

   D) −100 to −20

3. Suctioning should be performed for no longer than _____ seconds per attempt.

   A) 5

   B) 10

   C) 15

   D) 20

4. Which of the following tubes or catheters do not require surgical insertion?

   A) Gastric feeding tube, peripherally inserted central catheter.

   B) Gastrostomy tube, tracheostomy tube.

   C) Tunneled central venous catheter, implanted port.

   D) Peripherally inserted central catheter, tunneled central venous catheter.

5. Select the incorrect statement regarding CPAP and BiPap.

    A)   CPAP and BiPAP may be used in spontaneously breathing patients.

    B)   Use of CPAP or BiPAP does not require a tracheal tube or tracheostomy.

    C)   CPAP provides two levels of positive pressure; one level of positive pressure during inspiration and a lower pressure during expiration.

    D)   BiPAP is used in the treatment of patients with chronic respiratory failure.

Chapter Quiz Answers

1. Although many types of vascular access devices exist, they can be classified into one of these three general categories:

    A)   Central venous catheters (CVC).

    B)   Implanted ports.

    C)   Peripherally inserted central catheters (PICC).

2. B. When suctioning an infant or child, a suction pressure of –60 to –100 mm Hg is recommended to avoid trauma to the tracheal mucosa.

3. B. Insertion of the suction catheter and suctioning should take no longer than 10 seconds per attempt.

4. A. A gastric feeding tube and peripherally inserted central catheter (PICC) do not require surgical insertion. A gastrostomy tube, tracheostomy tube, tunneled central venous catheter, and implanted port require surgical placement.

5. C. CPAP and BiPAP may be used in spontaneously breathing patients. Use of CPAP or BiPAP does not require a tracheal tube or tracheostomy. BiPap (not CPAP) provides two levels of positive pressure; one level of positive pressure during inspiration and a lower pressure during expiration. BiPAP is used in the treatment of patients with chronic respiratory failure and may be helpful in the transition from invasive to noninvasive respiratory support.

16 Resuscitation of the Newly Born Outside the Delivery Room

Case Study

A 19-year-old-woman has just given birth. Your patient is the term infant.

During your visual assessment of the newborn, what questions should you ask yourself to determine if routine care is appropriate or if resuscitation must be initiated?

Objectives

1. Discuss the physiologic changes that occur in the transition from intrauterine life to extrauterine life.
2. Discuss antepartum and intrapartum factors associated with an increased risk for neonatal resuscitation.
3. Discuss the assessment findings associated with primary and secondary apnea in the neonate.
4. Discuss the treatment plan for apnea in the neonate.
5. Differentiate when a woman in labor should be transported and when to prepare for delivery in the field.
6. Describe the steps for performing a vaginal delivery and the steps performed immediately after delivery for every newborn.
7. Identify equipment that should be readily available for resuscitation of the newly born.
8. Identify the primary signs used for evaluating a newborn during resuscitation.
9. Formulate an appropriate treatment plan for providing initial care to a newborn.
10. Determine when the following interventions are appropriate for a newborn:
    A) Blow-by oxygen delivery
    B) Ventilatory assistance

C) Chest compressions

D) Tracheal intubation

E) Vascular access

11. Discuss the routes of medication administration for a newborn.

Principles of Resuscitation of the Newly Born

The term *newly born* refers to the infant in the first minutes to hours after birth.

Successful resuscitation of the newly born presents a challenge that requires the following:

- An understanding of the newborn transitional physiology
- The ability to anticipate high-risk situations in which the newborn may require resuscitation
- Adequate preparation with appropriate equipment and medications for newborn resuscitation
- The ability to initiate resuscitative efforts in a timely and effective manner.

Newborn Transitional Physiology (Adjustments to Extrauterine Life)

In utero, all of the oxygen used by the fetus diffuses across the placenta from the mother's blood to the baby's blood (Figure 16-1). The alveoli of the fetus are open and filled with fetal lung liquid instead of air and the pulmonary blood vessels are constricted. Before labor, the production of fetal lung fluid decreases dramatically, decreasing the volume by about one third. During vaginal delivery, the baby's thorax is squeezed, further reducing the volume of fetal lung fluid by approximately one third.

Unless the lungs are immature, absorption of fetal lung liquid is usually complete within 24 hours of birth.

With the first breath, the newborn must pull air into his or her fluid-filled airways and alveoli. When the alveoli begin to fill with air for the first time, surfactant helps them remain partially open and keeps the walls of the alveoli from sticking together when the newborn exhales. As air enters the lungs, pressure drives the remaining fetal lung fluid into the interstitium, where one half is absorbed by pulmonary lymphatics and the other half is absorbed by the interstitium and then carried away by the pulmonary vasculature. Breathing becomes easier and easier as the air sacs fill even more and then remain full of air.

The newborn's initial cries and deep breaths help move the fetal lung fluid out of the airways.

As the lungs fill with air, the pulmonary blood vessels relax, significantly increasing blood flow to the lungs. At about the same time, the umbilical arteries and vein constrict, increasing systemic blood pressure. Blood flow through the ductus arteriosus decreases and the newborn's skin turns from gray/blue to pink as oxygen-enriched blood enters the newborn's systemic circulation. Possible problems that may disrupt the newborn's transition to extrauterine life are shown in Table 16-1.

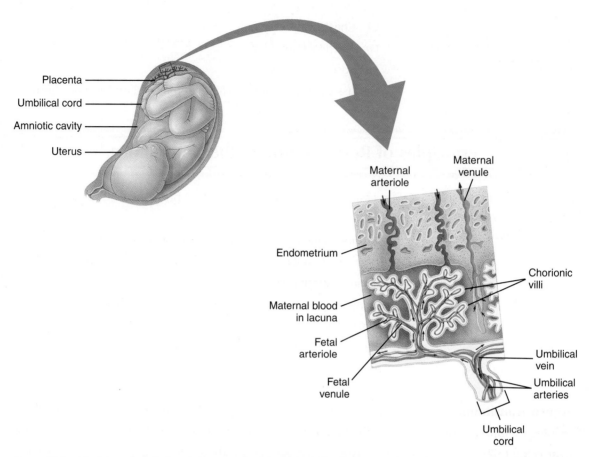

Figure 16-1   **The placenta: interface between maternal and fetal circulation. A,** Relationship of uterus, developing infant, and placenta. **B,** The close placement of the fetal blood supply and the maternal blood in the lacunae of the placenta permits diffusion of nutrients and other substances.

TABLE 16-1 *Problems That May Disrupt the Normal Transition to Extrauterine Life*

Problem	Possible Result
Newborn does not breathe sufficiently to force fluid from alveoli	Lungs do not fill with air; oxygen is not available to blood circulating through the lungs → hypoxia, cyanosis
Meconium blocks air from entering alveoli	
Insufficient blood return from placenta before or during birth	Systemic hypotension
Poor cardiac contractility	
Bradycardia due to insufficient delivery of oxygen to heart or brainstem	
Lack of oxygen or failure to distend lungs with air may result in sustained constriction of pulmonary arterioles	Persistent pulmonary hypertension
Insufficient oxygen delivery to brain	Depressed respiratory drive
Insufficient oxygen delivery to brain and muscles	Poor muscle tone

TABLE 16-2 *Factors Associated with Increased Risk for Neonatal Resuscitation*

Antepartum Risk Factors	Intrapartum Risk Factors
• Maternal age older than 35 y or younger than 16 y • Maternal diabetes • Maternal bleeding in second or third trimester • Maternal drug therapy (e.g., magnesium, adrenergic-blocking drugs, lithium carbonate) • Maternal substance abuse (e.g., heroin, methadone) • Chronic or pregnancy-induced hypertension • Chronic maternal illness (e.g., cardiovascular, thyroid, neurologic, pulmonary, renal) • Maternal anemia or isoimmunization • Maternal infection • Polyhydramnios • Oligohydramnios • Premature rupture of membranes • Previous fetal or neonatal death • Postterm gestation • Multiple gestation • Size-dates discrepancy • No prenatal care • Diminished fetal activity • Fetal malformation	• Abruptio placentae • Placenta previa • Premature labor • Precipitous labor • Chorioamnionitis • Prolonged rupture of membranes (more than 18 h before delivery) • Prolonged labor (longer than 24 h) • Prolonged second stage of labor (longer than 2 h) • Use of general anesthesia • Emergency cesarean delivery • Forceps or vacuum-assisted delivery • Uterine tetany • Narcotics administered to mother within 4 h of delivery • Breech or other abnormal presentation • Fetal bradycardia • Nonreassuring fetal heart rate patterns • Prolapsed cord • Meconium-stained amniotic fluid

Factors Associated with Increased Risk for Neonatal Resuscitation

During the birth process, a newborn may experience some asphyxia. A variety of circumstances can exaggerate the degree of asphyxia, resulting in a depressed newborn and the need for neonatal resuscitation (see Table 16-2). Identifying patients who may require intervention at birth based on the antepartum or intrapartum history is important and facilitates having the appropriate equipment and trained personnel available at the time of delivery. However, a detailed maternal history is impractical when delivery is imminent in the field or emergency department. Answers to the questions in Table 16-3 may be helpful in preparing for the birth.

Depending on gestational age, a premature baby may not have sufficient lung development for survival (Table 16-4). Premature babies are at higher risk of needing resuscitative efforts because of the following factors:

- The lungs may lack sufficient surfactant and be more difficult to ventilate.
- The brain substance is soft, gelatinous, easily torn and has fragile capillaries that may bleed during stress.
- They are more likely to be born with an infection.
- They are predisposed to problems with temperature regulation due to their thin skin, large surface area to body mass ratio, and lack of subcutaneous fat.

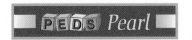

PEDS *Pearl*

Fewer than 10% of newly born infants require therapeutic measures to establish a vigorous cry or regular respirations, maintain a heart rate above 100 beats per minute, and achieve good color and tone.

TABLE 16-3 *Focused Maternal History*

Risk Factor	Question	Possible Risk	Preparation/Action
Estimate gestational age	When is your baby due?	Prematurity	Assisted ventilation Ensure availability of size-appropriate equipment
Multiple gestation	How many babies are there?	If more than one, newborns at greater risk for prematurity	Additional personnel and equipment needed
Meconium in amniotic fluid	Did your bag of waters rupture? What was the color of the water?	Respiratory distress Hypoxemia Aspiration pneumonia	Immediate suction Possible tracheal intubation
Maternal medications	Have you taken any medications or drugs?	Narcotic use within 4 hours of delivery may result in neonatal respiratory depression	Assisted ventilation
Maternal diabetes	Do you have high blood sugar or diabetes?	Neonatal hypoglycemia Congenital anomalies Large for gestational age	Assisted ventilation Vascular access
Breech position	Has your doctor told you if the baby is coming head first or feet first?	Birth trauma Prematurity Umbilical cord prolapse	Assisted ventilation Additional personnel and equipment needed
Vaginal bleeding	Have you experienced any vaginal bleeding? How long ago? Did you have any pain with the bleeding?	Maternal/placental hemorrhage—increased likelihood of hypovolemic shock and respiratory distress in neonate	Vascular access Fluid/blood administration
Fetal movement	When was the last time you felt the baby move?	Fetal distress	Assisted ventilation

TABLE 16-4 *Development and Growth of the Lung*

Stage	Period/Gestational Age	Structure Development
Intrauterine	Embryonic/conception to 7 wk	Lobar bronchi have begun development
	Pseudoglandular: 8 to 16 wk	Bronchial branching occurs; cartilage present in the trachea; lungs assume a glandular appearance; blood vessels begin to form
	Canalicular: 17 to 27 wk	Bronchioles begin to form, vascular supply develops and capillaries are brought closer to the airways
	Saccular: 28 to 35 wk	Terminal sacs form and increase in number; vascularization becomes more organized. At about 28 wk, differentiation into type I and type II alveolar epithelial cells has begun and a blood-gas barrier exists that is capable of permitting gas exchange. (Type II cells are the source of alveolar surfactant.)
	Alveolar: 36 wk to term	Continued proliferation of alveoli; actual number of alveoli at birth varies with measurements ranging from 10 million to almost 60 million.[3]
Postnatal	40 wk to 8 y	Continued proliferation of alveoli

Respirations are the first vital sign to cease when a newborn is deprived of oxygen.

In animal studies, this initial period of apnea typically lasts about 30 to 60 seconds.

Unlike adults, who develop tachycardia in response to hypoxia, the newly born responds initially with a reflex bradycardia.

PEDS *Pearl*

Because there is no definitive way to differentiate primary apnea from secondary apnea in the field or clinical setting, assume that any newborn who does not respond immediately to gentle stimulation and blow-by oxygen is experiencing secondary apnea. Provide positive-pressure ventilation with a bag-valve-mask device and high-concentration oxygen immediately.

When deprived of oxygen, a newborn's response follows a predictable pattern.

- Primary apnea
  - The newly born will initially respond to asphyxia by breathing faster in an attempt to maintain perfusion and oxygen delivery to vital organs.
  - The heart rate drops abruptly and skin color typically becomes progressively cyanotic and then blotchy because of vasoconstriction in an effort to maintain systemic blood pressure (blood pressure increases slightly).
  - If oxygen levels do not improve, respiratory efforts slow and eventually cease. This is called **primary apnea**.
  - If gently stimulated (e.g., drying, gently rubbing the back) during this period, the newborn will respond by resuming spontaneous breathing.

- Secondary apnea
  - Oxygen deprivation continues.
  - The newborn takes several gasping respirations.
  - The skin is cyanotic, bradycardia ensues, and blood pressure falls.
  - Gasping respirations become weaker and slower and then stop (**secondary apnea**).
    - During secondary apnea, the newborn will not respond to stimulation.
  - More vigorous and prolonged resuscitation is needed to reverse the process and restore adequate ventilation and circulation. Death will ensue unless resuscitation begins immediately.
  - Intervention requires bag-valve-mask ventilation with high-concentration oxygen.
  - "If gasping has already ceased, the first sign of recovery with initiation of positive-pressure ventilation is an increase in heart rate. The blood pressure then rises, rapidly if the last gasp has only just passed, but more slowly if the duration of asphyxia has been longer. The skin then becomes pink, and gasping ensues. Rhythmic spontaneous respiratory efforts become established after a further interval. For each 1 minute past the last gasp, 2 minutes of positive-pressure breathing is required before gasping begins and 4 minutes to reach rhythmic breathing. Not until some time later do the spinal and corneal reflexes return. Muscle tone gradually improves over the course of several hours." [1]

Preparation for Delivery

Table 16-5 presents a list of suggested supplies, medications, and equipment that should be readily available during delivery of a newborn. The availability of properly sized equipment is essential, particularly equipment used for airway management and ventilation, because it is most likely to be used.

Equipment

- Generally, transporting a woman in labor to the hospital is best unless delivery is expected within a few minutes
- Signs of imminent delivery
  - Consider delivering at the scene when
    - Delivery can be expected in a few minutes.
    - The patient feels the urge to push, bear down, or have a bowel movement.
    - Crowning is present (Figure 16-2).
    - Contractions are regular, lasting 45 to 60 seconds, and are 1 to 2 minutes apart.
      - Intervals are measured from the beginning of one contraction to the beginning of the next.
      - If contractions are more than 5 minutes apart, there is generally time to transport the mother to an appropriate receiving facility.
    - No suitable transportation is available.
    - The hospital cannot be reached (e.g., heavy traffic, bad weather, natural disaster).

Prehospital Predelivery Considerations

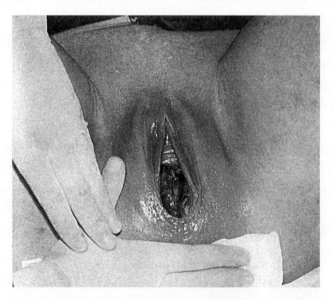

Figure 16-2   Crowning refers to the presence of a fetal body part or umbilical cord during uterine contraction.

TABLE 16-5 *Prehospital and Emergency Department Equipment List for Newborn Delivery*

Obstetrics Kit

Sterile gloves	Two or more baby blankets
Scalpel or surgical scissors	Sanitary napkins
Two hemostats or cord clamps	Identification bands for mother and neonate (hospital)
Bulb syringe	Footprint kit (optional: hospital)
Four or more clean, dry towels	
Gauze sponges	

Suction Equipment

Bulb syringe	Suction catheters in sizes 5-French or 6-French, 8-French, and 10-French or 12
Suction source and tubing	Meconium aspirator
8-French feeding tube and 20-mL syringe	

Bag–Mask Equipment

Oxygen source and tubing
Bag-valve-mask (200 to 750 mL) with pressure-release valve; must have oxygen reservoir
Anesthesia bag (hospital)
Transparent face mask with soft inflatable rim (sizes for preterm and term babies)

Tracheal Intubation Equipment

Pediatric laryngoscope handle with extra batteries	Tape or securing device for tracheal tube
Straight laryngoscope blades in sizes 0 (preterm) and 1 (term) with extra bulbs	End-tidal carbon dioxide detector (optional)
	Laryngeal mask airway (optional)
Tracheal tubes in sizes 2.5, 3.0, 3.5, and 4.0 mm	Stethoscope
Tracheal tube stylets (small)	5-French feeding tube (optional: for tracheal medications)

Intraosseous Equipment

18-gauge intraosseous needle and syringe	Normal saline

Umbilical Vessel Catheterization Equipment

Povidone-iodine solution	Three-way stopcock
Scalpel with blade	Mosquito clamp
Sterile gauze sponges, 5 cm or 10 cm square	Fine forceps without teeth
Sizes 3.5-French and 5-French umbilical catheters	Umbilical tape

Medications

Epinephrine 1:10,000	Normal saline for flushes and sterile water if dilution of bicarbonate or hypertonic glucose solutions is necessary
Sodium bicarbonate 4.2%	
Naloxone 0.4 mg/mL	
Dextrose 10%, 250 mL	Normal saline for volume expansion

Gastric Decompression Equipment

8-French gastric or feeding catheter	20-mL syringe

Additional Supplies

Personal protective equipment	Tape ($1/2$ or $3/4$ inch)
Oropharyngeal airways (0, 00, and 000 sizes)	1-, 3-, 5-, 10-, 20-, and 50-mL syringes
Cardiac monitor and electrodes (optional)	Pulse oximeter and probe (optional)
Clock	
18-, 21-, 25-gauge needles or puncture device for needleless systems	

- ◦ If there is time to transport the patient to the hospital
  - ▪ Place the patient on her left side.
  - ▪ Remove any undergarments that might obstruct delivery.
  - ▪ Transport promptly.
- If the decision is made to deliver on the scene
  - ◦ Consider the need for additional personnel and equipment (e.g., multiple birth).
  - ◦ Use personal protective equipment, including gloves, mask, eye protection, and a gown. Blood and amniotic fluid are expected and may splash.
  - ◦ Contact medical direction
    - ▪ If complications are anticipated. Medical direction may recommend expedited transport of the patient to an appropriate receiving facility.
    - ▪ If delivery does not occur within 10 minutes.
      - • Do not let the mother go to the bathroom. The mother will feel as if she needs to move her bowels. This sensation is caused by the head of the fetus in the vagina pressing against the walls of the patient's rectum.
      - • Do not hold the mother's legs together or attempt to delay or restrain delivery.

Delivery Procedure

- Use appropriate personal protective equipment (e.g., gloves, mask, gown, eye protection).
- Position the patient.
- Remove the patient's undergarments.
- The mother may be positioned in one of three ways for delivery:
  - ◦ Supine with good support for her head and a firm, stable surface under her lower body (e.g., bed) (Figure 16-3). Position the mother with her knees drawn up and spread apart. Elevate the patient's buttocks with a towel or blanket. Make sure sufficient space exists in front of the mother, at the end of the stretcher or bed, to accommodate the newborn after delivery. This position provides easy access to the infant's mouth and nares for suctioning.
  - ◦ Recumbent on her left side with her back toward you and her knees drawn up to her chest (Sims position). This position also provides easy access to the infant's mouth and nares for suctioning.
  - ◦ Supine with her buttocks at the edge of the bed or stretcher, legs apart, and her feet supported on chairs positioned at either side of

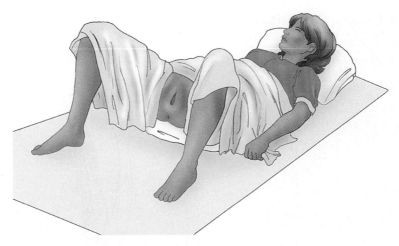

Figure 16-3 Position the mother with her knees drawn up and spread apart. Elevate the patient's buttocks with a towel or blanket. Make sure sufficient space exists in front of the mother, at the end of the stretcher or bed, to accommodate the newborn after delivery.

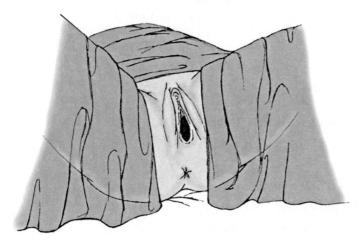

Figure 16-4 Create a sterile field around the vaginal opening using sterile towels or sterile packaged paper drapes.

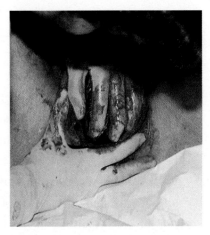

Figure 16-5 When the infant's head appears during crowning, place your gloved fingers on the bony part of the infant's skull and apply very gentle palm pressure to prevent an explosive delivery.

her body. This position provides less support for the mother, lacks a stable surface under the perineum for the newborn, and increases the risk of dropping the infant as delivery progresses.

- Organize the obstetrics kit and create a sterile field around the vaginal opening using sterile towels or sterile packaged paper drapes (Figure 16-4). Prepare oxygen and blankets for the newborn.
- Controlling the head
  - When the infant's head appears during crowning:
    - Place your gloved fingers on the bony part of the infant's skull and apply very gentle palm pressure to prevent an explosive delivery (Figure 16-5). Do not apply pressure to the infant's face or fontanelles.

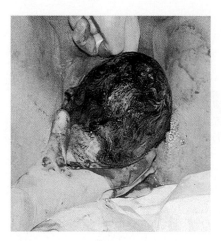

Figure 16-6   As the infant's head appears, determine if the umbilical cord is around the infant's neck.

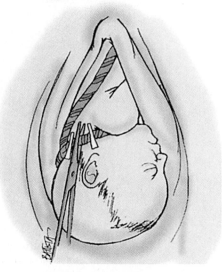

Figure 16-7   If the umbilical cord is around the baby's neck and cannot be removed, clamp the cord in two places, and carefully cut the cord between the two clamps. Remove the cord from the infant's neck.

- ○ If the amniotic sac does not break, or has not broken, use a clamp or your gloved fingers to puncture the sac and push it away from the infant's head and mouth as they appear.
- ○ As the infant's head appears, determine if the umbilical cord is around the infant's neck ("nuchal cord") (Figure 16-6).
  - ■ If the cord is around the neck, try to free it by gently pushing it over the newborn's head. If the cord cannot be removed, place two umbilical clamps on the cord, carefully cut the cord between the two clamps with sterile scissors, and remove the cord from the infant's neck (Figure 16-7).
  - ■ If the cord is *not* wrapped around the infant's neck, or if it can be freed easily, do not cut it until the infant is fully delivered.
- ○ When the infant's head is delivered, support the head with one hand and suction the mouth and then the nose with a bulb syringe (Figure 16-8).
- • After the head is delivered
  - ○ Support the baby's head as it rotates to line up with the shoulders (Figure 16-9).
  - ○ Guide the head downward to deliver the anterior (top) shoulder (Figure 16-10).
  - ○ Guide the head upward to deliver the posterior (bottom) shoulder (Figure 16-11).
  - ○ Tell the mother not to push during this time.

When meconium is observed in the amniotic fluid, deliver the head and suction meconium from the mouth and nose of the newborn as soon as the head is delivered.

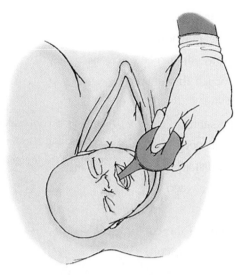

Figure 16-8 After the head is delivered, support the head and suction the baby's mouth, and then the nose, with a bulb syringe.

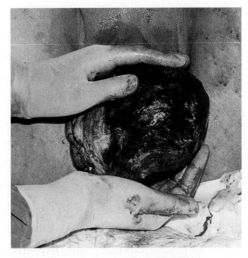

Figure 16-9 Support the baby's head as it rotates to line up with the shoulders.

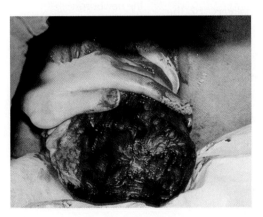

Figure 16-10 Guide the infant's head downward to deliver the anterior (top) shoulder.

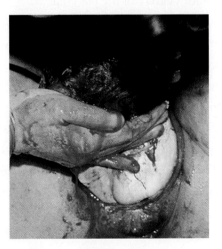

Figure 16-11 Guide the infant's head upward to deliver the posterior (bottom) shoulder.

- As the torso and full body are born, support the newborn with both hands. As the feet are born, grasp the feet.
- Wipe blood and mucus from the newborn's mouth and nose with sterile gauze. Suction the mouth and nose again with a bulb syringe as necessary.
- Dry, warm, and position the newborn (see next section Initial Steps of Resuscitation of the Newly Born).
    - It is important to position the newborn at the same level as the mother's vaginal opening until the cord has been clamped because blood can continue to flow between the newborn and the placenta.
    - If the infant is positioned above the level of the mother's vaginal opening (as when the baby is placed on the mother's abdomen or chest), blood may drain from the newborn's circulation into the placenta, decreasing the newborn's blood volume.

◦ If the infant is placed below the level of the mother's vaginal opening, blood may drain from the placenta into the newborn's circulation. This may cause the newborn to develop polycythemia, a condition characterized by an elevated hematocrit, which thickens the blood.

Polycythemia can lead to stroke.

• Clamp and cut the umbilical cord after the cord stops pulsating.

◦ Place the first clamp approximately 4 inches from the newborn's belly. Place the second clamp approximately 2 inches distally from the first. If the clamps are firmly in place, cut the cord between the two clamps with sterile scissors (Figure 16-12).

◦ Periodically check the cut ends of the cord for bleeding. If the cut end of the cord attached to the newborn is bleeding, clamp the cord proximal to the existing clamps. Do not remove the first clamp.

The umbilical cord usually stops pulsating 3 to 5 minutes after delivery of the newborn.

• Observe for delivery of the placenta.

◦ While preparing mother and newborn for transport, continue to warm and assess the newborn and watch for delivery of the placenta. (It is not necessary to wait for the placenta to deliver before transporting the mother and newborn.)

◦ Signs of placental separation include a gush of blood, lengthening of the umbilical cord, contraction of the uterus, and an urge to push.

◦ Encourage the mother to push to help deliver the placenta. Do **not** pull on the umbilical cord to deliver the placenta. Pulling can cause the uterus to invert.

The placenta is usually delivered within 20 minutes of the newborn.

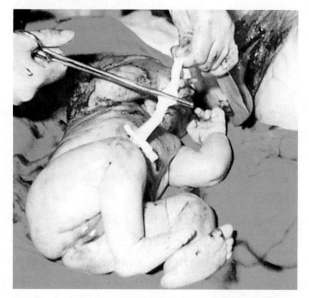

Figure 16-12 Clamp and cut the umbilical cord after the cord stops pulsating. Place the first clamp approximately 4 inches from the newborn's belly. Place the second clamp approximately 2 inches distally from the first. If the clamps are firmly in place, cut the cord between the two clamps with sterile scissors.

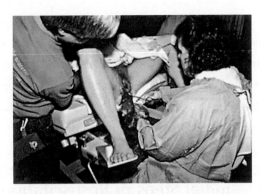

Figure 16-13 Wrap the placenta in a towel and place it in a plastic bag or an appropriate container with a lid for transportation to the hospital.

Retained pieces of placenta in the uterus will cause persistent bleeding.

- After delivery of the placenta
  - Put the newborn to the mother's breast to nurse. This stimulates the uterus to contract, thus constricting blood vessels within its walls and decreasing bleeding.
  - Wrap the placenta in a towel and put in a plastic bag or in an appropriate container with a lid (Figure 16-13). Transport the placenta to the hospital with the mother. Hospital personnel will examine the placenta for completeness.
- Examine the skin between the anus and the vagina (the perineum) for tears. Apply pressure to any bleeding tears with a sanitary napkin.
- Record the time of delivery and transport the mother, newborn, and placenta to the hospital.

Vaginal Bleeding Following Delivery

Up to 500 mL of blood loss is normal after delivery.

- If blood loss appears excessive
  - Administer oxygen to the mother by nonrebreather mask.
  - Massage the uterus.
    - With the fingers fully extended, place one hand horizontally across the abdomen, just above the symphysis pubis (pubic bone) to help prevent downward displacement of the uterus during the massage.
    - Cup the other hand around the uterus at the level of the umbilicus. Press down into the abdomen and, using a kneading motion, gently massage the uterus until it becomes firm (it should become approximately the size of a softball). Continue massaging until the uterus feels firm. This should take from 3 to 5 minutes. Bleeding should lessen as the uterus becomes firm.
  - If the newborn is stable, allowing the mother to breast-feed the infant also increases uterine muscle tone, which may decrease bleeding.
  - Reassess the patient every 5 minutes.

- If bleeding continues to appear excessive
  - Reassess your massage technique.
  - Transport immediately, continuing uterine massage en route.
  - Whatever the amount of blood loss, if the mother appears to be in shock, treat her for shock, and transport immediately. Uterine massage can be performed en route to the hospital.

Initial Steps of Resuscitation of the Newly Born

First Impression

Ask yourself five questions at the time of birth:
1. Clear of meconium?
2. Breathing or crying?
3. Good muscle tone?
4. Color pink?
5. Term gestation?

These questions can be answered by visual assessment of the newborn. If the answer to *all* of these questions is "Yes," proceed with routine newborn care (i.e., provide warmth, clear the airway, dry). If the answer to *any* question is "No," continue to the initial steps of resuscitation (see Initial Steps of Resuscitation of the Newly Born Algorithm). The inverted pyramid reflects the relative frequency with which various steps are performed in resuscitation of the newly born infant (Figure 16-14).

> **ABCs of Resuscitation of the Newly Born**
>
> - *A*irway—Position and clear
> - *B*reathing—Stimulate to breathe
> - *C*irculation—Assess heart rate and color

Provide Warmth

- Whenever possible, deliver the newborn in a warm, draft-free area.
- Methods to minimize heat loss
  - Placing the newborn under a radiant warmer (ideal)
  - Rapidly drying the skin
  - Removing wet linens immediately from the newborn
  - Wrapping the newborn in prewarmed blankets or towels, insulating film blankets, or using an infant chemical warming mattress
  - Covering the newborn's body and top of the head
  - Placing the dried newborn against the mother's chest (skin-to-skin contact)
  - Increasing room temperature

Care must be taken to maintain the newborn's body temperature.

Position and Suction

- Positioning
  - Dry the newborn quickly and place supine or on his or her side with the neck in a neutral or slightly extended (i.e., "sniffing") position.
  - The newborn has a relatively large occiput and anterior airway. Hyperextension or flexion of the neck may produce airway obstruction.

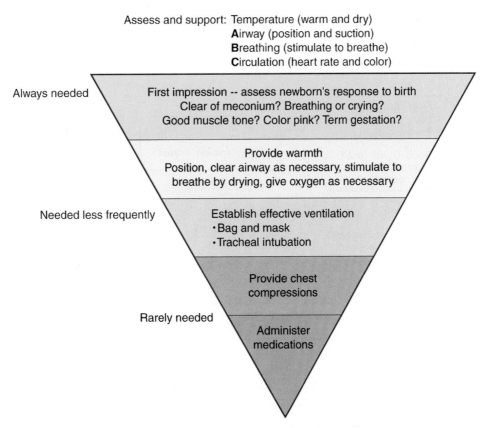

Assess and support: Temperature (warm and dry)
Airway (position and suction)
Breathing (stimulate to breathe)
Circulation (heart rate and color)

Always needed

First impression -- assess newborn's response to birth
Clear of meconium? Breathing or crying?
Good muscle tone? Color pink? Term gestation?

Provide warmth
Position, clear airway as necessary, stimulate to
breathe by drying, give oxygen as necessary

Needed less frequently

Establish effective ventilation
• Bag and mask
• Tracheal intubation

Provide chest
compressions

Rarely needed

Administer
medications

Figure 16-14 The inverted pyramid reflects the relative frequency with which various steps are performed in resuscitation of the newly born infant.

PEDS Pearl

The newly born infant is at risk for heat loss because of its relatively large surface-to-volume area, wet amniotic fluid covering, and exposure to a relatively cool environment, especially in contrast to intrauterine temperature. Furthermore, the newly born cannot generate heat by shivering and cannot retain heat because of low fat stores. Preventing heat loss in the newly born is important because cold stress can lead to increased oxygen consumption, metabolic acidosis, hypoglycemia, and apnea.

Cold stress can increase oxygen consumption and impede effective resuscitation. Increased oxygen consumption in a poorly oxygenated newborn can precipitate a change from aerobic to anaerobic metabolism. This change may lead to tissue hypoxia and acidosis because of the buildup of metabolic byproducts, such as lactate.

Hypoglycemia may develop in response to cold stress because the infant uses up glucose and glycogen reserves rapidly during anaerobic metabolism. Signs and symptoms of hypoglycemia include apnea, color changes, respiratory distress, lethargy, jitteriness, and seizures.

INITIAL STEPS OF RESUSCITATION OF THE NEWLY BORN

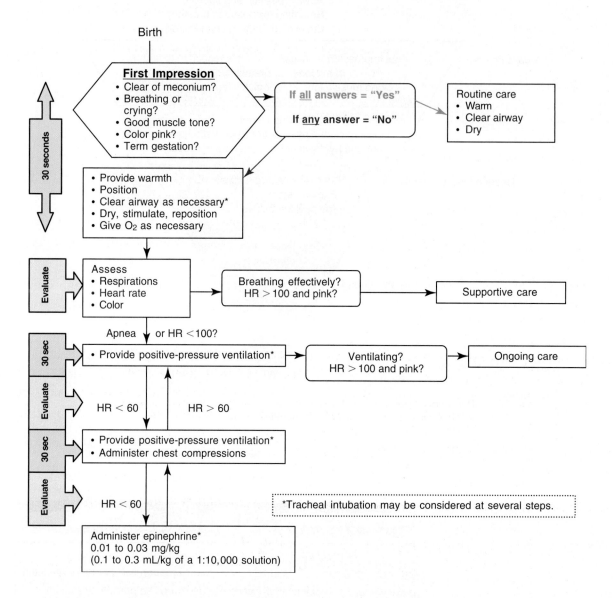

- ° Proper positioning may be facilitated by placing a rolled washcloth, blanket, or towel under the newborn's shoulders.
- ° If copious secretions are present, place the newborn on his/her side with the neck slightly extended.
- Suctioning
  - ° If the amniotic fluid is clear of meconium
    - Suction the mouth and then the nose with a bulb syringe or an 8-French or 10-French suction catheter connected to mechanical suction (negative pressure must not exceed −100 mm Hg).
      - Newborns are primarily "nose breathers." The mouth should be suctioned first to be sure there is nothing for the newborn to aspirate if he or she should gasp when the nose is suctioned.

Mouth before nose—M comes before N in the alphabet.

- When using a bulb syringe, squeeze the bulb of the syringe before inserting it into the newborn's mouth or nose. Gentle suctioning is usually adequate to remove secretions.
- Be careful how far the bulb syringe or suction catheter is inserted. Stimulation of the back of the throat can cause severe reflex bradycardia or apnea when performed within the first few minutes of delivery.
  - Meconium-stained fluid (Figure 16-15)
    - If the newborn is vigorous (strong respiratory effort, good muscle tone, heart rate above 100 beats per minute), suction the mouth and nose as for a newborn with clear fluid.
    - If the newborn is depressed (poor respiratory effort, decreased muscle tone, and/or a heart rate less than 100 beats per minute), delay drying and stimulation.
    - Examine the posterior pharynx with a laryngoscope and suction residual meconium with a 12-French or 14-French suction catheter.
    - Insert a tracheal tube into the trachea and attach the tracheal tube to suction. Apply suction as the tube is slowly withdrawn.
    - Repeat intubation and suctioning until little additional meconium is obtained or until the newborn's heart rate indicates that resuscitation must proceed immediately.
      - If the newborn's heart rate or respiration is severely depressed, it may be necessary to begin positive-pressure ventilation despite the presence of some meconium in the airway.

Do not suction for more than 3 to 5 seconds per attempt. Administer blow-by oxygen throughout the suctioning procedure.

Stimulate

- In most cases, the stimulation received during drying, warming, and suctioning is sufficient to cause the newborn to breathe effectively and may be the only resuscitative measures needed. However, if adequate respirations are not present, provide additional stimulation by rubbing the newborn's back, trunk, or extremities or tapping or flicking the

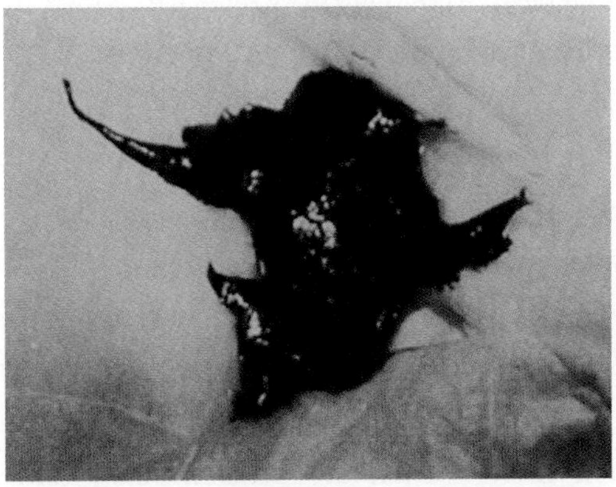

Figure 16-15 Meconium.

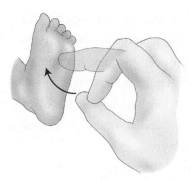

Figure 16-16 If adequate respirations are not present, provide additional stimulation by rubbing the newborn's back, trunk, or extremities or tapping or flicking the soles of the feet.

soles of the feet (Figure 16-16). These methods may be tried for 5 to 10 seconds to stimulate breathing.

- If a brief period of tactile stimulation is not effective in initiating respirations, the newborn is in secondary apnea and positive-pressure ventilation with a bag-valve-mask device is required.

Early administration of 100% oxygen is important if signs of distress (e.g., cyanosis, bradycardia) are observed in the newly born during the initial steps of stabilization. The goal of supplemental oxygen therapy is to administer sufficient oxygen to achieve pink color in the mucous membranes.

Blow-by oxygen can be delivered by means of a face mask and flow-inflating (anesthesia) bag (Figure 16-17), simple face mask held firmly (but not too tightly) to the newborn's face, or by means of a hand cupped around oxygen tubing. The oxygen source should be set to deliver at least 5 L per minute and held close to the face to maximize oxygen flow to the newborn's nose and mouth. Avoid administering unheated and unhumidified oxygen to a newborn at high flow rates (i.e., above 10 L per minute) because convective heat loss can become a problem.

Assessment of the newborn begins immediately after birth and focuses on three areas: respirations, heart rate, and color (Figure 16-18). These signs are important indicators of hypoxia. Further resuscitative efforts are required if the newborn's respiratory effort is inadequate, the heart rate is less than 100 beats per minute, or central cyanosis is present.

- Respiratory rate and effort (e.g., crying, adequate, gasping, apneic)
  - The term newborn's respiratory rate is normally between 30 and 60 breaths per minute in the first 12 hours of life.

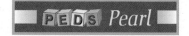

PEDS Pearl

When stimulating a newborn, avoid methods that are too vigorous because they will not help initiate respirations and may harm the newborn. Examples of methods that should not be used include the following:
- Slapping the back
- Forcing the thighs onto the abdomen
- Using hot or cold compresses
- Blowing cold oxygen onto the face or body
- Squeezing the rib cage
- Dilating the anal sphincter
- Shaking
- Putting the newborn into a hot or cold bath

Oxygen Administration

Blow-by oxygen refers to the administration of oxygen over the newborn's nose to enhance breathing of oxygen-enriched air.

PEDS Pearl

Many bag-valve-mask devices will not passively deliver sufficient oxygen flow (i.e., when not being squeezed) for effective use in blow-by oxygen administration.

Evaluate Respirations, Heart Rate, and Color

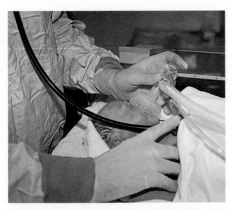

Figure 16-17 Blow-by oxygen can be delivered by means of a face mask and flow-inflating (anesthesia) bag (as shown here), simple face mask held firmly to the newborn's face, or by means of a hand cupped around oxygen tubing. The oxygen source should be set to deliver at least 5 L per minute and held close to the face to maximize oxygen flow to the newborn's nose and mouth.

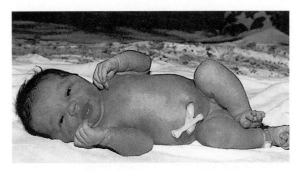

Figure 16-18 Assessment of the newborn begins immediately after birth and focuses on three areas: respiration, heart rate, and color.

In an uncompromised newborn, the heart rate should be consistently above 100 beats per minute. An increase or decrease in heart rate can provide evidence of improvement or deterioration in the newborn's condition.

Pulse oximetry is another method that may be used to monitor heart rate.

- The presence of gasping respirations or apnea requires intervention with positive-pressure ventilation.
- Heart rate
  - The term newborn's heart rate is normally 100 to 180 beats per minute in the first 12 hours of life.
  - Heart rate may be evaluated by the following:
    - Listening to the apical beat with a stethoscope
    - Feeling the pulse by lightly grasping the base of the umbilical cord
      - Palpation of the umbilical pulse allows assessment of heart rate without interruption of ventilation for auscultation
      - If pulsations cannot be felt at the base of the cord, auscultate the apical pulse.
  - In general, a spontaneously breathing newborn with effective respirations, pink color, and a heart rate over 100 beats per minute will require no further intervention.
  - If the heart rate is less than 100 beats per minute, begin positive-pressure ventilation. A heart rate below 60 beats per minute indicates that additional resuscitative measures are needed.

If cardiopulmonary compromise is not present, most newborns will be able to maintain a pink color without supplemental oxygen. If central cyanosis is present, administration of 100% oxygen is indicated.

- Color
  - Assess for central cyanosis, which is best evaluated in the face, trunk, and mucous membranes.
  - Acrocyanosis (cyanosis of the extremities) is a common finding

immediately after delivery and is not a reliable indicator of hypoxemia.

- Acrocyanosis may be an indicator of cold stress.
- Pallor may indicate decreased cardiac output, severe anemia, hypothermia, acidosis, or hypovolemia.
- Give blow-by oxygen if the newborn has spontaneous respirations and an adequate heart rate, but central cyanosis is present.

Apgar Scoring System

An Apgar scoring system is a numeric method of rating five specific signs pertaining to the newborn's condition after birth. Each sign is assigned a value of 0, 1, or 2 and added for a total Apgar score (Table 16-6). In general, the higher the score, the better the condition of the newborn.

Although the Apgar score is an important tool used in the assessment of a newborn, it is not recorded until 1 and 5 minutes after birth. If resuscitation of the newborn is needed, waiting until the first Apgar score (which reflects the need for immediate resuscitation) is obtained could be disastrous. The decision to begin resuscitative efforts and the newborn's response to resuscitation can be more accurately determined by evaluating the newborn's respiratory effort, heart rate, and color.

- Components of the Apgar scoring system:
  - **A**ppearance (color)
  - **P**ulse (heart rate)
  - **G**rimace (irritability)
  - **A**ctivity (muscle tone)
  - **R**espirations
- Apgar scores:
  - Seven to 10 indicates a newborn in mild distress or one with no distress; no assistance needed other than nasopharyngeal suctioning.
  - Four to 6 indicates a newborn in moderate distress (i.e., depressed respirations, flaccidity, and pallor or cyanosis).

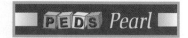

Count the heart rate for 6 seconds and multiply by 10 to estimate the beats per minute. Because the rate is rapid, it may be helpful to tap out the newborn's heart rate as you count it. This technique also enables an assistant to help listen for changes in the rate.

Do not delay resuscitative efforts to obtain an Apgar score.

TABLE 16-6 *The Apgar Scoring System*

	0	1	2
Appearance	Blue, pale	Body pink Extremities blue	Completely pink
Pulse	Absent	Less than 100	100 or more
Grimace/reflex irritability	No response	Grimaces, cries	Cough, sneeze, vigorous cry
Activity/muscle tone	Limp, flaccid	Some flexion of extremities	Active motion
Respiratory effort	Absent	Slow, irregular	Good, crying

◦ Zero to 3 indicates a newborn in severe distress; immediate resuscitation is necessary.

Ventilation

Most newborns requiring ventilatory support can be effectively ventilated with a bag and mask. If bag-valve-mask ventilation is required for more than 2 minutes, consider placement of an orogastric tube to prevent respiratory compromise from gastric distention.

- Indications for positive-pressure ventilation
  - ◦ Apnea or gasping respirations
  - ◦ Heart rate less than 100 beats per minute
  - ◦ Persistent central cyanosis despite administration of 100% oxygen
- Face mask and resuscitation bag size
  - ◦ Select a properly sized face mask.
    - ▪ Face masks are available in a variety of sizes and shapes. The preferred mask is equipped with a cushioned rim and is anatomically shaped. This type of mask offers several advantages:
      - • Low dead space (less than 5 mL)
      - • Less pressure required to maintain a tight seal than with a round or noncushioned mask
      - • Less chance of injury to the newborn's eyes if the mask is improperly positioned
    - ▪ A properly sized mask avoids the eyes, and covers the nose, mouth, and tip of the chin. Masks fitting preterm, term, and large newborns should be available.
      - • A mask that is too large will not seal well and may damage the newborn's eyes.
      - • A mask that is too small will not cover the mouth and nose (and may occlude the nose).
  - ◦ For a term newborn, select a resuscitation bag with a minimum volume of 450 to 500 mL and a maximum volume of 750 mL.
    - ▪ A term newborn requires approximately 15 to 25 mL with each ventilation (5 to 8 mL/kg). A preterm baby requires even less volume—some require as little as 5 to 10 mL per ventilation. Using a 750-mL volume (or larger) bag makes it difficult to provide such small tidal volumes and increases the risk of complications (e.g., hyperinflation).
    - ▪ If the bag-valve-mask has a pop-off valve, it should release at approximately 30 to 35 cm H_2O pressure and should have an override feature to permit delivery of higher pressures if necessary to achieve good chest expansion.
    - ▪ To open the alveoli in the newly born, pressures of 30 to 40 cm H_2O may be needed during the first few ventilations. This may

necessitate temporary disabling of the pop-off valve. After the first few breaths, pressure requirements typically drop to 20 to 30 cm H_2O.

- Assisting ventilation
  - One hundred percent oxygen is recommended for assisted ventilation; however, if supplemental oxygen is unavailable, positive-pressure ventilation should be initiated with room air.
  - Ventilate the newborn at a rate of 40 to 60 breaths per minute (i.e., slightly less than 1 breath per second). (The rate is 30 breaths per minute when chest compressions are also being delivered.)
  - The first breaths delivered to an apneic newborn may need to be longer (1 to 2 seconds) and use higher inspiratory pressures than subsequent breaths.
- Signs of adequate ventilation
  - Gentle chest rise
  - Presence of bilateral breath sounds
  - Improvement in color and heart rate
- A poor response to ventilation efforts may be the result of the following:
  - A poor seal between the newborn's face and the mask. Corrective action: Reapply the mask to the face. Check the seal when you reapply the mask, particularly between the cheek and the bridge of the nose.
  - Poor alignment of the head and neck. Corrective action: Reposition the head.
  - Insufficient ventilation pressure. Corrective action: Increased inflation pressure may be required. If adequate chest rise is still not achieved, tracheal intubation may be required.
  - Improper tracheal tube position (if intubated). Corrective action: Reassess tube placement; remove if the tube is improperly positioned or position is uncertain.
  - Blocked airway. Corrective action: Reposition the head, suction as needed, ventilate with the mouth slightly open.
  - Gastric distention. Corrective action: Insert an 8-French or 10-French orogastric tube and leave the end open to air. Periodically aspirate the tube with a syringe.
- Once adequate ventilation with 100% oxygen has been established for 30 seconds, reassess the newborn's heart rate, color, and respirations.
  - If the newborn is spontaneously breathing and the heart rate is greater than 100 beats per minute, positive-pressure ventilation may be gradually discontinued.
    - Observe the newborn for signs of adequate spontaneous breathing before ceasing ventilation.

Breathe, two, three = Squeeze, release, release.

- Gentle tactile stimulation may help maintain spontaneous breathing.
- If spontaneous breathing is adequate, administer blow-by oxygen.
  ○ If spontaneous breathing is inadequate, continue assisted ventilation.
  ○ If the newborn is unresponsive to positive-pressure ventilation and the heart rate is less than 60 beats per minute, continue positive-pressure ventilation and begin chest compressions. Consider tracheal intubation.

Chest Compressions

- Indications
  ○ Chest compressions are indicated if the newborn's heart rate is less than 60 beats per minute despite adequate ventilation with 100% oxygen for 30 seconds.
  ○ Because chest compressions may diminish the effectiveness of ventilation, they should not be initiated until ventilation has been established.
- Compression technique
  ○ Two compression techniques can be used, both of which should be delivered on the lower third of the sternum.
  ○ Thumb technique (preferred)
    - The thumbs are placed on the sternum side by side just below the nipple line unless the infant is small (or the rescuer's hands are extremely large), in which case the thumbs may be placed one over the other (Figure 16–19). The fingers encircle the chest and support the back.
    - This technique may be used in newly born infants and older infants whose size permits its use.
    - Studies suggest that this technique may offer some advantages in generating peak systolic and coronary perfusion pressure. Some healthcare providers prefer this technique to the two-finger method because it is less tiring and permits better control of the depth of compressions.
  ○ Two-finger method
    - The ring and middle fingers of one hand are placed on the sternum just below the nipple line (Figure 16-20). The other hand should support the infant's back.

Compression to ventilation ratio is 3:1.

    - Compression-ventilation ratio
      - Compressions and ventilations are coordinated to avoid simultaneous delivery. Deliver compressions smoothly, compressing approximately one third the depth of the chest or to a depth adequate to produce a palpable pulse.

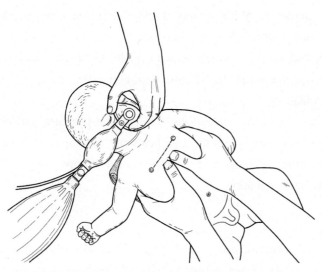

Figure 16-19 Newborn cardiopulmonary resuscitation using the thumb technique. The thumbs are placed on the sternum side by side just below the nipple line unless the infant is small (or the rescuer's hands are extremely large), in which case the thumbs may be placed one over the other. The fingers encircle the chest and support the back.

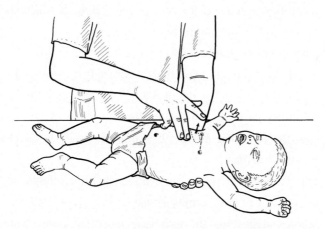

Figure 16-20 Two-finger method of cardiopulmonary resuscitation. The ring and middle fingers of one hand are placed on the sternum just below the nipple line. The other hand should support the baby's back.

- The compression to ventilation ratio is 3:1. Three chest compressions should be followed by a brief pause to deliver one ventilation. It is helpful for the compressor to count aloud, "One-and-two-and-three-and-bag-and..."
- Provide one complete cycle (three compressions and one ventilation) every 2 seconds. This results in 90 compressions and 30 breaths (approximately 120 events) per minute.
- After 30 seconds of chest compressions with assisted ventilation, reassess the newborn's heart rate.

Reassess the heart rate every 30 seconds.

- Discontinue chest compressions when the heart rate reaches 60 beats per minute or more.
- If the heart rate remains slower than 60 beats per minute, continue compressions and administer epinephrine via the intravenous (IV), intraosseous (IO), umbilical, or tracheal route.

Tracheal Intubation

Intubation attempts should be limited to 20 seconds to minimize the risk of hypoxia.

- Tracheal intubation may be indicated at several points during neonatal resuscitation:
  - When tracheal suctioning for meconium is required
  - If bag-mask ventilation is ineffective (i.e., inadequate chest expansion, persistent low heart rate) or prolonged
  - When chest compressions are performed
  - When tracheal administration of medications is desired
  - Special resuscitation circumstances (e.g., congenital diaphragmatic hernia or extremely low birth weight)
- Blade size
  - A straight blade should be used for tracheal intubation of the newborn.
  - Use size 0 for a preterm infant and size 1 for a term newborn.
- Tracheal tube size (Table 16-7)
- Vocal cord guide

Changes in the newborn's head position will alter the depth of insertion and may predispose to unintentional extubation or right mainstem bronchus intubation.

  - Most tracheal tubes intended for newborn use have a vocal cord line (a black line) near the distal tip of the tracheal tube. The tip of the tracheal tube should be inserted until the vocal cord guide is at the level of the cords. In this position, the tip of the tube should be between the vocal cords and carina.
  - After placement of the tube, note the centimeter marking on the tube at the newborn's upper lip. The tube should be located 7 cm at the lip for a 1000-g infant, 8 cm for a 2000-g infant, and 9 cm for a

TABLE 16-7 *Estimation of Laryngoscope Blade and Tracheal Tube Size Based on Infant Gestational Age and Weight*

Weight (g)	Gestational Age (wk)	Laryngoscope Blade Size	Laryngoscope Blade Type	Tracheal Tube Size (mm)	Depth of Tracheal Tube Insertion from Upper Lip (cm)
Less than 1000	Less than 28	0	Straight	2.5	6.5 to 7.0
1000 to 2000	28 to 34	0	Straight	2.5 to 3.0	7.0 to 8.0
2000 to 3000	34 to 38	0 to 1	Straight	3.0 to 3.5	8.0 to 9.0
More than 3000	More than 38	1	Straight	3.5 to 4.0	More than 9.0

3000-g infant. After proper tube position is confirmed, document and maintain this depth of insertion.

- A guide to determining proper distance for insertion of the tracheal tube is the "tip to lip" measurement: 6 cm + weight in kilograms = distance (in centimeters) from tracheal tube tip to infant's lips.

- Confirm the position of the tube
  - Watch for symmetric rise and fall of the chest.
  - Listen high in the axillae for equal breath sounds and for an absence of sounds over the stomach.
  - Confirm absence of gastric distention with ventilation.
  - Note improvement in color, heart rate, and activity of the newborn.
  - Detection of exhaled carbon dioxide
    - These devices are most useful if there is a perfusing rhythm and the newborn weighs more than 2 kg.
    - There is higher incidence of false-negative results with exhaled carbon dioxide detectors in extremely low–birthweight newborns or asphyxiated newborns who are failing to respond to resuscitative efforts.
  - Chest radiograph.

- Acute deterioration (bradycardia, decreased oxygen saturation) after intubation suggests one of the following problems (DOPE):
  - *Dislodgement:* The tube is no longer in the trachea (right mainstem bronchus or esophagus).
  - *Obstruction:* Secretions are obstructing airflow through the tube. Suspect obstruction of the tube when there is resistance to bagging and no chest wall movement.
  - *Pneumothorax*
  - *Equipment:* Oxygen is not being delivered to the patient (check equipment).

PEDS Pearl

Possible causes for a newborn's failure to respond to intubation and ventilation include mechanical difficulties, profound asphyxia with myocardial depression, or an inadequate circulating blood volume. If the patient acutely deteriorates after intubation, quickly check the equipment. If no explanation is obvious, remove the tracheal tube and ventilate the patient with a bag-valve-mask. If the patient is bradycardic, do not waste time adjusting or suctioning the endotracheal tube.

PEDS Pearl

The laryngeal mask airway (LMA) has been shown to be effective for ventilating newly born full-term infants. The LMA, when used by appropriately trained providers, may be an effective alternative for establishing an airway in resuscitation of the newly born infant, especially in the case of ineffective bag-mask ventilation or failed endotracheal intubation (class indeterminate). However, the reviewers for the 2000 Neonatal Resuscitation Guidelines "do not recommend routine use of the LMA at this time and the device cannot replace endotracheal intubation for meconium suctioning."[2]

Medications and Fluids

The Broselow tape has a section for newborns that can be used to determine equipment size and medication dosages for newborn resuscitation.

The 1-mL dilutional volume for tracheal epinephrine reflects the small size of the newborn.

If timely assessment and rapid response to a newborn with cardiopulmonary compromise are initiated, medications are rarely indicated for resuscitation. Bradycardia in the newborn is usually secondary to inadequate lung inflation and hypoxia, so ensuring adequate ventilation is the most important step in correcting a low heart rate. Medications should be administered if the heart rate remains less than 60 beats per minute despite adequate ventilation with 100% oxygen and chest compressions.

Routes of Medication Administration

- Tracheal
  - The tracheal route is frequently the most rapidly accessible route for medication administration during newborn resuscitation and may be used for administration of epinephrine and naloxone, but should not be used for administration of sodium bicarbonate.
    - Administration of epinephrine via the tracheal route may result in a more variable response than the IV route
  - Medications given via the tracheal route may be placed directly into the tracheal tube or given through a 5-French feeding tube inserted in the tracheal tube.
    - Medications may be given undiluted and followed with a 0.5- to 1-mL saline flush or may be diluted to a total volume of 1 mL in normal saline before administration.
    - After administration, provide several positive-pressure ventilations to distribute the medication throughout the tracheobronchial tree.

Umbilical vein catheterization may be attempted by those specially trained in this technique, usually after attempts at IV and IO access prove unsuccessful.

- Umbilical vein
  - Although rarely used as a means of vascular access outside the delivery room, cannulation of the umbilical vein is the preferred means of vascular access during resuscitation of the newly born because it is easily located and easily cannulated.
  - Anatomy
    - Two arteries and one vein readily identified in the umbilical cord stump.
    - The vein is a thin-walled vessel. The arteries are thicker-walled, paired, and often constricted.
  - Cannulation
    - A 3.5-French or 5-French umbilical catheter is attached to a three-way stopcock flushed with heparinized saline.
    - The catheter is inserted into the umbilical vein until the tip of the catheter is just below the skin and there is a good blood return (Figure 16-21).
  - Complications
    - Infection.

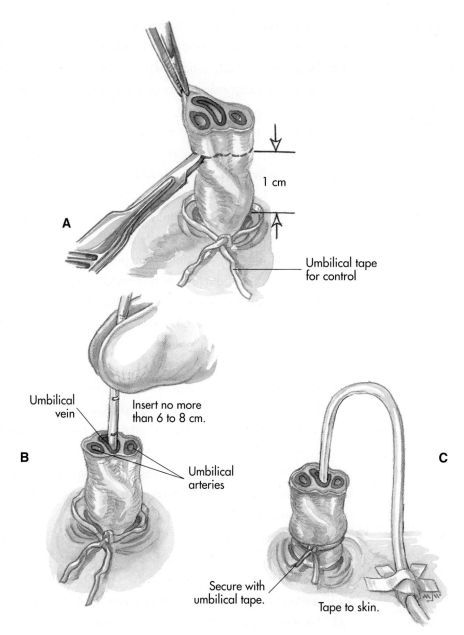

Figure 16-21 Cannulation of the umbilical vein. A, Identify the umbilical vein after trimming the cord. **B,** Insert the umbilical catheter into the vein. **C,** Secure the base of the cord to hold the catheter in place and stabilize the catheter with tape.

- A fatal air embolus can result if air enters the umbilical venous catheter.
- Advancing the catheter too far into the umbilical vein may cause infusion of medications directly into the liver with the potential for hepatic damage.
- Peripheral vascular access
  - Veins of the scalp and extremities are acceptable routes for administration of fluids and medications but are difficult to access during resuscitation.

- If you cannot establish peripheral IV access, attempt IO access. Insert an 18-gauge needle in the medial aspect of the tibia, just below the tibial tuberosity. Keep in mind that the newborn's bones are small and fragile and the IO space is small in a preterm infant.

Volume Expanders

Suspect hypovolemia in any infant who fails to respond to resuscitation.

- Indications
  - Volume expanders are indicated when acute bleeding is evident with signs of hypovolemia
    - Pallor that persists despite oxygenation
    - Weak pulses with a heart rate above 100 beats per minute
    - Poor response to resuscitative efforts, including effective ventilation
- Fluid choice
  - Fluid of choice for volume expansion is an isotonic crystalloid solution (e.g., normal saline or Ringer's lactate).
  - O-negative red blood cells may be indicated for replacement of large-volume blood loss.
- Dosage
  - Initial volume expander dosage is 10 mL/kg given slow IV push over 5 to 10 minutes.
  - Boluses may be repeated several times, guided by patient assessment.

Caution.

  - Care must be taken to minimize the use of rapid boluses of volume expanders or hyperosmolar solutions (e.g., sodium bicarbonate), when administering medications to a preterm newborn because portions of the brain are particularly vulnerable to bleeding when subjected to rapid changes in vascular pressure and osmolarity.

Medications

Table 16-8 lists medications that may be used during newborn resuscitation. Table 16-9 lists other medications that may be administered to newborns.

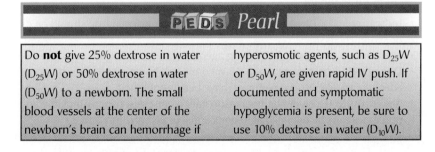

PEDS *Pearl*

Do **not** give 25% dextrose in water ($D_{25}W$) or 50% dextrose in water ($D_{50}W$) to a newborn. The small blood vessels at the center of the newborn's brain can hemorrhage if hyperosmotic agents, such as $D_{25}W$ or $D_{50}W$, are given rapid IV push. If documented and symptomatic hypoglycemia is present, be sure to use 10% dextrose in water ($D_{10}W$).

TABLE 16-8 *Medications Used in Neonatal Resuscitation*

Epinephrine

- **Indications**: Asystole or when the heart rate remains below 60 beats per minute after a minimum of 30 sec of adequate ventilation and chest compressions
- **Mechanism of action**: Has both α- and β-adrenergic stimulating properties. In cardiac arrest, α-adrenergic–mediated vasoconstriction may be the more important action. Vasoconstriction elevates the perfusion pressure during chest compressions, enhancing delivery of oxygen to the heart and brain. Epinephrine also enhances myocardial contractility, stimulates spontaneous contractions, and increases heart rate.
- **Dosage**: IV/IO/ET: 0.01 to 0.03 mg/kg (0.1 to 0.3 mL/kg of a 1:10,000 solution), repeated every 3 to 5 min as indicated.
- **Notes**: Available data regarding effects of high-dose epinephrine for resuscitation of newly born infants are inadequate to support routine use of higher doses of epinephrine.

Naloxone

- **Indications**: Reversal of respiratory depression in a newly born infant whose mother received narcotics within 4 h of delivery
- **Mechanism of action**: Competes with opioid receptor sites in the central nervous system, displacing previously administered narcotic analgesics.
- **Dosage**: IV/IO/IM/SubQ: 0.1 mg/kg of a 0.4-mg/mL or 1.0-mg/mL solution
- **Notes**: Establish and maintain adequate ventilation before administration. Avoid if mother is suspected of having recently abused narcotics. Administration of naloxone to these newborns may precipitate abrupt withdrawal signs. Repeated doses of naloxone may be necessary to prevent recurrent apnea because the duration of action of narcotics may exceed that of naloxone. Endotracheal naloxone is not recommended; preferred routes are IV and IM.

ET, endotracheal; IM, intramuscular; IO, intraosseous; IV, intravenous; SubQ, subcutaneous.

TABLE 16-9 *Other Medications*

Glucose

- **Indications**: Documented and symptomatic hypoglycemia
- **Mechanism of action**: Rapidly increases serum glucose concentration; reverses CNS effects of hypoglycemia.
- **Dosage**: IV/IO: 200 mg/kg (2 mL/kg of a D10W solution) slow IV push.
- **Notes**: Hypoglycemia = glucose level less than 40 mg/dL if less than 2.5 kg, or less than 30 mg/dL if less than 2.5 kg. Higher concentrations of glucose (e.g., D25W) are hyperosmolar and should be avoided. Repeated glucose measurement should be obtained 10 to 20 min after glucose administration.

Sodium Bicarbonate

- **Indications**: Persistent metabolic acidosis or hyperkalemia (use should be directed by arterial blood gas results or serum chemistries)
- **Mechanism of action**: Alkalinizing agent.
- **Dosage**: IV: 1 to 2 mEq/kg of a 0.5-mEq/mL solution may be given by slow IV push (over at least 2 min) after adequate ventilation and perfusion have been established.
- **Notes**: Do NOT use during brief resuscitation episodes; hyperosmolarity and carbon dioxide–generating properties may be detrimental to myocardial or cerebral function.

CNS, central nervous system; $D_{10}W$, 10% dextrose in water; $D_{25}W$, 25% dextrose in water; IO, intraosseous; IV, intravenous.

Postresuscitation Care

Continued monitoring, supportive care, and appropriate diagnostic evaluation are indicated in any newly born infant requiring stabilization and resuscitation. Postresuscitation monitoring should include the following:

- Monitoring of heart rate, respiratory rate, blood pressure, temperature, administered oxygen concentration and arterial oxygen saturation, with blood gas analysis as indicated.
- Determination of blood sugar level and treatment of hypoglycemia.
- Consider ongoing blood glucose screening and documentation of calcium.
- Obtaining a chest radiograph to evaluate lung expansion, assess placement of tubes and catheters, identify possible underlying causes of the arrest, or detect complications, such as pneumothorax.
- Treatment of hypotension with volume expanders, vasopressors, or both.
- Treatment of possible infection or seizures.
- Initiation of vascular access and appropriate fluid therapy.
- Documentation of observations and actions.
- Transport of the infant to the most appropriate unit (newborn nursery, level II nursery, or neonatal intensive care unit) for further care. A transport team with personnel skilled in neonatal resuscitation should be used.

Case Study Resolution

Ask yourself the following five questions at the time of birth:

1. Clear of meconium?
2. Breathing or crying?
3. Good muscle tone?
4. Color pink?
5. Term gestation?

These questions can be answered by visual assessment of the newborn. If the answer to *all* of these questions is "Yes," proceed with routine newborn care (i.e., provide warmth, clear the airway, dry). If the answer to *any* question is "No," begin the initial steps of resuscitation.

References

1. Rosenberg AA. The neonate. In: Gabbe SG, Niebyl JR, Simpson JL, eds. *Obstetrics: normal and problem pregnancies,* 4th ed. New York: Churchill Livingstone, 2002:653–692.
2. Contributors and Reviewers for the Neonatal Resuscitation Guidelines. International Guidelines for Neonatal Resuscitation: an excerpt from the Guidelines 2000 for Cardiopulmonary Resuscitation and Emergency Cardiovascular Care: International Consensus on Science. *Pediatrics* 2000;106:e29.
3. Langston C, Kida K, Reed M, et al. Human lung growth in late gestation and in the neonate. *Am Rev Respir Dis* 1984;129:607-613.

Chapter Quiz

1. Which of the following signs are associated with secondary apnea?
    A) Pink skin, increasing heart rate, normal blood pressure.
    B) Cyanotic skin, falling heart rate, falling blood pressure.
    C) Pink skin, falling heart rate, falling blood pressure.
    D) Cyanotic skin, increasing heart rate, normal blood pressure.

2. Which of the following signs are the **MOST** important when determining if additional resuscitative efforts are needed in the newly born?
    A) Heart rate, muscle tone, and color.
    B) Absence of meconium, muscle tone, and color.
    C) Heart rate, respiratory effort, and color.
    D) Respiratory effort, absence of meconium, and muscle tone.

3. The heart rate of the newly born should be assessed by palpating:
    A) The carotid pulse.
    B) The femoral pulse.
    C) The umbilical pulse.
    D) The brachial pulse.

4. When delivering positive-pressure ventilations with a bag-valve mask device to a newborn, the assisted ventilation rate should be _____ breaths/minute and _____ breaths/minute when chest compressions are also being delivered.
    A) 10 to 20; 30
    B) 20 to 40; 20
    C) 30 to 40; 40
    D) 40 to 60; 30

5. What is the initial recommended dosage of naloxone for the newly born infant?
   A) 10 mL/kg
   B) 1.0 mEq/kg
   C) 0.1 mg/kg
   D) 0.01 mg/kg

6. Assessment of a newly born infant one minute after delivery reveals the infant is crying vigorously on light tapping of the foot. Her heart rate is 130 beats/minute and some flexion of the extremities is noted. Respirations are regular at approximately 40 breaths/minute. The body is pink and the extremities are blue. You would assign an Apgar score of:
   A) 7
   B) 8
   C) 9
   D) 10

7. Volume expansion with normal saline or lactated Ringer's solution should begin with an initial bolus of _____ in a newborn and _____ in an infant or child.
   A) 10 mL/kg; 20 mL/kg
   B) 20 mL/kg; 30 mL/kg
   C) 10 mL/kg; 10 mL/kg
   D) 20 mL/kg; 40 mL/kg

8. When delivering blow-by oxygen during resuscitation of the newly born, the oxygen flow rate should be at least _____ L/min.
   A) 3
   B) 5
   C) 10
   D) 15

9. True or False: Neonates often demonstrate tachycardia in response to hypoxemia; older children will initially demonstrate bradycardia.

10. Acceptable methods of stimulating the newly born include:
    A) Squeezing the rib cage.
    B) Dilating the anal sphincter.
    C) Rubbing the back.
    D) Shaking the infant.

Chapter Quiz Answers

1. B. In secondary apnea, oxygen deprivation persists. The newborn takes several gasping respirations. The skin is cyanotic, bradycardia ensues, and blood pressure falls. Gasping respirations become weaker and then stop (secondary apnea).

2. C. Heart rate, respiratory effort, and color are the most important assessment parameters during resuscitation of the newly born.

3. C. Because central and peripheral pulses in the neck and extremities are often difficult to feel in newborns, heart rate should be assessed either by auscultating the apical pulse with a stethoscope or by palpating the base of the umbilical cord. The umbilical pulse is readily accessible in the newly born and permits assessment of heart rate without interruption of ventilation for auscultation.

4. D. The assisted ventilation rate should be 40 to 60 breaths per minute and 30 breaths per minute when chest compressions are also being delivered.

5. C. The recommended initial dosage of naloxone for the newly born is 0.1 mg/kg IV/IO/ET or, if perfusion is adequate, IM or SC.

6. B. An Apgar score of 8 is assigned based on the following: Some flexion of the extremities (1 point), regular respirations (2 points), blue extremities/pink body (1 point), heart rate > 100 (2 points), and vigorous crying on stimulation (2 points).

7. A. Volume expansion with normal saline or lactated Ringer's solution should begin with an initial bolus of 10 mL/kg in a newborn and 20 mL/kg in an infant or child.

8. B. When delivering blow-by oxygen during resuscitation of the newly born, the oxygen flow rate should be at least 5 L/min.

9. False. Neonates often demonstrate bradycardia in response to hypoxemia; older children may initially demonstrate tachycardia.

10. C. If adequate respirations are not present, stimulate the newly born infant by rubbing the infant's back, trunk, or extremities or tapping the soles of the feet. These methods may be tried for 5 to 10 seconds to stimulate breathing. Avoid methods that are too vigorous because they will not help initiate respirations and may harm the newborn. Examples of methods that should not be used include slapping the back, squeezing the rib cage, forcing the thighs onto the abdomen, dilating the anal sphincter, using hot or cold compresses, shaking, blowing cold oxygen onto the newborn's face or body, and putting the newborn into a hot or cold bath.

Posttest

Questions

1. A 6-year-old child has been intubated and a colorimetric $ETCO_2$ detector is being used as a secondary method of confirming proper placement of the tracheal tube. A pulse is present. Select the INCORRECT statement regarding the use of colorimetric capnography.
   A) Disposable colorimetric devices provide CO_2 readings by chemical reaction on pH-sensitive litmus paper housed in the detector.
   B) If a normal amount of CO_2 is detected, the color will change noticeably from its original color (i.e., confirms tracheal placement of the tube).
   C) The paper in the devices is unaffected by exposure to secretions, medications, or the environment.
   D) A small amount of CO_2 may be detected if the tube is in the correct position but the patient is not ventilating or perfusing adequately.

2. Which of the following is the most useful for removing thick secretions and particulate matter from the pharynx?
   A) Oropharyngeal airway.
   B) Rigid plastic suction catheter.
   C) Flexible plastic suction catheter.
   D) Nonrebreather mask.

3. Under optimum conditions, blow-by oxygen administered by means of a face mask can deliver an oxygen concentration of _____ at a flow rate of 10 L/min.
   A) 25 to 45%
   B) 35 to 40%
   C) 50 to 60%
   D) 60 to 95%

4. The initial energy dose for synchronized cardioversion for an infant or child is:
   A) 0.2 to 0.4 J/kg
   B) 0.5 to 1 J/kg
   C) 2 to 4 J/kg
   D) 5 to 10 J/kg

5. In which of the following situations would chest compressions be indicated?
   A) A 3-year-old with a pulse rate of 100.
   B) An apneic 18-month-old with a pulse rate of 50.
   C) An apneic 4-year-old with a pulse rate of 84.
   D) An 11-year-old with a pulse rate of 78.

6. When performing chest compressions on an infant, compress the chest approximately
   _____ at a rate of _____ times per minute.
   A) $1/3$ to $1/2$ the depth of the chest, about 100.
   B) 1 to $1^1/2$ inches, about 100.
   C) $1/3$ to $1/2$ the depth of the chest, at least 120.
   D) 2 to $2^1/2$ inches, about 120.

7. After opening the airway of an unresponsive infant, how many breaths should be delivered after determining she is not breathing?
   A) 1
   B) 2
   C) 3
   D) 4

8. A bradycardia that causes severe cardiopulmonary compromise in an infant or child is initially treated with:
   A) Effective oxygenation and ventilation.
   B) Transcutaneous pacing.
   C) Synchronized cardioversion.
   D) Administration of atropine.

9. Synchronized cardioversion:
   A) Is used in the treatment of pulseless ventricular tachycardia.
   B) Delivers a shock between the peak and end of the T wave.
   C) Is timed to avoid the vulnerable period of the cardiac cycle.
   D) Is used only for rhythms with a ventricular response of less than 100 beats/min.

10. A child has a 3.0 mm tracheostomy tube in place. What size catheter should be used to suction the tracheostomy tube?
    A) 3-French
    B) 4-French
    C) 6-French
    D) 8-French

11. A patient with a malfunctioning VP shunt may present with irritability, headache, neck pain, vomiting, a bulging or full fontanelle in infants, new seizures or a change in the child's seizure pattern, behavioral changes, or "just not acting right." These signs are most suggestive of:

    A) Congenital heart disease.

    B) Chronic pulmonary disease.

    C) Increased intracranial pressure.

    D) Congenital neuromuscular disease.

12. Activated charcoal may be used in the management of an ingestion involving:

    A) Hydrochloric acid.

    B) Bleach.

    C) Acetaminophen.

    D) Kerosene.

13. The pediatric age group at greatest risk for unintentional poisoning is:

    A) Less than 2 years of age.

    B) More than 12 years of age.

    C) Less than 6 years of age.

    D) More than 8 years of age.

14. The most common type of shock in the pediatric patient is:

    A) Septic.

    B) Hypovolemic.

    C) Cardiogenic.

    D) Anaphylactic.

15. What is meant by the term pulseless electrical activity (PEA)?

    A) PEA refers to a flat line on the cardiac monitor.

    B) PEA refers to a chaotic dysrhythmia that is likely to degenerate into cardiac arrest.

    C) PEA refers to an organized rhythm on the cardiac monitor, though a pulse is not present.

    D) PEA refers to a slow, wide–QRS ventricular rhythm.

16. A 44-pound child presents with fever, irritability, mottled color, cool extremities, and a prolonged capillary refill time. The appropriate initial fluid bolus for administration to this child is:

    A) 100 mL of normal saline over 30 to 60 minutes.

    B) 200 mL of 5% dextrose in water in less than 20 minutes.

    C) 800 mL of normal saline or Ringer's lactate infused over 30 to 60 minutes.

    D) 400 mL of normal saline or Ringer's lactate in less than 20 minutes.

17. Assessment of a newly born infant reveals central and peripheral cyanosis. The infant's heart rate is 140 beats/min. He has shallow, spontaneous respirations at a rate of 40/min. Your best course of action will be to:
    A) Perform immediate tracheal intubation.
    B) Reassess in 5 minutes.
    C) Begin chest compressions.
    D) Administer blow-by oxygen.

18. Assessment of the newborn begins immediately after birth and focuses on three areas. These areas are:
    A) Respirations, heart rate, and color.
    B) Muscle tone, respiratory effort, and heart rate.
    C) Reflex irritability, color, and respirations.
    D) Muscle tone, reflex irritability, and heart rate.

Questions 19 through 24 pertain to the following scenario.

A 9-month-old infant presents with a history of poor feeding. You note the infant appears pale and limp in her mother's arms. Intercostal retractions are present. She does not respond when her mother speaks her name.

19. From the information provided, complete the following documentation regarding the Pediatric Assessment Triangle.
    Appearance:
    Breathing:
    Circulation:

20. The normal respiratory rate range for an infant at rest is:
    A) 40 to 70 breaths/minute.
    B) 20 to 40 breaths/minute.
    C) 30 to 60 breaths/minute.
    D) 15 to 30 breaths/minute.

21. The normal heart rate range for an infant at rest is:
    A) 80 to 140 beats/minute.
    B) 100 to 160 beats/minute.
    C) 120 to 220 beats/minute.
    D) 150 to 250 beats/minute.

22. Your initial assessment reveals clear lung sounds and a respiratory rate of 40/min. Peripheral pulses are difficult to palpate. Capillary refill is > 5 seconds. The infant's heart rate is 250 beats/min. Oxygen saturation: 94%. Based on this information, your **first** action should be to:
    A) Begin chest compressions.
    B) Establish vascular access.
    C) Administer high concentration oxygen.
    D) Place the infant in a position of comfort.

23. The infant responds only to painful stimulation, and has no history of fever, vomiting, or diarrhea. The cardiac monitor displays the following rhythm.

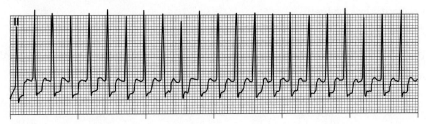

This rhythm is:
A) Sinus tachycardia.
B) Supraventricular tachycardia.
C) Ventricular tachycardia.
D) Ventricular fibrillation.

24. Vascular access has not been established. Your best course of action will be to:
A) Defibrillate immediately with 0.5 J/kg.
B) Insert an IV and administer atropine.
C) Insert an IV and administer adenosine.
D) Perform synchronized cardioversion with 0.5 to 1 J/kg.

25. Select the **incorrect** statement regarding defibrillation and synchronized cardioversion:
A) Before delivering a shock, ensure everyone is clear of the patient, bed, and any equipment connected to the patient.
B) Defibrillation is indicated for pulseless ventricular tachycardia, ventricular fibrillation, and supraventricular tachycardia.
C) If VF occurs during the course of synchronization, check the patient's pulse and rhythm, turn off the sync control, and defibrillate.
D) Before delivering a shock, ensure oxygen is not flowing over the patient's torso.

26. Select the incorrect statement regarding vagal maneuvers and the pediatric patient:
A) Application of external ocular pressure is the preferred vagal maneuver for terminating dysrhythmias in the pediatric patient.
B) If the child is able to follow instructions, ask the child to blow through a straw or take a deep breath and bear down as if having a bowel movement.
C) Ensure oxygen, suction, a defibrillator, and emergency medications are available before attempting the procedure.
D) In general, a vagal maneuver should not be continued for more than 10 seconds.

27. List three indications for intraosseous vascular access:
A)
B)
C)

28. True or False: Proper insertion of an oropharyngeal airway in a child is performed by inserting the airway upside down until it reaches the back of the throat. The device is then rotated 180 degrees until the flange rests on the patient's lips or teeth.

29. A 6-year-old suffered burns to his anterior chest, abdomen, and the anterior portion of both legs. What percentage of body surface area was burned?
    A) 18%
    B) 27%
    C) 32%
    D) 36%

30. Which of the following findings would **NOT** be expected in the early (hyperdynamic) phase of septic shock?
    A) Bounding peripheral pulses
    B) Mottled, cool extremities
    C) Brisk capillary refill
    D) Tachycardia

31. Select the incorrect statement regarding pain management and the pediatric patient:
    A) In general, pain in the pediatric patient is adequately treated by healthcare professionals.
    B) Some healthcare professionals do not view pain relief as important or do not want to "waste time" assessing pain.
    C) The *patient*, not the healthcare professional, is the authority regarding his or her pain.
    D) Methods for assessing pain in the pediatric patient will vary according to the age of the child.

32. The preferred intramuscular injection site in infants and children under three years of age is the:
    A) Vastus lateralis.
    B) Ventrogluteal.
    C) Dorsogluteal.
    D) Deltoid.

33. True or False: When cervical spine injury is suspected, traction should be applied to the neck while waiting to immobilize the child to a spine board.

34. Select the incorrect statement regarding assessment of blood pressure:
    A) Use of a blood pressure cuff that is too large will result in a falsely low reading.
    B) Blood pressure is one of the least sensitive indicators of adequate circulation in children.
    C) Blood pressure should be measured only after assessing pulse and respiration.
    D) To ensure an accurate patient assessment, it is essential to obtain serial blood pressure measurements in children younger than 3 years.

35. True or False: Needle cricothyroidotomy is preferred over surgical cricothyroidotomy in a child under 10 years of age.

36. List four reasons why a rigid cervical collar is used.
    A)
    B)
    C)
    D)

37. Which of the following statements is **incorrect** when assessing the abdomen of a pediatric patient?
    A) The abdomen of a young child is naturally protuberant and may appear somewhat distended.
    B) A toddler may scream throughout the examination.
    C) It is abnormal for an infant to tense his or her abdominal muscles when palpated.
    D) It may be necessary to evaluate the abdomen more than once for a more accurate assessment.

38. List four possible contraindications for spinal immobilization.
    A)
    B)
    C)
    D)

39. True or False: Spontaneous emesis in the first 30 to 60 minutes following head injury is common in children.

40. Which of the following may result from a sudden impact to the anterior chest wall and cause cessation of normal cardiac function?
    A) Pericardial tamponade.
    B) Traumatic asphyxia.
    C) Beck's triad.
    D) Commotio cordis.

41. If a properly fitting rigid cervical collar is not available, which of the following items should **NOT** be used when immobilizing the head and neck of a pediatric patient?
    A) Towels.
    B) Blanket rolls.
    C) Wash cloths.
    D) Sandbags.

42. Which of the following is true of the characteristics of neurogenic and hypovolemic shock?
    A) Neurogenic shock is characterized by a decreased blood pressure (BP) and normal or decreased heart rate. Hypovolemic shock is characterized by an increased BP and increased heart rate.
    B) Neurogenic shock is characterized by an increased BP and decreased heart rate. Hypovolemic shock is characterized by an increased BP and normal or decreased heart rate.
    C) Neurogenic shock is characterized by a decreased BP and normal or decreased heart rate. Hypovolemic shock is characterized by a decreased BP and increased heart rate.
    D) Neurogenic shock is characterized by an increased BP and increased heart rate. Hypovolemic shock is characterized by a decreased BP and decreased heart rate.

43. True or False: Analgesics used to manage severe pain usually cause sedation, but most sedatives do not provide analgesia.

44. True or False: If you observe a change in mental status in a febrile child (inconsolable, inability to recognize parents, unarousable), *immediately* consider the possibility of septic shock.

45. True or False: Medications administered via a peripheral vein during CPR should be followed with a saline flush of 15 to 20 mL to facilitate delivery of the medication to the central circulation.

46. What is the recommended rate and energy level when performing transcutaneous pacing in a pediatric patient?

47. Bradypnea can result from ingestion of all of the following **except:**
    A) Sedative/hypnotics.
    B) Lily of the valley, oleander.
    C) Theophylline or ephedrine.
    D) Licking of toads.

48. Which of the following statements is **incorrect** regarding Sudden Infant Death Syndrome (SIDS)?
    A) Most victims have suffered tissue hypoxia for some time before death.
    B) In the northern hemisphere, up to 95% of deaths occur between October and April.
    C) SIDS occurs more often in infant girls than in boys.
    D) The SIDS rate has declined since 1992.

49. Which of the following statements is **incorrect** regarding PICC lines?
    A) A PICC line is inserted directly into a central vein.
    B) PICC lines are small single or double lumen catheters.
    C) A PICC line does not require surgical placement; it can be inserted at the bedside.
    D) PICC lines are less expensive and are associated with fewer complications than central venous catheters.

50. Which of the following statements is **incorrect** regarding cerebrospinal fluid shunts?
    A) The proximal catheter is usually inserted into one of the ventricles of the brain.
    B) The distal catheter is tunneled under the skin and is most often placed in the peritoneal cavity (ventriculoperitoneal [VP] shunt).
    C) Shunts are named for the position of their proximal and distal catheters.
    D) A child with a malfunctioning shunt will always present with a fever.

Answers

1. C. Disposable colorimetric devices provide CO_2 readings by chemical reaction on pH-sensitive litmus paper housed in the detector. The paper in the $ETCO_2$ detector changes according to the amount of CO_2 detected. In a patient with a pulse, a lack of color change during exhalation suggests esophageal tube placement. If there is a small amount of CO_2 detected, the color will change slightly from its original color. Possible causes for this finding: 1) the tube may be in the correct position, but the patient may not be ventilating or perfusing adequately (e.g., shock, cardiopulmonary arrest) or 2) the tube may be in the esophagus and the CO_2 detector is reading CO_2 retained in the esophagus from bag–valve–mask ventilation, ingestion of a carbonated beverage, or alcohol. If a normal amount of CO_2 is detected during exhalation, the color will change noticeably from its original color (i.e., confirms tracheal placement of the tube). Colorimetric capnography is susceptible to inaccurate results due to exposure of the paper to medications, the environment, patient secretions (e.g., vomitus), and the age of the paper.

2. B. A rigid (also called a "hard," "tonsil tip," or "Yankauer") suction catheter is made of hard plastic and is angled to aid in the removal of thick secretions and particulate matter from the mouth and oropharynx.

3. B. Under optimum conditions, blow-by oxygen administered by means of a face mask can deliver an oxygen concentration of 35% to 40% at a flow rate of 10 L/min.

4. B. The initial energy dose for synchronized cardioversion for an infant and child is 0.5 to 1 J/kg.

5. B. Begin chest compressions if there is no pulse or if the heart rate is less than 60 beats/min with signs of poor perfusion.

6. A. When performing chest compressions on an infant, compress the chest approximately $1/3$ to $1/2$ the depth of the chest at a rate of about 100/minute.

7. B. If the patient is not breathing or if breathing is inadequate, maintain a patent airway with a chin-lift or jaw thrust without head-tilt. Deliver two breaths (1 second per breath) with sufficient volume to cause gentle chest rise. Allow for exhalation between breaths.

8. A. A bradycardia that causes severe cardiopulmonary compromise in an infant or child is initially treated with effective oxygenation and ventilation. If the heart rate is < 60/min and poor systemic perfusion persists despite oxygenation and ventilation, establish vascular access, identify and treat possible causes, and give epinephrine. Synchronized cardioversion is not indicated in the treatment of a bradycardia. Give atropine before epinephrine if the bradycardia is due to suspected increased vagal tone or any type of AV block. If no response, consider pacing.

9. C. Synchronized cardioversion is the delivery of a shock to the heart to terminate a rapid dysrhythmia that is timed to avoid the vulnerable period during the cardiac cycle. On the ECG, this period occurs during the peak of the T wave to approximately the end of the T wave. Synchronized cardioversion may be used to treat the "sick" (unstable) patient in SVT, atrial flutter with a rapid ventricular response, or ventricular tachycardia with a pulse. Signs of hemodynamic compromise include poor perfusion, hypotension, or heart failure. This procedure may also be performed electively in a child with stable SVT or VT at the direction of a pediatric cardiologist.

10. C. The suction catheter should be no more than 1/2 the internal diameter of the tube being suctioned. To determine the correct size suction catheter, use a length-based resuscitation tape or multiply the external diameter of the tracheostomy tube (in millimeters) by two. In this case, the tracheostomy tube is 3 mm in diameter. Use a 6-French suction catheter.

11. C. Irritability, headache, neck pain, vomiting, a bulging or full fontanelle in infants, new seizures or a change in the child's seizure pattern, behavioral changes, or "just not acting right" are signs suggestive of increased intracranial pressure.

12. C. Activated charcoal is contraindicated in poisonings involving ingestion of caustics (e.g., hydrochloric acid, bleach, ammonia) or hydrocarbons (e.g., gasoline, kerosene). Activated charcoal is ineffective for iron, lithium, heavy metals, and most solvents and is not recommended for poisonings involving these substances.

13. C. Children under the age of six are at the greatest risk for unintentional poisoning.

14. B. Hypovolemic shock is the most common type of shock in the pediatric patient.

15. C. In pulseless electrical activity (PEA), organized electrical activity is visible on the ECG, but central pulses are absent. The mnemonic "4 H's and 4 T's" can be used to memorize the possible causes of PEA. PEA has a poor prognosis unless the underlying cause can be rapidly identified and appropriately managed.

16. D. Administer a bolus of 20 mL/kg of isotonic crystalloid solution (NS or LR) over 5 to 20 minutes. 44 pounds = 20 kilograms. For this child, the appropriate initial fluid bolus is 400 mL of normal saline or Ringer's lactate.

17. D. Early administration of 100% oxygen is important if signs of distress (e.g., cyanosis, bradycardia) are observed in the newly born during the initial steps of stabilization. The goal of supplemental oxygen therapy is to administer sufficient oxygen to achieve pink color in the mucous membranes. Blow-by oxygen can be delivered by means of a face mask and flow-inflating (anesthesia) bag, simple face mask held firmly (but not too tightly) to the newborn's face, or by means of a hand cupped around oxygen tubing. The oxygen source should be set to deliver at least 5 L/min and held close to the face to maximize oxygen flow to the newborn's nose and mouth. Avoid administering unheated and unhumidified oxygen to a newborn at high flow rates (i.e., > 10 L/min) because convective heat loss can become a problem.

18. A. Assessment of the newborn begins immediately after birth and focuses on three areas: respirations, heart rate, and color. These signs are important indicators of hypoxia. Further resuscitative efforts are required if the newborn's respiratory effort is inadequate, the heart rate is less than 100 beats/minute, or central cyanosis is present.

19. Pediatric Assessment Triangle (first impression)
    Appearance: Unresponsive to verbal stimuli; limp
    Breathing: Increased work of breathing evident
    Circulation: Pale

20. C. The normal respiratory rate range for an infant at rest is 30 to 60 breaths/minute.

21. B. The normal heart rate range for an infant at rest is 100 to 160 beats/minute.

22. C. Your first action must be to ensure effective oxygenation and ventilation. Administer high concentration oxygen.

23. B. The rhythm displayed is supraventricular tachycardia.

24. D. Because vascular access has not been established, perform synchronized cardioversion beginning with 0.5 to 1 J/kg. If cardioversion does not terminate the dysrhythmia, increase the energy level to 2 J/kg.

25. B. Before delivering a shock, ensure everyone is clear of the patient, bed, and any equipment connected to the patient. Ensure oxygen is not flowing over the patient's torso (oxygen flow over the patient's torso during electrical therapy increases the risk of spark/fire). Defibrillation is indicated for pulseless ventricular tachycardia and ventricular fibrillation. Synchronized cardioversion may be used to treat the "sick" (unstable) patient in SVT, atrial flutter with a rapid ventricular response, or ventricular tachycardia with a pulse. This procedure may also be performed electively in a child with stable SVT or VT at the direction of a pediatric cardiologist. If VF occurs during the course of synchronization, check the patient's pulse and rhythm (verify all electrodes and cable connections are secure), turn off the sync control, and defibrillate.

26. A. Application of external ocular pressure may be dangerous and should not be used because of the risk of retinal detachment. Ensure oxygen, suction, a defibrillator, and crash cart are available before attempting the procedure. Obtain a 12-lead ECG before and after the vagal maneuver. Continuous monitoring of the patient's ECG is essential. Note the onset and end of the vagal maneuver on the ECG rhythm strip. In general, a vagal maneuver should not be continued for more than 10 seconds. Carotid massage is less effective in children than in adults and is not recommended. Application of a cold stimulus to the face (e.g., a washcloth soaked in iced water, cold pack, or crushed ice mixed with water in a plastic bag or glove) for up to 10 seconds is often effective in infants and young children. When using this method, do not obstruct the patient's mouth or nose or apply pressure to the eyes. Valsalva's maneuver is also an effective vagal maneuver. Instruct the child to blow through a straw or take a deep breath and bear down as if having a bowel movement for 10 seconds. This strains the abdominal muscles and increases intrathoracic pressure. In the younger child, abdominal palpation may be used to create the same effect. Abdominal palpation causes the child to bear down in an attempt to resist the pressure.

27. Indications for intraosseous vascular access include:
    A) Cardiopulmonary arrest or decompensated shock where vascular access is essential and venous access is not readily achieved.
    B) Multi-system trauma with associated shock and/or severe hypovolemia.
    C) Unresponsive patient in need of immediate medications or fluid resuscitation (e.g., burns, sepsis, near-drowning, anaphylaxis, status epilepticus).
    D) Presence of burns or a traumatic injury preventing access to the venous system at other sites.

28. False. The preferred technique for oropharyngeal airway insertion in an infant or child requires the use of a tongue blade. Depress the tongue with a tongue blade and gently insert the oropharyngeal airway with the curve downward. Place the airway over the tongue down into the mouth until the flange of the airway rests against the patient's lips.

29. C. Using the rule of nines, the child's anterior chest is 9%, abdomen 9%, and the anterior portion of each leg is approximately 7% (14% for the anterior portion of both legs).

30. B. Septic shock occurs in two clinical stages. The early (hyperdynamic) phase is characterized by peripheral vasodilation (warm shock) due to endotoxins that prevent catecholamine-induced vasoconstriction. The late (hypodynamic or decompensated) phase is characterized by cool extremities (cold shock) and resembles hypovolemic shock.

31. A. Pain is a subjective experience that is underestimated and inadequately treated by many healthcare professionals despite the availability of effective medications and other therapies. Many factors contribute to the inadequate treatment of pain including the attitudes, beliefs, and behaviors of healthcare professionals. Some do not view pain relief as important or do not want to "waste time" assessing pain. The safe and effective relief of pain should be a priority in the management of a patient of **any** age.

32. A. The vastus lateralis is the preferred intramuscular injection site for infants and children < 3 years, but may be used in all ages.

33. False. Do NOT apply traction to the neck. In a child with possible cervical spine trauma, the application of traction can exacerbate an existing injury or convert a stable cervical fracture to an unstable fracture.

34. D. Use of a blood pressure cuff that is too large will result in a falsely low reading. Blood pressure is one of the least sensitive indicators of adequate circulation in children. Blood pressure should be measured only after assessing pulse and respiration. Children often become agitated during this procedure, which increases their pulse and respiratory rate. Measure blood pressure in children more than 3 years of age. In children less than 3 years of age, a strong central pulse is considered an acceptable sign of adequate blood pressure.

35. True. Needle cricothyroidotomy is preferred over surgical cricothyroidotomy in a child under 10 years of age.

36. When used alone, a rigid cervical collar does not immobilize. For effective immobilization, a rigid collar must be used with manual stabilization or mechanical immobilization provided by a suitable spine immobilization device. A rigid collar is used to:
    A) Temporarily splint the head and neck in a neutral position.
    B) Limit movement of the cervical spine.
    C) Support the weight of the head while the patient is in a sitting position.
    D) Help maintain alignment of the cervical spine when the patient is in a supine position.
    E) Remind the patient and healthcare professionals that the integrity of the patient's cervical spine is questionable because of the mechanism of injury.

37. C. Assessment of an infant or young child's abdomen can be difficult. The abdomen of a young child is naturally protuberant and may appear somewhat distended. An infant will naturally tense his or her abdominal muscles when palpated, simulating guarding. A toddler may scream throughout the examination. It may be necessary to evaluate the abdomen more than once for a more accurate assessment.

38. Possible contraindications for spinal immobilization include:
    A) Combative child. Efforts to forcefully immobilize a combative child with a possible head or spinal injury may result in further manipulation of the spine and exacerbate the injury. If the risks of agitation and increased spinal movement from full spinal immobilization are greater than the benefits, defer the immobilization procedure and consider other immobilization options. For example, enlist the assistance of the child's parent or caregiver to hold the child in a position the child can tolerate that has a neutral effect on the spine and minimizes movement.
    B) Penetrating foreign body to the neck with hemorrhage.
    C) Massive cervical swelling.
    D) Presence of a tracheal stoma that is integral to the management of the patient's airway.
    E) Requirement for any maneuver to ensure adequate oxygenation and ventilation.
    Manual immobilization is better in these situations. If full spinal immobilization is indicated but not performed, be sure to clearly document the circumstances in the patient's medical record.

39. True. Spontaneous emesis in the first 30 to 60 minutes following head injury is common in children.

40. D. Commotio cordis is a disorder described in the pediatric population that results from sudden impact to the anterior chest wall (e.g., baseball injury) that causes cessation of normal cardiac function. The patient may have an immediate dysrhythmia or ventricular fibrillation that is refractory to resuscitation efforts.

41. D. If a properly fitting device is not available, use towels, washcloths, or blanket rolls (depending on the child's size) and adhesive tape across the forehead to immobilize the head as best as possible. Avoid the use of IV bags or sandbags; their weight may push the cervical spine out of alignment.

42. C. Neurogenic shock: ↓ blood pressure, normal or ↓ heart rate. Hypovolemic shock: ↓ blood pressure, ↑ heart rate.

43. True. Analgesics used to manage severe pain usually cause sedation, but most sedatives do not provide analgesia.

44. True. If you observe a change in mental status in a febrile child (inconsolable, inability to recognize parents, unarousable), *immediately* consider the possibility of septic shock.

45. False. Medications administered via a peripheral vein during CPR should be followed with a saline flush of 5 to 10 mL to facilitate delivery of the medication to the central circulation.

46. Set the initial rate at 100 pulses per minute. Then increase the output (milliamps) until the pacer spikes are visible before each QRS complex. Verify capture. The final mA setting should be slightly above where capture is obtained to prevent the loss of capture.

47. C. Bradypnea can result from ingestion of alcohols and ethanol, barbiturates (late), clonidine, opiates, and sedative/hypnotics. Acute poisoning can result from toad toxins or the licking of toads. Some aphrodisiacs intended for topical application contain toad venoms that cause vomiting, bradycardia, and other dysrhythmias when ingested. Tachypnea may result from ingestion of amphetamines, barbiturates (early), caffeine, cocaine, ethylene glycol, methanol, and salicylates.

48. C. SIDS occurs more often in infant boys than girls.

49. A. Peripherally inserted central catheters (PICC) are not inserted directly into a central vein. Instead, a PICC line is inserted into an antecubital vein and then advanced into the subclavian vein so that the tip lies in the superior vena cava or right atrium.

50. D. The child with a malfunctioning shunt may present with irritability, headache, neck pain, vomiting, a bulging or full fontanelle in infants, new seizures or a change in the child's seizure pattern, behavioral changes, or "just not acting right." These are signs of increased intracranial pressure, due to fluid

accumulation within the brain. Abdominal pain may be present because of infected CSF draining into the peritoneal cavity, causing peritoneal inflammation. If infection is present, redness, edema, or tenderness may be observed along the path of the shunt tubing. A child with a shunt infection is usually, but not always, febrile.

Illustration Credits

Chapter One

Fig 1-2.   EMSC Slide Set (CD-ROM). 1996. Courtesy of the Emergency Medical Services for Children Program, administered by the U.S. Department of Health and Human Service's Health Resources and Services Administration, Maternal and Child Health Bureau.

Chapter Two

Fig 2-1.   Courtesy Paul Vincent Kuntz.

Fig 2-2.   Courtesy Paul Vincent Kuntz.

Fig 2-3.   Hockenberry M, Wilson D, Winkelstein M, Kline N, Wong's Nursing Care of Infants and Children, 7e. St. Louis, 2002, Mosby.

Fig 2-4.   Hockenberry M, Wilson D, Winkelstein M, Kline N, Wong's Nursing Care of Infants and Children, 7e. St. Louis, 2002, Mosby.

Fig 2-5.   Hockenberry M, Wilson D, Winkelstein M, Kline N, Wong's Nursing Care of Infants and Children, 7e. St. Louis, 2002, Mosby.

Fig 2-6.   Hockenberry M, Wilson D, Winkelstein M, Kline N, Wong's Nursing Care of Infants and Children, 7e. St. Louis, 2002, Mosby.

Fig 2-7.   Hockenberry M, Wilson D, Winkelstein M, Kline N, Wong's Nursing Care of Infants and Children, 7e. St. Louis, 2002, Mosby.

Fig 2-8.   Hockenberry M, Wilson D, Winkelstein M, Kline N, Wong's Nursing Care of Infants and Children, 7e. St. Louis, 2002, Mosby.

Chapter Three

Fig 3-1.   Hockenberry M, Wilson D, Winkelstein M, Kline N, Wong's Nursing Care of Infants and Children, 7e. St. Louis, 2002, Mosby.

Fig 3-3.   Zitelli B, Davis H, Atlas of Pediatric Physical Diagnosis, 4e. St. Louis, 2002, Mosby.

Fig 3-4.   Hockenberry M, Wilson D, Winkelstein M, Kline N, Wong's Nursing Care of Infants and Children, 7e. St. Louis, 2002, Mosby.

Fig 3-5.   Zitelli B, Davis H, Atlas of Pediatric Physical Diagnosis, 4e. St. Louis, 2002, Mosby.

Fig 3-6.   Hockenberry M, Wilson D, Winkelstein M, Kline N, Wong's Nursing Care of Infants and Children, 7e. St. Louis, 2002, Mosby.

Fig 3-7.   Aehlert B, Pediatric Advanced Life Support Study Guide, 1e. St. Louis, 1994, Mosby.

Fig 3-8.   Hockenberry M, Wilson D, Winkelstein M, Kline N, Wong's Nursing Care of Infants and Children, 7e. St. Louis, 2002, Mosby.

Fig 3-9.   Seidel H, Ball J, Dains J, Benedict GW, Mosby's Guide to Physical Examination, 5e. St. Louis, 2003, Mosby.

Fig 3-10.   Courtesy Mead Johnson and Co., Evansville, Indiana.

Fig 3-11.   Seidel H, Ball J, Dains J, Benedict GW, Mosby's Guide to Physical Examination, 5e. St. Louis, 2003, Mosby.

Fig 3-12.   Beattie T: Pediatric Emergencies, London: Mosby-Wolfe, 1997.

Fig 3-13.   Hockenberry M, Wilson D, Winkelstein M, Kline N, Wong's Nursing Care of Infants and Children, 7e. St. Louis, 2002, Mosby.

Fig 3-15.   Hockenberry M, Wilson D, Winkelstein M, Kline N, Wong's Nursing Care of Infants and Children, 7e. St. Louis, 2002, Mosby.

Fig 3-16.   EMSC Slide Set (CD-ROM). 1996. Courtesy of the Emergency Medical Services for Children Program, administered by the U.S. Department of Health and Human Service's Health Resources and Services Administration, Maternal and Child Health Bureau.

Fig 3-17.   Courtesy Gary Quick, M.D.

Fig 3-18.   EMSC Slide Set (CD-ROM). 1996. Courtesy of the Emergency Medical Services for Children Program, administered by the U.S. Department of Health and Human Service's Health Resources and Services Administration, Maternal and Child Health Bureau.

Fig 3-19.   Seidel H, Ball J, Dains J, Benedict GW, Mosby's Guide to Physical Examination, 5e. St. Louis, 2003, Mosby.

Fig 3-20.   Seidel H, Ball J, Dains J, Benedict GW, Mosby's Guide to Physical Examination, 5e. St. Louis, 2003, Mosby.

Chapter Four

Fig 4-1 A&B.   EMSC Slide Set (CD-ROM). 1996. Courtesy of the Emergency Medical Services for Children Program, administered by the U.S. Department of Health and Human Service's Health Resources and Services Administration, Maternal and Child Health Bureau.

Fig 4-2.   Hazinski M, Manual of Pediatric Critical Care, 1e. St. Louis, 1999, Mosby.

Fig 4-3.   EMSC Slide Set (CD-ROM). 1996. Courtesy of the Emergency Medical Services for Children Program, administered by the U.S. Department of Health and Human Service's Health Resources and Services Administration, Maternal and Child Health Bureau.

Fig 4-4.   EMSC Slide Set (CD-ROM). 1996. Courtesy of the Emergency Medical Services for Children Program, administered by the U.S. Department of Health and Human Service's Health Resources and Services Administration, Maternal and Child Health Bureau.

Fig 4-5.   Hockenberry M, Wilson D, Winkelstein M, Kline N, Wong's Nursing Care of Infants and Children, 7e. St. Louis, 2002, Mosby.

Fig 4-6.   Zitelli B, Davis H, Atlas of Pediatric Physical Diagnosis, 4e. St. Louis, 2002, Mosby.

Fig 4-7.   Hockenberry M, Wilson D, Winkelstein M, Kline N, Wong's Nursing Care of Infants and Children, 7e. St. Louis, 2002, Mosby.

Fig 4-8.   Zitelli B, Davis H, Atlas of Pediatric Physical Diagnosis, 4e. St. Louis, 2002, Mosby.

Fig 4-9.   Behrman R, Kliegman R, Jenson H, Nelson Textbook of Pediatrics, 17e. Philadelphia, 2004, WB Saunders.

Fig 4-10.   Seidel H, Ball J, Dains J, Benedict GW, Mosby's Guide to Physical Examination, 5e. St. Louis, 2003, Mosby.

Fig 4-11.   Zitelli B, Davis H, Atlas of Pediatric Physical Diagnosis, 4e. St. Louis, 2002, Mosby.

Fig 4-12.   Behrman R, Kliegman R, Jenson H, Nelson Textbook of Pediatrics, 17e. Philadelphia, 2004, WB Saunders.

Fig 4-13.   EMSC Slide Set (CD-ROM). 1996. Courtesy of the Emergency Medical Services for Children Program, administered by the U.S. Department of Health and Human Service's Health Resources and Services Administration, Maternal and Child Health Bureau.

Fig 4-14.   Behrman R, Kliegman R, Jenson H, Nelson Textbook of Pediatrics, 16e. Philadelphia, 1999, WB Saunders.

Fig 4-15.   Behrman R, Kliegman R, Jenson H, Nelson Textbook of Pediatrics, 17e. Philadelphia, 2004, WB Saunders.

Fig 4-16.   Behrman R, Kliegman R, Jenson H, Nelson Textbook of Pediatrics, 16e. Philadelphia, 1999, WB Saunders.

Fig 4-17.   Gould B, Pathophysiology for the Health Professions, 2e. Philadelphia, 2002, WB Saunders.

Fig 4-18.   Huether S, McCance K, Understanding Pathophysiology, 2e. St. Louis, 1999, Mosby.

Fig 4-19.   Courtesy R.W. Shaw, M.D.

Fig 4-20.   Gould B, Pathophysiology for the Health Professions, 2e. Philadelphia, 2002, WB Saunders.

Fig 4-21.   Modified from Wilson, Thompson, 1990.

Chapter Five

Fig 5-1.   Prehospital Trauma Life Support Committee of the NAEMT, PHTL: Basic and advanced Prehospital Trauma Life Support, 5e. St. Louis, 2003, Mosby.

Fig 5-2.   Aehlert B, Pediatric Advanced Life Support Study Guide, 1e. St. Louis, 2005, Mosby.

Fig 5-3.   Aehlert B, Pediatric Advanced Life Support Study Guide, 1e. St. Louis, 2005, Mosby.

Fig 5-4.   Chapleau W: Emergency First Responder: Making the Difference, St. Louis, 2004, Mosby.

Fig 5-5   Chapleau W: Emergency First Responder: Making the Difference, St. Louis, 2004, Mosby.

Fig 5-6.   Aehlert B, Pediatric Advanced Life Support Study Guide, 1e. St. Louis, 2005, Mosby.

Fig 5-7.   Henry M, Stapleton E: EMT Prehospital Care, ed 3, St. Louis, 2004, Mosby.

Fig 5-9.   Stoy W/Center for Emergency Medicine, Mosby's EMT-Basic Textbook, St. Louis, 1996, Mosby-Year Book.

Fig 5-10.   French J, Pediatric Emergency Skills, 1e. St. Louis, 1995, Mosby.

Fig 5-11.   EMSC Slide Set (CD-ROM). 1996. Courtesy of the Emergency Medical Services for Children Program, administered by the U.S. Department of Health and Human Service's Health Resources and Services Administration, Maternal and Child Health Bureau.

Fig 5-12.   Sanders M, Mosby's Paramedic Textbook, revised 2e. St. Louis, 2001, Mosby.

Fig 5-13.   Aehlert B, ACLS Quick Review Study Guide, 2e. St. Louis, 2002, Mosby.

Fig 5-14 A.   American College of Emergency Physicians (Editor: Krohmer J), EMT-Basic Field Care: A Case Based Approach, St. Louis, 1999, Mosby.

Fig 5-14 B.   McSwain N, Paturas J, The Basic EMT: Comprehensive Prehospital Patient Care, 2e. St. Louis, 2003, Mosby.

Fig 5-15.   McSwain N, Paturas J, The Basic EMT: Comprehensive Prehospital Patient Care, 2e. St. Louis, 2003, Mosby.

Fig 5-16.   McSwain N, Paturas J, The Basic EMT: Comprehensive Prehospital Patient Care, 2e. St. Louis, 2003, Mosby.

Fig 5-17.   McSwain N, Paturas J, The Basic EMT: Comprehensive Prehospital Patient Care, 2e. St. Louis, 2003, Mosby.

Fig 5-18.   Aehlert B, ACLS Quick Review Study Guide, 2e. St. Louis, 2002, Mosby.

Fig 5-19.   American College of Emergency Physicians (Editor: Krohmer J), EMT-Basic Field Care: A Case Based Approach, St. Louis, 1999, Mosby.

Fig 5-20.   McSwain N, Paturas J, The Basic EMT: Comprehensive Prehospital Patient Care, 2e. St. Louis, 2003, Mosby.

Fig 5-21.   Sanders M, Mosby's Paramedic Textbook, revised 2e. St. Louis, 2001, Mosby.

Fig 5-22.   Dieckmann R, Fiser D, Selbst, Illustrated Textbook of Pediatric Emergency & Critical Care Procedures, 1e. St. Louis, 1997, Mosby.

Fig 5-23.   Dieckmann R, Fiser D, Selbst, Illustrated Textbook of Pediatric Emergency & Critical Care Procedures, 1e. St. Louis, 1997, Mosby.

Fig 5-24.   Aehlert B, Pediatric Advanced Life Support Study Guide, 2e. St. Louis, 2005, Mosby.

Fig 5-25.   Aehlert B, Pediatric Advanced Life Support Study Guide, 2e. St. Louis, 2005, Mosby.

Fig 5-26.   EMSC Slide Set (CD-ROM). 1996. Courtesy of the Emergency Medical Services for Children Program, administered by the U.S. Department of Health and Human Service's Health Resources and Services Administration, Maternal and Child Health Bureau.

Fig 5-27.   EMSC Slide Set (CD-ROM). 1996. Courtesy of the Emergency Medical Services for Children Program, administered by the U.S. Department of Health and Human Service's Health Resources and Services Administration, Maternal and Child Health Bureau.

Fig 5-28.   Aehlert B, Pediatric Advanced Life Support Study Guide, 1e. St. Louis, 1994, Mosby

Fig 5-29.   Hockenberry M, Wilson D, Winkelstein M, Kline N, Wong's Nursing Care of Infants and Children, 7e. St. Louis, 2002, Mosby.

Fig 5-30.   EMSC Slide Set (CD-ROM). 1996. Courtesy of the Emergency Medical Services for Children Program, administered by the U.S. Department of Health and Human Service's Health Resources and Services Administration, Maternal and Child Health Bureau.

Fig 5-31.   Mack D: Mosby's Comprehensive EMT-B Refresher & Review (CD-ROM), St. Louis, 2002, WB Saunders.

Fig 5-32.   Henry M, Stapleton E, EMT Prehospital Care, 3e. St. Louis, 2004, Mosby.

Fig 5-33.   McSwain N, Paturas J, The Basic EMT: Comprehensive Prehospital Patient Care, 2e. St. Louis, 2003, Mosby.

Fig 5-34.   McSwain N, Paturas J, The Basic EMT: Comprehensive Prehospital Patient Care, 2e. St. Louis, 2003, Mosby.

Fig 5-35.   Henry M, Stapleton E, EMT Prehospital Care, 3e. St. Louis, 2004, Mosby.

Fig 5-36.   EMSC Slide Set (CD-ROM). 1996. Courtesy of the Emergency Medical Services for Children Program, administered by the U.S. Department of Health and Human Service's Health Resources and Services Administration, Maternal and Child Health Bureau.

Fig 5-37.   Aehlert B, ACLS Quick Review Study Guide, 2e. St. Louis, 2002, Mosby.

Fig 5-38.   Mack D: Mosby's Comprehensive EMT-B Refresher & Review (CD-ROM), St. Louis, 2002, WB Saunders.

Fig 5-39.   Aehlert B, ACLS Quick Review Study Guide, 2e. St. Louis, 2002, Mosby.

Fig 5-40.   Aehlert B, ACLS Quick Review Study Guide, 2e. St. Louis, 2002, Mosby.

Fig 5-41.   Aehlert B, ACLS Quick Review Study Guide, 2e. St. Louis, 2002, Mosby.

Fig 5-42.   American College of Emergency Physicians (Editors: Pons P, Carson D), Paramedic Field Care: A Complaint-Based Approach, St. Louis, 1997, Mosby.

Fig 5-43.   McSwain N, Paturas J, The Basic EMT: Comprehensive Prehospital Patient Care, 2e. St. Louis, 2003, Mosby.

Fig 5-44.   EMSC Slide Set (CD-ROM). 1996. Courtesy of the Emergency Medical Services for Children Program, administered by the U.S. Department of Health and Human Service's Health Resources and Services Administration, Maternal and Child Health Bureau.

Fig 5-45.   Aehlert B, Pediatric Advanced Life Support Study Guide, 2e. St. Louis, 2005, Mosby.

Fig 5-46.   Roberts, Clinical Procedures in Emergency Medicine, 3e. Philadelphia, 1998, WB Saunders.

Fig 5-47.   Thibodeau G, Patton K, Anatomy and Physiology, 5e. St. Louis, 2003, Mosby.

Fig 5-48.   Aehlert B, ACLS Quick Review Study Guide, 2e. St. Louis, 2002, Mosby.

Fig 5-49.   Aehlert B, ACLS Quick Review Study Guide, 2e. St. Louis, 2002, Mosby.

Fig 5-50.   McSwain N, Paturas J, The Basic EMT: Comprehensive Prehospital Patient Care, 2e. St. Louis, 2003, Mosby.

Fig 5-51.   Thibodeau G, Patton K, Anatomy and Physiology, 5e. St. Louis, 2003, Mosby.

Fig 5-52.   Dieckmann R, Fiser D, Selbst, Illustrated Textbook of Pediatric Emergency & Critical Care Procedures, 1e. St. Louis, 1997, Mosby.

Fig 5-53.   Dieckmann R, Fiser D, Selbst, Illustrated Textbook of Pediatric Emergency & Critical Care Procedures, 1e. St. Louis, 1997, Mosby.

Fig 5-54.   Dieckmann R, Fiser D, Selbst, Illustrated Textbook of Pediatric Emergency & Critical Care Procedures, 1e. St. Louis, 1997, Mosby.

Chapter Six

Fig 6-1.   Herlihy B, Meabius N, The Human Body in Health and Illness, 2e. St. Louis, 2003, WB Saunders.
Fig 6-2.   Herlihy B, Meabius N, The Human Body in Health and Illness, 2e. St. Louis, 2003, WB Saunders.

Fig 6-3.   Herlihy B, Meabius N, The Human Body in Health and Illness, 2e. St. Louis, 2003, WB Saunders.
Fig 6-4.   Herlihy B, Meabius N, The Human Body in Health and Illness, 2e. St. Louis, 2003, WB Saunders.
Fig 6-5.   Herlihy B, Meabius N, The Human Body in Health and Illness, 2e. St. Louis, 2003, WB Saunders.
Fig 6-6.   Gould B, Pathophysiology for the Health Professions, 2e. Philadelphia, 2002, WB Saunders.
Fig 6-7.   Gould B, Pathophysiology for the Health Professions, 2e. Philadelphia, 2002, WB Saunders.
Fig 6-8.   Gould B, Pathophysiology for the Health Professions, 2e. Philadelphia, 2002, WB Saunders.
Fig 6-9.   Gould B, Pathophysiology for the Health Professions, 2e. Philadelphia, 2002, WB Saunders.
Fig 6-10.   Gould B, Pathophysiology for the Health Professions, 2e. Philadelphia, 2002, WB Saunders.
Fig 6-11.   Gould B, Pathophysiology for the Health Professions, 2e. Philadelphia, 2002, WB Saunders.
Fig 6-12.   Aehlert B, ACLS Quick Review Study Guide, 2e. St. Louis, 2002, Mosby.
Fig 6-13.   Dieckmann R, Fiser D, Selbst, Illustrated Textbook of Pediatric Emergency & Critical Care
                Procedures, 1e. St. Louis, 1997, Mosby.
Fig 6-14.   Aehlert B, ACLS Quick Review Study Guide, 2e. St. Louis, 2002, Mosby.
Fig 6-15.   Aehlert B, ACLS Quick Review Study Guide, 2e. St. Louis, 2002, Mosby.
Fig 6-16.   Sanders M: Mosby's Paramedic Textbook, St. Louis, 1994, Mosby.
Fig 6-17.   Sanders M: Mosby's Paramedic Textbook, St. Louis, 1994, Mosby.
Fig 6-18.   Aehlert B, ECGs Made Easy Study Cards, 2e. St. Louis, 2004, Mosby.
Fig 6-19.   Aehlert B, ECGs Made Easy Study Cards, 2e. St. Louis, 2004, Mosby.
Fig 6-20.   Aehlert B, ECGs Made Easy Study Cards, 2e. St. Louis, 2004, Mosby.
Fig 6-21.   Aehlert B, ECGs Made Easy Study Cards, 2e. St. Louis, 2004, Mosby.
Fig 6-22.   Aehlert B, ECGs Made Easy Study Cards, 2e. St. Louis, 2004, Mosby.
Fig 6-23.   Park MK, Guntheroth WG: How to read Pediatric ECGs, 3e. St. Louis, 1992, Mosby.
Fig 6-24.   Aehlert B, ECGs Made Easy, 2e. St. Louis, 2002, Mosby.
Fig 6-25.   Aehlert B, ECGs Made Easy Study Cards, 2e. St. Louis, 2004, Mosby.
Fig 6-26.   Aehlert B, ECGs Made Easy Study Cards, 2e. St. Louis, 2004, Mosby.
Fig 6-27.   Park MK, Guntheroth WG: How to read Pediatric ECGs, 3e. St. Louis, 1992, Mosby.
Fig 6-28.   Aehlert B, ECGs Made Easy, 2e. St. Louis, 2002, Mosby.
Fig 6-29.   Aehlert B, ECGs Made Easy Study Cards, 2e. St. Louis, 2004, Mosby.
Fig 6-30.   Aehlert B, ACLS Quick Review Study Guide, 2e. St. Louis, 2002, Mosby.
Fig 6-31.   Zitelli B, Davis H, Atlas of Pediatric Physical Diagnosis, 4e. St. Louis, 2002, Mosby.
Fig 6-32.   Hockenberry M, Wilson D, Winkelstein M, Kline N, Wong's Nursing Care of Infants and
                Children, 7e. St. Louis, 2002, Mosby.
Fig 6-33.   Hockenberry M, Wilson D, Winkelstein M, Kline N, Wong's Nursing Care of Infants and
                Children, 7e. St. Louis, 2002, Mosby.
Fig 6-34.   Hockenberry M, Wilson D, Winkelstein M, Kline N, Wong's Nursing Care of Infants and
                Children, 7e. St. Louis, 2002, Mosby.
Fig 6-35.   Hockenberry M, Wilson D, Winkelstein M, Kline N, Wong's Nursing Care of Infants and
                Children, 7e. St. Louis, 2002, Mosby.
Fig 6-36.   Hockenberry M, Wilson D, Winkelstein M, Kline N, Wong's Nursing Care of Infants and
                Children, 7e. St. Louis, 2002, Mosby.
Fig 6-37.   Hockenberry M, Wilson D, Winkelstein M, Kline N, Wong's Nursing Care of Infants and
                Children, 7e. St. Louis, 2002, Mosby.

Fig 6-38.   Hockenberry M, Wilson D, Winkelstein M, Kline N, Wong's Nursing Care of Infants and Children, 7e. St. Louis, 2002, Mosby.

Fig 6-39.   Zitelli B, Davis H, Atlas of Pediatric Physical Diagnosis, 4e. St. Louis, 2002, Mosby.

Fig 6-40.   Hockenberry M, Wilson D, Winkelstein M, Kline N, Wong's Nursing Care of Infants and Children, 7e. St. Louis, 2002, Mosby.

Fig 6-41.   Chaudhry B, Harvey D, Mosby's Color Atlas and Text of Pediatrics & Child Health, London, 2001, Mosby.

Fig 6-42.   Hockenberry M, Wilson D, Winkelstein M, Kline N, Wong's Nursing Care of Infants and Children, 7e. St. Louis, 2002, Mosby.

Fig 6-43.   Aehlert B, ECGs Made Easy, 2e. St. Louis, 2002, Mosby.

Question 10. Aehlert B, ECGs Made Easy, 2e. St. Louis, 2004, Mosby.

Question 11. Aehlert B, ECGs Made Easy Study Cards, 2e. St. Louis, 2002, Mosby.

Question 12. Aehlert B, ECGs Made Easy Study Cards, 2e. St. Louis, 2004, Mosby.

Question 13. Aehlert B, ECGs Made Easy, 2e. St. Louis, 2002, Mosby.

Question 14. Aehlert B, ECGs Made Easy Study Cards, 2e. St. Louis, 2004, Mosby.

Question 15. Aehlert B, ECGs Made Easy Study Cards, 2e. St. Louis, 2004, Mosby.

Question 16. Aehlert B, ECGs Made Easy Study Cards, 2e. St. Louis, 2004, Mosby.

Chapter Seven

Fig 7-1.   Stoy W/Center for Emergency Medicine, Mosby's EMT-Basic Textbook, St. Louis, 1996, Mosby-Year Book.

Fig 7-2.   Aehlert B, Pediatric Advanced Life Support Study Guide, 1e. St. Louis, 1994, Mosby.

Fig 7-3.   Aehlert B, Pediatric Advanced Life Support Study Guide, 2e. St. Louis, 2005, Mosby.

Fig 7-4.   Aehlert B, Pediatric Advanced Life Support Study Guide, 2e. St. Louis, 2005, Mosby.

Fig 7-5.   Dieckmann R, Fiser D, Selbst, Illustrated Textbook of Pediatric Emergency & Critical Care Procedures, 1e. St. Louis, 1997, Mosby.

Fig 7-6.   Shade B, Rothenberg M, Wertz E, Jones S, Collins T. Mosby's EMT-Intermediate Textbook, 2e. St. Louis, 2002, Mosby.

Fig 7-7.   Aehlert B, ACLS Quick Review Study Guide, 2e. St. Louis, 2002, Mosby.

Fig 7-8 A.   Aehlert B, ACLS Quick Review Study Guide, 2e. St. Louis, 2002, Mosby.

Fig 7-8 B.   EMSC Slide Set (CD-ROM). 1996. Courtesy of the Emergency Medical Services for Children Program, administered by the U.S. Department of Health and Human Service's Health Resources and Services Administration, Maternal and Child Health Bureau.

Fig 7-9.   Hockenberry M, Wilson D, Winkelstein M, Kline N, Wong's Nursing Care of Infants and Children, 7e. St. Louis, 2002, Mosby.

Fig 7-10 A.   Aehlert B, Pediatric Advanced Life Support Study Guide, 2e. St. Louis, 2005, Mosby.

Fig 7-10 B&C. EMSC Slide Set (CD-ROM). 1996. Courtesy of the Emergency Medical Services for Children Program, administered by the U.S. Department of Health and Human Service's Health Resources and Services Administration, Maternal and Child Health Bureau.

Fig 7-11.   Aehlert B, Pediatric Advanced Life Support Study Guide, 2e. St. Louis, 2005, Mosby.

Fig 7-12.   Sanders M, Mosby's Paramedic Textbook, revised 2e. St. Louis, 2001, Mosby.

Fig 7-13.   Aehlert B, Pediatric Advanced Life Support Study Guide, 2e. St. Louis, 2005, Mosby.

Fig 7-14.   Sanders M, Mosby's Paramedic Textbook, revised 2e. St. Louis, 2001, Mosby.

Fig 7-15.   Sanders M, Mosby's Paramedic Textbook, revised 2e. St. Louis, 2001, Mosby.

Fig 7-16.   Aehlert B, Pediatric Advanced Life Support Study Guide, 2e. St. Louis, 2005, Mosby.

Fig 7-17.   Dieckmann R, Fiser D, Selbst, Illustrated Textbook of Pediatric Emergency & Critical Care Procedures, 1e. St. Louis, 1997, Mosby.

Fig 7-18.   Aehlert B, Pediatric Advanced Life Support Study Guide, 2e. St. Louis, 2005, Mosby.

Fig 7-19.   Dieckmann R, Fiser D, Selbst, Illustrated Textbook of Pediatric Emergency & Critical Care Procedures, 1e. St. Louis, 1997, Mosby.

Fig 7-20 A.   Dieckmann R, Fiser D, Selbst, Illustrated Textbook of Pediatric Emergency & Critical Care Procedures, 1e. St. Louis, 1997, Mosby.

Fig 7-20 B.   EMSC Slide Set (CD-ROM). 1996. Courtesy of the Emergency Medical Services for Children Program, administered by the U.S. Department of Health and Human Service's Health Resources and Services Administration, Maternal and Child Health Bureau.

Fig 7-21.   EMSC Slide Set (CD-ROM). 1996. Courtesy of the Emergency Medical Services for Children Program, administered by the U.S. Department of Health and Human Service's Health Resources and Services Administration, Maternal and Child Health Bureau.

Fig 7-22.   Dieckmann R, Fiser D, Selbst, Illustrated Textbook of Pediatric Emergency & Critical Care Procedures, 1e. St. Louis, 1997, Mosby.

Fig 7-23.   Dieckmann R, Fiser D, Selbst, Illustrated Textbook of Pediatric Emergency & Critical Care Procedures, 1e. St. Louis, 1997, Mosby.

Fig 7-24.   Dieckmann R, Fiser D, Selbst, Illustrated Textbook of Pediatric Emergency & Critical Care Procedures, 1e. St. Louis, 1997, Mosby.

Fig 7-25 A-E.   Roberts JR, Hedges JR, Clinical Procedures in Emergency Medicine, 3e. Philadelphia, 1998, WB Sanders.

Fig 7-26.   Courtesy of Medtronic, Inc.

Fig 7-27 A&B.   Courtesy of Medtronic, Inc.

Fig 7-28 A.   EMSC Slide Set (CD-ROM). 1996. Courtesy of the Emergency Medical Services for Children Program, administered by the U.S. Department of Health and Human Service's Health Resources and Services Administration, Maternal and Child Health Bureau.

Fig 7-28 B.   Aehlert B, Pediatric Advanced Life Support Study Guide, 2e. St. Louis, 2005, Mosby.

Fig 7-29.   American College of Emergency Physicians (Editors: Pons P, Carson D), Paramedic Field Care: A Complaint-Based Approach, St. Louis, 1997, Mosby.

Fig 7-30 A&B.   Images provided courtesy of Philips Medical Systems.

Fig 7-31.   Aehlert B, ECGs Made Easy, 2e. St. Louis, 2002, Mosby.

Fig 7-32.   Aehlert B, ECGs Made Easy, 2e. St. Louis, 2002, Mosby.

Question 4.   Aehlert B, ECGs Made Easy, St. Louis, 2002, Mosby.

Question 13.   Aehlert B, ACLS Quick Review Study Guide, 2e. St. Louis, 2002, Mosby.

Chapter Eight

Fig 8-1.   Herlihy B, The Human Body in Health and Illness, 2e. St. Louis, 2003, WB Saunders.

Fig 8-2.   Hockenberry M, Wilson D, Winkelstein M, Kline N, Wong's Nursing Care of Infants and Children, 7e. St. Louis, 2002, Mosby.

Fig 8-3.   Hockenberry M, Wilson D, Winkelstein M, Kline N, Wong's Nursing Care of Infants and Children, 7e. St. Louis, 2002, Mosby.

Fig 8-4.   Dieckmann R, Fiser D, Selbst, Illustrated Textbook of Pediatric Emergency & Critical Care Procedures, 1e. St. Louis, 1997, Mosby.

Fig 8-5.   Dieckmann R, Fiser D, Selbst, Illustrated Textbook of Pediatric Emergency & Critical Care Procedures, 1e. St. Louis, 1997, Mosby.

Fig 8-6.   Hockenberry M, Wilson D, Winkelstein M, Kline N, Wong's Nursing Care of Infants and Children, 7e. St. Louis, 2002, Mosby.

Fig 8-7.   Hockenberry M, Wilson D, Winkelstein M, Kline N, Wong's Nursing Care of Infants and Children, 7e. St. Louis, 2002, Mosby.

Fig 8-8.   Hockenberry M, Wilson D, Winkelstein M, Kline N, Wong's Nursing Care of Infants and Children, 7e. St. Louis, 2002, Mosby.

Fig 8-9.   Hockenberry M, Wilson D, Winkelstein M, Kline N, Wong's Nursing Care of Infants and Children, 7e. St. Louis, 2002, Mosby.

Fig 8-10.   Hockenberry M, Wilson D, Winkelstein M, Kline N, Wong's Nursing Care of Infants and Children, 7e. St. Louis, 2002, Mosby.

Fig 8-11.   Hockenberry M, Wong's Essentials of Pediatric Nursing, 7e. St. Louis, 2005, Mosby.

Fig 8-12.   Hockenberry M, Wilson D, Winkelstein M, Kline N, Wong's Nursing Care of Infants and Children, 7e. St. Louis, 2002, Mosby.

Chapter Nine

Fig 9-1.   EMSC Slide Set (CD-ROM). 1996. Courtesy of the Emergency Medical Services for Children Program, administered by the U.S. Department of Health and Human Service's Health Resources and Services Administration, Maternal and Child Health Bureau.

Fig 9-2.   American College of Emergency Physicians (Editors: Pons P, Carson D), Paramedic Field Care: A Complaint-Based Approach, St. Louis, 1997, Mosby.

Fig 9-3.   McSwain N, Paturas J, The Basic EMT: Comprehensive Prehospital Patient Care, 2e. St. Louis, 2003, Mosby.

Fig 9-4.   McSwain N, Paturas J, The Basic EMT: Comprehensive Prehospital Patient Care, 2e. St. Louis, 2003, Mosby.

Fig 9-5.   McSwain N, Paturas J, The Basic EMT: Comprehensive Prehospital Patient Care, 2e. St. Louis, 2003, Mosby.

Fig 9-6.   Prehospital Trauma Life Support Committee of the NAEMT, PHTLS: Basic and Advanced Prehospital Trauma Life Support, 5e. St. Louis, 2003, Mosby.

Fig 9-7.   Prehospital Trauma Life Support Committee of the NAEMT, PHTLS: Basic and Advanced Prehospital Trauma Life Support, 5e. St. Louis, 2003, Mosby.

Fig 9-8.   Prehospital Trauma Life Support Committee of the NAEMT, PHTLS: Basic and Advanced Prehospital Trauma Life Support, 5e. St. Louis, 2003, Mosby.

Fig 9-9.   Zitelli B, Davis H, Atlas of Pediatric Physical Diagnosis, 4e. St. Louis, 2002, Mosby.

Fig 9-10.   Courtesy Ernest W. Beck.

Fig 9-11.   Gould B, Pathophysiology for the Health Professions, 2e. Philadelphia, 2002, WB Saunders.

Fig 9-12.   Gould B, Pathophysiology for the Health Professions, 2e. Philadelphia, 2002, WB Saunders.

Fig 9-13.   Zitelli B, Davis H, Atlas of Pediatric Physical Diagnosis, 4e. St. Louis, 2002, Mosby.

Fig 9-14.   Zitelli B, Davis H, Atlas of Pediatric Physical Diagnosis, 4e. St. Louis, 2002, Mosby.

Fig 9-15.   Sheehy S, Emergency Nursing, 3e. St. Louis, 1992, Mosby.

Fig 9-16.   Gould B, Pathophysiology for the Health Professions, 2e. Philadelphia, 2002, WB Saunders.

Fig 9-17.   Prehospital Trauma Life Support Committee of the NAEMT, PHTLS: Basic and Advanced Prehospital Trauma Life Support, 5e. St. Louis, 2003, Mosby.

Fig 9-18.   Prehospital Trauma Life Support Committee of the NAEMT, PHTLS: Basic and Advanced Prehospital Trauma Life Support, 5e. St. Louis, 2003, Mosby.

Fig 9-19.   Prehospital Trauma Life Support Committee of the NAEMT, PHTLS: Basic and Advanced Prehospital Trauma Life Support, 5e. St. Louis, 2003, Mosby.

Fig 9-20.   Prehospital Trauma Life Support Committee of the NAEMT, PHTLS: Basic and Advanced Prehospital Trauma Life Support, 5e. St. Louis, 2003, Mosby.

Fig 9-21 A-C.   Shade B, Rothenberg M, Wertz E, Jones S, Collins T, Mosby's EMT-Intermediate Textbook, 2e. St. Louis, 2002, Mosby.

Fig 9-22 A&B. Shade B, Rothenberg M, Wertz E, Jones S, Collins T, Mosby's EMT-Intermediate Textbook, 2e. St. Louis, 2002, Mosby.

Fig 9-23 A-D.   Shade B, Rothenberg M, Wertz E, Jones S, Collins T, Mosby's EMT-Intermediate Textbook, 2e. St. Louis, 2002, Mosby.

Fig 9-24.   Courtesy Kristen Burke.

Fig 9-25.   Gould B, Pathophysiology for the Health Professions, 2e. Philadelphia, 2002, WB Saunders.

Fig 9-26.   Gould B, Pathophysiology for the Health Professions, 2e. Philadelphia, 2002, WB Saunders.

Fig 9-27.   Gould B, Pathophysiology for the Health Professions, 2e. Philadelphia, 2002, WB Saunders.

Fig 9-28.   Sanders M, Mosby's Paramedic Textbook, revised 2e. St. Louis, 2001, Mosby.

Fig 9-29.   Gould B, Pathophysiology for the Health Professions, 2e. Philadelphia, 2002, WB Saunders.

Fig 9-30.   Courtesy Kristen Burke.

Fig 9-31.   American College of Emergency Physicians (Editor: Krohmer J), EMT-Basic Field Care: A Case Based Approach, St. Louis, 1999, Mosby.

Fig 9-32.   Gould B, Pathophysiology for the Health Professions, 2e. Philadelphia, 2002, WB Saunders.

Fig 9-33.   McSwain N, Paturas J, The Basic EMT: Comprehensive Prehospital Patient Care, 2e. St. Louis, 2003, Mosby.

Chapter Ten

Fig 10-1 A.   Zitelli B, Davis H, Atlas of Pediatric Physical Diagnosis, 4e. St. Louis, 2002, Mosby.

Fig 10-1 B.   Courtesy Robert Hickey, M.D.

Fig 10-1 C.   Courtesy Michael Sherlock, M.D.

Fig 10-2 A,B,E. Habif T: Clinical Dermatology, 4e. St. Louis, 2004, Mosby.

Fig 10-2 C&D.   Gershon A, et al, Krugman's Infectious Diseases of Children, 11e. St. Louis, 2004, Mosby.

Fig 10-3 A.   Gershon A, et al, Krugman's Infectious Diseases of Children, 11e. St. Louis, 2004, Mosby.

Fig 10-3 B.   Courtesy Michael Sherlock, M.D.

Fig 10-4 A&B.   Habif T: Clinical Dermatology, 4e. St. Louis, 2004, Mosby.

Fig 10-5 A&B.   Habif T: Clinical Dermatology, 4e. St. Louis, 2004, Mosby.

Fig 10-6 A-C.   Habif T: Clinical Dermatology, 4e. St. Louis, 2004, Mosby.

Fig 10-7.   Cohen J, Powderly W: Infectious Diseases, 2e. Philadelphia, 2004, WB Saunders.

Fig 10-8 A&B.   Cohen J, Powderly W: Infectious Diseases, 2e. Philadelphia, 2004, WB Saunders.

Fig 10-9 A-D.   Zitelli B, Davis H, Atlas of Pediatric Physical Diagnosis, 4e. St. Louis, 2002, Mosby.

Fig 10-10.   Zitelli B, Davis H, Atlas of Pediatric Physical Diagnosis, 4e. St. Louis, 2002, Mosby.

Fig 10-11.   Herlihy B, The Human Body in Health and Illness, St. Louis, 2000, WB Saunders.

Fig 10-12.   Gould B, Pathophysiology for the Health Professions, 2e. Philadelphia, 2002, WB Saunders.

Fig 10-13.   Gould B, Pathophysiology for the Health Professions, 2e. Philadelphia, 2002, WB Saunders.

Fig 10-14.   Behrman R, Kliegman R, Jenson H, Nelson Textbook of Pediatrics, 17e. Philadelphia, 2004, WB Saunders.

Chapter Eleven

Fig 11-1.   McSwain N, Paturas J, The Basic EMT: Comprehensive Prehospital Patient Care, 2e. St. Louis, 2003, Mosby.

Fig 11-2.   American College of Emergency Physicians (Editors: Pons P, Carson D), Paramedic Field Care: A Complaint-Based Approach, St. Louis, 1997, Mosby.

Chapter Twelve

Fig 12-1.   McSwain N, Paturas J, The Basic EMT: Comprehensive Prehospital Patient Care, 2e. St. Louis, 2003, Mosby.

Fig 12-2.   Henry M, Stapleton E, EMT Prehospital Care, 3e. St. Louis, 2004, Mosby.

Fig 12-3.   Henry M, Stapleton E, EMT Prehospital Care, 3e. St. Louis, 2004, Mosby.

Fig 12-4.   Henry M, Stapleton E, EMT Prehospital Care, 3e. St. Louis, 2004, Mosby.

Chapter Thirteen

Fig 13-1.   Zitelli B, Davis H, Atlas of Pediatric Physical Diagnosis, 4e. St. Louis, 2002, Mosby.

Fig 13-2.   Zitelli B, Davis H, Atlas of Pediatric Physical Diagnosis, 4e. St. Louis, 2002, Mosby.

Fig 13-3.   Courtesy Dr. Kent Hymel.

Fig 13-4.   Zitelli B, Davis H, Atlas of Pediatric Physical Diagnosis, 4e. St. Louis, 2002, Mosby.

Fig 13-5.   Courtesy Dr. Thomas Layton.

Fig 13-6.   Zitelli B, Davis H, Atlas of Pediatric Physical Diagnosis, 4e. St. Louis, 2002, Mosby.

Fig 13-7.   Zitelli B, Davis H, Atlas of Pediatric Physical Diagnosis, 4e. St. Louis, 2002, Mosby.

Fig 13-8.   Zitelli B, Davis H, Atlas of Pediatric Physical Diagnosis, 4e. St. Louis, 2002, Mosby.

Fig 13-9.   Zitelli B, Davis H, Atlas of Pediatric Physical Diagnosis, 4e. St. Louis, 2002, Mosby.

Chapter Fifteen

Fig 15-1.   Copyright American College of Emergency Physicians and American Academy of Pediatrics. Permission to reprint is granted with acknowledgement.

Fig 15-2.   Zitelli B, Davis H, Atlas of Pediatric Physical Diagnosis, 4e. St. Louis, 2002, Mosby.

Fig 15-3.   Smith E, Adirim T, Singh Tasmeen, Special Kids, Special Care: Emergency management of children with special health-care needs. MyWebCE.com, 1999.

Fig 15-4.   Chaudhry B, Harvey D, Mosby's Color Atlas and Text of Pediatrics and Child Health, London, 2001, Mosby.

Fig 15-5 A.   Wong DL: Nursing Care of Infants and Children, 5e. St. Louis, 1994, Mosby.

Fig 15-5 B.   Sanders M, Mosby's Paramedic Textbook, revised 2e. St. Louis, 2001, Mosby.

Fig 15-6.   Cohen J, Powderly W: Infectious Diseases, 2e. Philadelphia, 2004, WB Saunders.

Fig 15-7.   Cohen J, Powderly W: Infectious Diseases, 2e. Philadelphia, 2004, WB Saunders.

Fig 15-8.   Cohen J, Powderly W: Infectious Diseases, 2e. Philadelphia, 2004, WB Saunders.

Fig 15-9.   Hockenberry M, Wilson D, Winkelstein M, Kline N, Wong's Nursing Care of Infants and Children, 7e. St. Louis, 2002, Mosby.

Fig 15-10.   American College of Emergency Physicians (Editors: Pons P, Carson D), Paramedic Field Care: A Complaint-Based Approach, St. Louis, 1997, Mosby.

Fig 15-11.   Henry M, Stapleton E, EMT Prehospital Care, 3e. St. Louis, 2004, Mosby.

Fig 15-12.   Chaudhry B, Harvey D, Mosby's Color Atlas and Text of Pediatrics and Child Health, London, 2001, Mosby.

Fig 15-13 A.   Sanders M, Mosby's Paramedic Textbook, revised 2e. St. Louis, 2001, Mosby.

Fig 15-13 B.   Hockenberry M, Wilson D, Winkelstein M, Kline N, Wong's Nursing Care of Infants and Children, 7e. St. Louis, 2002, Mosby.

Fig 15-14 A.   Courtesy Smiths Medical ASD, Inc.

Fig 15-14 B.   Courtesy Smiths Medical ASD, Inc.

Fig 15-14 C.   Courtesy Smiths Medical ASD, Inc.

Fig 15-15.   Reprinted by permission of Nellcor Puritan Bennett Inc., Pleasanton, California.

Fig 15-16.   Roberts JR, Hedges JR, Clinical Procedures in Emergency Medicine, 3e. Philadelphia, 1998, W. B. Saunders.

Fig 15-17.   Reprinted by permission of Nellcor Puritan Bennett Inc., Pleasanton, California.

Fig 15-18.   Henry M, Stapleton E, EMT Prehospital Care, 3e. St. Louis, 2004, Mosby.

Fig 15-19.   McSwain N, Paturas J: The Basic EMT, Comprehensive Prehospital Patient Care, St. Louis, 2003, Mosby.

Fig 15-20.   Reprinted by permission of Nellcor Puritan Bennett Inc., Pleasanton, California.

Fig 15-21.   Dieckmann R, Fiser D, Selbst, Illustrated Textbook of Pediatric Emergency & Critical Care Procedures, 1e. St. Louis, 1997, Mosby.

Fig 15-22.   Dieckmann R, Fiser D, Selbst, Illustrated Textbook of Pediatric Emergency & Critical Care Procedures, 1e. St. Louis, 1997, Mosby.

Fig 15-23.   Hockenberry M, Wilson D, Winkelstein M, Kline N, Wong's Nursing Care of Infants and Children, 7e. St. Louis, 2002, Mosby.

Fig 15-24.   Hockenberry M, Wilson D, Winkelstein M, Kline N, Wong's Nursing Care of Infants and Children, 7e. St. Louis, 2002, Mosby.

Fig 15-25.   Hockenberry M, Wilson D, Winkelstein M, Kline N, Wong's Nursing Care of Infants and Children, 7e. St. Louis, 2002, Mosby.

Fig 15-26.   Courtesy Cook Incorporated, Bloomington, Indiana.

Chapter Sixteen

Fig 16-1.   Courtesy Kevin A. Somerville.

Fig 16-2.   American College of Emergency Physicians (Editors: Pons P, Carson D), Paramedic Field Care: A Complaint-Based Approach, St. Louis, 1997, Mosby.

Fig 16-3.   McSwain N, Paturas J, The Basic EMT: Comprehensive Prehospital Patient Care, 2e. St. Louis, 2003, Mosby.

Fig 16-4.   Stoy W/Center for Emergency Medicine, Mosby's EMT-Basic Textbook, St. Louis, 1996, Mosby-Year Book.

Fig 16-5.   Al-Azzawi F, Color Atlas of Childbirth and Obstetrics, London, 1995, Mosby-Wolfe.

Fig 16-6.   Al-Azzawi F, Color Atlas of Childbirth and Obstetrics, London, 1995, Mosby-Wolfe.

Fig 16-7.   Stoy W/Center for Emergency Medicine, Mosby's EMT-Basic Textbook, St. Louis, 1996, Mosby-Year Book.

Fig 16-8.   Stoy W/Center for Emergency Medicine, Mosby's EMT-Basic Textbook, St. Louis, 1996, Mosby-Year Book.

Fig 16-9.   Al-Azzawi F, Color Atlas of Childbirth and Obstetrics, London, 1995, Mosby-Wolfe.

Fig 16-10.   Al-Azzawi F, Color Atlas of Childbirth and Obstetrics, London, 1995, Mosby-Wolfe.

Fig 16-11.   Al-Azzawi F, Color Atlas of Childbirth and Obstetrics, London, 1995, Mosby-Wolfe.

Fig 16-12.   Sanders M, Mosby's Paramedic Textbook, revised 2e. St. Louis, 2001, Mosby.

Fig 16-13.   Bobak I, Lowdermilk D, Jensen M: Maternity Nursing, 4e. St. Louis, 1995, Mosby.

Fig 16-14.   Reproduced with permission, PALS Provides Manual © 2002, American Heart Association.

Fig 16-15.   Reprinted by permission of Nellcor Puritan Bennett Inc., Pleasanton, California.

Fig 16-16.   McSwain N, Paturas J, The Basic EMT: Comprehensive Prehospital Patient Care, 2e. St. Louis, 2003, Mosby.

Fig 16-17.   Chaudhry B, Harvey D, Mosby's Color Atlas and Text of Pediatrics & Child Health, London, 2001, Mosby.

Fig 16-18.   Courtesy Marjorie M. Pyle.

Fig 16-19.   Dieckmann R, Fiser D, Selbst, Illustrated Textbook of Pediatric Emergency & Critical Care Procedures, 1e. St. Louis, 1997, Mosby.

Fig 16-20.   Dieckmann R, Fiser D, Selbst, Illustrated Textbook of Pediatric Emergency & Critical Care Procedures, 1e. St. Louis, 1997, Mosby.

Fig 16-21.   Sanders M, Mosby's Paramedic Textbook, revised 2e. St. Louis, 2001, Mosby.

Glossary

Adrenergic   Having the characteristics of the sympathetic division of the autonomic nervous system.

Afterload   The pressure or resistance against which the ventricles must pump to eject blood.

Agonist   A drug or substance that produces a predictable response (stimulates action).

ALTE   Apparent life-threatening event, a nonfatal condition characterized by apnea continuing for more than 20 seconds, especially when accompanied by cyanosis, atony, or unresponsiveness.

Amnesia   Lack of memory about events occurring during a particular period.

Analgesia   Absence of pain in response to stimulation that would normally be painful.

Anaphylaxis   A severe allergic response to a foreign substance with which the patient has had prior contact.

Anemia   A condition in which oxygen-transporting material in the blood (such as erythrocytes) is abnormally low.

Anesthesia   A state of unconsciousness.

Antagonist   An agent that exerts an opposite action to another (blocks action).

Antepartum   The maternal period before delivery.

Anticholinergic   Antagonistic to the action of parasympathetic (cholinergic) nerve fibers.

Antidote   A substance that neutralizes a poison.

Anxiolysis   Relief of apprehension and uneasiness without alteration of awareness.

Arrhythmia   Term often used interchangeably with "dysrhythmia"; any disturbance or abnormality in a normal rhythmic pattern; any cardiac rhythm other than a sinus rhythm.

Artifact   Distortion of an electrocardiogram (ECG) tracing by electrical activity that is noncardiac in origin (e.g., electrical interference, poor electrical conduction, patient movement).

Assistive technology   A term used to describe devices that are used by children and adults with a disability to compensate for functional limitations and to enhance and increase learning, independence, mobility, communication, environmental control, and choice.

Asystole   Absence of cardiac electrical activity viewed as a straight (isoelectric) line on the ECG.

Atelectasis   The absence of air in part or the entire lung; may be chronic or acute; may be caused by secretions, obstruction by foreign bodies, or compression.

Atony   Lack of muscle tone; flaccidity.

Attention deficit/hyperactivity disorder (ADHD)   A behavioral syndrome characterized by a persistent pattern of inattention/easy distractibility, behavioral and emotional impulsivity, and *sometimes* hyperactivity or severe restlessness.

Bacteremia   The presence of viable bacteria in the blood.

Baroreceptors   Specialized nerve tissue (sensors) located in the internal carotid arteries and the aortic arch that detect changes in blood pressure and cause a reflex response in either the sympathetic or the parasympathetic division of the autonomic nervous system; pressoreceptors.

Barotrauma   Lung damage due to excessive ventilatory pressure.

Bpm   Abbreviation for beats per minute. The abbreviation bpm usually refers to an intrinsic heart rate, while pulses per minute (ppm) usually refers to a paced rate.

BiPAP   Bilevel positive airway pressure; a form of noninvasive, positive-pressure mechanical ventilation.

Blood pressure   The force exerted by the blood on the inner walls of the blood vessels.

Blunt trauma   Any mechanism of injury that occurs without actual penetration of the body; typically results from motor vehicle crashes, falls, or assaults with a blunt object.

Bronchiole   A small air passage in the lower airway.

Bronchiolitis   Inflammation of the bronchioles.

Bronchomalacia   Degeneration of elastic and connective tissue of the bronchi and trachea, causing collapse and relative upper airway obstruction during inhalation.

Bronchopulmonary dysplasia   A chronic lung disease characterized by persistent respiratory distress.

Bronchospasm   An abnormal contraction of the smooth muscle of the bronchi, resulting in acute narrowing and obstruction.

Brudzinski's sign   Involuntary flexion of the patient's lower extremities (hips and knees) when the neck is flexed constitutes a positive sign of meningeal irritation; thought to be caused by the irritation of motor nerve roots passing through inflamed meninges as the roots are brought under tension.

Capacitor   A device for storing an electrical charge.

Capnography   The continuous analysis and recording of carbon dioxide concentrations in respiratory gases.

Capnometer   A device that measures the concentration of carbon dioxide at the end of exhalation

Capnometry   The measurement of carbon dioxide concentrations without a continuous written record or waveform.

Carboxyhemoglobin   The resultant product when the oxygen in hemoglobin is displaced by carbon monoxide so that red blood cells cannot transport oxygen from the lungs to the tissues.

Cardiac arrest   The cessation of cardiac mechanical activity, confirmed by the absence of a detectable pulse, unresponsiveness, and apnea or agonal, gasping respiration.

Cardiac output   The amount of blood pumped into the aorta each minute by the heart. It is calculated as the stroke volume (amount of blood ejected from a ventricle with each heart beat) times the heart rate.

Cardiomyopathy   A disease of the heart muscle that affects the heart's pumping ability.

Carina   The point where the trachea bifurcates into the right and left mainstem bronchi (approximately the level of the fifth or sixth thoracic vertebra).

Caustic   Capable of burning or destroying tissue by chemical action.

Cerebral resuscitation   A term used to emphasize the need to preserve the cerebral viability of the cardiac arrest victim.

Chance fracture   A horizontal fracture of the thoracic or lumbar spine caused by hyperflexion injuries with little or no compression of the vertebral body; also called a seat-belt fracture, because they are commonly associated with the wearing of lap-type seat belts.

Chelation   Use of a chemical compound that combines with a heavy metal for rapid, safe excretion.

Chronotrope   A substance affecting heart rate.

Clonic   Rhythmic muscle contraction and relaxation.

Cognitive disability   An impairment that affects an individual's awareness, memory, and ability to learn, process information, communicate, and make decisions.

Compensated shock   Inadequate tissue perfusion without hypotension (i.e., shock with a "normal" blood pressure).

Compliance   The resistance of the patient's lung tissue to ventilation.

Continuous positive airway pressure (CPAP)   The delivery of a steady, gentle flow of air by means of a medical device through a soft mask worn over the nose or over the mouth and nose.

Costochondritis   An inflammation of the cartilage that connects the inner end of each rib to the sternum.

Crackles   High-pitched breath sounds (formerly referred to as rales) that indicate lower airway pathology, such as pneumonia or asthma.

Crepitation   A fine crackling sound resembling that of a hair rubbed between the fingers or a grating sensation felt over a fracture or an area of subcutaneous air.

Cricoid pressure   The use of gentle, continuous downward pressure on the cricoid cartilage of the larynx; intended to aid in protection from aspiration by compressing the larynx against the esophagus.

Cricothyroid membrane   A fibrous membrane located between the cricoid and thyroid cartilage; site for surgical and alternative airway placement.

Croup   Respiratory distress caused by narrowing below the glottis characterized by hoarseness, inspiratory stridor, and a barklike cough.

Crowing   Abnormal respiratory sound that suggests narrowing of the tracheal opening and laryngeal spasm.

Cullen's sign   A bluish discoloration around the umbilicus that may indicate intraabdominal or retroperitoneal hemorrhage.

Cushing's triad   Hypertension, bradycardia, and abnormal respirations resulting from increased intracranial pressure.

Cystic fibrosis   A hereditary disease of the exocrine glands characterized by production of viscous mucus that obstructs the bronchi.

Dactylitis   "Hand-foot syndrome"; symmetric, nonpitting swelling of the hands and/or feet, accompanied by warmth and tenderness, in a patient with sickle cell disease.

Decannulation   The removal of a cannula; in the case of a child with a tracheostomy, the removal of the tracheostomy tube.

Decannulation cap   A cap located in the outer cannula of a fenestrated tracheostomy tube that blocks airflow through the stoma.

Decompensated shock   A clinical state of tissue perfusion that is inadequate to meet the body's metabolic demands accompanied by hypotension; also called progressive or late shock.

Defasciculation agent   A medication that is given to inhibit muscle twitching.

Defibrillation   The therapeutic delivery of unsynchronized electrical current through the myocardium over a very brief period to terminate a cardiac dysrhythmia.

Defibrillation threshold   The least amount of energy in joules or volts delivered to the heart that reproducibly converts ventricular fibrillation to a perfusing rhythm.

Defibrillator   A device used to administer an electrical shock at a preset voltage to terminate a cardiac dysrhythmia.

Delusions   False, strongly held beliefs not influenced by logical reasoning or explained by a person's usual cultural concepts.

Diaphoresis   Profuse sweating.

Diarrhea   An alteration in a normal bowel movement characterized by an increase in the water content, volume, or frequency of stools.

Distraction   In pain management, the strategy of focusing one's attention on stimuli other than pain or the accompanying negative emotions.

Diuretic   A medication that increases urine output; used to treat hypertension, congestive heart failure, and edema.

Dromotrope   A substance that affects atrioventricular (AV) conduction velocity.

Drowning   Death from suffocation in a liquid.

Drug   Any chemical compound that produces an effect on a living organism.

Dyspnea   Difficulty breathing; shortness of breath.

Endocarditis   An infection of the heart valves and the inner lining of the heart muscle.

Endotracheal   Within or through the trachea.

Endotracheal intubation   An advanced airway procedure in which a tube is placed directly into the trachea.

Epiglottis   A small, leaf-shaped cartilage located at the top of the larynx that prevents food from entering the respiratory tract during swallowing.

Epiglottitis   A bacterial infection of the epiglottis and supraglottic structures; also called acute supraglottitis.

Epithelium   The cellular, avascular layer covering tissue surfaces.

ET   Endotracheal.

ETT   Endotracheal tube.

Extravasation   The actual (unintentional) escape or leakage of an agent that is irritating and causes blistering (a vesicant) from a vessel into the surrounding tissue.

Fasciculations   Involuntary muscle twitches.

Gasp   Inhaling and exhaling with quick, difficult breaths.

Gastrostomy   A surgically created passageway between the skin and the stomach through which a tube is placed to provide nutrients or medication.

General anesthesia   A controlled state of unconsciousness accompanied by partial or complete loss of protective reflexes, including inability to maintain an airway independently and inability to respond purposefully to physical stimulation or verbal command.

Glottis   The true vocal cords and the space between them.

Gravida   Refers to the number of a woman's current and past pregnancies.

Grey-Turner's sign   Bruising of the flanks that may indicate intraabdominal hemorrhage, often splenic (retroperitoneal) in origin.

Grunting   A short, low-pitched sound heard at the end of exhalation that represents an attempt to generate positive end-expiratory pressure (PEEP) by exhaling against a closed glottis, prolonging the period of oxygen and carbon dioxide exchange across the alveolar-capillary membrane; a compensatory mechanism to help maintain patency of small airways and prevent atelectasis.

Gurgling   Abnormal respiratory sound associated with collection of liquid or semisolid material in the patient's upper airway.

Hallucination   Hearing, seeing, or otherwise sensing the presence of things not actually there.

Hard palate   The bony portion of the roof of the mouth that forms the floor of the nasal cavity.

Head bobbing   Indicator of increased work of breathing in infants; the head falls forward with exhalation and comes up with expansion of the chest on inhalation.

Hemoglobin   The red oxygen-binding protein of erythrocytes.

Hemoptysis   Expectoration of blood that originates in the lungs or bronchi.

Hemorrhage   An acute loss of circulating blood.

Herniation   Protrusion of a structure through tissues normally containing it.

His-Purkinje system   The portion of the conduction system consisting of the bundle of His, bundle branches, and Purkinje fibers.

Hypoperfusion   The inadequate circulation of blood through an organ or a part of the body; shock.

Hypotonia   Decreased muscle tone.

Hypoxemia   In adults, children, and infants older than 28 days, hypoxemia is defined as an arterial oxygen tension (PaO_2) of less than 60 torr or arterial oxygen saturation (SaO_2) of less than 90% in an individual breathing room air or with a PaO_2 and/or SaO_2 below the desirable range for a specific clinical situation.

Hypoxia   A deficiency of oxygen reaching the tissues of the body.

Hyperpnea   Abnormally deep breathing.

Iatrogenic   A response to a medical or surgical treatment induced by the treatment itself.

Immersion syndrome   Death following submersion in extremely cold water.

Impedance   Resistance to the flow of current. Transthoracic impedance (resistance) refers to the resistance of the chest wall to current.

Induction   The use of pharmacologic agents, whether it be intravenous solutions or inhaled gases, that act on the brain to quickly move from consciousness to unconsciousness; to create a plane or level of anesthesia.

Infectious diarrhea   Diarrhea due to an infectious cause, often accompanied by symptoms of nausea, vomiting, or abdominal cramps.

Infiltration   The intentional or unintentional process in which a substance enters or infuses into another substance or a surrounding area.

Inherent   Natural, intrinsic.

Inotrope   A substance that affects myocardial contractility.

Inotropic effect   Refers to a change in myocardial contractility.

Interval   A waveform and a segment; in pacing, the period, measured in milliseconds, between any two designated cardiac events.

Intraosseous infusion (IOI)   The infusion of fluids, medications, or blood directly into the bone marrow cavity.

Intravenous cannulation   The placement of a catheter into a vein to gain access to the body's venous circulation.

Intrinsic rate   Rate at which a pacemaker of the heart normally generates impulses.

Intubation   Passing a tube into a body opening. When used alone, the term implies endotracheal intubation (placement of a tube into the trachea).

Ischemia   A decreased supply of oxygenated blood to a body part or organ.

Isoelectric line   An absence of electrical activity observed on the ECG as a straight line.

J point   The point where the QRS complex and ST-segment meet.

Joule   The basic unit of energy; equivalent to watt-seconds.

Kawasaki disease   An inflammation of the walls of small and medium arteries throughout the body; the leading cause of acquired heart disease in children.

Kehr's sign   Left upper quadrant pain with radiation to the left shoulder suggests injury to the spleen or liver (pain occurs because of blood or bile irritating the diaphragm).

Kernig's sign   Patient's leg is flexed 90 degrees at the hip and then extended; the inability to extend the patient's knees beyond 135 degrees without causing pain constitutes a positive test (sign of meningeal irritation); thought to be caused by the irritation of motor nerve roots passing through inflamed meninges as the roots are brought under tension.

Kinematics   The process of predicting injury patterns.

KVO   Abbreviation meaning, "keep the vein open." Also known as TKO, "to keep open."

Laryngoscope   An instrument used to examine the interior of the larynx. During endotracheal intubation, the device is used to visualize the glottic opening.

Laryngotracheobronchitis   Croup.

Lead   An electrical connection attached to the body to record electrical activity.

Learning disability   A general term that refers to a group of disorders manifested by significant difficulties in the acquisition and use of listening, spelling, reading, writing, reasoning, or mathematic skills.

Ligation   Tying.

Medication   Drugs used in the practice of medicine as a remedy.

Membrane potential   A difference in electrical charge across the cell membrane.

Mental impairment   Any mental or psychological disorder, such as mental retardation, organic brain syndrome, emotional or mental illness, and specific learning disabilities.

Milliampere (mA)   The unit of measure of electrical current needed to elicit depolarization of the myocardium.

Minute volume   The amount of air moved in and out of the lungs in one minute; determined by multiplying the tidal volume by the respiratory rate.

Monomorphic   Having the same shape.

Moro reflex (also called startle response, startle reflex, embrace reflex)   A primitive reflex present at birth that typically disappears by the age of about 4 to 6 months. When an infant is startled by a loud noise or sudden movement, the arms are thrown apart with the palms up and the thumbs flexed, the legs extend, and the head is thrown back. As the reflex ends, the infant draws the arms back to the body, elbows flexed, and then relaxes. The reflex should be brisk and symmetric. Absence of this reflex in an infant is abnormal. Presence of a Moro reflex in an older infant, child, or adult is also abnormal. Absence of this reflex on one side suggests a fractured clavicle or injury to the brachial plexus, possibly due to birth trauma. Two-sided absence of this reflex suggests damage to the brain or spinal cord.

Multiple organ dysfunction syndrome (MODS)   The progressive failure of two or more organ systems after a very severe illness or injury.

mV   Abbreviation for millivolt.

Myocardial cells   Working cells of the myocardium that contain contractile filaments and form the muscular layer of the atrial walls and the thicker muscular layer of the ventricular walls.

Myocarditis   Inflammation of the heart muscle with or without involvement of the endocardium or pericardium.

Myocardium   The middle and thickest layer of the heart; contains the cardiac muscle fibers that cause contraction of the heart and contains the conduction system.

Myoclonus   Shocklike contraction of a muscle.

Nasal flaring   Widening of the nostrils on inhalation; an attempt to increase the size of the airway and increase the amount of available oxygen.

Near-drowning   Survival, at least temporarily, after suffocation in a liquid.

Needle thoracostomy   Insertion of an over-the-needle catheter into the chest to relieve a tension pneumothorax.

Neglect   Failure to provide for a child's basic needs. Neglect can be physical, educational, or emotional.

Neurogenic shock   A type of shock that occurs because of a spinal cord injury that disrupts sympathetic control of vascular tone.

Neuromuscular relaxing agent   A medication that produces chemical paralysis of skeletal muscle; also called paralytic agent, neuromuscular blocker.

Neurotransmitter   A chemical responsible for transmission of an impulse across a synapse.

Oliguria   Scanty urine production.

Orthopnea   Difficulty breathing brought on or aggravated by lying flat; changing to a sitting or standing position typically permits deeper and more comfortable breathing.

Orthostatic hypotension   An inappropriate fall in blood pressure on assumption of an upright posture.

Pacemaker cells   Specialized cells of the heart's electrical conduction system capable of spontaneously generating and conducting electrical impulses.

Pain   An unpleasant sensory and emotional experience associated with actual or potential tissue damage, or described in terms of such damage.

Pain tolerance level   The greatest level of pain that a subject is prepared to tolerate.

Pain threshold   The least experience of pain that a subject can recognize.

Para   Refers to the number of a woman's past pregnancies that have remained viable to delivery; a woman who is pregnant for the first time is gravida 1, para 0; para can be further divided into four categories: number of term infants, number of premature infants, number of abortions/miscarriages, number of living children.

Paradoxic irritability   Irritable when held and lethargic when left alone; may be seen in infants and small children with neurologic infections.

Partial seizure   A seizure confined to one area of the brain.

Patent ductus arteriosus   A heart defect that occurs when the ductus arteriosus, a blood vessel present during fetal development that connects the pulmonary artery to the descending aorta, fails to close after birth.

Penetrating trauma   Any mechanism of injury that causes a cut or piercing of skin.

Perfusion   The circulation of blood through an organ or a part of the body.

Pericardium   A double-walled sac that encloses the heart and helps to anchor the heart in place, preventing excessive movement of the heart in the chest when body position changes, and protect it from trauma and infection.

Pericarditis   Inflammation of the pericardium that results in an increase in the volume of pericardial fluid that surrounds the heart.

Perinatal   Occurring at or near the time of birth.

Peripheral vascular resistance Resistance to the flow of blood determined by blood vessel diameter and the tone of the vascular musculature.

Petechiae Reddish-purple nonblanchable discolorations in the skin less than 0.5 cm in diameter.

Pocket mask A transparent semirigid mask designed for mouth-to-mask ventilation of an adult, child, or infant.

Poison A substance that, on ingestion, inhalation, absorption, application, injection, or development within the body in relatively small amounts, may cause structural damage or functional disturbance.

Poisoning Exposure to a substance that is harmful in any dosage.

Polarized state Period following repolarization of a myocardial cell (also called the "resting state") when the outside of the cell is positive and the interior of the cell is negative.

Polymorphic Varying in shape.

Preload The force exerted by the blood on the walls of the ventricles at the end of diastole.

Prenatal Existing or occurring before birth.

Preoxygenate The administration of oxygen to a patient before attempting a procedure (e.g., intubation).

Presyncope An episode in which the patient experiences signs and symptoms that precede actual syncope; presyncope does not include loss of consciousness.

Primary apnea The newly born's initial response to hypoxemia consisting of initial tachypnea, then apnea, bradycardia, and a slight increase in blood pressure; if stimulated, responds with resumption of breathing.

Primary bradycardia Bradycardia caused by structural heart disease.

Primipara A woman who has given birth only once.

Prodrome Symptoms that precede the patient's present chief complaint; an early warning symptom that may mark the beginning of a disease or illness.

Prolonged QT syndrome Cardiac disorder in which the interval between the QRS complex and the T wave is unusually long.

Pulse oximetry The use of the light absorption characteristics of oxygenated and deoxygenated hemoglobin to display an indirect measurement of the percentage of hemoglobin saturated with oxygen.

Pulse pressure The difference between the systolic and diastolic blood pressure; an indicator of stroke volume.

Pulseless electrical activity (PEA) Organized electrical activity observed on a cardiac monitor (other than ventricular tachycardia or ventricular fibrillation) without a palpable pulse.

Purkinje fibers An elaborate web of fibers distributed throughout the ventricular myocardium.

Purpura Red-purple nonblanchable discolorations larger than 0.5 cm in diameter. Large purpura lesions are called ecchymoses.

PVC Abbreviation for premature ventricular complex.

R wave On an ECG, the first positive deflection in the QRS complex, representing ventricular depolarization.

Rapid sequence intubation The use of medications to sedate and paralyze a patient to rapidly achieve tracheal intubation.

Reentry The propagation of an impulse through tissue already activated by that same impulse.

Refractoriness The extent to which a cell is able to respond to a stimulus.

Repolarization Movement of ions across a cell membrane in which the inside of the cell is restored to its negative charge.

Respiratory distress Increased work of breathing (respiratory effort).

Respiratory failure   A clinical condition in which there is inadequate blood oxygenation and/or ventilation to meet the metabolic demands of body tissues.

Retractions   Sinking in of the soft tissues above the sternum or clavicle or between or below the ribs during inhalation.

Retrograde   Moving backward; moving in the opposite direction to that which is considered normal.

Schizoaffective disorder   A major psychiatric disorder in which the individual experiences symptoms of both schizophrenia and an affective disorder (either bipolar disorder or depression).

Schizophrenia   A group of psychotic disorders characterized by disturbances in thought, mood, behavior, sense of self, and interaction with others.

Seat-belt sign   Abdominal contusion consisting of ecchymosis and bruising in a band that corresponds to the position of the seat belt across the abdomen.

Secondary apnea   When asphyxia is prolonged, a period of deep, gasping respirations with a concomitant fall in blood pressure and heart rate; gasping becomes weaker and slower and then ceases.

Secondary bradycardia   A slow heart rate due to a noncardiac cause.

Secondary drowning   Death occurring longer than 24 hours after submersion secondary to severe respiratory decompensation (e.g., acute respiratory distress syndrome, pulmonary edema).

Sedation   Depression of an individual's awareness of the environment and reduction of his or her responsiveness to external stimulation.

Seizure   A temporary alteration in behavior or consciousness caused by abnormal electrical activity of one or more groups of neurons in the brain.

Sellick maneuver   Technique used to compress the cricoid cartilage causing occlusion of the esophagus, thereby reducing the risk of aspiration; also called cricoid pressure.

Sequence of survival   A concept that represents the ideal sequence of events that should take place immediately following the recognition of an injury or the onset of sudden illness; early access to care, early cardiopulmonary resuscitation, early defibrillation, and early advanced care.

Sepsis   The systemic response to an infection.

Septicemia   An infection of the blood.

Septic shock   Sepsis with hypotension, despite adequate fluid resuscitation, along with the presence of perfusion abnormalities that may include, but are not limited to, lactic acidosis, oliguria, or an acute alteration in mental status.

Severe sepsis   Sepsis associated with organ dysfunction, hypoperfusion, or hypotension.

Shock   A clinical syndrome resulting from the failure of the cardiovascular system to deliver sufficient oxygen and nutrients to sustain vital organ function.

Sniffing position   In this position, the neck is flexed at the fifth and sixth cervical vertebrae, and the head is extended at the first and second cervical vertebrae. This position aligns the axes of the mouth, pharynx, and trachea, opening the airway and increasing airflow.

Snoring   Noisy breathing through the mouth and nose during sleep, caused by air passing through a narrowed upper airway.

Soft palate   Composed of mucous membrane, muscular fibers, and mucous glands and is suspended from the posterior border of the hard palate, forming the roof of the mouth.

ST-segment   The portion of the ECG representing the end of ventricular depolarization (end of the R wave) and the beginning of ventricular repolarization (T wave).

Status epilepticus   A single seizure lasting longer than 30 minutes or repeated seizures without full recovery of responsiveness between seizures and lasting longer than 30 minutes.

Stridor   A harsh, high-pitched sound heard on inspiration associated with upper airway obstruction. It is frequently described as a high-pitched crowing or "seal-bark" sound.

Stroke volume   The amount of blood ejected by either ventricle during one contraction; can be calculated as cardiac output divided by heart rate

Stylet   A malleable plastic-covered wire used for molding and maintaining the shape of an endotracheal tube.

Suicide attempt   Lethal self-destructive behavior for the purpose of ending one's life.

Suicide gesture   Nonlethal self-destructive behavior performed with the conscious or subconscious intent of obtaining attention, rather than ending life.

Synchronized cardioversion   Delivery of a shock to the heart to terminate a rapid dysrhythmia that is timed to avoid the vulnerable period during the cardiac cycle.

Syncope   A brief loss of consciousness caused by transient cerebral hypoxia.

Systemic inflammatory response syndrome (SIRS)   A response to infection manifested by derangement in two or more of the following: temperature, heart rate, respiratory rate, or white blood cell count.

Tachycardia   In adults, a heart rate above 100 beats per minute. In the pediatric patient, the term is used to describe a significant and persistent increase in heart rate. In infants, a tachycardia is a heart rate of more than 200 beats per minute. In a child older than 5 years, a tachycardia is a heart rate of more than 160 beats per minute.

Tachypnea   Abnormally rapid breathing.

Therapeutic effect   A beneficial action of a drug that corrects a bodily dysfunction.

Tidal volume   The amount of air exchanged with each breath.

TKO   Abbreviation meaning "to keep open." Also known as KVO, "keep the vein open."

Toxidrome   A constellation of signs and symptoms useful for recognizing a specific class of poisoning.

Toxin   A poisonous substance of plant or animal origin.

Tracheitis   Inflammation of the mucous membrane of the trachea.

Tracheobronchial   Pertaining to the trachea and bronchi.

Tracheomalacia   Degeneration of the elastic and connective tissue of the trachea.

Tragus   A tonguelike projection of cartilage anterior to the external opening of the ear.

Transthoracic impedance (resistance)   The resistance of the chest wall to current.

Tripod position   Position used to maintain airway patency: sitting upright and leaning forward with the neck slightly extended, chin projected, and mouth open and supported by the arms.

Turgor   Elasticity.

Vagal maneuver   Methods used to stimulate the vagus nerve in an attempt to slow conduction through the AV node, resulting in slowing of the heart rate.

Vallecula   The space (or "pocket") between the base of the tongue and the epiglottis; an important landmark when performing endotracheal intubation with a curved laryngoscope blade.

Vascular resistance   The amount of opposition that blood vessels give to the flow of blood.

Venous return   The amount of blood flowing into the right atrium each minute from the systemic circulation.

Waddell's triad   The injury pattern experienced by a child involved in a pedestrian injury; extremity trauma, thoracic and abdominal trauma, and head trauma.

Watt-second   A unit of energy equivalent to the joule.

Waveform   Movement away from the baseline in a positive or negative direction.

Wheezes   High-pitched "whistling" sounds produced by air moving through narrowed airway passages.

Subject Index